# Psychosocial, Educational, and Economic Impacts of COVID-19

*Edited by Brizeida Hernández-Sánchez, José Carlos Sánchez-García, António Carrizo Moreira and Alcides A. Monteiro*

Published in London, United Kingdom

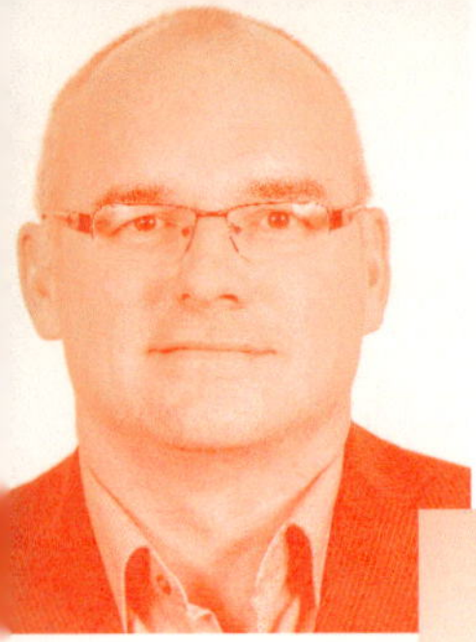
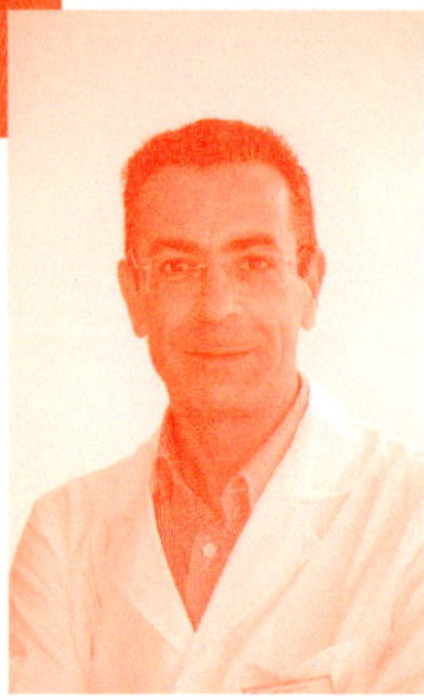
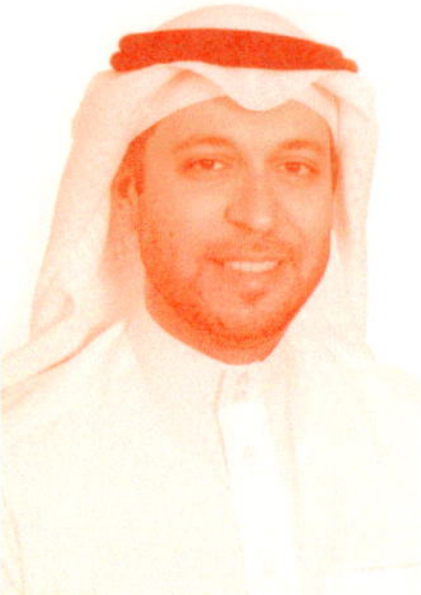
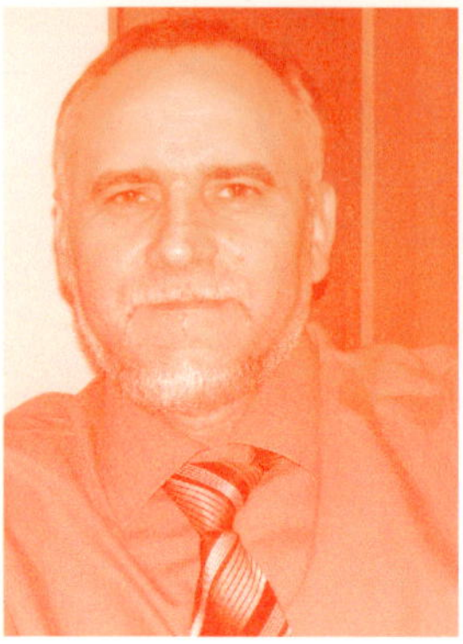
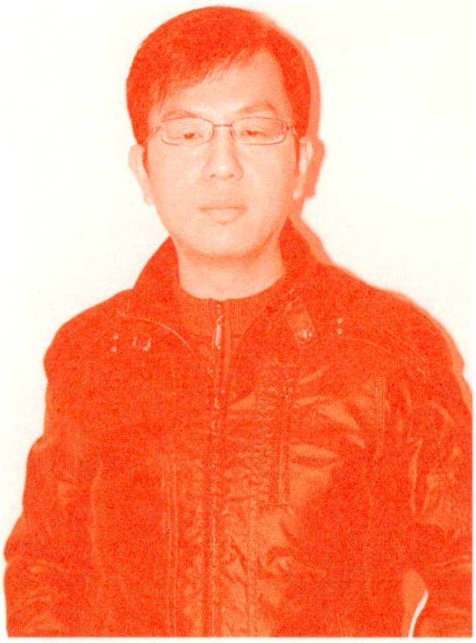
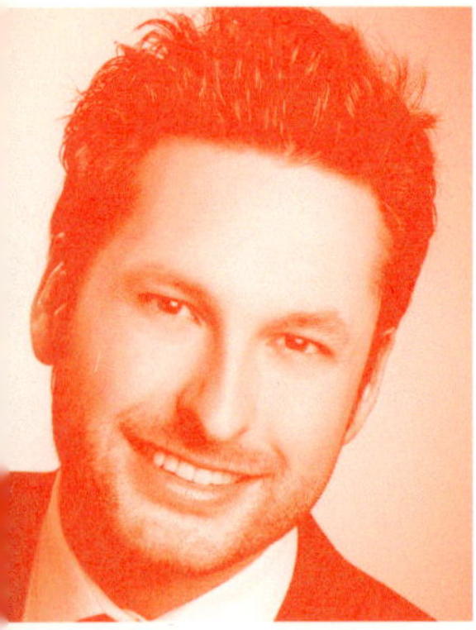
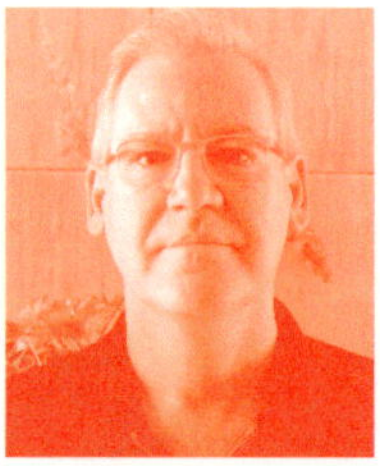

IntechOpen

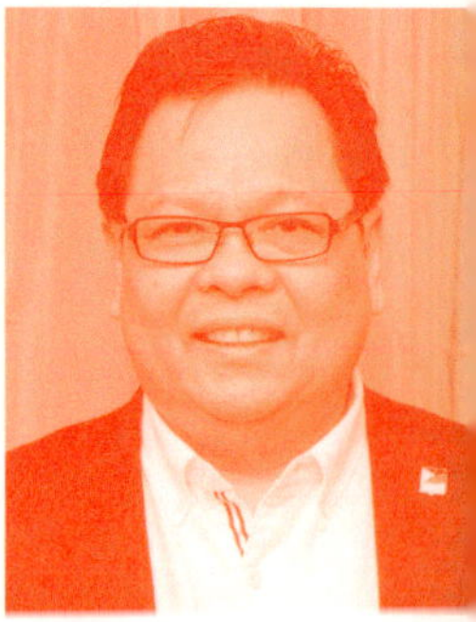
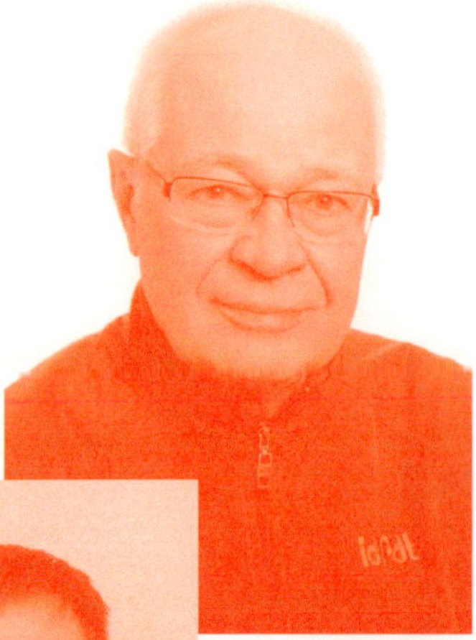
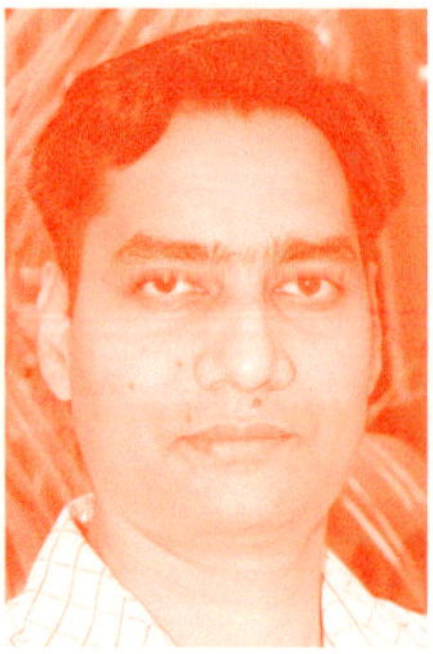
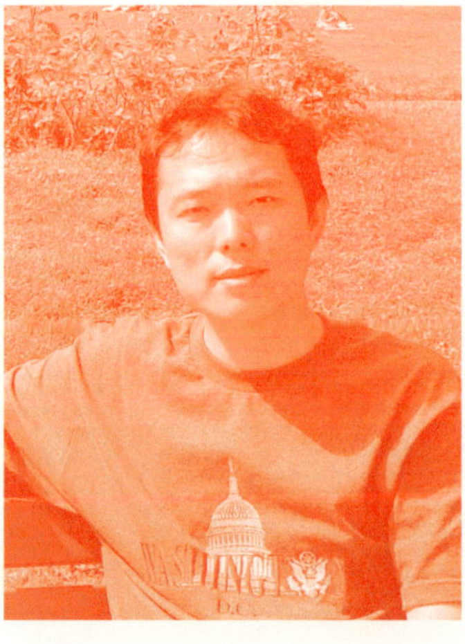
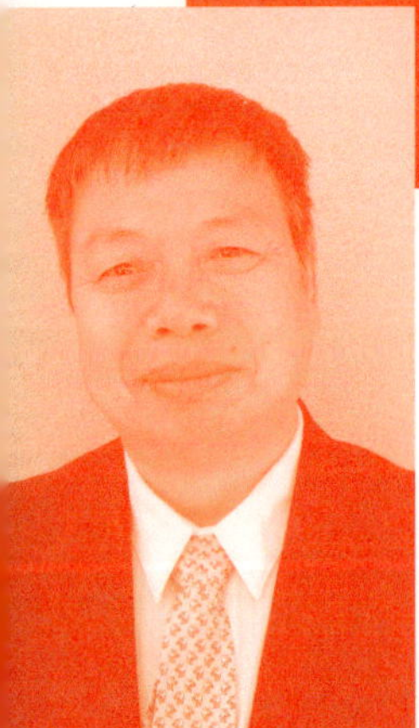
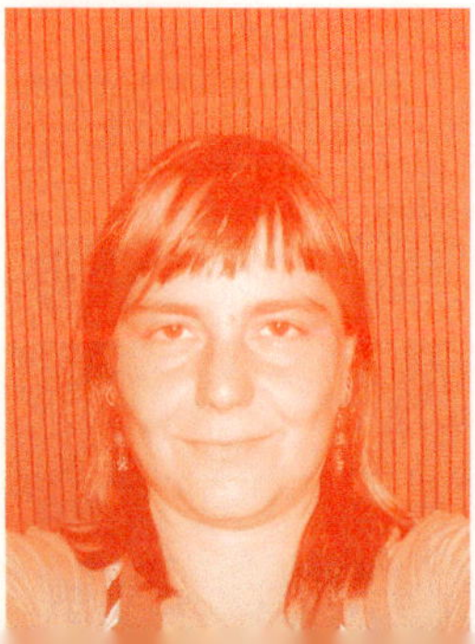

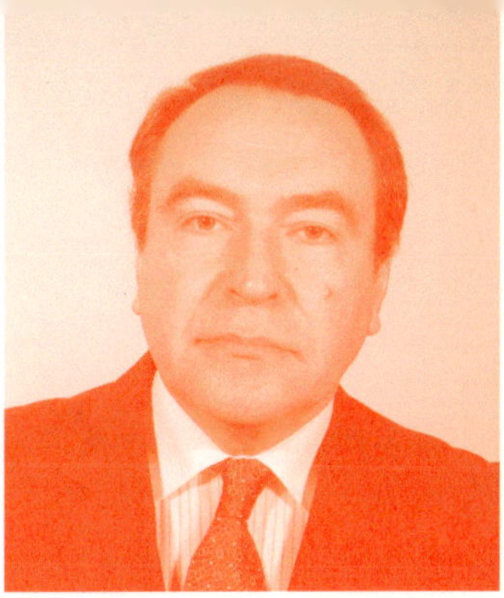

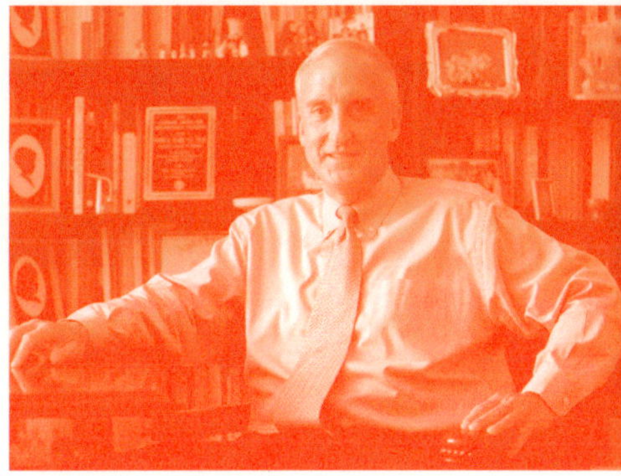

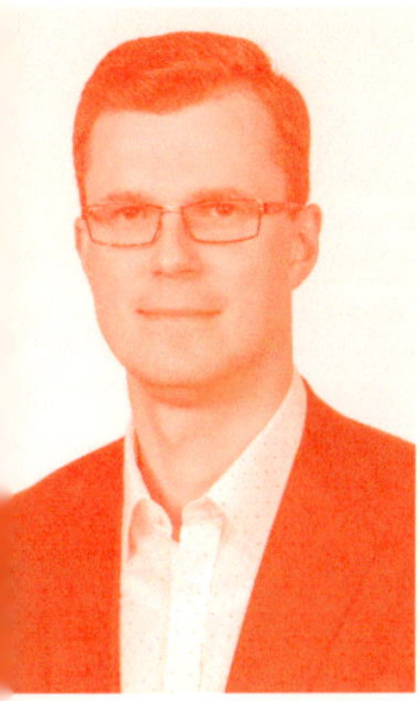

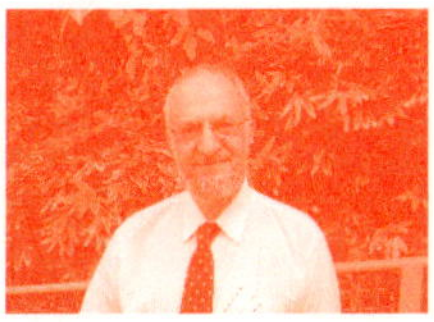

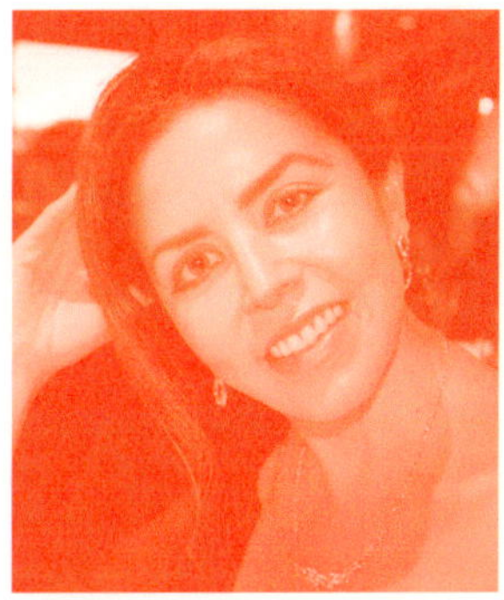

*Supporting open minds since 2005*

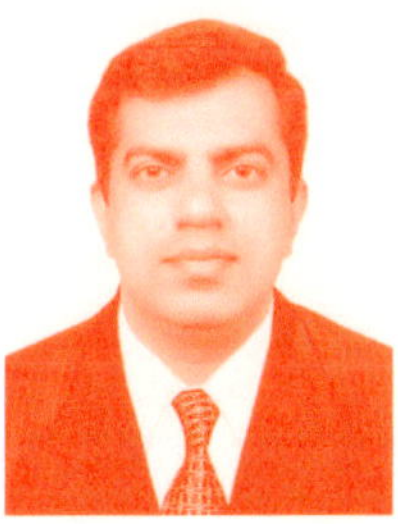

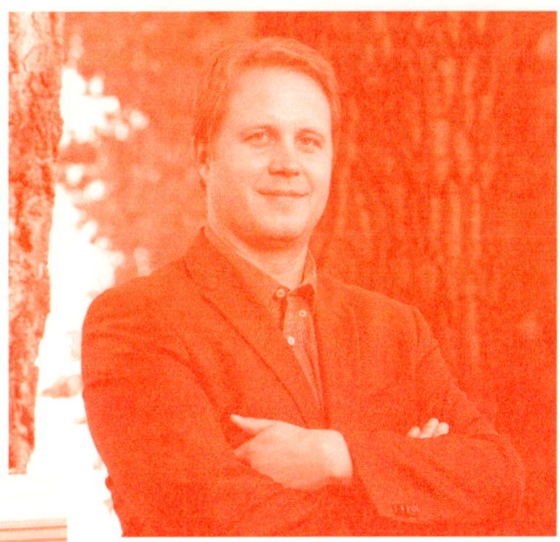

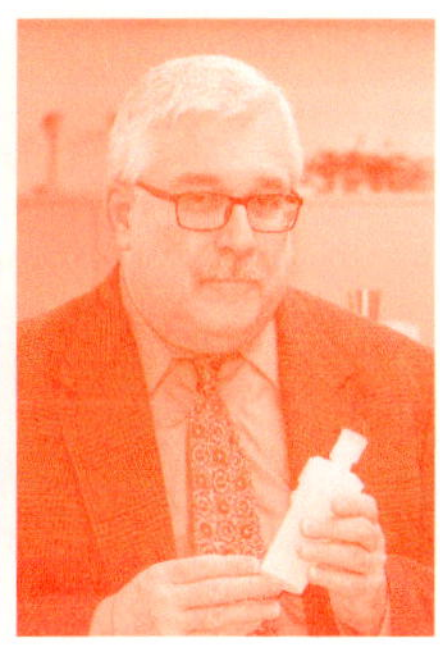

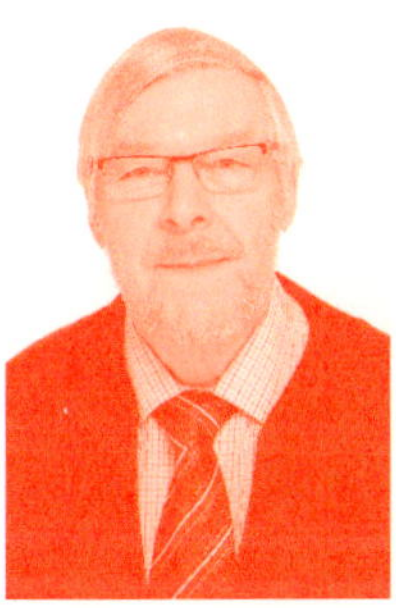

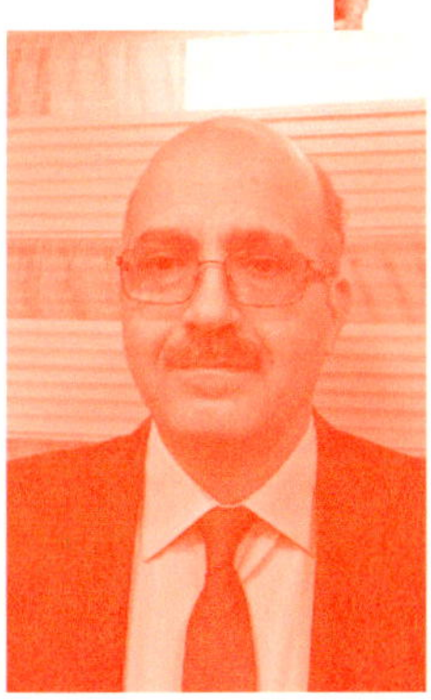

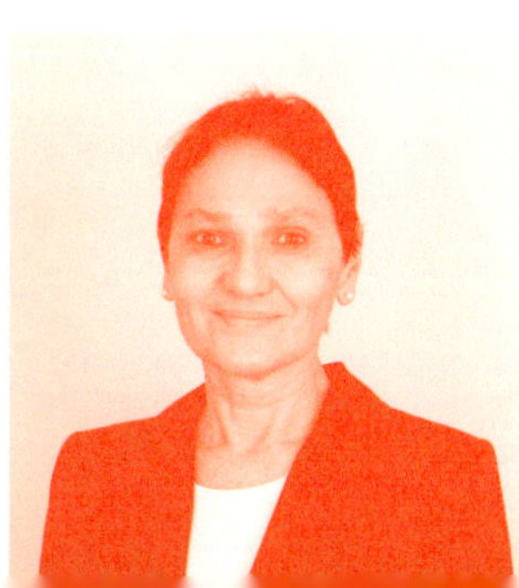

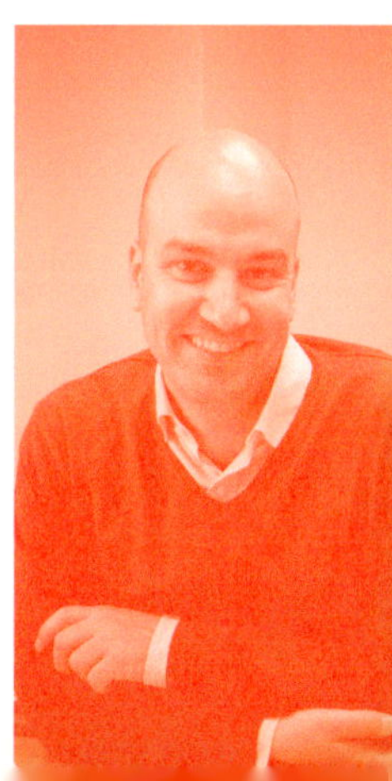

Psychosocial, Educational, and Economic Impacts of COVID-19
http://dx.doi.org/10.5772/intechopen.95221
Edited by Brizeida Hernández-Sánchez, José Carlos Sánchez-García, António Carrizo Moreira and Alcides A. Monteiro

Contributors
Gabriela Rubilar Donoso, Caterine Galaz Valderrama, Catherine A. LaBrenz, Anil Gumber, Prasan Kumar Panda, Ashwin Parchani, Vijay Krishnan, Bani Koumachi, Willy H. Engelbrecht, Cicek Hocaoglu, Dogancan Sonmez, Jia Yu, Priyanka Choudhary, Kishor Kunal, Jiwesh Kumar, Ravi Prakash, Anita Singh, Kirti Kanchan, Madireng Monyela, Prabha Pandey, Kavita Batra, Ravi Batra, Rutuja Sunil Patankar, Bongani Sibusiso Mchunu, Tharcisio Leone, Adamu Mumini, Ashim Gupta, Grace Koehler, Saadiq F. El-Amin III, Salman Sharif, Faridah Amin, Rabeeya Saeed, Samer Hammoudeh, Raghad Burjaq, Adalberto Rangone, Fitzgerald Witika, Vasfiye Bayram Değer, Goodluck A.K. Anthony Kelechi Ohanube, Uchejeso M. Mark Obeta, Mariana Cernicova-Buca, Jaime González Maiz Jiménez, Adán Reyes Santiago, Declan Lyons, Aisling Collins, Eleanor O'Driscoll, Alenka Lipovec, Blaž Zmazek, Igor Pesek, Nikos Christo Secchi Nicolás, Ángel de Jesús Gómez Alarcón, Chia-Hao Hsu, Chung-Hwan Chen, Hsuan-Ti Huang, Dibya Sundar Panda, Kei Aoki, Margaret Nampijja, Lilian Ayiro, Ruth Nalugya, Bulelwa Makena, Thandiswa Mpiti



First published in London, United Kingdom, 2023 by IntechOpen
IntechOpen is the global imprint of INTECHOPEN LIMITED, registered in England and Wales, registration number: 11086078, 5 Princes Gate Court, London, SW7 2QJ, United Kingdom
Printed in Croatia

British Library Cataloguing-in-Publication Data
A catalogue record for this book is available from the British Library

Additional hard and PDF copies can be obtained from orders@intechopen.com

Psychosocial, Educational, and Economic Impacts of COVID-19
Edited by Brizeida Hernández-Sánchez, José Carlos Sánchez-García, António Carrizo Moreira and Alcides A. Monteiro
p. cm.
Print ISBN 978-1-80355-039-8
Online ISBN 978-1-80355-040-4
eBook (PDF) ISBN 978-1-80355-041-1

For EU product safety concerns:
IN TECH d.o.o., Prolaz Marije Krucifikse Kozulić 3, 51000 Rijeka, Croatia, info@intechopen.com or visit our website at intechopen.com.

# Meet the editors

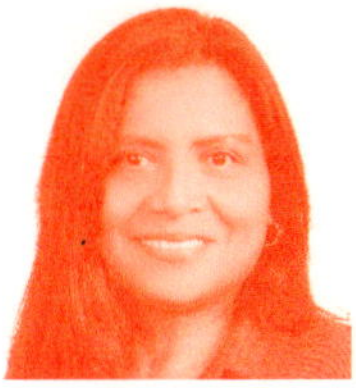

Professor Brizeida Hernández Sánchez has extensive training and pedagogical experience, with a focus on curricular design and teaching, specializing in project management and educational quality processes for different academic levels. She is an expert in Information and Communication Technologies (ICT) applied to education, social pedagogy, special education, educational technology, and management of public policies and educational institutions (supervising training in different master's degrees). This training trajectory is combined with a wide and extensive experience, both academic and professional, in pedagogy. She is the academic coordinator of the training program in the Chair of Entrepreneurship at the University of Salamanca and a member of the academic committee for international postgraduate programs. She is also a member of the Department of Scientific Research and Technological Development (SENACYT) Panama.

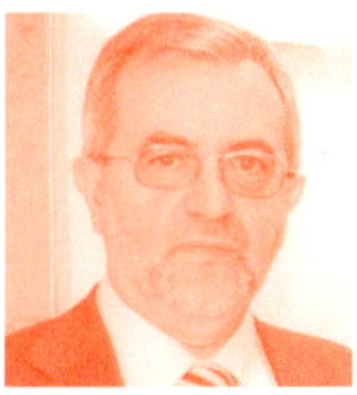

José Carlos Sánchez Garcia is a full professor in the Social Psychology Department, University of Salamanca, Spain, where is also the director of the Chair of Entrepreneurship. His main scientific interests are entrepreneurship, innovation, and regional development. He also carries out research in evaluation and participation methodologies, public policies, associations and volunteering, social innovation and social entrepreneurship, social inequalities, and lifelong learning. He is an active member of several civil society networks, including the United States Association for Small Business and Entrepreneurship (USASBE) and the Association of Former United Nations Industry and Development Experts (AFIDE). He is also a director of training programs on entrepreneurship.

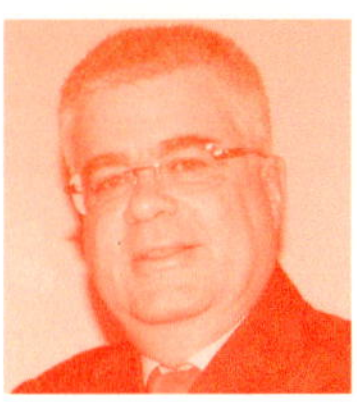

António Carrizo Moreira is an associate professor with habilitation in the Department of Economics, Management, Industrial Engineering, and Tourism (DEGEIT), University of Aveiro, Portugal, where he lectures courses on international business, strategy, marketing, entrepreneurship, innovation, and statistics. He received his master's degree in Management from the University of Porto, Portugal, an MBA from Porto Business School, and a Ph.D. from the University of Manchester, England. Dr. Moreira received scholarships from the Science and Technology Research National Board (JNICT) and Science and Technology Foundation (FCT).

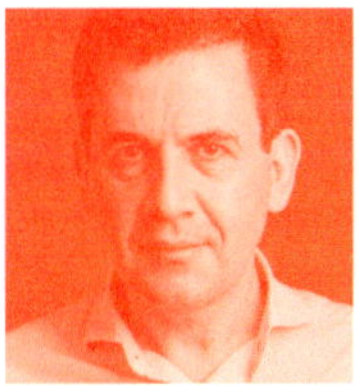

Alcides A. Monteiro is a full professor in the Sociology Department, University of Beira Interior (UBI), Portugal. He is currently the director of the Ph.D. course in sociology. His main scientific interest is local and regional development. He also carries out research in evaluation and participation methodologies, public policies, associations and volunteering, social innovation and social entrepreneurship, social inequalities, gender studies, adult education, and lifelong learning. He is an active member of several civil society networks, including the European Anti-Poverty Network (EAPN), Portuguese Association for Local Development (ANIMAR), Gender Equality Network (Citizenship Roadmap in Portugal), and European Network for Social Policy Analysis (ESPANET).

# Contents

# Preface

This book analyzes the psychosocial, educational, and economic impacts of COVID-19 worldwide.

*Psychosocial Impacts:*

One of the most observed effects of the COVID-19 pandemic is psychological stress. If we consider the student population, who already face stressful conditions such as assessments and social pressure to succeed daily, we quickly realize that they are one of the most vulnerable social groups. This is confirmed in Chapter 1, "Perspective Chapter: Impact of Pandemic Situation on Students Psychology and Support to Combat", by Rutuja Patankar, based on an analysis of online surveys of student populations during the pandemic in countries as diverse as India, Nigeria, and Ethiopia. In addition to confirming the worsening of stressful situations, the chapter also discusses the work done by organizations that tried to mitigate these situations.

The issue of psychological effects is also addressed in Chapter 2, "Perspective Chapter: Psychological Effects of COVID-19 Pandemic", by Vasfiye Bayram Değer. This chapter presents evidence of the psychological problems generated by the pandemic, namely, negative emotions, depression, anxiety, and distress. The chapter also addresses how quarantine and isolation situations, using masks, and social distancing during the pandemic generated trauma and examines the effects of this trauma across different age groups.

In Chapter 3, "Perspective Chapter: Psychosocial Impact of COVID-19 – A Global Scenario", Kishor Kunal et al. examine the social, socioeconomic, socio-political, social, professional, and healthcare effects of the COVID-19 pandemic. The chapter seeks to delineate the process of impact by looking into its pathophysiology, thus drawing lessons from the present situation and anticipating future impacts.

During the pandemic, a significant part of the world population experienced unprecedented isolation and social distance. Faced with the obligatory behaviors that were not natural to them, people naturally began to experience depression, anxiety, and stress. It was even observed that cases of suicidal ideation increased during this time. Chapter 4, "Perspective Chapter: The Psychosocial Effects of Isolation and Social Distancing during the Coronavirus Disease 2019 Pandemic – An Overview and Mitigation Strategies", by Raghad Burjaq and Samer Hammoudeh, analyzes the psychosocial effects of isolation and social distancing as well as strategies to mitigate their effects, such as exercise, limiting media exposure, counseling, and maintaining social networks.

The deployment of emergency remote education (ERE) is not an innovation brought by searching for responses to the COVID-19 crisis. However, the pandemic forced its use on a larger scale, with varying degrees of success and satisfaction around the world. Chapter 5, "Perspective Chapter: Perspectives on the Emergency Remote Assessment during the COVID-19 Pandemic", by Mariana Cernicova-Buca draws attention to the debate on the relevance and soundness of remote assessment activities, both for students and for society in general. Some voices enthusiastically champion the technological innovation and point to the benefits brought by computer-assisted assessment, while others warn against a "one-size-fits-all" approach and insist that emergency measures need careful examination and, while lessons can be taken from the situation, traditional patterns should be kept in place.

Grouping of language learners has been proven to lead to progress and success in academic achievement. However, the pandemic imposed the closure of schools and thus it was not possible for students to meet in person. In examining the effects of this situation on language learning proficiency, Bulelwa Makena and Thandiswa Mpiti in Chapter 6, "Social Distancing Disbanding Learner Groupings: A Case on Language Development", conduct a qualitative case study of selected English language teachers from three different primary schools in one district of the Eastern Cape Province in South Africa. Their findings suggest that reading levels and learner attitudes were negatively affected, with students feeling isolated from their peers.

Chapter 7, "Perspective Chapter: Psychosocial Impact of COVID-19 – Stigma and Xenophobia", by Dogancan Sonmez and Cicek Hocaoglu, focuses on the rise of stigma and feelings of xenophobia caused by the pandemic. Based on a literature review, the authors note the growth of fear, prejudice, and hateful attitudes, particularly towards certain groups, such as older people and foreigners. Faced with this escalation of stigmatizing and xenophobic attitudes during the pandemic, the authors stress the importance of reparative and preventive measures to ensure social cohesion in society.

Chapter 8, "COVID-19 Sends the Bill: Socially Disadvantaged Workers Suffer the Severest Losses in Earnings", by Tharcisio Leone, presents a nationally representative household survey conducted by phone during the COVID-19 pandemic to estimate the short-term impacts of lockdown measures on employment and income in Brazil. The results obtained point to visible negative effects on employment rates and people's income levels.

Chapter 9, "Why Knowledge Sharing Increases Well-Being – The Case of Adult Fans of LEGO", by Kei Aoki, reveals the relationship between knowledge sharing and well-being. Starting from his own thesis that participation in knowledge sharing has a significant positive impact on contributor well-being, the author seeks to understand the reasons underlying this advantage. He presents the results of in-depth interviews conducted by LEGO users who share their original creations. The study finds that contributors increased their wellbeing by deepening their knowledge and experience via competitive co-creation.

In times of crisis, minority and disadvantaged social groups tend to feel the effects more quickly and more intensely. In Chapter 10, "Perspective Chapter: Impact of COVID-19 on the Health of Ethnic Minorities in the UK – Salient Features and Recouping Strategies", Anil Gumber presents a study analyzing the exposure of Black, Asian and Ethnic Minorities (BAME) living in the United Kingdom to the impact of COVID-19. Promoting a multidimensional analysis, the author notes that BAME experienced not only health consequences but also economic and social consequences. In terms of health, there is, for example, a higher mortality rate among BAME patients as well as greater difficulty in accessing specialist health services (e.g., organ transplants). The chapter concludes by recommending both short- and long-term strategies to mitigate the devastating impact of COVID on BAME health and quality of life.

In Chapter 11, "Mental Impact of COVID-19 – Fear, Stress, Anxiety, Depression and Sequels", Parchani, Panda, et al., analyze how the pandemic and the public health measures used to tackle it gave rise to psychological reactions such as fear, stress, anxiety, and depression in both patients and healthcare workers. Many patients and healthcare workers report prolonged symptoms and aftereffects, which justifies investment in preventive actions to regulate and prevent mental illnesses. The authors highlight that research is urgently needed to evaluate the amount of anxiety, worry, helplessness and other mental health concerns related to COVID-19 as a way to develop tailored mental health initiatives.

In Chapter 12, "From Face-to-Face to Face-to-Screen: A Correlational Analysis of Psychological Impacts and Perception of Achievement of Ibn Tofail University Students during COVID-19 Times", Bani Koumachi presents the results of a survey of 297 students at the School of Languages, Letters, and Arts, Ibn Tofail University, Morocco. Using both descriptive and inferential statistics, the author shows that students' achievement is affected by all the factors composing the bio-ecological environment, revealing that the COVID-19 pandemic confinement had negative impacts on every sphere of life and education.

*Educational Impacts:*

The COVID-19 pandemic enacted a paradigm shift in education worldwide. Teaching and assessment methods have been greatly modified in online teaching. Online lecture delivery can be considered effective to the extent that the outcome domain is limited to knowledge, but for other domains such as cognitive, psychomotor, interpersonal, and communication, it is questionable. In Chapter 13, "Perspective Chapter: Impact of COVID-19 on Learning Outcomes of Students", Dibya Sundar Panda examines the impact of COVID-19 on learning outcomes of students. The author suggests that to ensure the achievement of learning outcomes, a careful approach must be taken to identify learning gaps in online teaching along with implementing corrective measures to address them.

Adamu Mumini In Chapter 14, "Psychosocial Educational and Economic Impact of COVID-19: Implication for Girl Child Education through Social Studies in Northeast Nigeria", examines the educational and economic psychosocial impact of COVID-19. The sudden economic collapse had a major impact on the socioeconomic lives of many people around the world. A Nigerian education system with over twelve million (12,000,000) students of which 36,400,000 primary and secondary students did not attend school.

Margaret Nampijja, Lillian Ayiro and Ruth Nalugya the authors of Chapter 15, "Perspective Chapter: Pedagogical Approaches and Access to Education among Early Childhood Education Learners with Disabilities in Africa during the COVID-19 Pandemic – Review of Available Literature", discuss pedagogical approaches and access to education among early childhood education learners with disabilities in Africa during the COVID-19 pandemic. The pandemic led to a shift from traditional face-to-face learning to remote online learning using modern technology, but this was not accessible for many students with disabilities, particularly in early childhood education, who rely primarily on individualized instruction. The available literature shows that the pandemic severely aggravated difficulties in accessing learning programs among students with disabilities in Africa and has widened the gap between them and their normally functioning counterparts.

Countries responded to the pandemic by introducing remote ways of delivering education to learners through radio, television, and other means. However, there was a lack of inclusion of strategies to serve young students with disabilities. Concerted efforts are needed at all levels to support effective learning for children with disabilities during the current pandemic and future crises. Future research that focuses on understanding the barriers to equitable education provision from the perspective of decision-makers will be useful. These aspects are analyzed in chapter 16, "Unveiling the Uncertainty-Revolutionizing Medical Education in COVID-19 Era", by Sharif Salman et al.

In Chapter 17, "COVID-19 and the Dynamic Role of Telemedicine", Grace Koehler, Saadiq F. El-Amin III, and Ashim Gupta examine the use of telemedicine during the pandemic. Before March 2020, telemedicine was in use but on a limited scale. As 2020 progressed, the use of telemedicine expanded rapidly, especially in the United States, presenting advantages such as safety and convenience and disadvantages such as loss of patient contact/physical examination and concern over new inequities. Adaptation of increased use of telehealth in primary care specifically appears to have the potential for long-term sustainability and patient use.

Chapter 18, "Education Equity in Times of Emergency Remote Teaching: The Case of Slovenia", by Alenka Lipovec, Blaž Zmazek and Igor Pesek presents empirical results from a study in Slovenia that indicate that the situation in schools in Slovenia was very diverse, which led to a lack of guarantee of the principle of equity in the education. The teaching methods used by teachers in teaching in crisis. The results show differences between the emergency remote teaching strategies of the mentor-teachers. Furthermore, they suggest that secondary school teachers have more effectively adopted and integrated different distance learning strategies into their work.

In Chapter 19, "Approaches to Teach Cataloguing Modules during Emergencies", Madireng Monyela presents a study on teaching and learning cataloging modules in higher education institutions. Cataloging modules require face-to-face interactions between instructors and students for the explanation of concepts. The modules involve the practical use of manuals and the application of standards, which are skills that students must master.

Chapter 20, "Tensions, Challenges, and Resistance among Academic Mothers during the COVID-19 Pandemic", by Gabriela Rubilar Donoso, Catherine A. LaBrenz, and Caterine Galaz Valderrama reflects on the processes through which academic mothers have reconciled work and family life during the COVID-19 pandemic. During the pandemic, academic mothers faced heightened productive and reproductive responsibilities. The authors interviewed three academic mothers and analyzed their narratives at various points during the COVID-19 pandemic. Three main themes emerged from the analysis: (1) bodies that produce and reproduce, (2) the triple day of academic mothers, and (3) resistance and change.

In Chapter 21, "Perspective Chapter: Fallout from the Pandemic – A Social and Psychological Description of COVID-19 Related Traumatic Sequelae", Aishling Collins, Eleanor O'Driscoll and Declan Lyons examine the utility of interpreting psychological outcomes of the pandemic at the individual and societal levels through the lens of collective trauma.

Chapter 22, "Perspective Chapter: Transforming Continuing Medical Education in the COVID-19", by Nikos Christo Secchi Nicolás and Ángel de Jesús Gómez Alarcón discusses medical education during the pandemic. Unexpectedly, and at very short notice, people were no longer able to teach or learn alongside other people. Medical educators can take advantage of technology to enhance medical education at both the undergraduate and graduate levels. Although more recent initiatives, such as remote transmissions, have been around for a long time, traditional classes, lectures, and face-to-face didactic tutorials continue to be the most important pillar of medical education both at home and abroad.

Chapter 23, "A Doctor's Training in COVID Era", by Jiwesh Kumar, Priyanka Choudhary, Kishor Kunal, Anita Singh, Ravi Prakash, and Prabha Pandey examines the impact of COVID-19 on physician training programs and suggests that a hybrid model combining virtual and real-world training and assessment for medical education has optimal benefits.

Chapter 24, " "Deaths of Despair" among College Students Amidst COVID-19 Pandemic: A Call for Action", by Kavita Batra and Ravi Batra aims to reflect on the factors that contribute to "deaths of despair" among university students as a result of the COVID-19 pandemic. The authors advocate for the development of personalized interventions to promote post-traumatic growth among college students.

*Economic Impacts:*

In Chapter 25, "Consistency in Leadership during a Pandemic: Managing Academics at a Private Higher Education Institution in South Africa", Willy H. Engelbrecht finds that most managers required only minor adjustments to their leadership approaches to transition to remote work and that various leadership styles applied in specific contexts helped to enhance leader efficiency.

In Chapter 26, "Measuring the Systematic Risk of Sectors within the US Market via Principal Components Analysis: Before and during the COVID-19 Pandemic", Jaime González Maiz Jiméncz and Adán Reyes Santiago use a Principal Component Analysis (PCA) technique to examine how ten economic sectors evolved during the COVID-19 pandemic. The authors selected five stocks per sector with the greatest market capitalization from the American Stock Market to measure the systematic risk of each sector. The chapter shows that the restaurant, clothing, and insurance industries had the greatest increase in exposure to systematic risk during the pandemic. Conversely, the auto and tobacco industries showed the greatest decrease in terms of exposure to systematic risk.

In Chapter 27, "Cases of Principal Leadership Responses in a Volatile, Uncertain and Complex School Environment", Bongani Sibusiso Mchunu investigates how teachers and principals responded to the implementation of social distancing and COVID-19 regulations in a volatile, uncertain, complex, and ambiguous environment. The findings suggest that principals were able to achieve their goals, whereas teachers tended to leave their positions, thus contributing to teacher shortages.

In Chapter 28, "Challenges and Futures of Long-Term Care Industry after COVID-19 Pandemic", Jia Yu analyzes the impact and challenges of COVID-19 on residential care homes in the United Kingdom, United States, and Australia and addresses possible implications for the long-term care market post- pandemic.

In Chapter 29, "Companies and Covid-19: Emerging Challenges and Recovery Strategies through Technological Upgrading", Adalberto Rangone outlines the challenges faced by businesses and prescribes, based on the "poker strategy," possible solutions for rapid recovery of production and commercial activities. The author recommends businesses invest in innovation rather than give up, so that they can maintain the trust of all stakeholders and regain market share.

In Chapter 30, "Deciphering Economic Effects of COVID-19", Fitzgerald Witika provides a critical approach to understanding the nature of the positive and negative effects of COVID-19 on economies. He uses the Aggregate Supply and Aggregate Demand (AS-AD) model to decipher the economic effects of COVID-19 on economies worldwide with reference to theoretical literature in economics on the operationalization of market forces.

In Chapter 31, "Perspective Chapter: Impact of the COVID-19 Pandemic on the Field of Orthopedics", Chia-Hao Hsu, Chung-Hwan Chen and Hsuan-Ti Huang report on the pandemic's effects on the field of orthopedics. The rates of all surgeries and elective surgeries decreased by 15.6%–49.4% and 43.5%–100%, respectively, as a result of staff redeployment and training to training for regular telemedicine in response to the pandemic. Furthermore, other problems accounted for include the low service volume for users and heavy workload impact, personal practice change, and psychological impact for medical staff.

In Chapter 32, "Analysis of the Concept of Deaths per Million in the Impact Assessment of COVID-19 Pandemic in 2020", Goodluck A.K. Ohanube and Uchejeso M. Obeta address the need for accurate methods of assessing public health measures, especially because there is no effective, reliable international comparable index. This chapter analyzes the case fatality ratio and mortality rate, which are existing public health indices, and the deaths per million index. The authors suggest that deaths per million is a good tool to use to determine the most appropriate time to impose lockdowns and other public health measures.

Our thanks to all the chapter authors and the staff at IntechOpen for all their assistance throughout the publication process.

**José Carlos Sánchez-García**
Full Professor,
Social Psychology Department,
University of Salamanca,
Salamanca, Spain

**Brizeida Hernández-Sánchez**
Academic Coordinator of the Training Program,
Chair of Entrepreneurship,
University of Salamanca,
Salamanca, Spain

**António Carrizo Moreira**
Associate Professor,
Department of Economics, Management, Industrial Engineering,
and Tourism (DEGEIT),
University of Aveiro,
Aveiro, Portugal

**Alcides A. Monteiro**
Full Professor,
Sociology Department,
University of Beira Interior (UBI),
Covilhã, Portugal

# Section 1

# Psychosocial Impacts

Chapter 1

# Perspective Chapter: Impact of Pandemic Situation on Students Psychology and Support to Combat

*Rutuja Patankar*


## Abstract

The extensive spread of the COVID-19 virus has resulted in not only a high danger of death but also a lot of psychological stress. Since the start of the coronavirus disease 2019 (COVID-19) pandemic, the number of cases and deaths has risen globally, and the closure of schools, universities, limited access to research labs, as well as a wide range of preventive measures, has left students feeling impotent, disconnected, frustrated, and uncertain of what would happen with their academic progress. Much psychological research has been done regarding the mental stage of students and to combat such a situation during this phase lots of online sessions, videos, series, different counseling sessions are been organized by many countries. The chapter includes the effect of a pandemic on student psychology, the effect on career as well as how different organizations are having their helping hand in combating this situation.


**Keywords:** pandemic, psychological stress, student, counseling, academic

## 1. Introduction

SARS-CoV-2 is a novel coronavirus which was first observed in Wuhan, Hubei, China in the end of 2019 as the global COVID-19 pandemic [1]. Symptoms of COVID-19 are primarily respiratory with acute respiratory distress syndrome eventually leading to death [2]. It is clear from many studies that the novel coronavirus (SARS-CoV-2) and the disease it causes (COVID-19) have greatly affected people's mental health and behavior [3]. It has also been shown that COVID-19 can affect other organs, including the brain, and reports of neurological symptoms due to COVID-19 infections are emerging recently. People who are more sensitive to stress as a result of the COVID-19 pandemic appear to be at greater risk for anxiety, depression, and post-traumatic symptoms [4, 5]. Also the pandemic emergency dramatically changed the lives of university students, who have active social habits based on relationships, contacts, sports, and university activities [6]. In many cases, these inexorable circumstances lead to stress, anxiety, and a sense of helplessness. In comparison with adults, research indicates that this pandemic may continue to have negative effects on children and adolescents for quite some time to come. Children and parents within this age group can be vulnerable due to a variety of factors such as their young child's developmental stage, present educational level, disabilities, mental health issues, poverty, and being quarantined because of an infection are all factors [7]. In this chapter, we discuss the effects of COVID-19 on psychology of students, its impact on academia and how to address such situations at national and international levels.

## 2. Pandemic conditions and preventive measures

This virus spreads mainly from person to person, mainly through the respiratory secretions produced by an infected person when they cough or sneeze. It is possible for these droplets to land in the mouths or noses of nearby people or even to be inhaled into the lungs. Unfortunately, there are no medications that have been tested in controlled studies and have been approved by the FDA for this global pandemic [8]. As a result of prevention measures, cases are being limited as much as possible. The disease must be diagnosed, isolated, and treated early to avoid further spread. The best preventive strategies focus on the isolation of patients and the careful control of infection, including measures to adopt during diagnosis and treatment of an infected patient [9]. A summary of COVID-19 preventive measures is shown in **Table 1**.

| **Preventive measures** |
|---|
| Self-Quarantine |
| Closure of Institutions, Local shops, Malls, Temple, Transport etc. |
| No crowding |
| Strict use of Mask and sanitizer |
| Social distance |
| Work from home |
| No social gatherings like party, marriages, outing etc. |

**Table 1.**
*COVID-19 preventive measures.*

## 3. Impact of COVID-19 on students

COVID-19 has profoundly impacted children and adolescents around the world. In almost every country, strategies of social isolation and distancing have been implemented to prevent the spread of COVID 19 infection [10]. Accordingly, several countries began to implement containment or lockdown measures since January 2020. One of the primary measures taken during lockdown has been the closure of schools, educational institutes, and activity centers. Those inexorable circumstances leading to stress, anxiety, and the feeling of helplessness were beyond normal experience for all [11]. According to some studies, this pandemic is likely to have greater adverse effects on youth and children than on adults. This age range bears the brunt of large-scale health impacts because of several vulnerabilities like developmental age, educational status, learning disabilities, mental health conditions and being economically disadvantaged. Another vulnerability factor is having a child/parent quarantined for infection or fear of infection [8].

### 3.1 Impact on children education

It is difficult to imagine the potential losses that the young generation may suffer from their lack of learning, and for the development of this generation's human capital [12]. Children view school as both a place of learning and an outlet for their energy. In addition to pedagogy and scholastics, schools provide freedom, an opportunity to interact with peers and seniors, and psychological comfort. Education in schools has a great impact on promoting ethical behavior, good health habits, physical activity, and healthy eating [13]. Whether it will be a short-term or long-term shutdown, captivity of children at home or in schools may negatively affect their mental and physical health and rip that sense of normalcy that schools used to provide. These long-term physical inactivity, irregular sleeping patterns, unhealthy dietary plans and longer screen time while on lockdown/school closure will ultimately result in overweight children and reduced cardio-respiratory fitness [14]. In both the developed and developing world, school is also a place of nutrition for many children living in destitution, so shutting it down will exacerbate food insecurity, which can be correlated with low academic achievement and health risks for students as a whole [14].

As a result of prolonged shutdowns, educational inequalities arise as well. In the event of this closure, the learning gap will be widened between children from lower-income families. It is very difficult for children from low-income households to access the audio-visual equipment they need to homeschool and a good internet connection to do so [13]. Even in developed countries, millions of children lack basic amenities, including a stable residence, required reading material, and a place to do their homework, access to computers, smartphones, and media. A COVID-19 pandemic could have socio-economic consequences such as child abuse, drop-out from education, involvement in high-risk activities and a rise child labor [15]. This is a global crisis and, for some children, its effects will last a lifetime.

### 3.2 Impact on education of youth and college student

The loss of dormitories and peer groups resulted in many university and college students having to leave campus immediately often without their belongings and being expected to continue academic work as usual, virtually. This disruption caused any student to be unfamiliar with their routine. The stress caused by the prolonged threat and the rapid evolution of the pandemic makes the experience unique [16]. Many studies related to physiological effect of pandemic on students have been carried.

#### *3.2.1 National study*

Initially for 21 days, a national level "lockdown" was declared from midnight of March 25, 2020 to May 3, 2020, to tackle the rapid outbreak and control the spread to communities [17]. It is true that lockdown can be effective and significant strategies to distancing the population from the highly infectious and rapidly spreading COVID-19 virus, however, they also can have some psychological impact on the masses [18].

Online survey was carried out to study the mental health of Maharashtra students belonging to the age between 16 and 25 years, during pandemic situation. Study says that more affect was seen on rural students as the hope for future source of support to the family. Female students found to be more concern regarding future and male found to be helpless [19]. Cross-sectional study was done across India by online survey on depression, anxiety and stress under this situation on students. There were significant associations between the emotional states and less time spent with their friends, this also led to rise in violence, irregular sleep, financial crisis, etc. [20]. Another cross-sectional study with 131 respondents for Google forms was done to find the mental stage of Indian students. More anxiety and depression was seen among female students which was moderate [21].

*3.2.2 International study*

Changes in academic frameworks, tests, and a battle with limited resources have all been linked to anxiety, tension, frustration, and depressive illnesses during COVID-19's lockdown period [19]. Lots of international studies have been done regarding impact on student's education. 'Gap-year' concept is well known among different countries which got affected due to pandemic situation. Many students who planned to carry university education immediately after high school was unable to do so due to drop in a year or extension of degree [22]. 127 students among Smolensk State University were surveyed regarding the issues they faced while admitting during pandemics. Students those having idea of interested course or training did not face any issue while taking an admission, while those who did not have any goals face an issue due to reasons like less score, finance, lack of knowledge, surrounding influence etc. So in this case self-determination played a role among students [23]. COVID-19 pandemic school closures affect approximately 1.5 billion pupils in 195 countries, according to UNESCO [14]. Parents, students, and teachers all benefit from distance learning solutions, which include platforms, educational software, and resources. Some countries use radio, television, and the internet to provide classes. However, many students are not able to attend any classes or learn digital course because of problem with net connection, financial crisis, no digital appliances, lack of handling knowledge etc. [24]. According to many research, university students have a high prevalence of depression, stress, and worry. According to research conducted in Pakistan and Bangladesh, the prevalence of depression among students was 34 and 82.4%, and of anxiety was 45 and 87.7% [25]. Students among Nigeria were also found to be under stress and depression. Similar study was done among the 350 students of University of Gondar, Ethiopia found to be under depression, worry and stress due to illness, sudden change in routine, isolation, no get-togethers, financial crisis, etc. [26]. Thus COVID-19 has an impact on the entire educational system, including examinations and assessments, the start of a new semester or term, and the possibility of extending the school year [27].

## 4. Impact of COVID-19 on psychology of students

COVID-19 became a pandemic almost shortly after its emergence and dissemination. Besides death from coronavirus infection, the pandemic put everyone under excruciating psychological strain. The COVID-19 pandemic's circumstances, including nationwide lockdown, isolation, as well as delays in the current educational system, such as delaying of examinations and unexpected shutdown of classes, are predicted to have an impact on the mental health of students at many schools, colleges, and universities across the country [28].

The types of situations a student has in the classroom have a significant impact on their academic success, psychological health, and well-being [29]. Adolescents and college students who do not feel like they belong in their academic contexts, for example, may experience more self-doubt, be less inspired, and perform poorly in school [30]. Those who reported a lesser sense of belonging at their university experienced increased anxiety, tension, and mood disorders, according to a study of graduate students from minority races and ethnicities [31]. Having a larger sense of connectedness and support from fellow postgraduates, on the other hand, has indeed been linked to lower stress and improved life satisfaction in prior studies [32]. The majority of graduate students struggle with career balance, employment instability, concerns about completing their research on time, and financial

| Sr. No | University or Country | Student/sampling number | Stress | Anxiety | Depression | Social interaction | Academic performance/ concentration | Reference |
|---|---|---|---|---|---|---|---|---|
| 1 | Large university system in Texas, United States | 195 | 71% | – | – | 86% | 82% | [41] |
| 2 | Arizona State University in Tempe, Clemson University in Clemson North Carolina State University in Raleigh Oregon State University in Corvallis Pennsylvania State University State College University of Montana in Missoula The University of Utah in Salt Lake City | 2534 | 14.6% | 17.4% | 5.7% | – | – | [42] |
| 3 | U.S. college students | 200 | | 60.8% | 59.8% | 34.1% | 60.9% | [43] |
| 4 | Changzhi medical college, China | 1143 | 30.1% | 38% | – | – | 76.6% | [44] |
| 5 | Public research university in Kentucky | 2691 | 88% | – | – | – | – | [45] |
| 6 | Public and private university of Bangladesh. | 15543 | 44.59% | – | – | – | – | [46] |
| 7 | Universities from Turkey | 358 | – | – | 63% | – | – | [47] |

**Table 2.**
*University and psychological factors affecting their students.*

worries [33]. Graduate students' mental health may deteriorate as a result of these challenges. Graduate students who said they suffered with work–life harmony also report greater levels of anxiety and depression [34]. Students' behaviors and attitudes toward education and school attendance might be affected by their absence from the study and learning environment.

At its peak, as per The United Nations Educational, Scientific and Cultural Organization (UNESCO 2021), the COVID-19 pandemic had a huge global impact on the lives and education of more over 1.6 billion students. The first country to be hit by the COVID-19 pandemic was China. As a result, various researches evaluating the effects of the outbreak on student's mental health have been published. Study explored the psychological problems and suicidal behavior among senior high students. A total of 859 middle school students participated in this study. Stress, worry, Trauma, suicidal thoughts, and suicide attempts were found to be 71, 54.5, 85.5, 31.3, and 7.5% [35]. Some other cross-sectional research of 532 Chinese school children employed three different types of surveys from previous studies and found that approximately 20% of the participants' mental health had been impaired [36]. Further research of 584 Chinese youngsters found that 40.4% were vulnerable to mental health issues and 14.4% experienced Post - traumatic stress disorder. Their findings in the context of COVID-19 revealed that mental health was linked to educational attainment, employment, and the use of negative behaviors [37]. Ecuadorian high school students participated in a cross-sectional survey. The participants were interviewed over the phone for their survey, which focused on themes connected to remote learning technologies and their effects. In their study, they discovered that 16% of those who took part had scores that indicated serious depression [38]. Similarly, after just 1 month of lockdowns, a longitudinal research including 442 students from last year's high school in Greece found a 15.3% increase in depression, a 17% increase in severe sadness, a 25.7% increase in worry, and a 16.7% increase in extreme anxiety [39].

Several studies examining factors linked to the COVID-19 outbreak among college students found high anxiety and concern regarding educational disruptions, as well as the impact of the epidemic on daily life, as a result of disruptions in students' daily routines in terms of events, goals, and social connections [40]. Some factors have been mention in **Table 2**.

## 5. Combating the psychological effects due to pandemic on students

College students suffer from a lot of anxiety. Educational attainment, pressure to win, and post-graduation planning are the top three concerns among students from all fields [48]. Students experience extreme anxiety as a result of economic uncertainties, family medical issues, infection concerns, the need to support and services for kids, and the challenges of distance learning [49].

Various combating techniques have been implemented to reduce the anxiety among students. Cross sectional study among nursing students were done, 244 students were selected to study their anxiety. Some methods to overcome students stress can be like staff helping students by maintaining stable syllabus, providing quality distance education, considering the students personal health issues, counseling them etc. [49]. To deal with the socio economic effects of the COVID-19 curfew on pupils in North-Eastern Nigeria, radio education initiatives were implemented, and solar radios were provided to villages in the region [50]. Furthermore, state governments used family fun performance and giving food to learners at home as coping strategies [51]. Students at Nigeria's University of Ibadan coped by viewing movies, using social media, and engaging in online skills training [52].

Other strategies reported states that, spending additional time indoors, apart from other obligations, had advantages such as investing quality time with the family. Furthermore, it has increased the rate at which productive activities and household duties such as preparing new dishes, housekeeping, parenting, and enjoying life have been accomplished. As a result, students will benefit from the pandemic's benefits as well [52]. Similarly, a poll conducted by University of Plymouth professors in revealed that the lockdown's impact to domestic life could be long-term, since it has aided parents and their students in finding the right balance among job, education, and home life. Also, doing domestic and household duties during COVID-19 lockdown is an excellent way to keep families on track, according to the report [53]. According to few studies, many students adapted by frequently spending time online, media platforms, and videophone chats with relatives, colleagues, and coworkers [54]. Moreover, while the pandemic was ongoing, many American students used meditation, relaxation, and workout as coping tactics. Spirituality, such as rereading their bibles, Religious books, and worshipping, were also used as coping mechanisms due to the pandemic's dread and uncertainty [55]. Importantly, asana and meditating have been proven to reduce stress, increase general wellness, and research has shown that exercise and yoga improve immunity [56]. As a result, employing these techniques to mitigate the effects of pandemic constraints can assist students in maintaining their health while still at homes.

## 6. Conclusion

The pandemic of COVID-19 brings people with it new challenges. The spread of viruses is not just affecting the health but also causing a psychological impact among students which further triggers stress, anxiety, worries, negative thoughts etc. Different studies related to psychological impact on students among different age groups have been done. Various combating strategies have also been implemented by universities and government. Many students have themselves diverted to some other work, meditation, yoga, exercise, cooking and learning other digital skills. The medical experts and administrations should devise a plan to ease the mental strain of the COVID-19 pandemic by giving emotional assistance to the entire population, but especially to students for further studies and better future during such situation.

## Acknowledgements

I would like to thanks all the researchers who did the survey on online basis under this pandemic situation. Also thanks to my family to support me to write this chapter with full concentration.

## Conflict of interest

No conflict of interest.

## Author details

Rutuja Patankar
Sandip University, Nashik, India

*Address all correspondence to: rutujapatankar19@gmail.com

## References

[1] Vindegaard N, Benros ME. COVID-19 pandemic and mental health consequences: Systematic review of the current evidence. Brain, Behavior, and Immunity. 2020;**89**:531-542. DOI: 10.1016/j.bbi.2020.05.048

[2] Huang C, Wang Y, Li X, Ren L, Zhao J, Hu Y, et al. Clinical features of patients infected with 2019 novel coronavirus in Wuhan, China. The Lancet. 2020;**395**(10223):497-506. DOI: 10.1016/S0140-6736(20)30183-5

[3] Fu L, Wang B, Yuan T, Chen X, Ao Y, Fitzpatrick T, et al. Clinical characteristics of coronavirus disease 2019 (COVID-19) in China: A systematic review and meta-analysis. Journal of Infection. 2020;**80**(6):656-665. DOI: 10.1016/j.jinf.2020.03.041

[4] Hawryluck L, Gold WL, Robinson S, Pogorski S, Galea S, Styra R. SARS control and psychological effects of quarantine, Toronto, Canada. Emerging Infectious Diseases. 2004;**10**(7):1206-1212. DOI: 10.3201/eid1007.030703

[5] Chen Y, Zhou H, Zhou Y, Zhou F. Prevalence of self-reported depression and anxiety among pediatric medical staff members during the COVID-19 outbreak in Guiyang, China. Psychiatry Research. 2020;**288**:113005. DOI: 10.1016/j.psychres.2020.113005

[6] Saladino V, Algeri D, Auriemma V. The psychological and social impact of Covid-19: New perspectives of well-being. Frontiers in Psychology. 2020;**11**:2550. DOI: 10.3389/fpsyg.2020.577684

[7] Villani L, Pastorino R, Molinari E, Anelli F, Ricciardi W, Graffigna G, et al. Impact of the COVID-19 pandemic on psychological well-being of students in an Italian university: A web-based cross-sectional survey. Globalization and Health. 2021;**17**(1):1-14. DOI: 10.1186/s12992-021-00680-w

[8] Kyrou I, Robbins T, Randeva H. COVID-19 and Diabetes: No time to drag our feet during an untimely pandemic. Journal of Diabetes and Its Complications. 2020;**1**(12):1-7. DOI: 10.1016/j.jdiacomp.2020.107621

[9] Güner R, Hasanoğlu İ, Aktaş F. Covid-19: Prevention and control measures in community. Turkish Journal of Medical Science. 2020; **50**(SI-1):571-577. DOI: 10.3906/sag-2004-146

[10] Shen K, Yang Y, Wang T, Zhao D, Jiang Y, Jin R, et al. Diagnosis, treatment, and prevention of 2019 novel coronavirus infection in children: Experts' consensus statement. World Journal of Pediatrics. 2020;**16**(3):223-231. DOI: 10.1007/s12519-020-00343-7

[11] Weisaeth L, Tonnessen A. Fear, information and control during a pandemic. Tidsskriftet Den Norske Laegeforening. 2020;**140**(10):30. [Online]. Available from: http://ovidsp.ovid.com/ovidweb.cgi?T=JS&CSC=Y&NEWS=N&PAGE=fulltext&D=prem&AN=32602307 http://sfx.library.cdc.gov/cdc?sid=OVID:medline&id=pmid:32602307&id=10.4045%2Ftidsskr.20.0346&issn=0029-2001&isbn=&volume=140&issue=10&spage=&pages=&date=2020&title=Tids

[12] Gupta S, Jawanda MK. The impacts of COVID-19 on children. Acta Paediatrica. 2020;**109**(11):2181-2183. DOI: 10.1111/apa.15484

[13] Viner RM et al. School closure and management practices during coronavirus outbreaks including COVID-19: A rapid systematic review. The Lancet Child & Adolescent Health. 2020;**4**(5):397-404. DOI: 10.1016/S2352-4642(20)30095-X

[14] Tadesse S, Muluye W. The impact of COVID-19 pandemic on education

system in developing countries: A review. Open Journal of Social Sciences. 2020;**08**(10):159-170. DOI: 10.4236/jss.2020.810011

[15] Watve MG, Yajnik CS. Evolutionary origins of insulin resistance : A behavioral switch hypothesis. BMC Evolutionary Biology. 2007;**13**:1-13. DOI: 10.1186/1471-2148-7-61

[16] Copeland WE, McGinnis E, Bai Y, Adams Z, Nardone H, Devadanam V, et al. Impact of COVID-19 pandemic on college student mental health and wellness. American Academy of Child and Adolescent Psychiatry. 2021;**60**(1):134-141.e2.

[17] The Lancet. India under COVID-19 lockdown. Lancet. 2020;**395**(10233):1315. DOI: 10.1016/S0140-6736(20)30938-7

[18] Grover S, Sahoo S, Reddy YCJ. Psychological impact of COVID-19 lockdown : An online survey from India. Indian J Psychiatry. 2020;**62**(4):354-362. DOI: 10.4103/psychiatry.IndianJPsychiatry_427_20

[19] Moghe K, Kotecha D, Patil M. COVID-19 and mental health: A study of its impact on students in Maharashtra, India .British Medical Journal. 2021;**5**(12):1-20. DOI: 10.1101/2020.08.05.20160499

[20] Purushothaman Ravichandran S, Kumaravel Palanichami M, Kumar Kalaiselvan K, Muthukumar A, Mahalingam G. Psychological impact of COVID-19 lock-down on college students across India- a cross sectional study. International Journal of Community Medicine and Public Health. 2020;7(12):4917. DOI: 10.18203/2394 6040.ijcmph20205163

[21] Verma K. The mental health impact of the COVID-19 epidemic on college students in India. Asian Journal of Psychiatry. 2020;**53**:102398

[22] Kremen S, Tsitsikashvili K. The representations of the regional university students about the 'gap year' in conditions of the Covid-19 pandemic. E3S Web of Conferences. 2021;**296**:08008. DOI: 10.1051/e3sconf/202129608008

[23] Kremen F, Kremen S. Features of career self-determination of regional university applicants in the context of the COVID-19 pandemic. E3S Web of Conferences. 2021;**291**:05020. DOI: 10.1051/e3sconf/202129105020

[24] Crawford J, Butler-Henderson K, Rudolph J, Malkawi B, Glowatz M, Burton R, et al. COVID-19 : 20 countries' higher education intra-period digital pedagogy responses. Journal of Applied Learning & Teaching. 2020;**3**(1):1-20. DOI: 10.37074/jalt.2020.3.1.7

[25] Akhtarul Islam M, Barna SD, Raihan H, Nafiul Alam Khan M, Tanvir Hossain M. Depression and anxiety among university students during the COVID-19 pandemic in Bangladesh: A web-based cross-sectional survey. PLoS One. 2020;**15**(8):1-12. DOI: 10.1371/journal.pone.0238162

[26] Mekonen EG, Workneh BS, Ali MS, Muluneh NY. The psychological impact of COVID-19 pandemic on graduating class students at the university of Gondar, northwest Ethiopia. Psychology Research and Behaviour Management. 2021;**14**:109-122. DOI: 10.2147/PRBM.S300262

[27] Tiruneh D. Covid-19 school closures may further widen the inequality gaps between the advantaged and the disadvantaged in Ethiopia. Education in Emergencies. 2020. DOI: 10.13140/RG.2.2.11243.57120

[28] Biswas S, Biswas A. Anxiety level among students of different college and universities in India during lock down in connection to the COVID-19 pandemic. Journal of Public Health. 2021

[29] Dennehy TC, Dasgupta N. Female peer mentors early in college increase women's positive academic experiences and retention in engineering. Proceedings of the National Academy of Sciences of the United States of America. 2017; **114**(23):1-6. DOI: 10.1073/pnas. 1613117114

[30] Neel CG, Fuligni A. A longitudinal study of school belonging and academic motivation across high school. Child Development. 2013;**842**:678-692. DOI: 10.1111/j.1467-8624.2012.01862.x

[31] Miller AN, Orsillo SM. Values, acceptance, and belongingess in graduate school : Perspectives from underrepresented minority students. Journal of Contextual Behavioral Science. 2020;**15**:197-206. DOI: 10.1016/ j.jcbs.2020.01.002

[32] Charles ST, Karnaze MM, Leslie FM, Charles ST, Karnaze MM, Positive FML. Positive factors related to graduate student mental health. Journal of American College Health. 2021;**69**(5):1-9

[33] Luchetti M, Lee JH, Aschwanden D, Sesker A, Strickhouser JE, Terracciano A, et al. The trajectory of loneliness in response to COVID-19. American Psychologist. 2020;**75**(7):897-908

[34] Evans TM, Bira L, Gastelum JB, Weiss LT, Vanderford NL. Evidence for a mental health crisis in graduate education. Nature Biotechnology. 2018;**36**:7-12

[35] Hou T, Mao X, Dong W, Cai W, Deng G. Prevalence of and factors associated with mental health problems and suicidality among senior high school students in rural China during the COVID-19 outbreak. Asian Journal of Psychiatry. 2020;**54**:102305. DOI: 10.1016/j.ajp.2020.102305

[36] Zhang C, Ye M, Fu Y, Yang M, Luo F, Yuan J, et al. The psychological impact of the COVID-19 pandemic on teenagers in China. Journal of Adolescent Health. 2020;**67**(6):747-755. DOI: 10.1016/j. jadohealth.2020.08.026

[37] Liang L, Ren H, Cao R, Hu Y, Qin Z, Li C, et al. The effect of COVID-19 on youth mental health. Psychiatric Quarterly. 2020;**91**(3):841-852

[38] Veit CT, Ware JE. The structure of psychological distress and well-being in general populations. Journal of Consulting and Clinical Psychology. 1983;**51**(5):730-742

[39] Neshat N, Mahlooji H, Kazemi A. An enhanced neural network model for predictive control of granule quality characteristics. Scientia Iranica. 2011;**18**(3):722-730. DOI: 10.1016/j. scient.2011.05.019

[40] Zurlo MC, Francesca M, Della C, Vallone F. COVID-19 student stress questionnaire: Development and validation of a questionnaire to evaluate students' stressors related to the coronavirus pandemic lockdown. Frontiers in Psychology. 2020;**11**:1-11. DOI: 10.3389/fpsyg.2020.576758

[41] Editor M, Eysenbach G, Fagherazzi G, Torous J. Effects of COVID-19 on college students' mental health in the United States : Interview survey study. Journal of Medical Internet Research. 2020;**22**(9):1-18. DOI: 10.2196/21279

[42] Browning MHEM, Larson LR, Sharaievska I, Rigolon A, McAnirlin O, Mullenbach L, et al. Psychological impacts from COVID-19 among university students : Risk factors across seven states in the United States. PLoS One. 2021;**16**(1):1-27

[43] Lee J, Solomon M, Stead T, Kwon B, Ganti L. Impact of COVID-19 on the mental health of US college students. BMC Psychology. 2021;**9**(1):1-10. DOI: 10.1186/s40359-021-00598-3

[44] Cao W, Fang Z, Hou G, Han M, Xu X, Dong J, et al. The psychological impact of the COVID-19 epidemic on college students in China. Psychiatry Research. 2020;**287**:112934. DOI: 10.1016/j.psychres.2020.112934

[45] Lee J, Ju H, Sujin J. Stress, anxiety, and depression among undergraduate students during the COVID-19 pandemic and their use of mental health services. Innovative Higher Education. 2021;**46**:519-538. DOI: 10.1007/s10755-021-09552-y

[46] Dhar BK, Ayittey FK, Sarkar SM. Impact of COVID-19 on psychology among the university students. Global Challenges. 2020;**4**(11):1-5. DOI: 10.1002/gch2.202000038

[47] Aslan I, Ochnik D, Çınar O. Exploring perceived stress among students in Turkey during the COVID-19 pandemic. International Journal of Environmental Research and Public Health. 2020;**17**(23):8961.

[48] Beiter R, Nash R, McCrady M, Rhoades D, Linscomb M, Clarahan M, et al. The prevalence and correlates of depression, anxiety, and stress in a sample of college students. Journal of Affective Disorders. 2015;**173**:90-96. DOI: 10.1016/j.jad.2014.10.054

[49] Savitsky B, Findling Y, Ereli A, Hendel T. Since January 2020 Elsevier has created a COVID-19 resource centre with free information in English and Mandarin on the novel coronavirus COVID- 19. The COVID-19 resource centre is hosted on Elsevier Connect, the company's public news and information. 2020.

[50] Obro S, Atubi FO. Social impact and coping strategies of Covid 19 pandemic: Insights from social studies undergraduates students. Journal of Research in Humanities and Social Science. 2021;**9**(7):61-68

[51] Nigeria EiE Working Group. Nigeria Education Sector COVID-19 Response Strategy in North East. 2020. Available from: https://inee.org/resources/nigeria-education-sector-covid-19-response-strategy-north-east

[52] Ojewale LY. Psychological state, family functioning and coping strategies among students of the University of Ibadan, Nigeria, during the COVID-19 lockdown. medRxiv. 2020;**1**(15):1-19. DOI: 10.1101/2020.07.09.20149997

[53] WVUTODAY. Ten tips for on keeping your family on track during the COVID-19. 2020. Available from: https://wvutoday.wvu.edu/media-center-blog/2020/03/20/expert-pitch-ten-tips-for-on-keeping-your-family-on-track-during-the-covid-19-pandemic

[54] Hussain W. Role of social media in COVID-19 pandemic. The International Journal of Frontier Sciences. 2020;**4**(2):59-60. DOI: 10.37978/tijfs.v4i2.144

[55] Cohut M. COVID-19 pandemic: Some top coping strategies and why they work. Medical News Today. 2020:1-6

[56] Whiteman H. Yoga, meditation counter gene expression changes that cause stress. 2017. Available from: https://www.medicalnewstoday.com/articles/317946#MBIs-reduce-production-of-pro-inflammatory-molecules

Chapter 2

# Perspective Chapter: Psychological Effects of COVID-19 Pandemic

*Vasfiye Bayram Değer*

## Abstract

COVID-19, the viral pneumonia seen in China towards the end of 2019, was declared a global pandemic in March 2020 since it spread almost all over the world. While such pandemic situations that are concerned with public health cause a sense of insecurity, confusion, loneliness and stigmatization among individuals, it can result in economic losses, closure of workplaces and schools, insufficient resources for medical needs and inadequate satisfaction of needs in societies. The economic crisis, which is one of the most important problems in pandemic periods, and the concomitant uncertainties can also cause suicidal thoughts. As a result, how the society responds psychologically during epidemics has an important role in shaping the spread of the disease, emotional difficulties and social problems during and after the epidemic. It often appears that no resources are allocated to manage, or at least mitigate the effects of epidemics on psychological health and well-being. In the acute phase of the epidemic, health system administrators prioritize testing, preventing contagion and providing patient care, but psychological needs should not be disregarded either.

**Keywords:** psychological impacts, covid 19, pandemic, adults, elderly, trauma

## 1. Introduction

COVID-19 global pandemic, caused by the severe acute respiratory syndrome coronavirus 2 (SARS-COV-2) virus, has precipitated government-mandated quarantines, social distancing, and other measures for the benefit of public health. Forced curfews have changed and disrupted people's daily routines, work, travel and leisure activities abruptly and dramatically in a way that most people living outside of war zones have not experienced. Moreover, this highly contagious virus has transformed situations such as social interaction, touching one's face, attending a concert, shaking someone's hand, and even hugging grandparents into those perceived as potentially dangerous [1].

The Covid-19 pandemic has been deemed as the most prevalent disease of our generation. This pandemic has affected people from almost all nations, continents, races and socioeconomic groups [2]. Mankind has been challenged with many undesirable and unexpected events including natural disasters such as earthquakes, floods, storms, volcanic eruptions, hurricanes, and tornadoes as well as human-induced conditions such as wars, terrorism, and accidents. These unforeseen and sudden events are considered as a crisis situation [3]. It is argued that the crisis as a term is the main subject and core concept of many scientific fields. In a broader definition, James and Gilliand states that a crisis is an event and situation that an individual encounters at an unexpected time, has difficulty tolerating and can disrupt their equilibrium [4]. On the other hand, Kaya and Yıldırım suggest that a crisis emanates from life events that occur in some periods of one's lifetime and can lead to pathological consequences unless rational decisions are taken [5].

Given different definitions, it can be argued that the crises affect individuals adversely with their unexpected nature threatening the life, and involve making quick and rational decisions. The crises can influence the individuals physically, socially and psychologically by provoking negative emotions and eliciting different reactions by creating pressure, distress, panic and insecurity on individuals [6] and it is emphasized that the mental balance of individuals is impaired in case of any crisis. All individuals are affected by such crises differently in proportion to their developmental period and may exhibit different reactions. For example, being a child, adolescent, adult or elderly person in the event of a crisis emerges as a different situation [7, 8]. It is contended that infectious diseases are highly associated with mental problems, which is clearly illustrated by the COVID-19 pandemic [9]. The COVID-19 pandemic is a process that needs to be addressed with its social, economic, political and spiritual consequences [10], threatening people's lives and causing traumatic distress [11]. It is widely known that the COVID-19 pandemic especially gives rise to psychological problems [12–14]. It is stated that the solution to overcome this critical process in a healthy way largely depends on the extensive research on the psychological effects of the pandemic [15]. During the pandemic process, people's psychological responses significantly influence the spread of the disease and increase the emotional distress and social dysfunctions that may occur in the next stage [16]. Therefore, the psychological effects of the pandemic must be thoroughly investigated. A recent study conducted by Wang et al. in China has shown that the pandemic process causes moderate and severe psychological effects among the public [14]. Due to the pandemic, people are experiencing psychological problems such as depression, anxiety and distress. Another study conducted by Li et al. has revealed that the COVID-19 pandemic causes a decrease in people's positive emotions and an increase in their negative emotions [17]. After the pandemic, which is inherently a stressful process, people may experience anxiety and discomfort. Stressful situations need to be handled effectively in order to prevent distress and anxiety from turning into more acute state. It is important to understand how people respond to and cope with the threats of the pandemic [15]. It is thought that psychological resilience especially plays a decisive role in coping effectively with this process [18].

Psychological resilience refers to the capacity of an individual to adapt to the challenges of life and maintain mental health despite exposure to adversity [19]. The reactions or coping strategies of individual who have been exposed to many adversities, shocking, traumatic and stressful life events throughout their lifetimes may vary. While some individuals react to stressful and traumatic situations in the form of mental problems such as anxiety and depression, others can recover from their negative mood in a short time and continue their normal lives. This phenomenon is termed as psychological resilience in the positive psychology [20]. It is stated that there are optimistic perspectives that most people become stronger by tackling the difficulties they face through resilience [21]. Psychological resilience, which is defined as the capability to adapt flexibly to the changes brought about by stressful events and to recover from negative emotional experiences [22], affects the course of disease and health conditions afterwards [23].

Moreover, it was reported that the psychological effects of the epidemic lasted longer and were more common than that of the physical, and it was very difficult to calculate psychosocial and economic effects in past epidemics [24, 25]. For example, it was stated that the fear experienced during the Ebola epidemic and the resulting behaviors intensified psychological symptoms, indirectly contributing to the increase in death rates due to reasons other than Ebola [26]. Similarly, easy access to mass media and other technologies along with spread of false and inconsistent information during the COVID-19 process can instigate harmful social reactions such as violent and aggressive behaviors in individuals [27]. During the recent SARS epidemic, both healthcare staff and surviving patients experienced various psychological disorders [28, 29]. A study conducted by Mak et al. has revealed that the most common psychological disorders among the public after the SARS epidemic included as post-traumatic stress and depressive disorders [30]. Similar results were observed after the MERS outbreak [31].

Isolation measures and quarantine practices taken to avoid getting sick or to prevent the spread of the disease arouse a great deal of fear, hopelessness and loneliness among the public [32, 33]. All these negative emotional states increase suicidal thoughts. During the pandemic process, death cases that were directly or indirectly associated with COVID-19 infection were reported in many countries including India, Saudi Arabia, England and Germany [34]. The spread and prolongation of the COVID-19 pandemic imposes deeper impact on financially and socially vulnerable groups. It is predicted that suicide cases will increase in this process, and therefore, necessary precautions should be taken immediately [35]. Following many natural disasters in the world, dramatic changes have been observed in suicide rates due to regional and social structure [36]. In a study investigating the suicide rates in the elderly population after the SARS-CoV-2 epidemic in Hong Kong in 2003, it was observed that suicide rates increased by 30% especially in women compared to 2002 [36]. In a survey conducted in Canada in 2003 on the individuals who were isolated due to SARS-CoV-2, it was found that they had been experiencing boredom, frustration, and anger, and their social life after isolation was adversely affected by this period [37]. In studies conducted among uninfected individuals during the SARS-CoV-2 infection process, it has been observed that there are many psychiatric morbidities that occur with the feeling of guilt at young age [38]. It will be revealed by future studies that the COVID-19 infection may also trigger suicidal thoughts and behaviors in individuals, and underlying factors at the individual and social level.

The major situations that contribute to psychological problems during the pandemic include quarantine and isolation, wearing masks and social distancing, and stigma.

## 2. The psychological effects of quarantine and isolation

In simple terms, quarantine means separation of people who are exposed to a potentially contagious disease from other individuals to detect whether they are sick and restricting their freedom of movement, thereby reducing the risk of transmission to others [39]. This definition differs from isolation during which people diagnosed with an infectious disease are separated from those who are not sick. However, the two terms are often used interchangeably, particularly in public communication [40]. Quarantine is often an unpleasant experience for those experiencing it. Separation from the beloved ones, loss of freedom, uncertainty about disease, and boredom can sometimes have dramatic effects. Suicide cases have been reported following quarantine practices in previous outbreaks. The potential benefits of mandatory mass quarantine must be carefully assessed against the possible psychological costs [41]. The successful implementation of quarantine as a public health measure requires that we reduce as much as possible the adverse effects associated with it [42]. In another study comparing the psychological states of the quarantined and non-quarantined, it was found that hospital staff who may have been in contact with SARS suffered from symptoms of acute stress disorder immediately after the end of the 9-day quarantine period. In the same study, it was found that the quarantined staff had significantly higher levels of fatigue, detachment from others, feeling anxious when dealing with patients with fever, irritability, insomnia, poor concentration and indecisiveness, poor job performance, and reluctance to work or considering to quit their job [43]. In another study [44], the effect of quarantine in hospital staff was found to cause symptoms of post-traumatic stress even after 3 years. Another study comparing the indicators of post-traumatic stress among the quarantined parents and children with those not quarantined, it was found that the post-traumatic stress mean scores of quarantined children were four times higher than those of non-quarantined. In this study, 28% of the quarantined parents and 6% of the non-quarantined parents had sufficient symptoms to be diagnosed with a trauma-related mental health disorder [45]. In other quantitative studies on this subject, psychological distress and disorder symptoms among the quarantined persons were highly prevalent.

Major psychological symptoms with a high prevalence include emotional discomfort [46], depression [47], stress [48], low mood, irritability, insomnia [49], post-traumatic stress [37], anger [50], and emotional burnout [51]. In two studies on the long-term effects of quarantine in healthcare staff, it was found that alcohol use or addiction were positively associated with quarantine 3 years after the SARS epidemic [52]. Therefore, recognizing the stressors in quarantine and taking measures against them is one of the most important points in mitigating the harmful effects of the quarantine process. The duration of quarantine, fears of infection, frustration and boredom, insufficient supplies, missing information are among the major stressors during quarantine while financial concerns are among the post-quarantine stressors [42].

### 2.1 Wearing masks and social distancing

The interpersonal space (IPS) refers to the area surrounding our own bodies where we comfortably interact with other individuals. Typically, individuals regulate IPS through two basic behavioral patterns: they extend their distance when they feel they are in dangerous and uncomfortable situations (i.e. avoidance behavior) or, conversely, they reduce their distance when they feel they are in friendly and safe situations (i.e. approach behavior). During the COVID-19 outbreak, holding larger-than-normal IPS and wearing a face mask is one of the most effective measures to curb the COVID-19 outbreak which is still highly recommended despite the possibility of vaccination [53].

The members of the society interact with each other. As a result of this interaction, it is known that social values, which are also described as shared values, coexist with human beings. These values are accepted, adopted and influential in people's lives. Love, respect, tolerance, freedom, justice and equality, fraternity, cooperation, honesty, industriousness, hospitality, compassion and mercifulness, and protecting cultural heritage, which are counted as social values, are important values to be handed down to future generations [54]. Being locked down, feeling like a captive, being separated from the beloved ones and close contacts have unexpectedly and radically changed our daily life and traditional values. When encountered with situations such as epidemics with unpredictable effects, it is considered natural for individuals to exhibit panic, fear, hopelessness, avoidance and protective behaviors [55]. When feelings such as anxiety, fear and uneasiness begin to spread among the public, the factors that create fear and anxiety begin to direct people, and with the weakening of traditional solidarity, individuals who are isolated in big cities feel more vulnerable and powerless, thereby promoting the feeling of insecurity. Staying indoors for a long time, being disconnected from social life and work have caused psychological problems. The social imbalance between those who have the opportunity to work at home and those who have to go to work has been clearly revealed. Consequently, we all experience that the social/physical isolation in our lives with the pandemic affects our interpersonal relations adversely. A study conducted among 145 participants on the subject drew attention to the psychological effects of the virus on themselves and their relationships in most of their responses. Participants reported that, in addition to the fear of contracting the disease, there was a lack of communication between them and their loved ones due to the social/physical distance in the process, that they distanced individuals from each other, and that they were worried about the fact that the traditional ties that bound the generations and the society together would disappear if the process continued like this [56].

### 2.2 Stigma

Public health strategies to deal with emerging outbreaks require a delicate balance between maintaining public health and initiating exclusionary practices and treatments that can lead to fear, stigma and discrimination against certain communities. Due to their evolving nature and inherent scientific ambiguity, emerging epidemics of infectious disease may be associated with fear in a significant way in the general population or in certain communities, particularly where the disease and death are significant. Reducing fear and discrimination against the infected and the affected by a contagious disease can be vitally important in controlling the transmission. Those people who are feared and stigmatized may delay seeking care, remaining unnoticed within the society [57]. Fear of being socially marginalized and stigmatized on account of a disease outbreak may contribute to individuals' denial of early clinical symptoms and failure to seek medical care on time [57]. Such fears can aggravate stigma when cases are detected at a later time. The stigma associated with discrimination often has social and economic consequences that exacerbate internalized stigma and feelings of fear [57].

Among those affected by the 2003 SARS epidemic, the stigma associated with the disease was found to be somewhat evident even years later, and resuming the usual rituals of daily life was very difficult for many [50, 57, 58]. Similarly, the COVID 19 pandemic, with all its social and economic consequences, can lead to stigmatizing factors such as fear of isolation, racism, discrimination and marginalization [58]. A stigmatized community tends to seek medical care late and conceal their important medical history related to travel in particular. In addition to the potential psychological problems caused by the Covid 19 pandemic, the stigma, discrimination and social rejection of the quarantined group, suspicion and avoidance by the neighbor, distrust of property, prejudice at workplace and withdrawal from sociocultural events even after the epidemic is under control are among other crucial issues [42]. Health care providers (HCPs), especially general practitioners, have been found to be more prone to stigma of those caring for patients affected by SARS [59]. Since health care staff are quarantined and constantly more psychologically affected, they are more subject to stigma than the general public.

During the period after the onset of the COVID-19 epidemic in China, the 'social media panic', characterized by an endless flux of false and manipulated information and misinformation, evolved into a metastatic condition more rapidly than the coronavirus itself [60, 61]. WHO defined it as "coronavirus infodemic" that fueled fear and panic by unleashing uncontrolled mind-blowing rumors, bombastic news propaganda, and sensationalism [62] From the onset of the COVID-19 pandemic, social media has played an integral role in generating anti-Chinese sentiments and opinions around the World [60]. Conspiracy theory, derogatory headlines about eating habits, biased comments on Chinese socio-cultural norms posted on social

| Social strata | Psychosocial issues | Intervention |
|---|---|---|
| COVID-19 positive patients and quarantined individuals | • Loneliness<br>• Anxiety<br>• Panic<br>• PTSD<br>• Depression | • Secure communication-channel between patient and family<br>• Delivery of progress-reports and discussion with families on further treatment plans through telephone, video-calls, WhatsApp, e-mail etc.<br>• Close monitoring of mental state of quarantined persons using tools like impact of event scale-revised (IES-R) and through smartphone technology<br>• In-time referral<br>• Psychotherapy by stress-adaptation model<br>• Psychiatric follow-up post-discharge, if needed |
| Health care providers | • Fear of worthlessness<br>• Guilt<br>• Overwhelming work-pressure<br>• Deprivation of family while being in quarantine<br>• Burnouts<br>• Depression<br>• Fear of infection and outcomes<br>• Uncertainty<br>• PTSD<br>• Substance abuse | • Support from Higher authority<br>• Clear communication and regular accurate updates regarding precautionary measures<br>• Sustained connection with family and friends through smartphone<br>• Shorter working duration, regular rest period, rotating shifts<br>• Sufficient supply of appropriate PPE<br>• Arrangements for well-equipped isolation wards specific for infected HCPs, insurance-system for work-related injuries<br>• Long term psychological follow-up |
| Children | • Boredom<br>• Anxiety related to educational development<br>• Irritability<br>• Developmental issues<br>• Fear of infection | • Proper parenting<br>• Online classes, online study material<br>• Clear, direct, open and detailed information about disease transmission and precautionary measures<br>• Maintenance of sleep cycle, physical exercise schedule<br>• Educate about proper hygiene practice |
| Old age | • Irritability, anger, fear, anxiety, cognitive decline<br>• Deprivation from pre-scheduled check-up and/or follow-up sessions<br>• Difficulties in accessing medicines due to travel restriction and lockdown | • Home-based physical exercise during quarantine<br>• Sessions via telephone, online video-conference for physician guidance and mental health services<br>• Essential drug-delivery system via online approach |
| Marginalized community | • Depression<br>• Stress<br>• Financial insecurity<br>• Stigma of discrimination<br>• Health crime | • Protection of basic human rights<br>• Providing proper accommodation<br>• Adequate food and waters supply from government and NGO<br>• Affordable health care delivery<br>• Education about social distancing, hygiene<br>• Deploy mental health social worker to address specific need and referral to psychiatrists, if needed |

| Social strata | Psychosocial issues | Intervention |
|---|---|---|
| Psychiatric patients | • Hampered routine psychiatric follow-up<br>• Addiction<br>• Violence | • Structured letter therapy<br>• Counseling via telephone, online chat<br>• Online based psycho-reduction therapies<br>• Proper supply of prescribed medications |

*Source: Dubey et al. [65].*

**Table 1.**
*Psychosocial impact o Covid 19 on different strata of society and suggested interventions.*

media, and news have paved the way for situations that could lead to discrimination, isolation of an entire nation, and a rise of racism [63].

Stigma and blaming targeted at the affected communities can hamper international trade, finance and relations, provoking further unrest. Due care should be taken to eliminate the stigma associated with disease, racism, religious propaganda and psychosocial impact. Furthermore, it should be implemented through regular evaluation with trained and specialized health staff by establishing a directly health-related task force and executive teams [64].

To avoid discrimination and stigma in the context of COVID-19, governmental institutions, political leaders and health officials must undertake an integral role in maintaining interracial harmony during and after the pandemic [65]. In addition to the aforementioned issues, the Covid 19 pandemic has effects on different segments of the society. Special attention should be paid to more vulnerable groups such as quarantined people, healthcare staff, children, the elderly, marginalized communities (including daily bookies, migrant workers, slum dwellers, inmates and homeless populations) and patients with pre-existing psychiatric conditions (**Table 1**) [64].

The **Figure 1** below illustrates the relevant psychosocial consequences and impact of COVID-19 in various segments of modern society [65].

Bearing in mind that psychopathology may differ across developmental stages, it is essential to address the psychological effects of the pandemic primarily on adults, children, adolescents and the elderly.

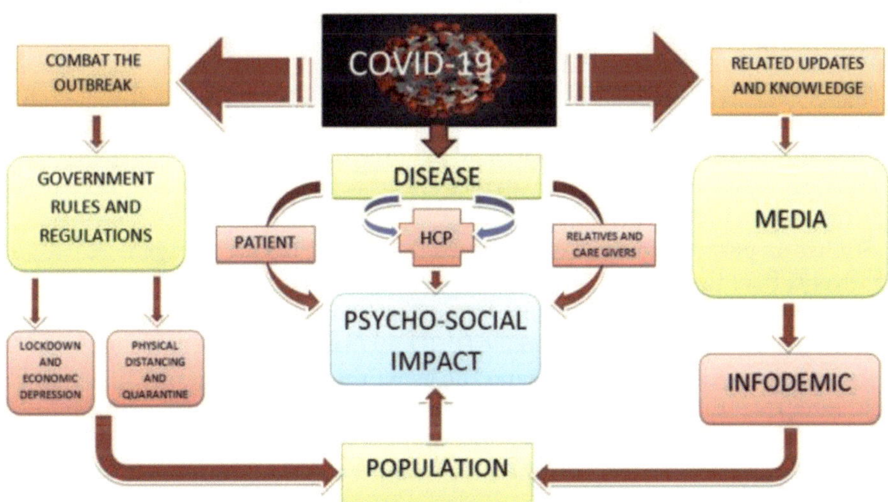


**Figure 1.**
*Intricate psychosocial relationship between the disease, health care providers, government and population. Source: Dubey et al. [65].*

## 3. The effects on psychological health of children and adolescents

The psychological impact of the COVID-19 pandemic on young children and adolescents is perhaps a crucial but apparently ignored aspect of this phenomenon [66, 67]. Developmental psychology literature has substantially revealed that experiences learned through environmental factors in early childhood lay the foundations for lifelong behavioral patterns and success, since it is a critical stage for cognitive, emotional, and psychosocial skills development [68]. During a severe pandemic like COVID-19, community-based mitigation programs such as the closure of schools, parks and playgrounds can disrupt children's usual lifestyles, potentially causing distress and confusion. The children who have to cope with these changes may display impatience, distress and hostility while both younger and older children are likely to become more demanding, which can lead to physical and mental violence by parents who are under extreme pressure. Stress factors such as monotonous Daily life, frustration, lack of face-to-face communication with classmates, friends, and teachers, inadequate personal space at home, and financial losses of the family during the quarantine can all trigger potentially distressing and even long-lasting adverse mental consequences among the children [66]. The interplay between changes in daily routine, house arrest, and fear of infection can further intensify these undesirable mental responses, leading to a vicious circle [66, 69]. A European study has also revealed that there are strikingly positive associations between children's fearful responses to the disease and parents' knowledge of H1N1 virus threat [70]. Likewise, children experiencing the COVID-19 pandemic may suffer from various phobias and PTSD after learning risk information and other depressing details through mass media, especially social media [66, 71]. The children with single parents, including healthcare staff caring for COVID-19 patients, may experience adjustment disorders if their parents are to be quarantined [72]. Immediate or temporary separation of parents from children can create tensions, thereby causing long-lasting psychological effects as the children fear for their life or his loved ones.

Adults should provide information to considering the children's age and level of intelligence when talking about the epidemic. It has been stated that having a sensitive and effective conversation about a life-threatening disease is an improving factor for the long-term psychological health of the child and family [73]. Given that the adolescents indicate less or no symptoms of coronavirus, not paying attention to the social distance rule and personal hygiene may accelerate spread of the infection [74]. Hence, curfews were enforced for those under the age of 20 in many countries in the first months of the epidemic. However, since adolescence is a period in which autonomy develops and peer relationships gain importance [75], this process, in which social distance rules are particularly emphasized, may affect adolescents psychologically negatively.

Studies on past epidemics have reported that public health emergencies negatively affect the psychological states of university students, and may lead to complaints such as anxiety, fear, and depression [76]. The main reasons why the university students are worried about COVID-19 may include the impact of the virus on their educational life [77] and the belief that they will be unemployed after graduation [14]. It is widely known that anxiety disorders occur or worsen in the absence of interpersonal communication, and the isolation of young people from their peers and social settings during the quarantine could be one of the reasons that increase their anxiety [78].

To put it briefly, it has been stated that the factors that escalate anxiety among the university students include the economic stressors emerging with the epidemic, the disruptive changes in daily life routine (travel restrictions, all mandatory measures to control the epidemic), academic delays (changes and reorganization of the academic calendar), distance education and decreased social support [79].

Considering the challenge of education during the pandemic, the only effective way to continue education is teaching online lectures and assignments. However, experts have warned about overloading on the web. Specific psychological needs, healthy lifestyles, appropriate hygiene advice and good parenting guidelines can be addressed through the same online platform [66].

## 4. The effects on adult psychological health

It is obvious that the current pandemic process will bring some drastic changes in human life such as reshaping of the economic and social system in the context of the transition to remote working systems [80]. It is also thought that the immediate effects of the pandemic period will be apparent in economical indicators in terms of visibility, followed by social and psychological issues depending on both economic and other factors [81]. It is argued that these problems will differ according to age groups, and in general, problems such as stress, anxiety, lowered motivation [3], fear at night, insomnia, pessimism and isolation from social environments, and demoralization, temporary memory loss, and irritability in some people can be observed [82]. Individuals may project their psychological problems on their families and private lives [81]. From this perspective, a sociological crisis may appear as a result of individuals projecting their problems on the family and then to the society since sudden changes in daily life can evolve into a social trauma [83].

Daily lifestyles and many routines of adults such as their relations with their environment, the way they go to work, and their social activities have been changed due to the epidemic. This phenomenon shows the extent of a crisis like the COVID-19 pandemic as well as challenges encountered by the adults in adapting to the new lifestyle. These changes, along with social isolation, have led to a dramatic surge of stress and anxiety in individuals. On the other hand, there are some uncertainties in social life that cause individuals to be afraid and panic. It can be argued that these uncertainties are primarily about how the epidemic is transmitted, how long it will end, whether a treatment or effective vaccine will be found, and how business and working life will be shaped in the future [84]. It is believed that the COVID-19 Pandemic may cause significant mental problems in individuals in the long term, and therefore it is important to address the psychological problems of individuals arising from the pandemic [3].

On the other hand, the pandemic process has also affected working patterns, requiring the use of the remote working system usually from home. However, remote working system can be perceived as normal by those individuals who are socially isolated or who have introverted +personality traits. This may also pose a problem for those individuals who are apt to using technological devices. However, for those sociable individuals with extroverted personality traits, this situation can actually pose a problem [3].

A report (2020) released by Inter-Agency Standing Committee (IASC) categorized the reactions of employed or unemployed adults to the epidemic crisis in the following [3];

- Fear of being infected and dying,
- Reluctance to apply to hospitals and other health facilities,
- Fear of losing one's job,

- Fear of being quarantined,
- Concerns about losing relatives due to the epidemic,
- Fear of being separated from relatives due to quarantine,
- Feeling helpless and alone due to social isolation.

It is clear that the mental reactions shown during the epidemic range from experiencing extreme fear to being indifferent. Therefore, it is plausible to contend that the responses to the epidemic are variable [8]. Given the reactions of employed adults to the crisis, it is seen that these reactions generally differ from each other in terms of mental and behavioral characteristics [8]. Considering the psychological status of adults [85], who work at risky conditions in the healthcare system for the benefit of society, it is seen that they also experience mental problems such as stress, anxiety, low motivation [3] in the lead, being afraid at night, insomnia, pessimism and being isolated from social environments while some may also suffer from moodiness, temporary memory loss, and irritability [82]. Therefore, it is considered important to create a safe and healthy working environment for the adults working in healthcare and to meet the psychological support needs of individuals with impaired mental health [86].

On the other hand, it can be suggested that the unemployed adults are negatively affected in terms of psychological resilience during the epidemic as much as those employed [87]. In this period, it is thought that parents who take care of their children at home are affected negatively from the epidemic both physically and psychologically as much as those employed. For instance, insomnia, muscle pain and joint problems and a constant state of fear and anxiety can be observed in parents. Considering that such a continuous state of fear and panic at home can have an adverse effect on children, it can be argued that the reactions of adults to the crisis are vitally important [88]. Now that it seems inevitable that adults who spend almost all of the day in isolation at home, they project their disrupted emotions on their children [89].

It is stated that the psychological resilience levels of adults who suffer from high levels of depression and anxiety and do not take adequate precautions against the epidemic are significantly lower than others. It is believed that the main reason lies in the fact that they feel insecure because of not taking measures. On the other hand, it is obvious that the psychological resilience of adults who have low depression and anxiety levels and take the necessary precautions against the epidemic is significantly high [90]. In addition, obsessive behaviors such as frequent hand washing can be observed in individuals with extremely high sensitivity to the epidemic. The major reason for this situation is thought to be the need for individuals to feel safe [91]. Living under the continuous threat of death can elicit feelings of helplessness and trauma in some adults. Psychological studies on natural disasters conclude that societies will experience emotional distress and therefore will be negatively affected psychologically. Particularly the economic crisis and the accompanying uncertainties may trigger suicidal thoughts [92].

Other studies have reported that patients with or suspected of being infected with COVID-19 exhibit intense emotional and behavioral responses such as fear, boredom, loneliness, anxiety, insomnia, or anger [12, 93]. Such responses have been associated with disorders such as panic and post-traumatic stress disorder, psychotic and paranoid symptoms, and even suicidal behavior [94]. These symptoms may be more prevalent especially among the quarantined patients [42]. Even in patients with conventional flu symptoms, stress and fear may emerge due to its similarity to COVID-19, creating psychological distress [95]. Despite the relatively low number of suspected cases, the majority of cases showing asymptomatic or mild symptoms, and the low mortality rate of the epidemic, the psychological effects of the epidemic can be much more serious [96].

In a study conducted in China on the COVID-19 epidemic, a high rate of generalized anxiety disorder and sleep quality problems are observed in the population. The anxiety disorders are found to be more prevalent in those younger than 35 years, particularly those who pay too much attention to the agenda on the epidemic [97]. In a study by Ho et al., it is stated that the failure of planned travel plans, social distance, continuous exposure to information about the epidemic from the media, and panic about meeting the household needs trigger anxiety and depression all over the world [98]. In another study conducted in China, the indirect traumatization levels of the society are found to be higher than the nurses working in the field [99]. In another survey, symptoms of post-traumatic stress disorder are observed among the participants in the first period after the outbreak. The same surveys are administered four weeks later and although the symptoms of post-traumatic stress disorder are decreased, it is revealed that this decrease was not clinically significant and the symptoms were severe. In the same study, moderate to severe levels of stress, anxiety, and depression are determined in the first evaluation, and it is observed that the same severe psychological distress persist in the evaluation made four weeks later [100]. According to a study conducted in Turkey, it is found that participants show significantly high levels of somatization, anxiety, phobic anxiety, obsessive–compulsive disorder, depression, hostility, and anger after COVID-19 [101]. In addition, when the pre- and post-coronavirus symptom scores are compared, it is determined that women differ significantly in all symptoms, indicating that they are much more affected psychologically by the coronavirus [101].

In addition, it is reported that the psychological symptoms of those who are anxious about their health and fear contracting the disease before COVID-19 have worsened considerably during the epidemic period. On the other hand, individuals with pre-epidemic obsessive–compulsive disorder (OCD) may be the most affected group by the epidemic due to obsession of contamination, hygiene compulsion, suspicion obsession, and control compulsion. The increase in symptoms, stress and disease anxiety in OCD patients due to the epidemic seem to be quite challenging [102]. In a large-scale study in China, 53.8% of the respondents reported the negative impact of the epidemic on their psychology as moderate or severe. 16.5% of them reported that they experienced moderate and severe depressive symptoms. 28.8% of them reported moderate and severe anxiety symptoms, and 8.1% experienced moderate and severe stress. 84.7% of them spent 20–24 hours a day at home while 75.2% of them were seriously worried about their family members. Variables such as being female, studying, experiencing physical symptoms like cold, dizziness and muscle pain, and evaluating the health status as poor were associated with experiencing more stress, anxiety and depression. It has been stated that obtaining epidemic-specific health information such as treatment protocols in the country and the number of appropriate beds in local hospitals, paying attention to hand hygiene, and taking precautions by wearing masks reduce the possible negative psychological effects of the epidemic [100]. In addition to the patients diagnosed with or suspected of having COVID-19, psychological disorders may also be observed in their families and close contacts. It has been stated that this may cause mass hysteria as the number of cases increases [42, 103, 104].

## 5. The effects on psychological health of elderly individuals

The elderly individuals, particularly those older than 80 years, are at higher risk of suffering from adverse effects which can lead to a mortality rate five times the global average [105]. More than 95% of deaths due to COVID-19 in Europe and about 80% in China involve people over 60 years of age [106, 107]. Although the effects of COVID-19 on all age groups are prominent, most of the confirmed cases and deaths in particular have occurred among the elderly [108]. According to a report published by the US Centers for Disease Control and Prevention (CDC) in March 2020, more than 80% of deaths are seen in patients older than 65 years, indicating that the elderly are more vulnerable to the virus [109, 110]. In addition, China has reported that the increase in serious infection and death rate from COVID-19 depend on age. Specifically, the incidence of severe infection was found to be 19.8%, 43.2% and 81.3% in 50–64 years, 65–79 years, and 80 years and older age groups, respectively, indicating a relationship between the incidence of severe infection and age. In addition, the mortality rate for these age groups rose 1.2%, 4.5% and 18.8%, respectively [111]. The mean age of death in Korea was found to be 75.7, and reports have shown that the death rate from COVID-19 increases with age [108]. The elderly are vulnerable to serious infections and death due to weakened immune function and comorbidities caused by aging [112, 113]. In a study, 50–75% of Korean patients had underlying comorbid medical conditions such as high blood pressure, diabetes, cardiovascular disease, chronic obstructive pulmonary disease, and cancer, so they were classified as vulnerable to COVID-19 and at a high-risk group [114, 115]. Health care, emergency response and quarantine measures for the elderly become mandatory since the elderly, especially those with comorbidities, are vulnerable to epidemics. The psychological and mental health problems caused by COVID-19 among the elderly should be discussed in a broader perspective and investigated thoroughly. In particular, the individuals over the age of 60 require more effort and attention and are classified as high-risk group [116] since they are physically and mentally more susceptible than other age groups. In a recent study of the general population in China, it was found that 53.8% of the participants were moderately or severely affected psychologically and it was reported that the most common problems were severe depression (16.5%), anxiety (28.8%), and stress (8.1%) [117]. Studies have highlighted that 37.1% of the elderly have experienced depression and anxiety during the pandemic [42] and that the emotional response of individuals over 60 years is more prominent compared to other age groups [118].

Recently, besides indicators of a prolongation of the pandemic, strict measures implemented around the world such as avoidance of social activities, social distancing and isolation to prevent the spread of COVID-19 have further raised mental health concerns among the elderly. These social measures will contribute immeasurably to combat against the spread of disease. However, the mental health of the elderly requires more attention and care as they constitute the demographic group that experiences social isolation for the longest period [119]. In addition, as shown by previous studies on the elderly, social isolation measures which increase the risk of cardiovascular, autoimmune, neurological and mental health problems, and the impact of COVID-19 on elderly mental health problems need to be discussed and addressed as a public health crisis.

## 6. Conclusion

The new type coronavirus disease (COVID-19) has become a pandemic affecting health and well-being at global scale. In addition to its effects on physical health and socioeconomic structures, its psychological effects are increasingly being reported in the literature. The current literature suggests that those affected by COVID-19 may have a high burden of mental health problems such as depression, anxiety disorders, stress, panic attacks, irrational anger, impulsivity, somatization, sleep disorders, emotional disturbance, post-traumatic stress, suicidal tendencies. Moreover; age, gender, marital status, educational level, occupation, income, place of residence, close contact with people diagnosed with COVID-19, accompanying physical and mental health problems, exposure to news and social media about COVID-19, coping styles, stigma, psychosocial support, health communication, safe healthcare, personal protective measures, risk of contracting COVID-19, and perceived probability of survival have been identified in the literature as the factors associated with mental health problems in COVID-19. Present evidence pinpoint that a psychiatric outbreak has emerged with the COVID-19 pandemic, which will warrant the attention of the global health community. Therefore, COVID-19 should be recognized as a global public health emergency with enormous mental health implications. Future epidemiological studies should focus on the psychopathological variations and temporariness of mental health problems in different populations. However, multifaceted interventions need to be developed and adopted to address current psychosocial challenges to support mental health during the COVID-19 pandemic [120].

## 7. Recommendations

Current evidence on the epidemiological burden of mental health problems in COVID-19 require the development and implementation of multifaceted interventions and strategies for promoting mental health. Furthermore, since face-to-face mental health services are largely disrupted, psychosocial interventions delivered via digital platforms like the world wide web, social media, mobile phones and applications are increasingly being popular. Again, special strategies should be provided in terms of access to mental health for disadvantaged groups such as those who cannot use these services, have limited access to these technologies, live in rural areas, have a low education level, and are in the elderly age group. In this context, mental health policies and programs should be reviewed and strengthened, taking into account the operational challenges of COVID-19.

While the high prevalence of mental health problems indicates a widespread need for mental health services, most countries lack adequate infrastructure and human resources to provide these services. In this sense, mental health services should be integrated into primary care, as it can significantly increase access to mental health services. Many studies have highlighted the fact that access to accurate information is associated with a lower risk of mental health problems. Rumors or misinformation have appeared on mass media and social media platforms since the beginning of the pandemic. In short, infodemic should be combated, and access to accurate information and mental health resources should be provided. Timely and effective health communication regarding factual information and preventive measures is essential to avoid public concern and fear of COVID-19. Moreover, access to resources that promote positive mental health can greatly assist in addressing and self-managing mental health issues among individuals. Online resources such as self-help meditation, mental health education, providing information and care about early symptoms can be helpful methods to consider for preventing COVID-19 and associated mental health problems. In addition, to address mental health inequalities in the combat against these problems, to mobilize social and community resources and organizations, factors such as strengthening mental health systems for COVID-19 and future public health emergencies should not be disregarded.

Consequently, one of the major lessons to be learned from the COVID-19 pandemic is to strengthen mental health systems that provide resilience to systemic shocks. Potential strategies to achieve such resilience involve establishing mental health policies, developing population-based programs, consolidating institutional capacities to develop the mental health workforce, reviewing health systems financing for mental health, addressing barriers to accessing mental health by communities and institutions, and promoting positive relationships among the communities and promoting mental health should be taken seriously.

## Author details

Vasfiye Bayram Değer
Faculty Health of Science, Mardin Artuklu Universıty, Mardin, Turkey

*Address all correspondence to: vasfiyedeg@gmail.com

## References

[1] Gloster AT, Lamnisos D, Lubenko J, Presti G, Squatrito V, Constantinou M, et al. Impact of COVID-19 pandemic on mental health: An İnternational study. PLoS One. 2020;**15**(12):e0244809. DOI: 10.1371/journal.pone.0244809

[2] Çiçek B, Almalı V. COVID-19 Pandemisi Sürecinde Kaygı Öz-yeterlilik ve Psikolojik İyi Oluş Arasındaki İlişki: Özel Sektör ve Kamu Çalışanları Karşılaştırması. Electronic Turkish Studies. 2020;**15**(4):242-260. DOI: 10.7827/TurkishStudies.43492

[3] Sargın N, Kutluca V. Covid-19 Salgını Sürecinde Yetişkinlerin Tepkileri. Bilge Uluslararası Sosyal Araştırmalar Dergisi. 2020;**4**(2):64-70

[4] James RK, Gilliland BE. Crisis İntervention Strategies. 7th ed. Pacific Grove. Belmont, CA: Brooks/Cole, Cengage Learning; 2013

[5] Kaya M, Yıldırım T. Liselerde Çalışan Psikolojik Danışmanların Okullarda Yaşanan Kriz Durumlarına İlişkin Algıları. İnsan ve Toplum Bilimleri Araştırmaları Dergisi. 2017;**6**(2):835-857

[6] Aslan Ş, Atabey A, Yörük E. Örgütsel Kriz Yönetim Tarzlarının ve Kriz Dönemlerindeki Yönetici Davranışlarının Araştırılması: Konya Örneği. Journal of Azerbaijan Studies; 2007;**10**(3-4):72-96. https://arastirmax.com/en/system/files/dergiler/91826/makaleler/12/1-2/arastrmx_91826_12_pp_72-96.pdf

[7] Erden G, Gürdil G. Savaş Yaşantılarının Ardından Çocuk ve Ergenlerde Gözlenen Travma Tepkileri ve Psiko-Sosyal Yardım Önerileri. Türk Psikoloji Yazıları. 2009;**12**(24):1-13

[8] Havva T. Olağanüstü Durumlar ve Hemşirelik. Anadolu Hemşirelik ve Sağlık Bilimleri Dergisi. 2017;**19**(4):278-282

[9] Erdoğan A, Hocaoğlu Ç. Enfeksiyon Hastalıklarının ve Pandeminin Psikiyatrik Yönü: Bir Gözden Geçirme. Klinik Psikiyatri Dergisi. 2020;**23**(1):72-80. DOI: 10.5505/kpd.2020.90277

[10] Akat M, Karataş K. Psychological effects of COVID-19 pandemic on society and its reflections on education. Turkish Studies. 2020;**15**(4):1-13. DOI: 10.7827/TurkishStudies.44336

[11] Kaya B. Pandeminin Ruh Sağlığına Etkileri. Klinik Psikiyatri Dergisi. 2020;**23**(2):123-124. DOI: 10.5505/kpd.2020.64325

[12] Li W, Yang Y, Liu ZH, Zhao YJ, Zhang Q, Zhang L, et al. Progression of mental health services during the COVID-19 outbreak in China. International Journal of Biological Sciences. 2020;**16**(10):1732-1738. DOI: 10.7150/ijbs.45120

[13] Stankovska G, Memedi I, Dimitrovski D. Coronavırus COVİD-19 disease, mental health and psychosocial support. Society Register. 2020;**4**(2):33-48. DOI: 10.14746/sr.2020.4.2.03

[14] Wang C, Pan R, Wan X, Tan Y, Xu L, Ho CS, et al. Immediate psychological responses and associated factors during the initial stage of the 2019 coronavirus disease (COVID-19) epidemic among the general population in China. International Journal of Environmental Research and Public Health. 2020;*17*(5):1729. DOI: 10.3390/ijerph17051729

[15] Arden MA, Chilcot J. Health psychology and the coronavirus (COVID-19) global pandemic: A call for research. British Journal of Health Psychology. 2020;**25**(2):231-232. DOI: 10.1111/bjhp.12414

[16] Cullen W, Gulati G, Kelly BD. Mental health in the Covid-19 pandemic. QJM: An International

Journal of Medicine. 2020;**113**(5):311-312. DOI: 10.1093/qjmed/hcaa110

[17] Li S, Wang Y, Xue J, Zhao N, Zhu T. The impact of COVID-19 epidemic declaration on psychological consequences: A study on active Weibo users. International Journal of Environmental Research and Public Health. 2020;**17**(6):2032. DOI: 10.3390/ijerph17062032

[18] Kluge HP. Statement – Physical and Mental Health Key to Resilience During COVID-19 Pandemic. World Health Organization; 2020 https://www.euro.who.int/en/media-centre/sections/statements/2020/statement-physical-and-mental-health-key-to-resilience-during-covid-19-pandemic

[19] Jackson D, Firtko A, Edenborough M. Personal resilience as a strategy for surviving and thriving in the face of workplace adversity: A literature review. Journal of Advanced Nursing. 2020;**60**(1):1-9. DOI: 10.1111/j.1365-2648.2007.04412.x

[20] Doğan T. Kısa Psikolojik Sağlamlık Ölçeği'nin Türkçe uyarlaması: Geçerlik ve güvenirlik çalışması. The Journal of Happiness & Well-Being. 2015;**3**(1):93-102 https://www.journalofhappiness.net/article/getpdf/154

[21] Polizzi C, Lynn SJ, Perry A. Stress and coping in the time of COVID-19: Pathways to resilience and recovery. Clinical Neuropsychiatry. 2020;**17**(2):59-62. DOI: 10.36131/CN20200204

[22] Tugade MM, Fredrickson BL. Resilient individuals use positive emotions to bounce back from negative emotional experiences. Journal of Personality and Social Psychology. 2004;**86**(2):320 333. DOI: 10.1037/0022-3514.86.2.320

[23] Naeem F, Irfan M, Javed A. Coping with COVID-19: Urgent need for building resilience through cognitive behaviour therapy. Khyber Medical University Journal. 2020;**12**(1):1-3. DOI: 10.35845/kmuj.2020.20194

[24] Reardon S. Ebola's mental-health wounds Linger in Africa: Health-care workers struggle to help people who have been traumatized by the epidemic. Nature. 2015;**519**(7541):13-15

[25] Shigemura J, Ursano RJ, Morganstein JC, Kurosawa M, Benedek DM. Public responses to the novel 2019 coronavirus (2019-nCoV) in Japan: Mental health consequences and target populations. Psychiatry and Clinical Neurosciences. 2020;**74**(4):281-282

[26] Shultz JM, Cooper JL, Baingana F, Oquendo MA, Espinel Z, Althouse BM, et al. The role of fear-related behaviors in the 2013-2016 West Africa Ebola virus disease outbreak. Current Psychiatry Reports. 2016;**18**(11):104

[27] Wang Y, McKee M, Torbica A, Stuckler D. Systematic literature review on the spread of health-related misinformation on social media. Social Science & Medicine. 2019;**240**(112552):1-12. DOI: 10.1016/j.socscimed.2019.112552

[28] Lee AM, Wong JG, McAlonan GM, Cheung V, Cheung C, Sham PC, et al. Stress and psychological distress among SARS survivors 1 year after the outbreak. The Canadian Journal of Psychiatry. 2007;**52**:233-240. DOI: 10.1177/070674370705200405

[29] Lu YC, Shu BC, Chang YY, Lung FW. The mental health of hospital workers dealing with severe acute respiratory syndrome. Psychotherapy and Psychosomatics. 2006;**75**:370-375. DOI: 10.1159/000095443

[30] Mak IW, Chu MC, Pan PC, Yiu MG, Chan VL. Long-term psychiatric morbidities among SARS survivors. General Hospital Psychiatry.

2009;**31**:318-326. DOI: 10.1016/j.genhosppsych.2009.03.001

[31] Lee SM, Kang WS, Cho AR, Kim T, Park JK. Psychological impact of the 2015 MERS outbreak on hospital workers and quarantined hemodialysis patients. Comprehensive Psychiatry. 2018;**87**:123-127. DOI: 10.1016/j.comppsych.2018.10.003

[32] Sher L. COVID-19, anxiety, sleep disturbances and suicide. Sleep Medicine. 2020;**70**:124

[33] Bhuiyan AI, Sakib N, Pakpour AH, Griffiths MD, Mamun MA. COVID-19-Related suicides in Bangladesh due to lockdown and economic factors: Case study evidence from media reports. International Journal of Mental Health and Addiction. 2020:1-6. DOI: 10.1007/s11469-020-00307-y

[34] Thakur V, Jain A. COVID 2019-suicides: A global psychological pandemic. Brain, Behavior, and Immunity. 2020;**88**:952-953

[35] Gunnell D, Appleby L, Arensman E, Hawton K, John A, Kapur N, et al. Suicide risk and prevention during the COVID-19 pandemic. The Lancet Psychiatry. 2020;**7**(6):468-471

[36] Chan SMS, Chiu FKH, Lam CWL, Leung PYV, Conwell Y. Elderly suicide and the 2003 SARS epidemic in Hong Kong. International Journal of Geriatric Psychiatry: A Journal of the Psychiatry of Late Life and Allied Sciences. 2006;**21**(2):113-118

[37] Reynolds DL, Garay J, Deamond S, Moran MK, Gold W, Styra R. Understanding, compliance and psychological impact of the SARS quarantine experience. Epidemiology & Infection. 2008;**136**(7):997-1007

[38] Sim K, Chan YH, Chong PN, Chua HC, Soon SW. Psychosocial and coping responses within the community health care setting towards a National outbreak of an infectious disease. Journal of Psychosomatic Research. 2010;**68**(2):195-202

[39] Centers for Disease Control and Prevention Quarantine and Isolation. https://www.cdc.gov/quarantine/index.html. 2017 [Accessed: January 30, 2020]

[40] Manuell ME, Cukor J. Mother nature versus human nature: Public compliance with evacuation and quarantine. Disasters. 2011;**35**(2):417-442. DOI: 10.1111/j.1467-7717.2010.01219.x

[41] Rubin GJ, Wessely S. The psychological effects of quarantining a city. BMJ. 2020;**368**:m313

[42] Brooks SK, Webster RK, Smith LE, Woodland L, Wessely S, Greenberg N, et al. The psychological impact of quarantine and how to reduce it: Rapid review of the evidence. Lancet. 2020; **395**(10227):912-920. DOI: 10.1016/S0140-6736(20)30460-8

[43] Bai Y, Lin CC, Lin CY, Chen JY, Chue CM, Chou P. Survey of stress reactions among health care workers involved with the SARS outbreak. Psychiatric Services. 2004;**55**:1055-1057

[44] Wu P, Fang Y, Guan Z, Fan B, Kong J, Yao Z, et al. The psychological impact of the SARS epidemic on hospital employees in China: Exposure, risk perception, and Altruistic acceptance of risk. Canadian Journal of Psychiatry. 2009;**54**(5):302-311. DOI: 10.1177/070674370905400504

[45] Liu X, Kakade M, Fuller CJ, Fan B, Fang Y, Kong J, et al. Depression after exposure to stressful events: Lessons learned from the severe acute respiratory syndrome epidemic. Comprehensive Psychiatry. 2012;**53**(1): 15-23. DOI: 10.1016/j.comppsych.2011.02.003

[46] Yoon MK, Kim SY, Ko HS, Lee MS. System effectiveness of detection, brief

intervention and refer to treatment for the people with post-traumatic emotional distress by MERS: A case report of community-based proactive intervention in South Korea. International Journal of Mental Health Systems. 2016;**10**:51. DOI: 10.1186/s13033-016-0083-5

[47] Hawryluck L, Gold WL, Robinson S, Pogorski S, Galea S, Styra R. SARS control and psychological effects of quarantine, Toronto, Canada. Emerging Infectious Diseases. 2004;**10**:1206-1212

[48] Di Giovanni C, Conley J, Chiu D, Zaborski J. Factors influencing compliance with quarantine in Toronto during the 2003 SARS outbreak. Biosecurity and Bioterrorism. 2004;**2**(4):265-272. DOI: 10.1089/bsp.2004.2.265

[49] Lee S, Chan LY, Chau AM, Kwok KP, Kleinman A. The experience of SARS-related Stigma at Amoy Gardens. Social Science & Medicine. 2005;**61**(9):2038-2046. DOI: 10.1016/j.socscimed.2005.04.010

[50] Marjanovic Z, Greenglass ER, Coffey S. The relevance of psychosocial variables and working conditions in predicting nurses' coping strategies during the SARS crisis: an online questionnaire survey. International Journal of Nursing Studies. 2007;**44**(6):991-998. DOI: 10.1016/j.ijnurstu.2006.02.012

[51] Maunder R, Hunter J, Vincent L, Bennett J, Peladeau N, Leszcz M, et al. The immediate psychological and occupational impact of the 2003 SARS outbreak in a teaching hospital. CMAJ. 2003;**168**(10):1245-1251

[52] Wu P, Liu X, Fang Y, Fan B, Fuller CJ, Guan Z, et al. Alcohol abuse/dependence symptoms among hospital employees exposed to a SARS outbreak. Alcohol and Alcoholism. 2008;**43**(6):706-712. DOI: 10.1093/alcalc/agn073

[53] Iachini T, Frassinetti F, Ruotolo F, Sbordone FL, Ferrara A, Arioli M, et al. Social distance during the COVID-19 pandemic reflects perceived rather than actual risk. International Journal of Environmental Research and Public Health. 2021;**18**(11):5504. DOI: 10.3390/ijerph18115504

[54] Kemal G. Toplumsal Değerler Bağlamında Yaşama Hürriyeti. İlahiyat Fakültesi Dergisi. 2014;**1**(1):85-101

[55] Beck U. Risk Society: Towards a New Modernity. London: Sage Publications; 1992

[56] Yurtkulu F, Miyase A. Hayatta Kalmanın Yeni Adı: Sosyal Mesafe. Sosyal Hizmet Uzmanları Derneği Yayını. Publication of Association of Social Workers. 2021:6-32

[57] Person B, Sy F, Holton K, Govert B, Liang A. National center for infectious diseases/SARS community outreach team. Fear and Stigma: The epidemic within the SARS outbreak. Emerging Infectious Diseases. 2004;**10**(2):358-363. DOI: 10.3201/eid1002.030750

[58] Siu JY. The SARS-associated stigma of SARS victims in the post-SARS era of Hong Kong. Qualitative Health Research; 2008;**18**(6):729-738. DOI: 10.1177/1049732308318372

[59] Verma S, Mythily S, Chan YH, Deslypere JP, Teo EK, Chong SA. Post-SARS psychological morbidity and stigma among general practitioners and traditional Chinese medicine practitioners in Singapore. Annals of the Academy of Medicine, Singapore. 2004;**33**(6):743-748

[60] Depoux A, Martin S, Karafillakis E, Preet R, Wilder-Smith A, Larson H. The pandemic of Social Media Panic Travels Faster than the COVID-19 outbreak. Journal of Travel Medicine. 2020;**27**(3): taaa031. DOI: 10.1093/jtm/taaa031

[61] Shimizu K. 2019-nCoV, fake news, and racism. Lancet. 2020;**395**(10225): 685-686. DOI: 10.1016/S0140-6736(20)30357-3

[62] Zarocostas J. How to fight an infodemic. Lancet. 2020;**395**(10225): 676. DOI: 10.1016/S0140-6736(20)30461-X

[63] Malta M, Rimoin AW, Strathdee SA. The coronavirus 2019-nCoV epidemic: Is Hindsight 20/20? EClinicalMedicine. 2020;**20**:100289. DOI: 10.1016/j.eclinm.2020.100289

[64] Liu S, Yang L, Zhang C, Xiang YT, Liu Z, Hu S, et al. Online mental health services in China during the COVID-19 outbreak. Lancet Psychiatry. 2020;**7**(4): e17-e18. DOI: 10.1016/S2215-0366(20)30077-8

[65] Dubey S, Biswas P, Ghosh R, Chatterjee S, Dubey MJ, Chatterjee S, et al. Psychosocial impact of COVID-19. Diabetes & Metabolic Syndrome: Clinical Research & Reviews. 2020; **14**(5):779-788

[66] Wang G, Zhang Y, Zhao J, Zhang J, Jiang F. Mitigate the effects of home confinement on children during the COVID-19 outbreak. Lancet. 2020; **395**(10228):945-947. DOI: 10.1016/S0140-6736(20)30547-X

[67] Ghosh R, Dubey MJ, Chatterjee S, Dubey S. Impact of COVID -19 on children: Special focus on the psychosocial aspect. Minerva Pediatrica. 2020;**72**(3):226-235. DOI: 10.23736/S0026-4946.20.05887-9

[68] Allen R, Kelly B. Committee on the Science of Children Birth to Age 8: Deepening and Broadening the Foundation for Success; Board on Children, Youth, and Families. Institute of Medicine; National Research Council; 2015

[69] Sprang G, Silman M. Posttraumatic stress disorder in parents and youth after health-related disasters. Disaster Medicine and Public Health Preparedness. 2013;**7**(1):105-110. DOI: 10.1017/dmp.2013.22

[70] Remmerswaal D, Muris P. Children's fear reactions to the 2009 Swine flu pandemic: The role of threat information as provided by parents. Journal of Anxiety Disorders. 2011;**25**(3): 444-449. DOI: 10.1016/j.janxdis.2010.11.008

[71] Muris P, Field AP. The role of verbal threat information in the development of childhood fear. "Beware The Jabberwock!". Clinical Child and Family Psychology Review. 2010;**13**(2):129-150. DOI: 10.1007/s10567-010-0064-1

[72] Dubey S, Dubey MJ, Ghosh R, Chatterjee S. Children of frontline coronavirus disease-2019 warriors: Our observations. The Journal of Pediatrics. 2020;**224**:188-189. DOI: 10.1016/j.jpeds.2020.05.026

[73] Dalton L, Rapa E, Ziebland S, Rochat T, Kelly B, Hanington L, et al. Communication with children and adolescents about the diagnosis of a life-threatening condition in their parent. Lancet. 2019;**393**(10176): 1164-1176. DOI: 10.1016/S0140-6736(18)33202-1

[74] Dong Y, Mo X, Hu Y, Qi X, Jiang F, Jiang Z, et al. Epidemiological characteristics of 2143 pediatric patients with 2019 Coronavirus disease in China. Pediatrics. 2020;**58**(4):712-713. DOI: 10.1542/peds.2020-0702 https://pediatrics.aappublications.org/content/pediatrics/early/2020/03/16/peds.2020-0702.full.pdf

[75] Smetana JG, Campione-Barr N, Metzger A. Adolescent development in interpersonal and societal contexts. Annual Review of Psychology. 2006;**57**: 255-284

[76] Mei SL, Yu JX, He BW, Li JY. Psychological investigation of University Students in a University in Jilin Province. Medicine and Society (Berkeley). 2011;**24**(05):84-86

[77] Cornine A. Reducing nursing student anxiety in the clinical setting: An integrative review. Nursing Education Perspectives. 2020;**41**(4): 229-234. DOI: 10.1097/01.NEP.0000000000000633

[78] Xiao C. A novel approach of consultation on 2019 Novel Coronavirus (COVID-19)-related psychological and mental problems: Structured letter therapy. Psychiatry Investigation. 2020;**17**(2):175-176

[79] Cao W, Fang Z, Hou G, Han M, Xu X, Dong J, et al. The psychological impact of COVID-19 epidemic on college students in China. Psychiatry Research. 2020;**287**:112934

[80] Bozkurt Y, Zeybek Z, Aşkın R. COVİD-19 Pandemisi: Psikolojik Etkileri ve Terapötik Müdahaleler. İstanbul Ticaret Üniversitesi Sosyal Bilimler Dergisi. 2020;**19**(37):304-318

[81] Kanberoğlu Z, Kara O. Küresel Krizlerin Sosyal Yaşam Üzerindeki Etkisi: Van İli Örneği. Muğla Üniversitesi Sosyal Bilimler Enstitüsü Dergisi. 2013;**31**:35-48

[82] Mustafayeva L, Dosaliyeva D. Sosyal hizmet işletmelerinde kriz yönetimi. Süleyman Demirel Üniversitesi Vizyoner Dergisi. 2015:148-175. Special Volume on Social Work.

[83] Aykut S, Aykut SS. Kovid-19 Pandemisi ve Travma Sonrası Stres Bozukluğu Temelinde Sosyal Hizmetin Önemi. Toplumsal Politika Dergisi. 2020;**1**(1):56-66

[84] Yıldız MA. Bir kriz durumu: Pandemi (covid-19) Günlerinde Ruh Sağlığımızı Korumak, Stres Ve Kaygıyla Baş Etme. Okul Psikolojik Danışmanlığı Dergisi. 2020;**10**(2):7-25

[85] Şahan C, Özgür EA, Arkan G, Alagüney ME, Demiral Y. COVID-19 Pandemisi'nde Meslek Hastalığı Tanı Kılavuzu. İş ve Meslek Hastalıkları Uzmanları Derneği ve Halk Sağlığı Uzmanları Derneği. https://korona.hasuder.org.tr/wp-content/uploads/Mesleksel-COVID_19_Tan%C4%B1_Rehberi_2020.pdf

[86] Polat ÖP, Coşkun F. COVID-19 Salgınında Sağlık Çalışanlarının Kişisel Koruyucu Ekipman Kullanımları İle Depresyon, Anksiyete, Stres Düzeyleri Arasındaki İlişkinin Belirlenmesi. Batı Karadeniz Tıp Dergisi. 2020;**4**(2):51-58

[87] Tönbül Ö. Koronavirüs (Covid-19) Salgını Sonrası 20-60 Yaş Arası Bireylerin Psikolojik Dayanıklılıklarının Bazı Değişkenler Açısından İncelenmesi. Humanistic Perspective. 2020;**2**(2): 159-174

[88] Demirbaş NK, Koçak SS. 2-6 Yaş Arasında Çocuğu Olan Ebeveynlerin Bakış Açısıyla Covıd-19 Salgın Sürecinin Değerlendirilmesi. Avrasya Sosyal ve Ekonomi Araştırmaları Dergisi. 2020;**7**(6):328-349

[89] Mazza C, Ricci E, Biondi S, Colasanti M, Ferracuti S, Napoli C, et al. A nationwide survey of psychological distress among Italian people during the COVID-19 pandemic: Immediate psychological responses and associated factors. International Journal of Environmental Research and Public Health. 2020;**17**:3165

[90] Bozdağ F. Pandemi Sürecinde Psikolojik Sağlamlık. Electronic Turkish Studies. 2020;**15**(6):247-257. DOI: 10.7827/TurkishStudies.44890

[91] Tükel R. COVID-19 Pandemi Sürecinde Ruh Sağlığı. In: Türk Tabipleri Birliği COVID-19 Pandemisi Altıncı Ay Değerlendirme Raporu. 2020. pp. 617-628. ISBN 978-605-9665-58-2. https://www.ttb.org.tr/kutuphane/covid19-rapor_6/covid19-rapor_6_Part71.pdf

[92] Pfefferbaum B, North CS. Mental health and the Covid-19 pandemic. The

New England Journal of Medicine. 2020;**383**(6):510-512. DOI: 10.1056/NEJMp2008017

[93] Ornell F, Schuch JB, Sordi AO, Kessler FHP. "Pandemic Fear" and COVID-19: Mental health burden and strategies. Brazilian Journal of Psychiatry. 2020;**42**(3):232-235. DOI: 10.1590/1516-4446-2020-0008

[94] Xiang YT, Yang Y, Li W, Zhang L, Zhang Q, Cheung T, et al. Timely mental health care for the 2019 novel coronavirus outbreak is urgently needed. The Lancet Psychiatry. 2020;**7**(3):228-229. DOI: 10.1016/S2215-0366(20)30046-8

[95] Park SC, Park YC. Mental health care measures in response to the 2019 Novel Coronavirus outbreak in Korea. Psychiatry Investigation. 2020;**17**(2):85. DOI: 10.30773/pi.2020.0058

[96] Wang Y, Wang Y, Chen Y, Qin Q. Unique epidemiological and clinical features of the emerging 2019 Novel Coronavirus pneumonia (COVID-19) implicate special control measures. Journal of Medical Virology. 2020; **92**(6):568-576. DOI: 10.1002/jmv.25748

[97] Huang Y, Zhao N. Generalized anxiety disorder, depressive symptoms and sleep quality during COVID-19 epidemic in China: A web based cross sectional study. Psychiatry Research. 2020;**288**:112954. DOI: 10.1016/j.psychres.2020.112954

[98] Ho CS, Chee CY, Ho RC. Mental health strategies to combat the psychological impact of Coronavirus disease 2019 (COVID-19) beyond paranoia and panic. Annals of the Academy of Medicine, Singapore. 2020;**49**(3):155-160

[99] Li Z, Ge J, Yang M, Feng J, Qiao M, Jiang R, et al. Vicarious traumatization in the general public, members, and non-members of medical teams aiding İn COVID-19 control. Brain, Behavior, and Immunity. 2020;**88**:916-919. DOI: 10.1016/j.bbi.2020.03.007

[100] Wang C, Pan R, Wan X, Tan Y, Xu L, McIntyre RS, et al. A longitudinal study on the mental health of general population during the COVID-19 epidemic in China. Brain, Behavior, and Immunity. 2020;**87**:40-48. DOI: 10.1016/j.bbi.2020.04.028

[101] Bilge Y, Bilge Y. Koronavirüs Salgını ve Sosyal İzolasyonun Psikolojik Semptomlar Üzerindeki Etkilerinin Psikolojik Sağlamlık ve Stresle Baş Etme Tarzları Açısından İncelenmesi. Klinik Psikiyatri Dergisi. 2020;**23**(1):38-51. DOI: 10.5505/kpd.2020.66934

[102] Banerjee D. The Other Side of COVID-19: Impact on Obsessive Compulsive Disorder (OCD) and Hoarding. Psychiatry Research. 2020;**288**:112966. DOI: 10.1016/j.psychres.2020.112966

[103] Duan L, Zhu G. Psychological interventions for people affected by the COVID-19 epidemic. The Lancet Psychiatry. 2020;**7**(4):300-302. DOI: 10.1016/S2215-0366(20)30073-0

[104] Yang Y, Peng F, Wang R, Guan K, Jiang T, Xu G. The deadly coronaviruses: The 2003 SARS pandemic and the 2020 novel coronavirus epidemic in China. Journal of Autoimmunity. 2020; **109**(102438). DOI: 10.1016/j.jaut.2020.102434

[105] World Health Organization. COVID-19 Strategy Up Date. World Heal Organ, Geneva, Switzerland; 2020 https://www.who.int/pubhcations-detail/covid-19-strategy-update—14-april-2020

[106] WHO. Statements, press and ministerial briefings. 2020. http://www.euro.who.int/en/health-topics/

health-emergencies/coronavirus-covid-19/statements

[107] Zazhi ZLX. The epidemiological characteristics of an outbreak of 2019 Novel Coronavirus Diseases (COVID-19) in China, Epidemiol Work Gr NCIP Epidemic Response, Chinese Cent Dis Control Prev. 2020;**41**(2):145-151

[108] Yazawa A, Inoue Y, Fujiwara T, Stickley A, Shirai K, Amemiya A, et al. Association between social participation and hypertension among older people in Japan: The JAGES study. Hypertension Research. 2016;**39**(11):818-824. DOI: 10.1038/hr.2016.78

[109] Douglas H, Georgiou A, Westbrook J. Social participation as an indicator of successful aging: An overview of concepts and their associations with health. Australian Health Review. 2017;**41**(4):455-462. DOI: 10.1071/AH16038

[110] Sepúlveda-Loyola W, Ganz F, Maciel RPT, et al. Social participation is associated with better functionality, health status and educational level in elderly women. Brazilian Journal of Development. 2020;**6**(4):S983-S992. DOI: 10.34117/bjdv6n4-299

[111] Smith GL, Banting L, Eime R, Sullivan GO, Van UJGZ. The association between social support and physical activity in older adults: A systematic review. Int. J. Behav. Nutr. Phys. Act. 2017,**14**(56).1-21. DOI. 10.1186/s12966-017-0509-8

[112] Chiao C, Weng LJ, Botticello AL. Social participation reduces depressive symptoms among older adults: An 18-year longitudinal analysis in Taiwan. BMC Public Health. 2011;**11**:292. DOI: 10.1186/1471-2458-11-292

[113] Wallace LMK, Theou O, Pena F, Rockwood K, Andrew MK. Social vulnerability as a predictor of mortality and disability: Cross-country differences in the survey of health, aging, and retirement in Europe (SHARE). Aging Clinical and Experimental Research. 2015;**27**(3):365-372. DOI: 10.1007/s40520-014-0271-6

[114] Holt-Lunstad J, Smith TB, Layton JB. Social relationships and mortality risk: A meta-analytic review. PLoS Medicine. 2010;**7**(7):1-22. e1000316. DOI: 10.1371/journal.pmed.1000316

[115] Choi NG, DiNitto DM, Marti CN. Social participation and self-rated health among older male veterans and non-veterans. Geriatrics & Gerontology International. 2016;**16**(8):920-927. DOI: 10.1111/ggi.12577

[116] Tomioka K, Kurumatani N, Hosoi H. Social participation and the prevention of decline in effectance among community-dwelling elderly: A population-based Cohort study. PLoS One. 2015;**10**(9):e0139065. DOI: 10.1371/journal.pone.0139065

[117] Croezen S, Avendano M, Burdorf A, van Lenthe FJ. Social participation and depression in old age: A fixed-effects analysis in 10 European countries. American Journal of Epidemiology. 2015;**182**(2):168-176. DOI: 10.1093/aje/kwv015

[118] Morley JE, Vellas B. COVID-19 and older adults. The Journal of Nutrition, Health & Aging. 2020;**24**(4):364-365. DOI: 10.1007/s12603-020-1349-9

[119] Armitage R, Nellums LB. COVID-19 and the consequences of isolating the elderly. The Lancet Public Health. 2020;**5**(5):e256. DOI: 10.1016/S2468-2667(20)30061-X

[120] Hossain MM, Tasnim S, Sultana A, Faizah F, Mazumder H, Zou L, et al. Epidemiology of mental health problems in COVID-19: A review. F1000 Res. 2020;**9**:636. DOI: 10.12688/f1000research.24457.1

Chapter 3

# Perspective Chapter: Psychosocial Impact of COVID-19 – A Global Scenario

*Kishor Kunal, Priyanka Choudhary, Jiwesh Kumar, Ravi Prakash, Anita Singh and Kirti Kanchan*

## Abstract

COVID-19 outbreak reminds us of nationwide lockdowns, home-confinement, overburdened hospitals, country wide curfews, violent and chaotic health-facilities and domestic scenario and gradual but steady rise of stigmatizing factors like fear of isolation, racism, discrimination and marginalization cumulatively intensifying the unavoidable stress, fear, anxiety, depression, poor life quality, substance abuse resulting in enhanced mortality risk particularly among the health-compromised population. With objectives to analyze the psychosocial impact of COVID19 and to delineate the process of impact, by looking into its pathophysiology a literature review was carried on. Various impacts and adaptations were found. With a proper mapping algorithm, their responses can be understood. Different states of individual showed different responses to the same stress creating a gamut of responses which led to different socio-economic, socio-political, professional and psychosocial impact. Identification of stress, mapping of response and a better preparedness from experience can all help us in preventing and controlling it next time.

**Keywords:** COVID-19, psychosocial, social, impact, risk factors, HCWs

## 1. Introduction

COVID-19 outbreak reminds us of nationwide lockdowns, home-confinement, overburdened hospitals, country wide curfews, violent and chaotic health-facilities and domestic scenario and gradual but steady rise of stigmatizing factors like fear of isolation, racism, discrimination and marginalization cumulatively intensifying the unavoidable stress, fear, anxiety, depression, poor life quality, substance abuse resulting in enhanced mortality risk particularly among the health-compromised population [1–3] . Survival through this turmoil highlighted the elemental role of mental health organizations, individual healthcare and research, social media, awareness programs at both personal and community levels in significantly combating the world's psychosocial distress [4–6]. Although, COVID-19 bears the brunt of rising mental illness, a clear understanding of world's disease response would certainly aid in improving our medical emergencies and coping skills around the world.

Psychosocial impact of COVID-19 has been widely discussed in literature but what remains untouched as with all other parts of psychiatry is that the cause of impact has not been discussed [2–4, 7]. It is often easy to label each and every disorder that a psychiatrist is seeing in COVID-19 patients or in patients or healthy beings having the effects somehow related to the pandemic to label as evidence. It thus becomes imperative to discuss the impact that a society is having through a unique lens that widens the perspective relating to the cause and consequence of each and every response that happens to the disease process. To help with this perspective, we shall use the model described by Kunal in his paper on hypothesis spanning the diversities of psychiatry and normalcy, in the section on pathophysiology [8]. But before we shall delve into this new perspective, we shall see what evidence has to say for the psychosocial impact of the pandemic.

## 2. Methodology

### 2.1 Objectives

i. To analyze the psychosocial impact of COVID19.

ii. To delineate the process of impact, by looking into its pathophysiology.

### 2.2 Data acquisition

Literature was reviewed from PubMed and Google Scholar to find out articles describing the psychosocial impact of COVID19. A search was also carried out to find the explanations pertaining to different behavior of an individual to a given stress in order to justify the impact and explore management options.

### 2.3 Data analysis

The compilation of effects was studied and a way was formulated to better understand the psychosocial impact (**Figure 1**).

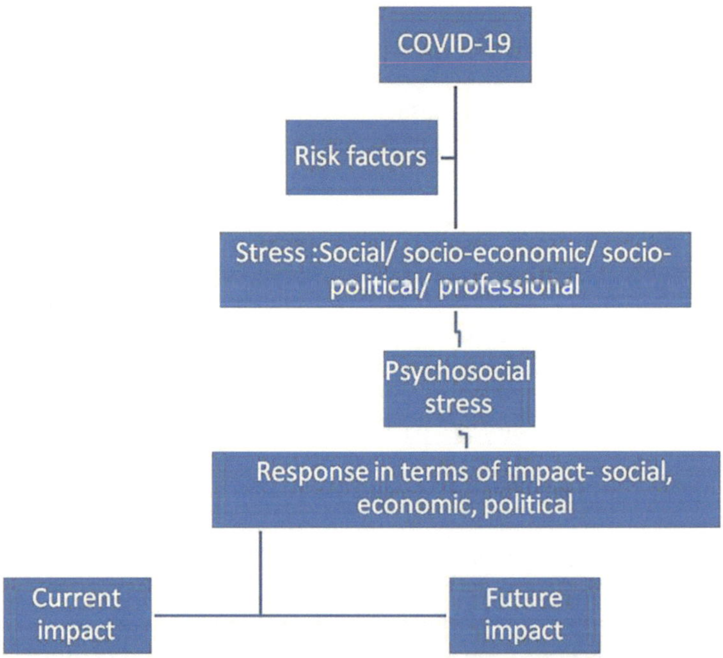


**Figure 1.**
*Algorithm to show mapping of psychosocial impact of COVID19 based on literature.*

## 3. Results and discussion

### 3.1 Social impact

When talking about social impact one needs to understand how a society is formed and functions. Society is like a big web of individuals who are inter-related because of friendship, families or workplace. There are visible and some invisible connections where a person relates to another person or set of person based on ideologies, principles or practice like in name of color, caste, creed or nationality. Invisible connections that often turn into sentiments of positivity or negativity. Stigmatization based on religion, social status and nationality has been a core of social discrimination in this pandemic [2, 9].

A revolution this pandemic brought was the strengthening of visible connections. Spending more time with families had both positive and negative impact. The bonding of families increased however spending too much of time together also had reportedly increased rates of divorce among couples [2, 10]. Veliyannoor coined this as 'return of the repressed' where old conflicts re-emerged during the lockdown due to prolonged forced togetherness between couples [10].

Joshi noticed in her review of psycho-social impact of COVID19 in India that adolescents and young people found it restricting and frustrating to be monitored by parents. Also, she pointed out how the conventional gender role expectations in an Indian society resulted in their overburdening leading to frustration and anger bursts. Family dynamics were also influenced by forced togetherness or separation [2].

Based on age, Dubey *et al.* showed various psychological issues that can happen in different groups and suggested intervention accordingly [7]. Authors showed that children are more prone to boredom, anxiety related to educational development, irritability and fear of infection. Indeed these fears might have been cultivated in them by their parents or guardians to prevent them from going outside. Though the psychological treatment should aim to control extreme fear, casual fear is indeed protective. Proper parenting, online education, and inculcation of healthy habits can provide a feasible solution but this can result in obsession for cleanliness sometimes which if not controlled earlier can get incorporated in psyche and lead to development of OCD (see section on pathophysiology). Young adults developed more anxiety due to low experience in coping with facing distress. Elderlies had irritability, anger issues, fear, anxiety and cognitive decline. Deprivation from pre-scheduled checkup or follow-up can lead to aggravation of their current conditions thus exacerbating the impact. Telepsychology or sessions via telephone or online consultations proved to be useful in all these cases [11]. Telemedicine has gained a lot of popularity during last 2 years and has almost replaced for physical visits except for emergencies at least at some point of time. Though it is not a true alternative to physical consultations it can have advantages in times of distress where risk–benefit ratio might be high for the physical visits for simple follow-ups or chronic illnesses.

Education builds society into a framework as we see and want to see. Conventional education has long been debated but has never been challenged at this scale. Pandemic showed the world a new perspective towards education in terms of online education system. The cellphones which were till an year back not allowed in many schools have become an integral part of education system and has also given food for thought as whether our thought process of keeping these at bay mattered? Long term effects are yet to be seen and short term reports have shown that not going to school may have psychologically affected children but again what impact it shall have on overall growth of a child is yet to be found out. Educational impact can be understood in three different ways- one on parents, one on children and one on teachers. While parents are still doubtful of new education system, it may be difficult for teachers too as maintaining the sanctity and discipline of class could not be strictly possible in addition to the fact that it is not possible to look after every student in classroom now. Also, teachers may face a constant struggle for validation as this technique of teaching is new for many and they might be under supervision of hundreds of parents who might be listening to what they speak. For students the learning experience has changed, as the way they interact with teachers and fellows have been changed. But not only the schools, even the crucial education deliveries have changed like that of medical training program even though examination patterns have remained nearly same. How this will change the social dynamics is yet to be seen in future [12–14].

The increasing role of social media cannot be overlooked in context of COVID19. The major role it played in pandemic has both positive and negative sides. Positive side includes spreading awareness, helping out friends and locals in times of need like shortage of supplies, finding hospitals etc. seeking help in times of distress (which inculcated a sense of hope in lockdown and quarantines) and enhance bonding among people. But nothing comes without a cost, like enhanced bonding promoted stigmatization of particular community or nationality, outbursts of racism and therapeutic misadventures tried by lay people misleading the general public about treatment or prophylaxis. Coronavirus 'infodemic' is another concern that was created on social media in which panic was created by laying out unchecked mind-boggling rumors [15]. Also it helped to promote the disobedience attitude among people who failed to recognize the disease as pandemic and labeled it as hoax created by world governments to divert the commoners from daily problems.

### 3.2 Socio-economic impact

Economic profiles can lead to formation of two groups in society- one whose livelihood has been greatly affected like those of laborers or small businessmen and another those whose work were less affected like those of HCPs, government servants, big businessmen and those working in private sector companies that still ran work-from home. The latter group had lesser financial implications, while former group went nearly bankrupt. Financial implications along with separation from families led migrant workers into great despair. Daily wage earners could not get enough wages to support family. Movement in groups and living in poor conditions predisposed them to infection and stigmatization of being carriers. The ill planned distribution of health services and expense of medical treatment led to hoarding of supplies, black marketing and other health crimes [9].

### 3.3 Socio-political impact

This section shall be incomplete without the mention of social and political revolutions. Revolution does not see the face of pandemic to break out. A very crucial aspect of any society is opposition to the laid rules. Protest is common in democracy as problems do not cease to exist in democracy. These people are marginalized and unheard, complicated by existence of pandemic, media often ignore either their plea or glorify their ignorance towards safety guidelines like wearing of masks, grouping together or following proper guidelines. The protestors may also have a feeling of vulnerability and learned helplessness as described for those people who have patients admitted in hospitals and must break social protocols to be able to provide proper care.

Social inequities like belonging to marginalized sections with poor health facilities often expose to chronic diseases leading to higher mortality when contracting COVID19 which has been reported by Osofsky *et al*. They also reported how poorer connectivity can affect seeking help in times of distress [16]. The solution to this cannot be made in a day but it points towards a poor preparedness for any such catastrophic event.

### 3.4 Social impact on health care

Based on health care the society was clearly divided into two strata during the pandemic- one providing health service and the other at receiving end. Patients developed anxiety, depression, panic, irritability, while the attendants developed a sense of uncertainty, helplessness, worthlessness and a fear of infection [1, 7, 17]. The kin of those who died developed prolonged grief, depression, substance abuse, and stigma related to spread of infection [7]. Inability to do a proper funeral further accentuated the problem. The visuals of ill treatment of dead bodies or mass funerals can further develop a sense of despair in individuals who could not say a proper good-bye to family and same could be for the families too. Another perspective could be for those persons who have their patients admitted in hospitals. They might develop fear of contracting the infection on one hand and on other might feel helpless in not being able to maintain social restrictions thus depicting learned helplessness [7].

Another special set of patients that needs special mention is psychiatric patients. Violence, addiction and disturbed routine follow-up were common issues faced by them. Xiao proposed novel approach of structure letter therapy while Saladino *et al.* and Zhou *et al.* emphasized the use of telepsychology and telehealth [11, 18, 19]. Another aspect for proper health care delivery to these patients would be to ensure that supply of prescribed medicines should be monitored and checked to prevent any lapse and family members or caretakers should also be looked for as they might develop their own set of problems.

On the other hand, psychological impact on HCWs could be very different. They felt overworked, unable to attend to family duties and guilt of not being able to save the patients. Those not involved in direct care of patients could have felt worthlessness for not being able to help [7]. Overwork can lead to burnouts, depression and anxiety [5]. Lack of facilities can also produce secondary traumatic stress disorder where HCWs have to decide who can access and who cannot access the facilities [20]. Lai *et al.* reported that nearly half of HCWs working in COVID wards had depression followed by anxiety and insomnia and nearly three-fourth had distress [21]. The problems faced by HCWs can be broadly labeled into three categories: those faced by them related to work and family needs, those faced by problems related to patient care and those faced by colleagues distress created by news of violence against doctors, work under poor safety guidelines, eviction of doctors from their rented house in various resident communities and death while providing services to patients. Though all three creates a similar type of stress pattern, psychotherapy shall aim at different roots when going for consultations. In most cases, these HCWs would not seek professional opinion and these distresses would be transient though theoretically affecting the patient care sometimes by reducing efficiency or indirectly affecting other colleagues or family member who might feel helpless in saving him or her.

### 3.5 Professional impact on training

Trainee doctors and medical graduates were also affected in their training. Reduced patient contact led to decrement in development of skills [22, 23]. Surgeons faced redeployment and decreased operation theater postings which in turn affected their surgical skill development [24]. Adaptation to online learning and problems with submission of dissertation was also a challenge and all these stress added to psychological impact on them [24–26]. A positive statement was that with online classes and posting in backup teams, these trainees got time to let the steam off and de-stress them. The training of not only health care workers but also every sector suffered tremendously thus also creating a question mark for not only training modules in past but also in future of the trainees trained during COVID19. Although, detailed discussion is out of scope of this chapter.

### 3.6 Risk factors for psychosocial impact

Romm *et al.* reported that females and sexual minorities were at risk for increased depression while males were at greater risk for decreased physical activity. Whites when compared to Blacks were at greater risk for increase in mental health impacts while Asians had greater chances of alcohol abuse. Hispanics were at greater risk for decreased relationship quality, physical activity, and increased sedentary activity [27]. Fteropoulli *et al.* found that factors associated with poorer outcomes for psychosocial impact include medical profession, female gender, frontline work and use of avoidance as coping skill [6]. They also reported depression and burnout to be strongest predictors of poor quality of life parameters, similar to findings reported by Suryavanshi *et al.* in Indian HCWs [28].

### 3.7 Pathophysiology- a fresh perspective

So what caused this impact? This is not a direct impact of the virus. Let us consider COVID-19 as a stress- a newly found one (**Figure 2**), according the "third-eye model' [8]. It is a new experience and in some way have affected every person even the dead who could not get proper funerals and good-byes. And indeed that too has affected the living. **Figure 3** shows normal response to stress. Whenever a stress strikes, it tends to push the brain cycle into NREM phase. A person always tries to end it and mount a REM response based on conditionings in brain. Conditionings are the coping skills that a person had learned during lifetime, so technically children will have lesser conditioning than adults and young will have lesser conditioning than elders. Thus problems with children will focus on what they do as in difficulty in concentrating, boredom, irritability, restlessness, nervousness, sense of loneliness, uneasiness, and worries, while adults would have anxiety, depression, burnouts, loneliness, panic, and substance use disorders.

But not all people suffer from psychological impact at a given time. If one believes that the stress shall be controlled and it is indeed controlled then the behavior is more towards normalcy like with those whose income was not affected- pensioners, HCPs and government employees. Even though many times they worked under the fear of getting infected sometimes this fear was casual but at times where situation was not under control like working with limited supplies or exposure to large number of COVID patients or working long shifts, this could turn into anxiety or panic.

Whenever the stress is identified as stress like a person believes that abnormal response to COVID19 is validated, a justification happens for stress. If this justification is for a process that just a mirror image of what a person usually saw this could lead to adjustment disorders giving sense of irritability or loneliness to the person but if it backed by emotional turmoil or magnification where COVID19 is seen to impact the lives of people like never before killing thousands, breaking families, blowing the finances of families or simply loss of very close one who had no disease otherwise can lead to PTSD. It is often the effect of COVID19 that tends to cause adjustment disorder and PTSD than itself. Multiplied by isolation and long stays at home it is not difficult to imagine that bereavement reaction can also be prolonged.

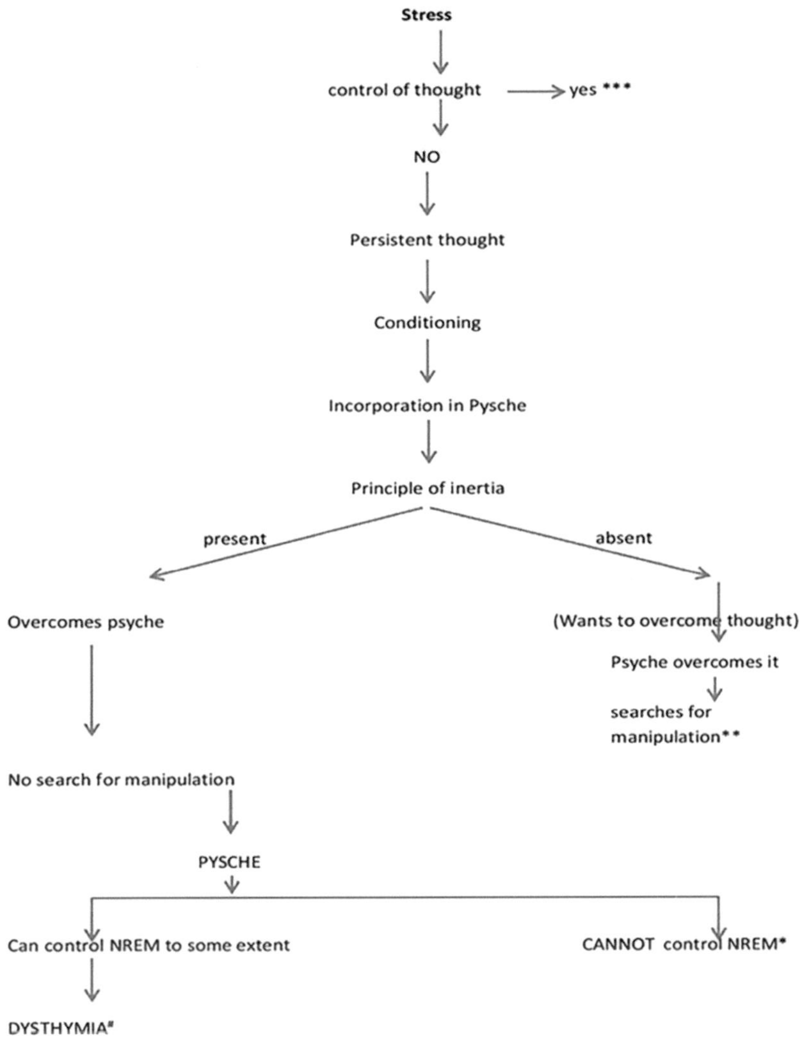


**Figure 2.**
*Algorithm showing basic response to any stress (further algorithm is given in* ***Figures*** *3–5).*

Now all of this may comprise a normal response to a pandemic because the person still has some control over thoughts of stress and often the problem would lay on impact of stress as in death of a person, inability to help others, financial breakdowns and social cut-offs rather than COVID19 itself. Once the stress is incorporated in psyche of an individual, the principle of inertia decides as to whether the psyche can overcome the persistence of thoughts. If it tries to overcome it, it searches for a manipulation (remember here the thoughts have persisted and cannot be simply overthrown by mounting a response as explained in above text). From **Figure 4**, we can see if the manipulation is specific to stress it can be lead to anxiety if the manipulation is feasible for psyche but patient cannot do that. Another common way to mount a response is to mount a response which is very feasible to psyche like washing hands repeatedly as in OCD or shifting to over smoking or over drinking for stress relief. Sometimes this substance abuse can be an excuse for stress where the patient may be trying to gain sympathy or needs a leave from workplace and do not want to malinger which indeed can be very common due to non-specific and objective complaints of COVID-19 which can be practically anything from myalgia to loose

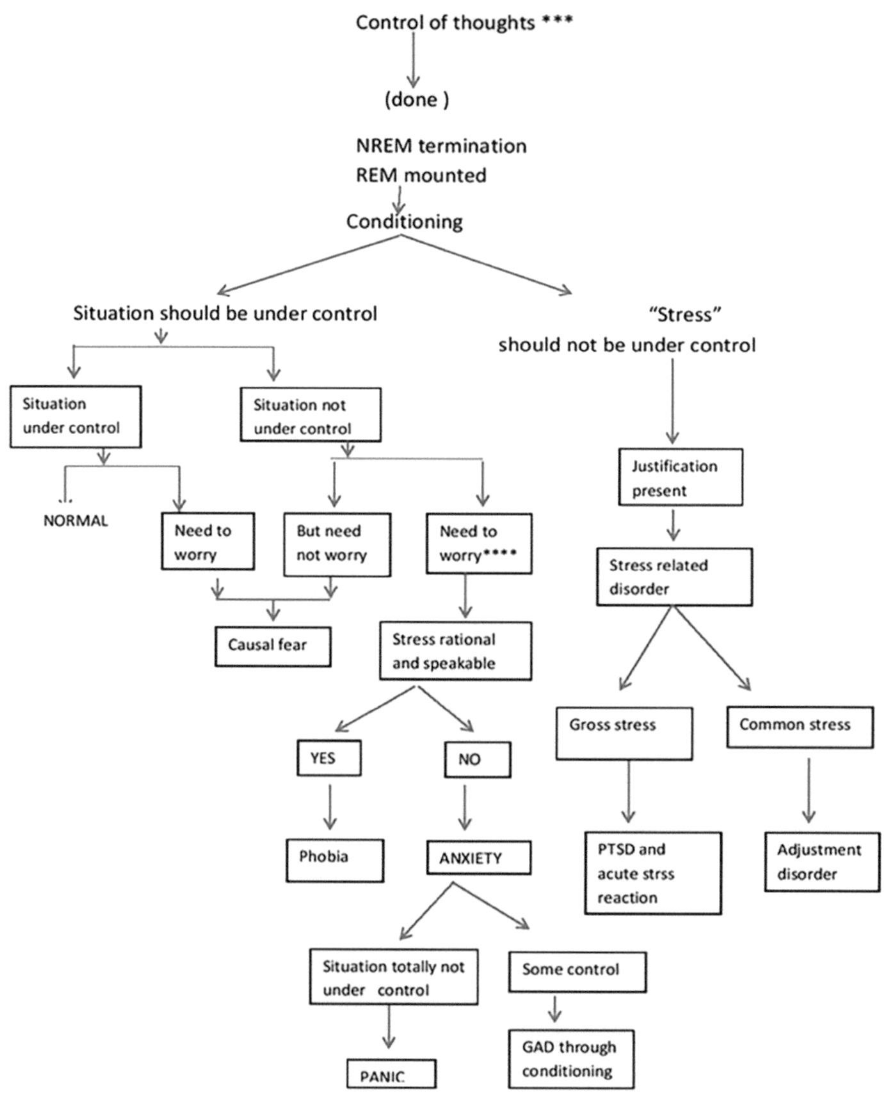


**Figure 3.**
*Algorithm showing response when a patient can control the thoughts provoking mental stress and possible responses.*

stools. If the patient is already not ill can present with a spectrum of somatization and this could be for same reason except for the fact that malingering or claiming false symptoms is not feasible to psyche, i.e. the person does not want to malinger or do substance abuse which can be due to ethics, emotions or rationality.

Although, the above pathologies are not uncommon but another common response pattern is where the NREM state induced by stress is only controlled to some extent or cannot be controlled at all (**Figures 2** and **5**). In any of these cases, giving up to brain cycle is difficult as these people would have otherwise stronger will to control the brain. COVID19 is a pandemic and has affected everyone in some extent and thus does not target any specific group and is a boon for others. This feeling helps the person to control rather than be controlled by brain. Dysthymia has a definition to fulfill and can be underreported or can be diagnosed as depression by many. Low mood is not uncommon as it does not require any specific action from the person, it is like 'going with the flow'.

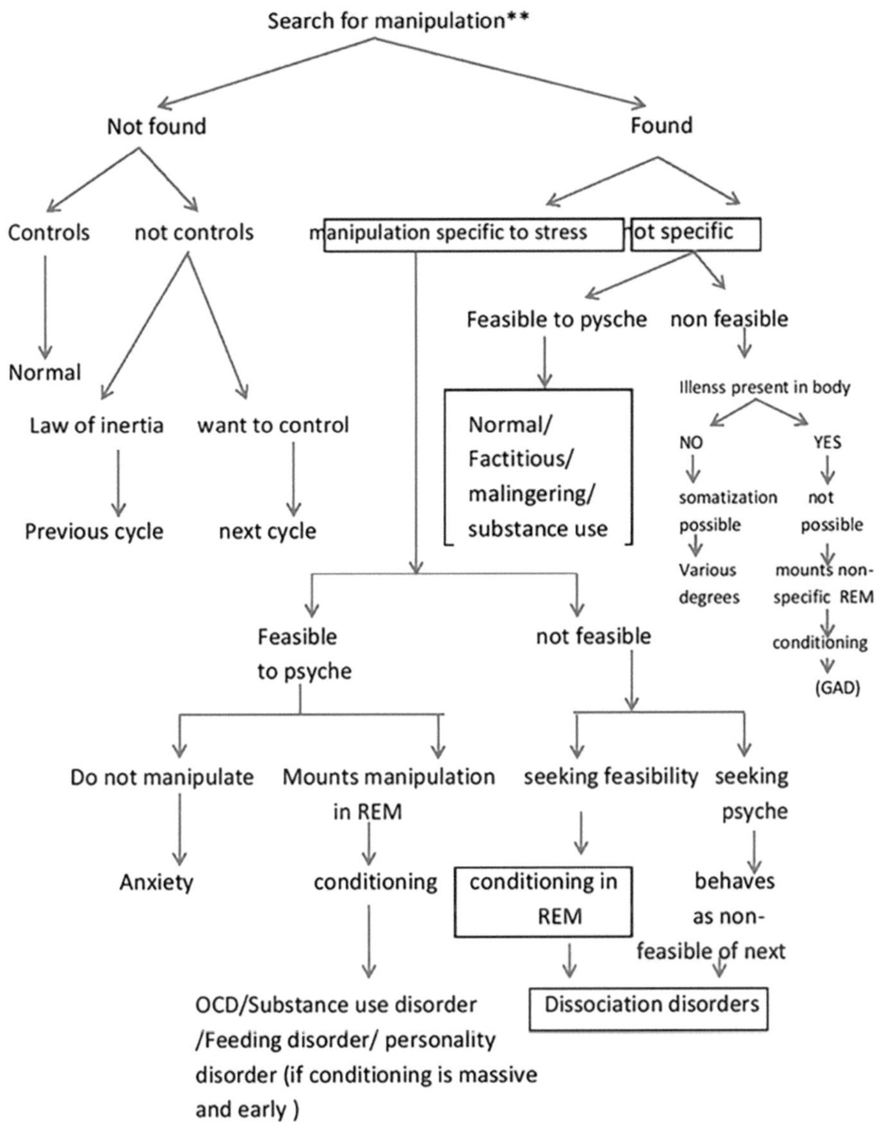


**Figure 4.**
*Algorithm showing response when a patient cannot control the thoughts provoking mental stress and still tries to find possible ways to control its inception in thought process.*

Each and every response can be mapped and the therapy oriented at that, however it is beyond the scope of this chapter to discuss every disease and intervention in detail [8].

### 3.8 Future prospects

Studying the impact can help us delineate the stress parameters and try to streamline treatment modalities. Saladino *et al.* recommended the same as primary prevention modality [11]. Under secondary prophylaxis, they recommended sensitizing the general populace on telepsychology, training next generation of psychotherapists in managing online devices and developing new tools of support and psychological treatment. However they mostly related to psychological issues needing treatment often the part unlooked is the iceberg below the tip. Those

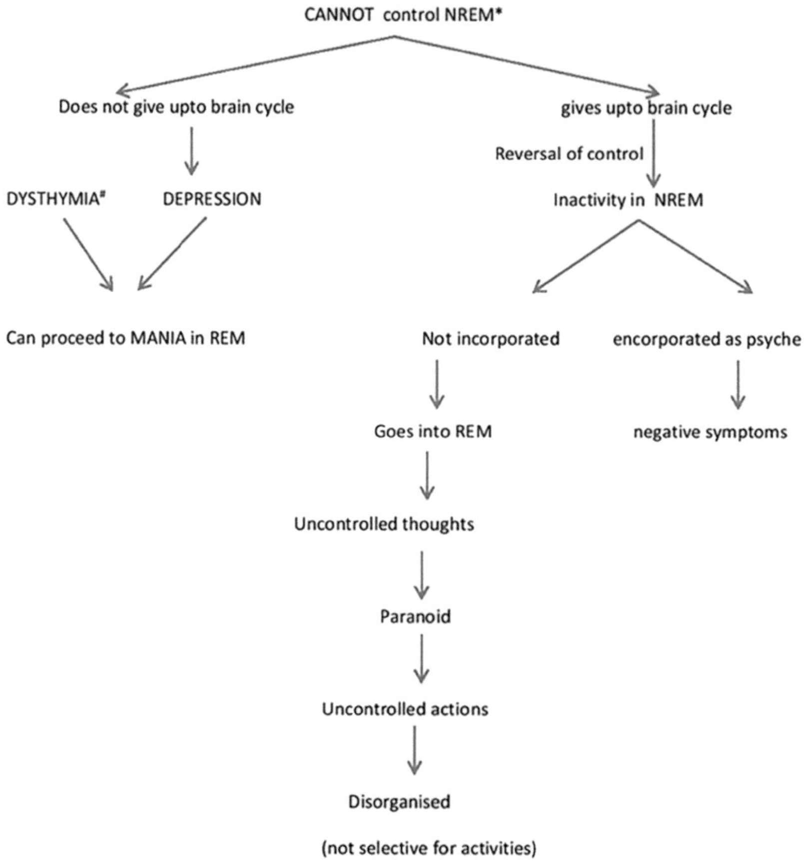


**Figure 5.**
*Algorithm showing response when a patient cannot control the thoughts provoking mental stress and cannot find possible ways to control its inception in thought process.*

unreported psychological impact can be overcome by better preparedness for next pandemic by government, people, and society in general. A change is inevitable so rather than resisting the change, we shall look at its brighter side: incorporate healthy habits, give time to family and friends, look at education in terms of learning and prepare for medical emergency.

## 4. Conclusions

The visuals of people dying despite best health facilities puts the question forward for us as to what are we in front of nature? How much have we learned and how much we are we prepared for catastrophe? The rapid response and adaptability of general population cannot be overlooked. But it has left a deep impact with long term unforeseen effects. We shall not only study the effects in its past form but also anticipate further damage it can cause in late future. Other than teaching us the fact that we need a lot of medical preparedness, it also taught us that healthy individuals can also become transiently stressed and show symptoms which may not be deemed as psychologically fit. This blemish had to be erased to bring people to talk about psychological issues with even non-medico or non-psychiatrist friends and colleagues. Ignorance had been a bliss for ignorant but not for those who suffered in silence. It is the awareness that has brought us together in the face of crisis.

COVID19 came as wave and swayed the humanity. Different states of individual showed different responses to the same stress creating a gamut of responses which led to different socio-economic, socio-political, professional and psychosocial impact. Identification of stress, mapping of response and a better preparedness from experience can all help us in preventing and controlling it next time.

## Conflict of interest

The authors declare no conflict of interest.



## Author details

Kishor Kunal[1], Priyanka Choudhary[2]*, Jiwesh Kumar[3], Ravi Prakash[4], Anita Singh[5] and Kirti Kanchan[6]

1 Department of Orthopaedics, AIIMS, Jodhpur, India

2 Department of Plant Pathology, BHU, Varanasi, India

3 Department of General Surgery, RIMS, Ranchi, India

4 Department of Anesthesia, Medanta, Gurugram, India

5 Travelling Veterinary Officer, Govt of Bihar, India

6 Department of General Surgery, SKMCH, Muzzafarpur, India

*Address all correspondence to: prinku30dec@gmail.com

## References

[1] Serafini G, Parmigiani B, Amerio A, Aguglia A, Sher L, Amore M. The psychological impact of COVID-19 on the mental health in the general population. QJM. 22 Jun 2020;**113**(8):531-537. DOI: 10.1093/qjmed/hcaa201. Epub ahead of print. PMID: 32569360; PMCID: PMC7337855

[2] Joshi A. COVID-19 pandemic in India: Through psycho-social lens. Journal of Social and Economic Development. Sep 2021;**23**(2):414-437

[3] Chawla N, Tom A, Sen MS, Sagar R. Psychological impact of COVID-19 on children and adolescents: A systematic review. Indian Journal of Psychological Medicine. 2021;**43**:294-299

[4] Dong F, Liu H, Yang M, Lu C, Dai N, Zhang Y, et al. Immediate psychosocial impact on healthcare workers during COVID-19 pandemic in China: A systematic review and Meta-analysis. Frontiers in Psychology. 2021;**12**:645460

[5] Sheraton M, Deo N, Dutt T, Surani S, Hall-Flavin D, Kashyap R. Psychological effects of the COVID 19 pandemic on healthcare workers globally: A systematic review. Psychiatry Research. 2020;**292**:113360

[6] Fteropoulli T, Kalavana TV, Yiallourou A, Karaiskakis M, Koliou Mazeri M, Vryonides S, et al. Beyond the physical risk: Psychosocial impact and coping in healthcare professionals during the COVID-19 pandemic. Journal of Clinical Nursing. 6 Jul 2021. DOI: 10.1111/jocn.15938. Epub ahead of print. PMID: 34231263; PMCID: PMC8447326

[7] Dubey S, Biswas P, Ghosh R, Chatterjee S, Dubey MJ, Chatterjee S, et al. Psychosocial impact of COVID-19. Diabetes & Metabolic Syndrome: Clinical Research and Reviews. 2020;**14**:779-788

[8] Kunal K. Third eye model: A hypothesis to span the diversities of psychiatry and normalcy. Neuropsychiatry (London). 2019;**9**: 2397-2418

[9] Caki N, Krupić D, Corr P ). Pyschosocial effects of the COVID-19 pandemic. In: Bozkurt V, Dawes G, Gulerce H, Westenbroek P, editors. The societal impacts of COVID-19: A transnational perspective. Istanbul, Turkey: Istanbul University Press. 2021. pp. 63-78. DOI: 10.26650/B/SS49.2021.006.05

[10] Veliyannoor P. The return of the repressed. COVID-19: The need for intervention at socio-cultural inscape. In: COVID-19 Pandemic: Challenges and Responses of Psychologists from India. Manickam LSS ed. Thiruvananthapuram: The Editor; 2020. pp. 108-129

[11] Saladino V, Algeri D, Auriemma V. The psychological and social impact of Covid-19: New perspectives of well-being. Frontiers in Psychology. 2020;**11**:577684

[12] Chick RC, Clifton GT, Peace KM, Propper BW, Hale DF, Alseidi AA, et al. Using technology to maintain the education of residents during the COVID-19 pandemic. Journal of Surgical Education. 2020;**77**:729-732

[13] Ahmed H, Allaf M, Elghazaly H. COVID-19 and medical education. The Lancet Infectious Diseases. 2020;**20**:777-778

[14] Daniel J. Education and the COVID-19 pandemic. Prospects. 2020;**49**:91-96

[15] Eysenbach G. How to fight an infodemic: The four pillars of infodemic management. Journal of Medical Internet Research. 2020;**22**:e21820

[16] Osofsky JD, Osofsky HJ, Mamon LY. Psychological and social impact of COVID-19. Psychological Trauma: Theory, Research, Practice, and Policy. 2020;**12**:468

[17] Saha K, Torous J, Caine ED, De Choudhury M. Psychosocial effects of the COVID-19 pandemic: Large-scale quasi-experimental study on social media. Journal of Medical Internet Research. 2020;**22**:e22600

[18] Xiao H, Zhang Y, Kong D, Li S, Yang N. The effects of social support on sleep quality of medical staff treating patients with coronavirus disease 2019 (COVID-19) in January and February 2020 in China. Medical Science Monitor: International Medical Journal of Experimental and Clinical Research. 2020;**26**:e923549-e923541

[19] Zhou X, Snoswell CL, Harding LE, Bambling M, Edirippulige S, Bai X, et al. The role of telehealth in reducing the mental health burden from COVID-19. Telemedicine and e-Health. 2020;**26**:377-379

[20] Orrù G, Marzetti F, Conversano C, Vagheggini G, Miccoli M, Ciacchini R, et al. Secondary traumatic stress and burnout in healthcare workers during COVID-19 outbreak. International Journal of Environmental Research and Public Health. 2021;**18**:337

[21] Lai J, Ma S, Wang Y, Cai Z, Hu J, Wei N, et al. Factors associated with mental health outcomes among health care workers exposed to coronavirus disease 2019. JAMA Network Open. 2020;**3**:e203976-e203976

[22] Edigin E, Eseaton PO, Shaka H, Ojemolon PE, Asemota IR, Akuna E. Impact of COVID-19 pandemic on medical postgraduate training in the United States. Medical Education Online. 2020;**25**:1774318

[23] Liang ZC, Ooi SBS, Wang W. Pandemics and their impact on medical training: Lessons from Singapore. Academic Medicine. 2020;**95**:1359-1361

[24] Upadhyaya GK, Jain VK, Iyengar KP, Patralekh MK, Vaish A. Impact of COVID-19 on post-graduate orthopaedic training in Delhi-NCR. Journal of Clinical Orthopaedics and Trauma. 2020;**11**:S687-S695

[25] Yuen J, Xie F. Medical education during the COVID-19 pandemic: Perspectives from UK trainees. Postgraduate Medical Journal. 2020;**96**:432-433

[26] Crosby DL, Sharma A. Insights on otolaryngology residency training during the COVID-19 pandemic. Otolaryngology and Head and Neck Surgery. 2020;**163**:38-41

[27] Romm KF, Patterson B, Wysota CN, Wang Y, Berg CJ. Predictors of negative psychosocial and health behavior impact of COVID-19 among young adults. Health Education Research. 2022;**36**(4):385-397. DOI: 10.1093/her/cyab026

[28] Suryavanshi N, Kadam A, Dhumal G, Nimkar S, Mave V, Gupta A, et al. Mental health and quality of life among healthcare professionals during the COVID-19 pandemic in India. Brain and Behavior. 2020;**10**:e01837

Chapter 4

# Perspective Chapter: The Psychosocial Effects of Isolation and Social Distancing during the Coronavirus Disease 2019 Pandemic – An Overview and Mitigation Strategies

*Raghad Burjaq and Samer Hammoudeh*


## Abstract

There is no doubt that the coronavirus disease 2019 pandemic has changed the world in unprecedented ways. Among its turbulent effects, it has impacted many aspects of the lives of individuals, ranging from their mental health to finances. As such, it is essential to determine the psychosocial factors at play and examine how they have impacted the lives of people around the world. This chapter examines psychosocial factors, such as depression, anxiety, and stress, which have been on the rise. Furthermore, the interplay of mental health factors and other stressors brought on by the pandemic has led to the concern that cases of suicidal ideation are also increasing. In response to the stay-at-home orders, family members spent unprecedented amounts of time in close contact with one another, which has had mental health repercussions. In addition, changes in the format of lesson delivery have been stress-inducing and have robbed many students of proper education. Another factor is unemployment, which has been on the rise since the start of the pandemic. Finally, rates of sexual and domestic violence have also increased, significantly impacting women. Exercise, limiting media exposure, counseling, and maintaining social networks are the strategies that have been identified to mitigate the effects of the psychosocial factors discussed in this chapter.


**Keywords:** pandemic, COVID-19, mental health, psychosocial factors, mitigation strategies

## 1. Introduction

The coronavirus disease 2019 (COVID-19) pandemic has undoubtedly changed the lives of individuals all around the world in profound ways. First identified in Wuhan, a city in Hubei Province in China, at the end of 2019, the pathogen responsible for the pandemic, severe acute respiratory syndrome 2 (SARS-CoV-2), has noticeably become the modern era's largest global health threat [1]. Although, Chinese authorities reported the country's first cluster of pneumonia cases related to this virus on December 31, 2019, it wasn't until January 30, 2020, that the World Health Organization (WHO) declared a global health emergency [2]. At the beginning of March 2020, the world essentially shut down, with countries closing their borders, schools closing their doors, and employees either laid off or directed to begin working from home. As the virus was confirmed to be capable of human-to-human transmission via respiratory droplets, individuals began to wear masks, social distance from one another, and quarantine to contain its spread [3]. Within weeks, the world effectively began to witness and experience the repercussions of the pandemic; beyond its disruption of the global economic and health care systems, it has impacted the physical health of individuals significantly, with the virus resulting in hundreds of millions of cases and, consequently, millions of deaths [4]. Those who became infected with SARS-CoV-2 experienced symptoms that ranged from fever, dry cough, fatigue, and loss of taste and smell to pneumonia, respiratory distress, septic shock, and organ failure [5–7]. Many individuals who recovered from COVID-19 have since reported experiencing lingering symptoms as part of a condition that came to be called long COVID [8]. The unique range of symptoms associated with COVID-19 and the consequential fear and anxiety associated with SARS-CoV-2 infection, including concerning the possibility of dying from it, led to the development of what is now termed "coronaphobia" [9]. This kind of state of prolonged fear and anxiety has been shown to increase the risk of major psychiatric disorders [10]. Furthermore, prolonged social isolation with minimal social contact, as was made necessary by the pandemic, has been shown to increase individuals' chances of developing mental health complications that include anxiety, depression, posttraumatic stress disorder (PTSD), and insomnia [11].

With the lives of individuals changing radically in all areas, including daily routines, work and family dynamics, income, leisure, and socialization, a global concern for the mental health of individuals has emerged [4]. According to Pfefferbaum and North [12], the uncertain prospects, resource shortages, the enforcement of public health measures that resulted in infringement on individual freedoms, the financial loss brought on by the economic crisis, and the contradicting information presented by authorities triggered an increase in the prevalence of stress which, in turn, led to a heightened risk of developing mental illness during the pandemic. Since mental health issues are the result of a dynamic interplay between mental, emotional, and social factors [13], identifying these psychosocial factors is crucial to helping those already affected, as well as for mitigating—or eliminating altogether—the effects of these factors. In addition, with no clear end to the pandemic in sight, despite the approval of vaccines and their subsequent rollout, this remains an ongoing issue [14].

Accordingly, this chapter will examine the psychosocial factors brought on by the COVID-19 pandemic, which include depression, anxiety, and stress and their association with substance abuse, and sleep disturbances, suicidal ideation, changes in family dynamics and education, an increase in unemployment rates, and the increase in sexual and domestic violence rates. This chapter will then go on to scrutinize mitigation techniques, such as exercise, limiting exposure to the media, counseling, and maintaining social networks.

## 2. Psychosocial factors

### 2.1 Depression, anxiety, and stress

It is no surprise that the spread of SARS-CoV-2 has resulted in a global mental health burden; the COVID-19 pandemic has both resulted in a substantial increase in psychiatric illnesses and further aggravated pre-existing psychiatric disorders [15]. The COVID-19 pandemic not only disrupted critical mental health services in more than 93% of countries globally but also increased the number of individuals suffering from mental health issues, thus further increasing the demand for mental health support services [16]. A survey conducted by the WHO in the summer of 2020 found that 70% of countries had adopted a telemedicine approach to therapy, forgoing in-person sessions, thus resulting in inconsistencies in the effectiveness of interventions. Furthermore, before the pandemic, countries were spending less than 2% of their health budgets on mental health and were falling short in meeting the demand for mental health services [16]. With the aftermath of the pandemic that encompasses the isolation, loss of income, bereavement, and fear; countries are expected to struggle further to meet their populations' need for access to mental health services. A study by Cambridge University investigated the global prevalence of anxiety and stress during the COVID-19 pandemic and documented high prevalence rates of both depression (24%) and anxiety (21.3%) worldwide. The study then went on to investigate the prevalence rates in different regions of the world. The report noted that, before the pandemic, the prevalence rates of depression and anxiety in Asian countries ranged from 1.3% to 3.4% and from 2.1% to 4.1%, respectively, while, post-pandemic onset, these numbers increased to ranges of 15.4–19.8% for depression and 15.4–20.3% for anxiety. For Europe, a large difference was witnessed, with the pre-pandemic prevalence rate ranging from 1.4% to 3.9% for depression and 3% to 7.4% for anxiety, while post-pandemic onset, the prevalence rate for depression reached 26% and that for anxiety reached 19.2%. Finally, the 2011 pre-pandemic prevalence rates for regions outside Asia and Europe were reported to range from 2.1% to 4.3% for depression and 2.8% to 7.1% for anxiety, but they increased to 29.2% and 28.6% for depression and anxiety, respectively [17].

Persistent uncertainty about the pandemic and the resulting significant changes in many areas of life created an environment in which stress can increase [18, 19]. The COVID-19 pandemic led to rising stress levels due to increased and prolonged worrying about issues such as finances, health, isolation, loneliness, and changes in daily routines [20]. A study conducted among the public in China found that stress and anxiety increased by 25% during the pandemic compared to before the pandemic [21]. Another study reported that 8.1–29.2% of individuals in China, 11.6% in India, 14.6% in Italy, and 0.6–9.2% of men and 1.2–8.9% in women in Spain reported experiencing stress [22]. In fact, with the exceptional economic circumstances, the hundreds of thousands of deaths, and the prolonged exposure to stressors brought about by the pandemic, current stress levels have surpassed normal ones attributed to the usual range of human experiences and have inflicted major psychological trauma that has led some individuals to experience PTSD [23, 24]. According to Xiao et al. [24], this trauma can be the sum of traumas from three distinct circumstances, the first being that experienced by those who suffer from the disease and experience traumatizing symptoms, such as respiratory distress and near-death experiences; the second being that experienced while watching someone suffer and/or die from the disease; and the third being that triggered by fears—whether realistic or not—about catching the virus, being alone, or being stigmatized because of the disease. A study in Italy investigated the prevalence of PTSD in individuals who suffered from acute COVID-19 and found that, among the 115 participants who survived COVID, the prevalence of PTSD was 30.2% [25]. Among health care workers, especially frontline workers, the toll of watching thousands of patients die from COVID-19 has been uniquely traumatizing. A study conducted by King's College London found that 45% of intensive care unit employees in the United Kingdom were suffering from severe anxiety, PTSD, or other psychological disorders [26]. Finally, in considering the isolation and fear of contracting the virus, Zhang et al. [27] reported the prevalence rate of PTSD in the general population during the pandemic to be 15%.

This increase in stress, due to the unprecedented changes in the lives of individuals worldwide, has manifested into negative health consequences, one of which is insomnia or sleep disturbances. A colloquial term, "coronasomnia," has been established to describe the array of sleep dysfunction symptoms—which include but are not limited to insomnia, disrupted sleep, alteration in the sleep-wake cycles, and reductions in sleep quality—brought about by the stress of the pandemic [28]. The global prevalence rates for insomnia symptoms have previously been reported to be 20–45% [29]; however, Voitsidis et al. [20] investigated the prevalence of insomnia in the Greek population during the COVID-19 pandemic and, based on the participation of 2427 individuals, detected sleep problems in 37.6% of participants. Another study explored the prevalence of insomnia in the general French population during the COVID-19 pandemic and reported that the prevalence of clinical insomnia was 19.1% [30]. Research has also examined the rates of insomnia specifically in health care workers [31]; this kind of work is crucial as frontline health care workers are a group that has remained highly vulnerable to developing mental health problems during the pandemic [32]. Ultimately, Stewart et al. found that nearly all individuals who took part in their study reported poor sleep, with almost half reporting moderate to severe insomnia [31].

Another health consequence brought about by the higher stress levels experienced by individuals during the pandemic is the increase in substance abuse. There is no denying that the COVID-19 pandemic has resulted in greater stress for individuals around the world, and this increase in stress has been correlated with the abuse of addictive substances [33]. In fact, according to a study done by Rogers et al. [34], the worry, fear, and stress associated with the pandemic have led to the use of substances as a coping mechanism; of the 160 participants who took part in their study, 8.8% reported they had started drinking during the pandemic, while 6.9% had started smoking cigarettes, 5% had started using cannabis, 4.4% had started using electronic cigarettes, 5.6% had started using stimulants, and 5.6% had started using opioids. In addition, in looking at the reason for this rise in substance abuse, the negative reinforcement models of substance use postulate that disasters, stress, worry, and/or anxiety, such as that brought on by the pandemic, trigger an increase in negative effects which, in turn, strengthens the motivation of individuals to use and even abuse substances to mitigate such effects [35–37]. In other words, individuals used or even abused substances as a maladaptive coping strategy during the pandemic because the isolation, social distancing, and stay-at-home measures limited the options for healthier forms of emotional regulation, such as social interaction or working out and being active [34]. Another reason suggested by existing research that could explain the maladaptive use of addictive substances as a strategy for coping with the increased levels of stress, anxiety, and depression brought on by the COVID-19 pandemic is the behavioral immune system (BIS) [12, 38, 39]. The BIS has been shown to increase interoceptive awareness and signals the body in case of a potential infection. In turn, this leads to the production of behaviors that help prevent an illness. However, this feedback is linked with anxiety, stress, trauma, and fear, which are all reactions that are associated with an increased risk of substance use and abuse [15, 40]. More specifically, research has shown that activation of the BIS and the consequential rise in anxiety levels due to interoceptive awareness can lead to higher usage rates of both alcohol and marijuana [41, 42].

In general, identifying the prevalence of psychosocial factors such as depression, anxiety, and stress is essential to better understand how to mitigate the effects of these factors. However, given the increased need and demand for mental services during the pandemic, it is crucial to identify those individuals who urgently need help to provide them with more support [43]. As such, determining the high-risk groups is essential. As it pertains to depression, anxiety, and stress, research has found that younger individuals are more vulnerable and have reported greater levels of depression, anxiety, and stress compared to their middle- and older-age counterparts [44]. Furthermore, the Centers for Disease Control and Prevention found that young adults are exhibiting worsening depression and anxiety during the COVID-19 pandemic [45]. In addition, they are also the group that has seen the largest increase in unmet mental health needs [46].

### 2.2 Suicidal ideation

Along with the anxiety, depression, stress, insomnia, and substance abuse discussed above, the financial stressors brought about by the global economic hardships and the social isolation brought on by the stay-at-home measures have created what psychologists have termed “the perfect storm,” leading to the concern that suicide rates may increase [47]. It has been found that suicidal ideation is on the rise, especially in young adults [48]. Fortgang et al. [49] investigated whether suicidal thoughts were predicted by an increase in social isolation and found that rates of suicidal ideation increased with greater feelings of isolation. However, another study conducted in the Spanish general population found that the overall prevalence of suicidal ideation did not change significantly between before and after the start of the pandemic [50]. With these variations in findings, no clear trends can yet be established, and such data on suicide rates still need to be compiled [51].

It has been indicated above that the prevalence of depression during the pandemic is on the rise. With that in mind, research has identified depression as a major risk factor for suicidal ideation [52]. The pandemic has resulted in closed businesses and stay-at-home directives to curb the spread of SARS-CoV-2. This has, in turn, led to employees being laid off and/or working reduced hours. In the past, economic declines such as this have been associated with a higher rate of suicide [53]. Another crucial side effect of the pandemic is social isolation. Social connection is a protective factor against suicidal ideation; however, the pandemic has made establishing and maintaining social connections difficult and has led to greater rates of loneliness. This social isolation and loneliness have been shown to lead to suicidal thoughts [54]. Interestingly, the Japanese government created what they termed the “Ministry of Loneliness” after 20,919 people took their lives in 2020 [55].

While the pandemic has had its toll, in one way or another, on individuals worldwide, some groups have been more heavily affected than others. As it pertains to suicidal ideation, health care workers fighting on the front lines are one of them. For example, health care workers reported higher rates of suicidal thoughts when they also suffered from PTSD. In addition, these individuals also reported higher rates of feeling isolated [56]. Another high-risk group is adolescents. With the lack of social connections and the upheaval of daily routines, navigating the pandemic has been particularly tough on adolescents. One study found that the suicide rates among adolescent girls aged 12–17 years increased by 51% during the pandemic [57]. These trends are an indication that these groups require urgent mental health services.

### 2.3 Changes in family dynamics and education

It is undeniable that the pandemic has led to the restructuring of relationships in ways that either pushed individuals to live in closer contact with each other or further apart from one another. With schools shutting down, shops and restaurants closing, and parents being asked to work from home, contact with the outside world was limited in unparalleled ways [58]. Often, families found themselves confined to their homes and isolated together for unprecedented amounts of time. Paired with financial troubles, stress, anxiety, and fear due to the pandemic, a situation has emerged in which a high-pressure confinement environment was created [59]. This has been associated with dysfunction in the lives of individuals and families. When Feinberg et al. examined the impact of the pandemic and its mitigation interventions on the mental health of parents, children, and overall family functioning, they found that, during the first month of the pandemic, children reported elevated levels of internalizing problems, such as depression, and of externalizing problems, like aggressive behaviors. As for the parents, they reported decreased quality levels of co-parenting and higher levels of depression [60].

The pandemic has disrupted the traditional methods by which education is delivered worldwide. Instead of the traditional in-person education, children were now left attending schools online via digital learning software programs, YouTube videos, and Zoom classes [61]. This arrangement has created several educational challenges for children [62]. Parents were also left needing to support their children more and, with the little warning they had, they did not have much time to prepare [63]. In response to the shift to online learning and the closure of childcare facilities, parents had to learn to allocate responsibilities. One study found that 67% of women assumed responsibility for the education of their children compared to 52% of men. While some parents have attempted to share this responsibility, women were rendered not only more likely to take charge of homeschooling but to also spend more time washing, dressing, and feeding their kids [64]. It was reported that 53% of women have been struggling with educating their children at home and that their mental health was negatively impacted as a result. In contrast, 43% of men reported the same struggles [64]. Along with this, many parents were dealing with other stressors brought on by the pandemic. It was reported that 74% of parents perceived a disruption had occurred in their daily routine and found the necessary adaptation to be a critical stressor [65]. In addition, children were significantly impacted too. It was reported that 52% of parents in Great Britain stated that their children were struggling with being educated at home. When looking at the major causative factors, it was determined that the absence of motivation, guidance, and support was an issue [64]. Another issue brought on by distance learning is that not all children have access to the equipment necessary to carry it out. According to the United Nations Educational, Scientific and Cultural Organization, 463 million around the world were no longer receiving an education during the pandemic because they could not access remote learning [62].

The COVID-19 pandemic, in addition to its many negative consequences, has brought with it the worst economic crisis since the Great Depression of 1930 [66]. With this came the loss of income due to a lack of employment or being laid off. This has particularly impacted children of low-income, less-educated parents. To better understand family dynamics following the consequences of the pandemic, responses were collected from 572 low-income families in Chicago; what was found was that the parents' job and income loss were strongly linked to their stress level, loss of a sense of hope, depression, and negative interactions with their children [67]. Yet, this does not apply to parents who have lost jobs but did not experience simultaneous income loss. On the contrary, positive parent-child interactions were seen among individuals who lost their jobs but did not experience any income loss. Another outcome that was observed in this study was that parents who spent more time taking care of their children reported more positive parent-child connections, while negative parent-child interactions were seen among parents who were exposed to SARS-CoV-2 [67].

### 2.4 Unemployment

The COVID-19 pandemic was not merely a public health crisis—it was an economic crisis as well [68]. With businesses closing and travel and hospitality businesses becoming obsolete, many individuals around the world lost their jobs and, consequently, their incomes [68, 69]. According to a survey conducted by the International Labour Organization, 30% of respondents lost their source of income, and 25% of respondents were unable to meet their basic needs. Furthermore, 5% reported not being able to pay their rent [70]. In addition to this, according to the United Nations labor agency, the COVID-19 pandemic has caused more than 100 million workers to be pushed into poverty. This means that families were surviving on less than 3.20 US dollars a day. This trend was caused by the job losses, reductions in job hours, and lack of access to good jobs brought on by the pandemic [71]. According to WHO, because of the economic and social disruption caused by the pandemic, tens of millions of people have been put at risk of falling into extreme poverty. In addition, there is an estimated 690 million undernourished people in the world, and this number was expected to increase by up to 132 million by the end of 2020. As for job losses, almost half of the world's workforce is at risk of losing their jobs [72].

With all this in mind, it should be noted that exposure to SARS-CoV-2 is not random. One of the highest-risk groups is those who live in poverty. It has been shown that individuals who are in low-paid, manual jobs in the retail, service, and care sectors are more highly and likely to be exposed to the virus as they hold jobs that cannot be performed remotely. In addition, poorer individuals are more likely to contract the virus as they have higher levels of pre-existing illnesses [73]. Another area in which lower-income families have been greatly affected by the pandemic is that of childcare. With community support programs and free services being halted, low-income families with children are having to put up with extra costs in food, heating, and housing [74]. According to Brewer and Patrick [75], in 2020, 36% of low-income families who had children saw an increase in their spending, while families without children saw a 40% reduction in their spending.

Previous studies have investigated the effects of unemployment on suicide rates in 63 countries around the world, without factoring in the extra stressors of the pandemic. What was found was that suicide rates increase by 20–30% when unemployment is factored in [76]. When trying to ascertain the rates of suicide due to unemployment while factoring in the health and psychiatric implications of the pandemic, the relationship is less clear, and a lot of the findings are speculative. When looking at similar situations in history, such as during the severe acute respiratory syndrome epidemic of 2003, it was found that suicide rates in the affected Asian countries increased together with unemployment, reaching historic levels in that year. However, since the severe acute respiratory syndrome pandemic occurred at the peak of the Asian financial crisis, it can be hard to separate that event from the larger findings [77]. Projections have been made, with the use of time-trend regression models, about the rate of suicides as it relates to unemployment during the COVID-19 pandemic. In Canada for example, the rate was projected to be 27% [78] while, in the United States, it was projected to be 3.3–8.4% [79].

### 2.5 Sexual and domestic violence

As a result of the emergency stay-at-home measures taken to curb the spread of SARS-CoV-2 and "flatten the curve," many individuals have been forced to spend unprecedented amounts of time indoors, and this trend has raised concerns about an increased risk for sexual violence [80]. According to data, the percentage of women worldwide who have had violence perpetrated against them by a partner or a non-partner is 35% [81]. It has been predicted that, due to the COVID-19 pandemic, the rate of domestic violence has increased by at least 25%, and this phenomenon has been termed the "shadow pandemic." However, it should be noted that this has yet to be fully confirmed, and further insight and monitoring of the issue are required [82]. The best way to learn about the present is to look at the past, and research from previous pandemics has shown that factors that most commonly increase the risk of violence include economic uncertainty, stress related to poverty, quarantine requirements, the loss of a job or a reduction in working hours, and the social isolation [83–86]. As previously discussed in the above sections, pandemics have been linked to depression, stress, PTSD, insomnia, and substance abuse, which are all factors that have been correlated with increased violence rates [87–89].

Another side effect of the pandemic's lockdowns is that they create the ideal environment for domestic violence. An exponential increase in domestic violence has been recorded since the start of the pandemic [90–92], including especially against women. According to WHO, this is in line with the current world circumstances as violence against women tends to increase in disaster situations such as the current pandemic we are living through. The environment that has been created by the pandemic, in which there are high levels of stress, increased economic turmoil, upheaval, and reduced access to social and protective networks that serve as protective factors, is ripe for domestic violence [93]. In Australia, a 5% increase in domestic violence has been recorded [94–96]. In a study in Portugal that consisted of 1062 participants, 13.7% reported experiencing some form of domestic violence [97]. In France, reports increased by 30%, while a 25% increase was seen in Argentina and a 30% increase was noted in Cyprus. In Singapore, a 33% increase was seen. Finally, this trend has also been seen in the United Kingdom, the United States, Canada, Germany, and Spain [90].

## 3. Mitigation strategies

### 3.1 Exercise

Exercise has been proven to reduce stress and anxiety. It was found that exercising during the pandemic reduces symptoms of stress, anxiety, depression, boredom, and frustration, and it renders individuals more mentally and physically resilient [98]. When we exercise, our brains release endorphins, and these are the hormones that help us deal with stress and reduce sensations of pain. As such, exercising on a regular schedule will facilitate a consistent release of endorphins, thus mitigating the effects of stress [99]. This is crucial, as prolonged stress can harm the body physically by negatively affecting our cardiovascular system, central nervous system, immune system, and central nervous system [100]. Prolonged stress has been shown to accelerate aging by increasing the rate at which telomeres shorten, and short telomeres have been linked to diseases like osteoporosis and coronary heart disease [101]. In addition, the constant stimulation and emotional arousal brought on by chronic stress have been shown to cause insomnia [102]. Furthermore, stress has been linked to depression and anxiety; as such, eliminating or at least minimizing stress can keep one from developing anxiety and depression [103].

Exercise not only benefits the mental health of individuals but also their physical health. Exercise has also been shown to improve the immunity of individuals. Since SARS-CoV-2 is a virus that attacks the respiratory and immune systems, strengthening our immune systems is crucial to ward it off [104]. According to da Silveira et al. [105], exercise stimulates cellular immunity; however, intensity plays a crucial role. Moderate-intensity exercise stimulates immunity, while high-intensity exercise has been shown to have the opposite effect. Furthermore, exercising consistently is a protective factor against both viral and bacterial infections and can also increase the immune system's response to vaccines [106]. In addition, regular moderate-intensity exercise minimizes respiratory infection and stimulates humoral and cellular immunity [107]. When looking at the types of exercises, one particularly beneficial mode is aerobic exercises. This kind of exercise increases the body's immunity by increasing neutrophils, macrophages, T-lymphocytes, and monocytes. The increase in these components is not only crucial for protecting against infection but also plays a particularly crucial role in increasing immunoglobulin levels, especially immunoglobulins A and G, which have a substantial role in fighting lung infections such as those caused by the COVID-19 virus [108]. This is of importance since the medical indication of COVID-19 is dominated by respiratory symptoms [109]. Another practice that has been proven successful in improving the mental health of individuals during the COVID-19 pandemic is yoga. Yoga is a practice that is widely used to lower stress and anxiety and has even been shown to improve immunity [110, 111]. A study by Nagarathna and colleagues [112] examined the effects of yoga on the physical health, mental health, lifestyle, and coping skills of individuals during the COVID-19 pandemic and what was found was that those who practiced yoga exhibited less anxiety, stress, and fear, as well as had better coping strategies. In addition, yoga practitioners had better physical health and endurance, were less likely to use substances, consume unhealthy food, and had better quality sleep. All these aspects are crucial when it comes to the strength of the immune system [112].

### 3.2 Minimizing media exposure

With the novelty of SARS-CoV-2 and the confusion brought on by it, individuals have turned to social media and news outlets to gain information. According to Garfin et al. [113], the extensive media coverage of the pandemic has magnified the distress caused by it. When individuals are exposed to too much stressful news, it can not only strengthen their fears but also preclude them from concentrating on regular everyday tasks and adopting protective behaviors [114]. A study conducted in China examined the association between media exposure about the COVID-19 pandemic and the stress response, and the study investigators found that prolonged exposure to the media was not only associated with higher levels of stress but also with acute stress disorder. This led to the recommendations that governments should be more conscious of the negative impacts that such exposure has on their citizens and should develop suitable mediation strategies that do not compromise citizen well-being but rather promote it in times of crisis [115].

It has been shown that, since the start of the pandemic, the rates of anxiety have tripled and those of depression have quadrupled in the United States, and research has suggested that the media has played a role in these trends [116]. This is fathomable as the media coverage of the pandemic has consisted of commentary on distress and death. Furthermore, the media's reporting of exaggerated numbers, inaccurate facts, and conspiracy theories have led to fear and confusion [116, 117]. Looi et al. [118] offered three recommendations that could mitigate the mental health effects of the pandemic; the first is that governments and health authorities should be responsible for communicating information clearly and correcting misinformation. Second is that these authorities should warn citizens of the likely adverse mental health effects of prolonged media exposure during the pandemic, and third is that limiting exposure to the media is essential. In fact, as per research recommendations, individuals should limit their exposure to COVID-19-related news to a maximum of 2 h per day. Spending more than 2 h a day focusing on COVID-19-related news has been associated with anxiety and depression [119, 120].

Furthermore, attending to the media should be avoided at least 1 h before bedtime to avoid experiencing insomnia [120, 121].

### 3.3 Counseling

The pandemic has left a psychic scar that still needs tending. With psychological pressures like depression, anxiety, and stress that then may manifest into health issues like insomnia and substance abuse, counseling is necessary to be able to support those who are affected [122]. Due to the social and physical distancing required by the COVID-19 pandemic, the usual means of support are no longer as accessible and have been disrupted immensely [123]. When looking at 130 countries, it was found that 67% of them saw disruptions to their counseling and psychotherapy services. Despite this, the pandemic is increasing the demand for mental health services [16]. In response, countries have begun to adopt electronic mental health tools and, while the acceptance of these tools was quite minimal before the pandemic, they have now become the best and highest-quality solutions available given the circumstances brought about by the need for physical distancing [124, 125]. As for how effective counseling during the pandemic is, research has shown that individuals who regularly attend counseling sessions experience lower levels of depression, anxiety, and stress [122].

One very salient effect of the pandemic is the transition from in-person to online therapy sessions. With the increasing rates of stress, anxiety, and depression and the lasting impact they are expected to have, it is essential to make sure that the adopted treatment methods alleviate the patient's distress and have lasting effects [126]. One technique that has been shown to alleviate stress, depression and anxiety is cognitive behavioral therapy (CBT). CBT psychotherapeutic approach aims to change the constant destructive and disturbing patterns of negative thoughts that result in stress, depression, and anxiety with ones that are more objective and realistic [127]. Weiner et al. [126] developed a protocol that is looking at how effective online cognitive behavioral therapy is for health care workers, a group that is at higher risk of developing mental health repercussions because of stressors of the pandemic. According to this study, similar protocols have been shown to improve resilience in high-stress scenarios, such as that of a pandemic, as well as to mitigate the chances that psychological disorders might emerge. While this protocol is still being implemented, the findings may prove significantly helpful in managing the long-term mental health effects of the COVID-19 pandemic [126]. Another study investigated the effectiveness of cognitive-behavioral therapy and found that computer-based cognitive behavioral therapy proved to be an effective treatment for patients with COVID-19 who suffered from anxiety, depression, and insomnia. In support of this Mahoney and colleagues decided to look at the effects of online CBT on anxiety and depression during the COVID-19 pandemic and found a sizeable reduction in anxiety and depression symptom severity, as well as a reduction in psychological distress [128]. Nevertheless, further research is needed to better understand the long-term effects of such a treatment approach [129]. On the other hand, a study conducted by Barker and Barker [130] found that face-to-face counseling sessions are more effective than online sessions. It was noted that individuals appeared more diverted and disengaged during virtual sessions. In addition, they were not as open or comfortable with confiding in their counselor.

### 3.4 Maintaining social connections

Humans are hard-wired to need social connection [131]. While the pandemic has altered all types of social norms, it does not mean these norms have to be eliminated; instead, they can be altered, and individuals can adapt to the alterations because maintaining a regular human connection in times like these is as important as ever [132]. Higher levels of social connectedness during the pandemic were associated with lower levels of stress and fatigue. In addition, the larger and more active their social networks are, the lower individuals' levels of distress and anxiety are [133]. Furthermore, social connections are crucial in building resilience in times of hardship by shielding individuals against any trying mental and physical outcomes brought on by those times [113]. On the other hand, chronic loneliness has been associated with negative health outcomes, like an addiction. As for the effects of loneliness, they are more harmful than hypertension and obesity [134, 135]. Captivatingly, social connections are not only beneficial to our mental health but also our physical health: they can help to fight off infections. It has been found that maintaining healthy social connections aids our immune system in creating more antibodies, which can then go on to fight diseases [136, 137]. All this research has clearly shown that maintaining social connectedness is crucial in not only fighting off mental health ailments but also physical ones.

Since the Internet has been the sole means of maintaining social connections in a socially distanced world, it is worth examining the effectiveness of using the Internet to maintain these social connections. With the pandemic, all aspects of life have become Internet-based, from counseling to religious services to parties [126, 138, 139]. A study conducted in Germany investigated the effects that Internet- and technology-based communication had on maintaining social connections during the pandemic. What was found was that, while the impact of audiovisual communication was minimal, that of text-based communication has been found to promote the maintenance of social distancing measures and increase life satisfaction and the feeling of being socially supported. However, when looking at the long-term effects, some of these findings changed. While the feeling of being socially supported increased, the desire to maintain communication and social distancing measures decreased [140]. On the other hand, another study compared social networking data pre-pandemic and during the pandemic and found that there were substantial decreases in network density and size [141]. This can be attributed to the fact that, with the prolonged lack of face-to-face communication, the familiar feeling of being close to family and friends begins to fade; more specifically, after a two-month period, the feeling decreases by 30% while, after a five-month period, the feeling decreases by 80% [141, 142]. Furthermore, when comparing the levels of loneliness, before the COVID-19 pandemic (June 2019) and during the COVID-19 pandemic (June 2020), face-to-face interactions, along with the duration and frequency, have been shown to be associated with smaller increases in levels of loneliness compared to other modes of communication during the COVID-19 pandemic [141].

## 4. Summary

It's needless to say that the COVID-19 pandemic has had seismic effects on the lives of individuals worldwide. With the documented impacts on mental health and financial well-being, it is crucial to determine the psychosocial factors at play to be able to mitigate their effects. The first psychosocial factors covered in this chapter were depression, anxiety, and stress. The research discussed in this chapter shows that depression, anxiety, and stress have increased during the pandemic. The next factor focused on was suicidal ideation, and preliminary research has indicated rates of this phenomenon are rising during the pandemic. In addition, some groups have documented higher rates than others, and frontline health care workers and adolescents may be particularly at risk. Then, changes in family dynamics and education were discussed. The pandemic has forced certain people to spend unprecedented amounts of time with one another, which has had its effects. The pandemic has proven to be particularly difficult on children and has made things hard on parents as well when it comes to cooperativity, which has also affected their mental health. As for education, adjusting to distance learning has been difficult for both parents and children. The shift to distance learning has also particularly affected low-income families. Furthermore, many children are no longer able to receive an education due to a lack of access to remote learning equipment. Unemployment was another factor discussed. Although, many individuals lost their jobs and source of income, this has again impacted low-income families more. In addition, their low-income status has left some individuals more at risk of SARS-CoV-2 infection as they have jobs that cannot be done remotely. The pandemic has also made childcare more expensive as the usual means of support that were relied upon are no longer available, and lower-income families were left taking on more costs for childcare. Unemployment has influenced mental health, leaving mental health providers worried about its effect on suicide rates. The last factor discussed was that of sexual and domestic violence, which the pandemic has created the ideal environment for. Rates for both have increased due to the pandemic, and a particularly stronger impact on women has been noted. Finally, mitigation strategies were discussed to ease the effects of these factors. The first was exercise, which has been shown to alleviate the depression, anxiety, and stress brought on by the pandemic. Limiting media exposure can also help ease the stress and anxiety created by the pandemic and its confusion. Counseling represents another mitigation strategy. The need for mental health services has increased in the wake of the pandemic; however, with the distancing measures, traditional counseling techniques have had to be altered and moved to a virtual setting. Nevertheless, those attending such sessions have shown improvements in mental health. The final mitigation strategy discussed was maintaining social connections. We are social beings, and social connections constitute not only a protective factor for mental health but also one for physical health. Connecting socially also aids in building the resilience that allows us to survive instances of adversity, such as what we are currently living through.

## Author details

Raghad Burjaq[1] and Samer Hammoudeh[2]*

1 Sidra Medicine, Doha, Qatar

2 Medical Research Center, Hamad Medical Corporation, Doha, Qatar

*Address all correspondence to: shammoudeh@hamad.qa

## References

[1] AlKhaldi M, James N, Chattu V, Ahmed S, Meghari H, Kaiser K, et al. Rethinking and strengthening the global health diplomacy through triangulated nexus between policy makers, scientists and the community in light of COVID-19 global crisis. Global Health Research and Policy. 2021;**6**(1)

[2] Who.int. Archived: WHO Timeline—COVID-19. 2021. Available from: https://www.who.int/news/item/27-04-2020-who-timeline---covid-19

[3] Katella K. Our Pandemic Year—A COVID-19 Timeline. Yale Medicine. 2021. Available from: https://www.yalemedicine.org/news/covid-timeline

[4] Ogrodniczuk J, Rice S, Kealy D, Seidler Z, Delara M, Oliffe J. Psychosocial impact of the COVID-19 pandemic: A cross-sectional study of online help-seeking Canadian men. Postgraduate Medicine. 2021;**133**(7):750-759

[5] Wang H, Li X, Yan Z, Sun X, Han J, Zhang B. Potential neurological symptoms of COVID-19. Therapeutic Advances in Neurological Disorders. 2020;**13**

[6] Dawson P, Rabold E, Laws R, Conners E, Gharpure R, Yin S, et al. Loss of taste and smell as distinguishing symptoms of coronavirus disease 2019. Clinical Infectious Diseases. 2020;**72**(4):682-685

[7] Shahbaz S, Ashraf M, Zakar R, Fischer F, Zakar M. Psychosocial effects of the COVID-19 pandemic and lockdown on university students: Understanding apprehensions through a phenomenographic approach. PLoS One. 2021;**5**(16):e0251641. DOI: 10.1371/journal.pone.0251641

[8] Sudre CH, Murray B, Varsavsky T, Graham MS, Penfold RS, Bowyer RC, et al. Attributes and predictors of long-COVID: Analysis of COVID cases and their symptoms collected by the COVID symptoms study app. MedRxiv. 2020. DOI: 10.1101/2020.10.19.20214494

[9] Arora A, Jha AK, Alat P, Das SS. Understanding coronaphobia. Asian Journal of Psychiatry. 2020;**54**:102384. DOI: 10.1016/j.ajp.2020.102384

[10] Mah L, Szabuniewicz C, Fiocco AJ. Can anxiety damage the brain? Current Opinion in Psychiatry. 2016;**29**(1):56-63. DOI: 10.1097/yco.0000000000000223

[11] Huremović D. Psychiatry of Pandemics: A Mental Health Response to Infection Outbreak. Switzerland AG: Springer Nature; 2019

[12] Pfefferbaum B, North CS. Mental health and the covid-19 pandemic. New England Journal of Medicine. 2020;**383**(6):510-512. DOI: 10.1056/nejmp2008017

[13] Cornah D. The Impact of Spirituality on Mental Health: A Review of the Literature. Mental Health Foundation; 2006

[14] World Health Organization. WHO director-general's opening remarks at the media briefing on covid-19. 2020. Available from: https://www.who.int/director-general/speeches/detail/who-director-general-s-opening-remarks-at-the-media-briefing-on-covid-19---21-august-2020

[15] McKay D, Asmundson G. COVID-19 stress and substance use: Current issues and future preparations. Journal of Anxiety Disorders. 2020;**74**:102274. DOI: 10.1016/j.janxdis.2020.102274

[16] World Health Organization. COVID-19 disrupting mental health

services in most countries. WHO survey. 2020. Available from: https://www.who.int/news/item/05-10-2020-covid-19-disrupting-mental-health-services-in-most-countries-who-survey

[17] Castaldelli-Maia J, Marziali M, Lu Z, Martins S. Investigating the effect of national government physical distancing measures on depression and anxiety during the COVID-19 pandemic through meta-analysis and meta-regression. Psychological Medicine. 2021;**51**(6):881-893. DOI: 10.1017/S0033291721000933

[18] Arslan G, Yıldırım M, Tanhan A, Buluş M, Allen KA. Coronavirus stress, optimism-pessimism, psychological inflexibility, and psychological health: Psychometric properties of the coronavirus stress measure. International Journal of Mental Health and Addiction. 2020;1-17. DOI: 10.1007/s11469-020-00337-6

[19] Talaee N, Varahram M, Jamaati H, Salimi A, Attarchi M, Kazempour dizaji M., et al. Stress and burnout in health care workers during Covid-19 pandemic: Validation of a questionnaire. Journal of Public Health. 2020;1-6. DOI: 10.1007/s10389-020-01313-z

[20] Voitsidis P, Gliatas I, Bairachtari V, Papadopoulou K, Papageorgiou G, Parlapani E, et al. Insomnia during the COVID-19 pandemic in a Greek population. Psychiatry Research. 2020;**289**:113076. DOI: 10.1016/j.psychres.2020.113076

[21] Qiu J, Shen B, Zhao M, Wang Z, Xie B, Xu Y. A nationwide survey of psychological distress among Chinese people in the COVID-19 epidemic: Implications and policy recommendations. General Psychiatry. 2020;**33**(2):19-21

[22] Lakhan R, Agrawal A, Sharma M. Prevalence of depression, anxiety, and stress during covid-19 pandemic. Journal of Neurosciences in Rural Practice. 2020;**11**(04):519-525. DOI: 10.1055/s-0040-1716442

[23] Belrose C, Duffaud AM, Dutheil F, Trichereau J, Trousselard M. Challenges associated with the civilian reintegration of soldiers with chronic PTSD: A new approach integrating psychological resources and values in action reappropriation. Frontiers in Psychiatry. 2018;**9**:737

[24] Xiao S, Luo D, Xiao Y. Survivors of COVID-19 are at high risk of posttraumatic stress disorder. Global Health Research and Policy. 2020;**5**:29. DOI: 10.1186/s41256-020-00155-2

[25] Janiri D, Carfì A, Kotzalidis GD, et al. Posttraumatic stress disorder in patients after severe COVID-19 infection. JAMA Psychiatry. 2021;**78**(5):567-569. DOI: 10.1001/jamapsychiatry.2021.0109

[26] Greenberg N, Weston D, Hall C, Caulfield T, Williamson V, Fong K. The mental health of staff working in intensive care during covid-19. Occup Med (Lond). 2021;**71**(2):62-67. DOI: 10.1093/occmed/kqaa220

[27] Zhang L, Pan R, Cai Y, Pan J. The prevalence of post-traumatic stress disorder in the general population during the COVID-19 pandemic: A systematic review and single-arm meta-analysis. Psychiatry Investigation. 2021;**18**(5):426-433. DOI: 10.30773/pi.2020.0458

[28] Bhat S, Chokroverty S. Sleep disorders and covid-19. Sleep Medicine. 2021. DOI: 10.1016/j.sleep.2021.07.021

[29] Cénat JM, Blais-Rochette C, Kokou-Kpolou CK. Prevalence of symptoms of depression, anxiety, insomnia, posttraumatic stress disorder, and psychological distress among populations affected by the COVID-19

pandemic: A systematic review and meta-analysis. Psychiatry Research. 2021;**295**:113599. DOI: 10.1016/j.psychres.2020.113599

[30] Kokou-Kpolou CK, Megalakaki O, Laimou D, Kousouri M. Insomnia during COVID-19 pandemic and lockdown: Prevalence, severity, and associated risk factors in French population. Psychiatry Research. 2020;**290**:113128. DOI: 10.1016/j.psychres.2020.113128

[31] Stewart NH, Koza A, Dhaon S, Shoushtari C, Martinez M, Arora VM. Sleep disturbances in frontline health care workers during the COVID-19 pandemic: Social media survey study. Journal of Medical Internet Research. 2021;**23**(5):e27331. DOI: 10.2196/27331

[32] Cabarkapa S, Nadjidai SE, Murgier J, Ng CH. The psychological impact of COVID-19 and other viral epidemics on frontline healthcare workers and ways to address it: A rapid systematic review. Brain, Behavior, & Immunity-Health. 2020;**8**:100144. DOI: 10.1016/j.bbih.2020.100144

[33] Sinha R. Chronic stress, drug use, and vulnerability to addiction. Annals of the New York Academy of Sciences. 2008;**1141**:105-130. DOI: 10.1196/annals.1441.030

[34] Rogers AH, Shepherd JM, Garey L, Zvolensky MJ. Psychological factors associated with substance use initiation during the COVID-19 pandemic. Psychiatry Research. 2020;**293**:113407. DOI: 10.1016/j.psychres.2020.113407

[35] Baker TB, Piper ME, McCarthy DE, Majeskie MR, Fiore MC. Addiction motivation reformulated: An affective processing model of negative reinforcement. Psychological Review. 2004;**111**:33-51. DOI: 10.1037/0033-295X.111.1.33

[36] Bravo M, Rubio-Stipec M, Canino GJ, Woodbury MA, Ribera JC. The psychological sequelae of disaster stress prospectively and retrospectively evaluated. American Journal of Community Psychology. 1990;**18**:661-680. DOI: 10.1007/BF00931236

[37] David D, Mellman TA, Mendoza LM, Kulick-Bell R, Ironson G, Schneiderman N. Psychiatric morbidity following Hurricane Andrew. Journal of Traumatic Stress. 1996;**9**:607-612. DOI: 10.1007/BF02103669

[38] Schaller M, Park JH. The behavioral immune system (and why it matters). Current Directions in Psychological Science. 2011;**20**:99-103. DOI: 10.1177/0963721411402596

[39] Wang C, Pan R, Wan X, Tan Y, Xu L, Ho CS. Immediate psychological responses and associated factors during the initial stage of the 2019 Coronavirus disease (COVID-19) epidemic among the general population in China. International Journal of Environmental Research and Public Health. 2020;**17**:1729

[40] McKay D, Yang H, Elhai J, Asmundson G. Anxiety regarding contracting COVID-19 related to interoceptive anxiety sensations: The moderating role of disgust propensity and sensitivity. Journal of Anxiety Disorders. 2020;**72**:102233. DOI:10.1016/j.janxdis.2020.102233

[41] Novak A, Burgess ES, Clark M, Zvolensky MJ, Brown RA. Anxiety sensitivity, self-reported motives for alcohol and nicotine use, and level of consumption. Journal of Anxiety Disorders. 2003;**17**:165-180

[42] Bonn-Miller MO, Zvolensky MJ, Bernstein A. Marijuana use motives: Concurrent relations to frequency of past 30-day use and anxiety sensitivity among young adult marijuana smokers. Addictive Behaviors. 2007;**32**:49-62

[43] Panchal N, Kamal R, Cox C, Garfield R. The implications of Covid-19

for mental health and substance use. KFF. 2021. Available from: https://www.kff.org/coronavirus-covid-19/issue-brief/the-implications-of-covid-19-for-mental-health-and-substance-use/

[44] Varma P, Junge M, Meaklim H, Jackson ML. Younger people are more vulnerable to stress, anxiety and depression during COVID-19 pandemic: A global cross-sectional survey. Progress in Neuro-Psychopharmacology & Biological Psychiatry. 2021;**109**:110236. DOI: 10.1016/j.pnpbp.2020.110236

[45] Vahratian A, Blumberg SJ, Terlizzi EP, Schiller JS. Symptoms of anxiety or depressive disorder and use of mental health care among adults during the COVID-19 pandemic. Morbidity and Mortality Weekly Report. 2021;**70**:490-494. DOI: 10.15585/mmwr.mm7013e2

[46] Stephenson J. Cdc study finds worsening anxiety and depression, especially in young adults, during covid-19 pandemic. JAMA Health Forum. 2021;**2**(4). DOI: 10.1001/jamahealthforum.2021.0724

[47] Reger MA, Stanley IH, Joiner TE. Suicide mortality and coronavirus disease 2019—A perfect storm? JAMA Psychiatry. 2020;**77**(11):1093-1094. DOI: 10.1001/jamapsychiatry.2020.1060

[48] O'Connor R, Wetherall K, Cleare S, McClelland H, Melson A, Niedzwiedz C, et al. Mental health and well-being during the COVID-19 pandemic: Longitudinal analyses of adults in the UK COVID-19 mental health & wellbeing study. The British Journal of Psychiatry. 2021;**218**(6):326-333. DOI: 10.1192/bjp.2020.212

[49] Fortgang RG, Wang SB, Millner AJ, Reid-Russell A, Beukenhorst AL, Kleiman EM, et al. Increase in suicidal thinking during covid-19. Clinical Psychological Science. 2021;**9**(3):482-488. DOI: 10.1177/2167702621993857

[50] Ayuso-Mateos J, Morillo D, Haro J, Olaya B, Lara E, Miret M. Changes in depression and suicidal ideation under severe lockdown restrictions during the first wave of the COVID-19 pandemic in Spain: A longitudinal study in the general population. Epidemiology and Psychiatric Sciences. 2021;**30**:E49. DOI: 10.1017/S2045796021000408

[51] Iapoce C. Covid-19 pandemic did not lead to significant suicide risk increase. HCPLive. 2021. Available from: https://www.hcplive.com/view/covid-19-pandemic-did-not-lead-significant-suicide-risk-increase

[52] Franklin JC, Ribeiro JD, Fox KR, Bentley KH, Kleiman EM, Huang, et al. Risk factors for suicidal thoughts and behaviors: A meta-analysis of 50 years of research. Psychological Bulletin. 2017;**143**(2):187-232. DOI: 10.1037/bul0000084

[53] Oyesanya M, Lopez-Morinigo J, Dutta R. Systematic review of suicide in economic recession. World Journal of Psychiatry. 2015;**5**(2):243-254. DOI: 10.5498/wjp.v5.i2.243

[54] Van Orden KA, Witte TK, Cukrowicz KC, Braithwaite SR, Selby EA, Joiner TE Jr. The interpersonal theory of suicide. Psychological Review. 2010;**117**(2):575-600. DOI: 10.1037/a0018697

[55] Melimopoulos E. How the COVID-19 pandemic is affecting mental health. 2021. Available from: https://www.aljazeera.com/news/2021/3/22/hold-coronavirus-and-mental-health

[56] Bayazit H, Ozel M, Arac S, Dulgeroglu-Bayazit D, Joshi A. Posttraumatic stress disorder among healthcare workers during COVID-19 era. APA Annual Meeting; May 1-3, 2021. Abstract/Poster 5224. 2021

[57] Yard E, Radhakrishnan L, Ballesteros MF, et al. Emergency department visits for suspected suicide attempts among persons aged 12-25 years before and during the COVID-19 pandemic. Morbidity and Mortality Weekly Report. 2021;**70**:888-894. DOI: 10.15585/mmwr.mm7024e1

[58] Liu Y-L. Is covid-19 changing our relationships? BBC Future. 2020. Available from: https://www.bbc.com/future/article/20200601-how-is-covid-19-is-affecting-relationships

[59] Henderson E. Research reveals the impact of COVID-19 pandemic on Families' well-being and functioning. 2021. Available from: https://www.news-medical.net/news/20210412/Research-reveals-the-impact-of-COVIDe2809019-pandemic-on-families-well-being-and-functioning.aspx

[60] Feinberg ME, Mogle JA, Lee JK, Tornello SL, Hostetler ML, Cifelli JA, et al. Impact of the COVID-19 pandemic on parent, child, and family functioning. Family Process. 2021. DOI: 10.1111/famp.12649

[61] Elahi T. The Impact of Homeschooling During Covid-19. Human Rights Pulse. 2021. Avaialable from: https://www.humanrightspulse.com/mastercontentblog/the-impact-of-homeschooling-during-covid-19

[62] Adverse consequences of school closures. UNESCO. 2020. Available from: https://en.unesco.org/covid19/educationresponse/consequences

[63] Lee SJ, Ward KP, Chang OD, Downing KM. Parenting activities and the transition to home-based education during the COVID-19 pandemic. Children and Youth Services Review. 2021;**122**:105585. DOI: 10.1016/j.childyouth.2020.105585

[64] Office for National Statistics. Coronavirus and homeschooling in Great Britain: April to June 2020. Coronavirus and homeschooling in Great Britain - Office for National Statistics. 2020. Available from: https://www.ons.gov.uk/peoplepopulationandcommunity/educationandchildcare/articles/coronavirusandhomeschoolingingreatbritain/apriltojune2020

[65] American Psychological Association. Stress in America™ 2020: Stress in the time OF COVID-19, volume one. American Psychological Association; 2020. Available from: https://www.apa.org/news/press/releases/stress/2020/report

[66] Mohesky V. FACT check: Covid-19 could be the worst economic crisis since the Great Depression. Columbia Missourian. 2020. Available from: https://www.columbiamissourian.com/news/politifact_missouri/fact-check-covid-19-could-be-the-worst-economic-crisis-since-the-great-depression/article_fb2640d2-3be3-11eb-ae53-5b24bac04ba5.html

[67] Khalil A, Mayer S, Shah R. Impact of the COVID-19 Crisis on Family Dynamics in Economically Vulnerable Households. Becker Friedman Institute working paper no. 2020-143. 2020. Available from: https://bfi.uchicago.edu/wp-content/uploads/2020/10/BFI_WP_2020143.pdf

[68] Pak A, Adegboye OA, Adekunle AI, Rahman KM, McBryde ES, Eisen DP. Economic consequences of the covid-19 outbreak: The need for epidemic preparedness. Frontiers in Public Health. 2020;**8**. DOI: 10.3389/fpubh.2020.00241

[69] Wallin B. How the death of business travel will change your next vacation. Travel. 2021. Available from: https://www.nationalgeographic.com/travel/

article/is-business-travel-a-thing-of-the-past

[70] International Labour Organization. Socio Economic Impact of COVID-19 towards People Living with HIV and Key Population. 2021. Available from: https://www.ilo.org/wcmsp5/groups/public/---asia/---ro-bangkok/---ilo-jakarta/documents/publication/wcms_794829.pdf

[71] International Labour Organization. World Employment and Social Outlook. 2021. Available from: https://www.ilo.org/wcmsp5/groups/public/---dgreports/---dcomm/documents/publication/wcms_794452.pdf

[72] World Health Organization. Impact of covid-19 on people's livelihoods, their health and our food systems. 2021. Available from: https://www.who.int/news/item/13-10-2020-impact-of-covid-19-on-people%27s-livelihoods-their-health-and-our-food-systems

[73] Whitehead M, Taylor-Robinson D, Barr B. Poverty, health, and covid-19. BMJ. 2021;**372**:n376. DOI: 10.1136/bmj.n376

[74] Hefferon C, Taylor C, Bennett D, Falconer C, Campbell M, Williams JG, et al. Priorities for the Child public health response to the COVID-19 Pandemic recovery in England. Archives of Disease in Childhood. 2020;**106**(6):533-538. DOI: 10.1136/archdischild-2020-320214

[75] Brewer M, Patrick R. Pandemic Pressures: Why families on a low income are spending more during Covid-19. Resolution Foundation. 2021. Available from: https://www.resolutionfoundation.org/publications/pandemic-pressures/

[76] Nordt C, Warnke I, Seifritz E, Kawohl W. Modelling suicide and unemployment: A longitudinal analysis covering 63 countries, 2000-11. The Lancet Psychiatry. 2015;**2**(3):239-245. DOI: 10.1016/s2215-0366(14)00118-7

[77] Chang SS, Gunnell D, Sterne JA, et al. Was the economic crisis 1997-1998 responsible for rising suicide rates in East/Southeast Asia? A time-trend analysis for Japan, Hong Kong, South Korea, Taiwan, Singapore and Thailand. Social Science & Medicine. 2009;**68**:1322-1331

[78] McIntyre RS, Lee Y. Projected increases in suicide in Canada as a consequence of COVID-19. Psychiatry Research. 2020;**290**:113104

[79] McIntyre RS, Lee Y. Preventing suicide in the context of the COVID-19 pandemic. World Psychiatry. 2020;**19**:250-251

[80] Stevens LM, Rockey JC, Rockowitz SR, Kanja W, Colloff MF, Flowe HD. Children's vulnerability to sexual violence During COVID-19 in Kenya: Recommendations for the future. Frontiers in Global Women's Health. 2021;**2**. DOI: 10.3389/fgwh.2021.630901

[81] World Health Organization. Global and regional estimates of violence against women: Prevalence and health effects of intimate partner violence and non-partner sexual violence. 2013. Available from: https://apps.who.int/iris/bitstream/handle/10665/85239/9789241564625_eng.pdf

[82] Cetin S. COVID-19 outbreak triggers violence against women. Anadolu Ajansı. 2020. Available from: https://www.aa.com.tr/en/latest-on-coronavirus-outbreak/covid-19-outbreak-triggers-violence-against-women/2055833

[83] Harville EW, Taylor CA, Tesfai H, Xiong X, Buekens P. Experience of Hurricane Katrina and reported intimate partner violence. Journal of Interpersonal Violence. 2011;**26**(4):833-845. DOI: 10.1177/0886260510365861

[84] Schumacher JA, Coffey SF, Norris FH, Tracy M, Clements K, Galea S. Intimate partner violence and

Hurricane Katrina: Predictors and associated mental health outcomes. Violence and Victims. 2010;**25**(5):588-603. DOI: 10.1891/0886-6708.25.5.588

[85] Rezaeian M. The association between natural disasters and violence: A systematic review of the literature and a call for more epidemiological studies. Journal of Research in Medical Sciences : The Official Journal of Isfahan University of Medical Sciences. 2013;**18**(12):1103-1107

[86] Johnson K, Asher J, Rosborough S, et al. Association of combatant status and sexual violence with health and mental health outcomes in post-conflict Liberia. Journal of the American Medical Association. 2008;**300**(6): 676-690

[87] Benson M, Fox G, DeMaris A, Van Wyk J. Neighbourhood disadvantage, individual economic distress and violence against women in intimate relationships. Journal of Quantitative Criminology. 2003;**18**:207-325

[88] Trevillion K, Oram S, Feder G, Howard L. Experiences of domestic violence and mental disorders: A systematic review and meta-analysis. PLoS One. 2012;**7**:e51740

[89] Boden J, Fergusson D, Horwood L. Alcohol misuse and violence behaviour: Findings from a 30-year longitudinal study. Drug and Alcohol Dependence. 2012;**122**:135-141

[90] United Nations. UNDP brief: Gender based violence and COVID19. 2020. Available from: https://www.undp.org/sites/g/files/zskgke326/files/publications/undp-gender-GBV_and_COVID-19_0.pdf

[91] Bradley NL, DiPasquale AM, Dillabough K, Schneider PS. Health care practitioners' responsibility to ADDRESS intimate partner violence related to the COVID-19 pandemic. Canadian Medical Association Journal. 2020;**192**(22). DOI: 10.1503/cmaj.200634

[92] Moreira DN, Pinto da Costa M. The impact of the Covid-19 pandemic in the precipitation of intimate partner violence. International Journal of Law and Psychiatry. 2020;**71**:101606. DOI: 10.1016/j.ijlp.2020.101606

[93] World Health Organization. Eastern Mediterranean region. 2021. Available from: http://www.emro.who.int/violence-injuries-disabilities/violence-news/levels-of-domestic-violence-increase-as-covid-19-pandemic-escalates.html

[94] Bradbury-Jones C, Isham L. The pandemic paradox: The consequences of COVID-19 on domestic violence. Journal of Clinical Nursing. 2020;**29**(13-14): 2047-2049. DOI: 10.1111/jocn.15296

[95] Usher K, Bhullar N, Durkin J, Gyamfi N, Jackson D. Family violence and COVID-19: Increased vulnerability and reduced options for support. International Journal of Mental Health Nursing. 2020;**29**(4):549-552. DOI: 10.1111/inm.12735

[96] van Gelder N, Peterman A, Potts A, O'Donnell M, Thompson K, Shah N, et al. COVID-19: Reducing the risk of infection might increase the risk of intimate partner violence. E Clinical Medicine. 2020;**21**:100348. DOI: 10.1016/j.eclinm.2020.100348

[97] Gama A, Pedro AR, de Carvalho MJL, Guerreiro AE, Duarte V, Quintas J, et al. Domestic violence during the Covid-19 pandemic in Portugal. Portuguese Journal of Public Health. 2020;**38**(suppl 1):32-40. DOI: 10.1159/000514341

[98] Amatriain-Fernández S, Murillo-Rodríguez ES, Gronwald T, Machado S, Budde H. Benefits of physical activity and physical exercise in

the time of pandemic. Psychological Trauma: Theory, Research, Practice, and Policy. 2020;**12**(S1):264-266

[99] Domonell K, Burn D. Why endorphins (and exercise) make you happy. CNN. 2016. Available from: https://edition.cnn.com/2016/01/13/health/endorphins-exercise-cause-happiness/index.html

[100] Anderson NB. Levels of analysis in health science: A framework for integrating sociobehavioral and biomedical research. Annals of the New York. 1998;**840**:563-576. DOI: 10.1111/j.1749-6632.1998.tb09595.x

[101] Choi J, Fauce SR, Effros RB. Reduced telomerase activity in human T lymphocytes exposed to cortisol. Brain, Behavior, and Immunity. 2008;**22**(4):600-605. DOI: 10.1016/j.bbi.2007.12.004

[102] Shaver JL, Johnston SK, Lentz MJ, Landis CA. Stress exposure, psychological distress, and physiological stress activation in midlife women with insomnia. Psychosomatic Medicine. 2002;**64**(5):793-802. DOI: 10.1097/01.psy.0000024235.11538.9a

[103] Ardayfio P, Kim KS. Anxiogenic-like effect of chronic corticosterone in the light-dark emergence task in mice. Behavioral Neuroscience. 2006;**120**(2):249-256. DOI: 10.1037/0735-7044.120.2.249

[104] Mousavizadeh L, Ghasemi S. Genotype and phenotype of COVID-19: Their roles in pathogenesis. Journal of Microbiology, Immunology and Infection. 2021;**54**(2):159-163. DOI: 10.1016/j. jmii.2020.03.022

[105] da Silveira MP, da Silva Fagundes KK, Bizuti MR, Starck É, Rossi RC, de Resende e Silva, D. T. Physical exercise as a tool to help the immune system against COVID-19: An integrative review of the current literature. Clinical and Experimental Medicine. 2021;**21**(1):15-28. DOI: 10.1007/s10238-020-00650-3

[106] Scheffer, D. da L., Latini, A. Exercise-induced immune system response: Anti-inflammatory status on peripheral and central organs. Biochimica et Biophysica Acta - Molecular Basis of Disease. 2020;**1866**(10):1-15. DOI: 10.1016/j.bbadis.2020.165823

[107] Furtado GE, Letieri RV, Caldo-Silva A, Sardão VA, Teixeira AM, de Barros MP, et al. Sustaining efficient immune functions with regular physical exercise in the COVID-19 era and beyond. European Journal of Clinical Investigation. 2021;**51**(5). DOI: 10.1111/eci.13485

[108] Mohamed AA, Alawna M. Role of increasing the aerobic capacity on improving the function of immune and respiratory systems in patients with coronavirus (COVID-19): A review. Diabetes and Metabolic Syndrome: Clinical Research and Reviews. 2020;**14**(4):489-496

[109] Huang C, Wang Y, Li X, Ren L, Zhao J, Hu Y, et al. Clinical features of patients infected with 2019 novel coronavirus in Wuhan, China. The Lancet. 2020;**395**(10223):497-506. DOI: 10.1016/S0140-6736(20)30183-5

[110] Hendriks T. The effects of Sahaja Yoga meditation on Mental Health: A Systematic Review. Journal of Complementary and Integrative Medicine. 2018;**15**(3). DOI: 10.1515/jcim-2016-0163

[111] Nair PMK, Joseph B, Nanda A. Effects of naturopathy and yoga intervention on CD4 count of the individuals receiving antiretroviral therapy-report from a human immunodeficiency virus sanatorium, Pune. International Journal of Yoga. 2015;**8**(2):122. DOI: 10.4103/0973-6131.158475

[112] Nagarathna R, Anand A, Rain M, Srivastava V, Sivapuram MS, Kulkarni R, et al. Yoga practice is beneficial for maintaining healthy lifestyle and endurance under restrictions and stress imposed by lockdown during COVID-19 pandemic. Frontiers in Psychiatry. 2021;**12**. DOI: 10.3389/fpsyt.2021.613762

[113] Garfin DR, Silver RC, Holman EA. The novel coronavirus (COVID-2019) outbreak: Amplification of public health consequences by media exposure. Health Psychology. 2020;**39**(5):355-357. DOI: 10.1037/hea0000875

[114] Fiorillo A, Gorwood P. The consequences of the COVID-19 pandemic on mental health and implications for clinical practice. European Psychiatry. 2020;**63**(1):E32. DOI: 10.1192/j.eurpsy.2020.35

[115] Luo Y, He X, Wang S, Li J, Zhang Y. Media exposure predicts acute stress and probable acute stress disorder during the early COVID-19 outbreak in China. PeerJ. 2021;**9**:e11407. DOI: 10.7717/peerj.11407

[116] First J, Shin H, Ranjit YS, Houston JB. COVID-19 stress and depression: Examining social media. Traditional Media, and Interpersonal Communication, Journal of Loss and Trauma. 2021;**26**(2):101-115. DOI: 10.1080/15325024.2020.1835386

[117] Romer D, Jamieson KH. Conspiracy theories as barriers to controlling the spread of COVID-19 in the U.S. Social Science & Medicine. 2020;**263**:113356. DOI: 10.1016/j.socscimed.2020.113356

[118] Looi JC, Allison S, Bastiampillai T, Maguire PA. Clinical update on managing media exposure and misinformation during COVID-19: Recommendations for governments and healthcare professionals. Australasian Psychiatry. 2021;**29**(1):22-25. DOI: 10.1177/1039856220963947

[119] Ni MY, Yang L, Leung C, Li N, Yao XI, Wang Y, et al. Mental health, risk factors, and social media use during the COVID-19 epidemic and cordon sanitaire among the community and health professionals in Wuhan, China: Cross-sectional survey. JMIR Mental Health. 2020;**7**(5):e19009. DOI: 10.2196/19009

[120] Sheek-Hussein M, Abu-Zidan FM, Stip E. Disaster management of the psychological impact of the COVID-19 pandemic. International Journal of Emergency Medicine. 2021;**14**:19. DOI: 10.1186/s12245-021-00342-z

[121] Geoffroy PA, Bénard V, Amad A, Royant-Parola S, Poirot I, Guichard K, et al. Advices from sleep experts to sleep well and keep regular rhythms for adults and children in this period of COVID-19 containment. Médecine Du Sommeil. 2020;**17**(2):113-117. DOI: 10.1016/j.msom.2020.04.002

[122] Kumari A, Singh P. Impact of counseling on psychological health during lockdown of Covid-19. Journal of Statistics and Management Systems. 2021;**24**(1):53-65. DOI: 10.1080/09720510.2020.1833448

[123] Feijt M, de Kort Y, Bongers I, Bierbooms J, Westerink J, Ijsselsteijn W. Mental health care goes online: Practitioners' experiences of providing mental health care during the COVID-19 pandemic. Cyberpsychology, Behavior and Social Networking. 2020;**23**(8):860-864. DOI: 10.1089/cyber.2020.0370

[124] Riva G, Wiederhold BK. How cyberpsychology and virtual reality can help us to overcome the psychological burden of coronavirus. Cyberpsychology, Behavior and Social Networking. 2020;**23**(5):277-279. DOI: 10.1089/cyber.2020.29183.gri

[125] Zhou X, Snoswell CL, Harding LE, Bambling M, Edirippulige S, Bai X, et al. The role of telehealth in reducing the mental health burden from COVID-19. Telemedicine and e-Health. 2020;**26**(4): 377-379. DOI: 10.1089/tmj.2020.0068

[126] Weiner L, Berna F, Nourry N, Severac F, Vidailhet P, Mengin AC. Efficacy of an online cognitive behavioral therapy program developed for healthcare workers during the Covid-19 pandemic: The reduction of STress (REST) study protocol for a randomized controlled trial. Trials. 2020;**21**(1). DOI: 10.1186/s13063-020-04772-7

[127] Cherry K. How cognitive behavior therapy works. Very well Mind. 2021. Retrieved December 17, 2021. Available from: https://www.verywellmind.com/what-is-cognitive-behavior-therapy-2795747

[128] Mahoney A, Li I, Haskelberg H, Millard M, Newby JM. The uptake and effectiveness of online cognitive behaviour therapy for symptoms of anxiety and depression during COVID-19. Journal of Affective Disorders. 2021;**292**:197-203. DOI: 10.1016/j.jad.2021.05.116

[129] Liu Z, Qiao D, Xu Y, Zhao W, Yang Y, Wen D, et al. The efficacy of Computerized cognitive behavioral therapy for depressive and anxiety symptoms in patients with COVID-19: Randomized controlled trial. Journal of Medical Internet Research. 2021;**23**(5). DOI: 10.2196/26883

[130] Barker GG, Barker EE. Online therapy: Lessons learned from the covid-19 health crisis. British Journal of Guidance & Counselling. 2021:1-16. DOI: 10.1080/03069885.2021.1889462

[131] Sukel K. In sync: How humans are hard-wired for social relationships. Dana Foundation. 2019. Available from: https://dana.org/article/in-sync-how-humans-are-hard-wired-for-social-relationships/

[132] Matys M. The importance of staying socially connected during the COVID-19 pandemic. Your Health Matters. 2020. Available from: https://health.sunnybrook.ca/covid-19-coronavirus/social-connections-covid-19-pandemic/

[133] Nitschke JP, Forbes PAG, Ali N, Cutler J, Apps MAJ, Lockwood PL, et al. Resilience during uncertainty? Greater social connectedness during COVID-19 lockdown is associated with reduced distress and fatigue. British Journal of Health Psychology. 2021;**26**:553-569. DOI: 10.1111/bjhp.12485

[134] American Psychological Association. Social isolation, loneliness could be greater threat to public health than obesity. ScienceDaily. 2017. Available from: www.sciencedaily.com/releases/2017/08/170805165319.htm

[135] Tate N. Loneliness rivals obesity, smoking as health risk. WebMD. 2018. Available from: https://www.webmd.com/balance/news/20180504/loneliness-rivals-obesity-smoking-as-health-risk

[136] Marchant J. How Happiness Boosts the Immune System. Scientific American. 2013. Available from: https://www.scientificamerican.com/article/how-happiness-boosts-the-immune-system/

[137] Pappas S. Loneliness is Bad for Your Health, Study Suggests. Live Science. 2013. Available from: https://www.livescience.com/26431-loneliness-harms-health-immune-system.html

[138] Napoleon C. Gary mayor, ministers preach creative church services with assist from technology during Coronavirus outbreak.

Chicago Tribune. 2020. Available from: https://www.chicagotribune.com/suburbs/post-tribune/ct-ptb-gary-churches-order-st-0326-20200325-rkvkzcndczdddddrtf5rxxmq7e-story.html

[139] Criddle C. Coronavirus: How to host a Christmas party on zoom. BBC News. 2020. Available from: https://www.bbc.com/news/technology-54894806

[140] Kluck JP, Stoyanova F, Krämer NC. Putting the social back into physical distancing: The role of digital connections in a pandemic crisis. International Journal of Psychology. 2021;**56**:594-606. DOI: 10.1002/ijop.12746

[141] Kovacs B, Caplan N, Grob S, King M. Social networks and loneliness during the COVID-19 pandemic. Socius. 2021;7:1-16. DOI: 10.1177/2378023120985254

[142] Roberts SGB, Dunbar RIM. Communication in social networks: Effects of kinship, network size, and emotional closeness. Personal Relationships. 2011;**18**:439-452. DOI: 10.1111/j.1475-6811.2010.01310.x

Chapter 5

# Perspective Chapter: Perspectives on the Emergency Remote Assessment during the COVID-19 Pandemic

*Mariana Cernicova-Buca*

## Abstract

The unprecedented health crisis triggered by the COVID-19 pandemic put on hold traditional educational practices. Emergency remote teaching was adopted as a response, with various degrees of success and satisfaction around the globe. This perspective chapter focuses on the remote emergency assessment as a measure to ensure the completion of the educational cycle for students caught in the 2020 crisis, after debates around the relevance and soundness of such activities both for students, and for society at large. Some voices enthusiastically champion the technological innovation and point to the benefits brought by the computer-assisted assessment, while others warn against the 'one-size-fit-all' approach and insist that the emergency measures need a careful examination and, although lessons can be taken away from the situation, the traditional patterns should be kept in place.

**Keywords:** assessment, emergency remote assessment, online, sustainability, COVID-19, student, change in education, higher education

## 1. Introduction

In the modern world, universities are living communities, immersed in the socio-economic and political environment of their residence, sharing the ideas, concerns, and major objectives of society at large. As Ernest Boyer [1] so adequately defined it, the university community, comprised of professors, students, administrative and support staff, is educationally purposeful, open, just, disciplined, caring and celebrative. The university community is *educationally purposeful*, in the sense that the community members work together to strengthen teaching and learning; it is *open* because freedom of expression is protected and affirmed; it strives to be *just*, in the sense that it believes in the sacredness of the person and champions diversity; it is a *disciplined* community, with individuals accepting their responsibilities and working towards the common good; the community is *caring*, in the sense that the well-being of each member is supported and service to others is encouraged; finally, it is a *celebrative* community, traditionally re-enacting rituals of passage that transform learners into professionals.

Universities face the same opportunities and threats as all the other types of communities and need to project plans ensuring their resilience during and after unexpected disruptions. They are not immune to natural or man-made disasters, the numerous examples in the 21st century – to limit the discussion only to these – offering ample food for thought. Hurricane Katrina in Louisiana (USA) in 2005, shooting on campus at Virginia Tech in 2007, earthquakes in Taiwan, 2019, extreme weather events in Australia, led to the adoption of guidebooks, emergency plans and training packages preparing the higher education system to manage the crisis and ensure the transition to the "business-as-usual" model. Region by region and country by country universities adopted the types of measures and documents suiting the specifics of their situation. Australian universities, for instance, constantly renew their internal regulations according to the nationally developed Emergency Planning Handbook [2], which emphasizes extreme weather events (2020). American universities base their crisis and emergency plans on the Department of Education's Guide of 2013 [3], preparing both for natural, and man-made disasters. Taiwan incorporated disaster literacy in school programs, to facilitate disaster prevention and recovery from the frequent earthquakes in the region. Resilience plan for earthquakes and tsunamis are also adopted in Japan, Indonesia, India, etc. [4]. Inland countries, such as Romania, are less exposed to extreme weather events. Apart from drills related to firefighting or earthquakes, no significant preparation was made in Romania, for example, to face potential threats posed to education since the most major crises in the past century did not affect this sector to the extent of disruption. Higher education institutions, therefore, treated crisis-related topics lightly. Emergency topics remain relevant on the global scale, with UNESCO, as the United Nations lead for education, unfolding ample processes to ensure crisis preparedness and the response of countries and regions facing armed conflict, refugee crisis, natural hazards, and other types of risks [5].

Despite the theoretical, practical and actional preparedness, reflected in the above-mentioned guidelines, handbooks, policy recommendations referring to disasters (natural, man-made or otherwise), crisis, emergencies, or other significant events, the magnitude and depth of the global health crisis triggered by the COVID-19 pandemic took the educational system by surprise. On March 11, 2020, the World Health Organization publicly declared COVID-19 a pandemic [6]. Social distancing, face masks wearing in public places and stay-at-home measures were recommended, to "flatten the curve" and slow the spread of COVID-19. Reportedly, the pandemic affected 94% of the world's student population, educational institutions struggling to diminish the impact of the crisis [7]. Buildings were untouched, the population was not displaced, but traditional educational face-to-face interactions were put on hold for an indefinite period. The solution resided in adopting emergency remote formats. The continuation of educational processes could not prevent regression in the recruitment and retention rates of students, many of the dropouts not having the intention to return to school even after "business as usual" is resumed. Hence, the importance of reflecting upon education during and in the aftermath of the crisis.

## 2. Emergency remote education

Emergency remote education (ERE) is not an innovation brought by searching for responses to the COVID-19 crisis. It received special attention with the creation of the Inter-agency Network for Education in Emergencies (INEE) [8], during a strategy session on Education in Emergencies held at the 2000 World Education Forum in Dakar. Since its' creation, INEE developed the concept of education in emergencies, understood as "quality learning opportunities for all ages (...). Education in emergencies provides physical, psychosocial, and cognitive protection that can sustain and save lives. Common situations of crisis in which education in emergencies is essential include conflicts, situations of violence, forced displacement, disasters, and public health emergencies". INEE develops standards, training packages and even publishes a *Journal on Education in Emergencies* (since 2015) which deals with academic research, but also with field notes addressing topics relating to emergency education response in natural disasters, conflict/fragile states and complex emergencies, resilience, transitions from emergency to recovery/post-conflict to development, forced migration and education, etc. The fact that emergency remote education does not automatically mean switching in-person education to online learning deserves emphasis, despite many researchers considering the technological intervention as automatic and online learning as the hallmark option in times of crisis [7, 9, 10]. In low-tech environments, emergency remote education can resort to low-tech solutions, but with higher education institutions, the focus of this chapter, technological affordances are presupposed as being present in the form of computers, telephones, some sort of digital devices, accompanied by ICT skills, shared by academia and students.

Higher education systems relied, at the peak of the COVID-19 crisis, on the pedagogical acquisitions of online learning experiences, even though for many stakeholders in the educational process online learning, e-learning or distance education represented entirely different cohorts from the in-campus education. One of the most referred to articles in the current literature on the educational response to the COVID-19 crisis is Charles Hodge's *The Difference Between Emergency Remote Teaching and Online Learning* [11]. Apart from the insights into the specificity of emergency remote education and its numerous challenges, Hodges rightfully highlights the fact that the learning outcomes should be carefully assessed, the pre-crisis models being almost impossible to apply. In his words, "a common misconception is that comparing a face-to-face course with an online version of the course constitutes a useful evaluation" [11]. Hodges's list of open questions to evaluating the outcomes of the emergency remote education is quite impressive, starting with normative and administrative aspects, going through technological affordances, and culminating in the shared, informed consensus between educational stakeholders on the way in which evaluation is to be performed and incorporated in the institutional memory and practice, in the aftermath of the crisis. At this point, the emergency remote assessment becomes a crucial concept [12, 13], especially because first-response studies on education during the COVID-19 crisis showed that "assessment was deprioritized in initial planning" and that "teachers saw assessment expectations as unstable or unfair during a crisis" [14]. Scenarios concerning the postponement or even cancelation of final assessment were under debate and the greatest fear was that society might be reluctant in accepting the results of assessment activities (especially for graduation exams) carried out during the unfamiliar global crisis triggered by the COVID-19 pandemic [15].

### 2.1 Assessment and emergency remote assessment

Assessment is a crucial element of the educational process, representing the segment during which professors evaluate, measure, and document the academic readiness, learning progress, skill acquisition, or educational needs of students after a teaching-learning sequence. It is often considered as a pivotal element for modernizing education systems, affecting how teaching and learning take place, but also as a tool for certification, enabling potential employers to understand the academic achievements of an individual [16]. Educational literature emphasizes the need to incorporate assessment provisions in the curriculum design and to ensure coherence and synergy between curriculum, pedagogy and learning outcomes [17]. In UNESCO's Education strategy 2014–2021 assessment is treated as an important part of action towards "more just, inclusive, and equitable learning societies" [18]. However, the crisis of 2020–2021 brought new meanings to the assessment-related concerns.

The traditional pen-and-pencil exam was replaced by new tools, and frenzic searches for reliable and acceptable forms of assessment were enacted. Studies from the field show mixed reactions: to some practitioners, COVID-19 was the modernizing driver, that accelerated the incorporation of technological tools and facilitated the qualitative leap forward [19]. Others looked more at the "dark side" of technologically mediated assessment activities, which leave ample room for cheating and academic dishonesty on the part of the students [20]. A third path, however, is more fruitful in terms of enhancing the reliability and acceptability of assessment activities: the path opened by David Boud in his conceptualization of *sustainable assessment*, launched in 2000 and constantly developed with new resources available for in higher education, presented on the website—www.assessmentfutures.com [21].

Due to social isolation measures and the remote delivery of educational content, assessment activities were organized also in a remote fashion. Emergency remote assessment could not take place without the mediation of technology. Therefore, depending on the taught subject-matter, on the technological affordances, the teacher's own capacity to innovate, students' consent to the proposed activity, the emergency remote assessment took the form of:

- self-assessment [22, 23]
- peer-assessment [22]
- take-home exams [24]
- portfolios [23, 25]
- e-assessment activities (exams), human-led or computer-based [26].

All the above have been already carefully documented by Boud and Soler [21] as paths towards sustainable assessment implementation, but the disruption caused by the pandemic accelerated these possibilities as viable alternatives to the traditional assessment activities and enrich the community of practice with new case studies, reflections, and recommendations regarding the modernization of assessment. The calls to experiment and change in assessment practices, long claimed for [21, 27] could not be ignored.

Evidence from the abundant literature on teaching amid the COVID-19 crisis points to the fact that teachers felt overwhelmed by the added responsibilities to the workload assumed before the outbreak of the pandemic, while students felt anxiety, anger, detachment, and a loss of purpose in their educational path. Universities succeeded at uneven rates to provide normative and instructional support mechanisms to ease the shift from in-campus education to emergency remote teaching and learning [11]. The whole higher education ecosystem was challenged, and the psychological factors had to be considered alongside pedagogical solutions, technical affordances and the commitment of teachers and students to keep educational processes functional.

The pandemic situation forced a change in the environment for assessment activities. Instead of face-to-face exams (be those pen-and-pencil, oral, or computer-assisted, but with the physical presence of instructors in the exam room), a virtual environment had to be created, affecting the very medium of the exam conditions. It was *terra incognita* for both participants in the exam, professors, and students alike. Some of the elements in this new setting did not allow for familiar mechanisms of control. So, professors tried to cope with the novelty by negotiating new rules of engagement with the students, adapting assessment techniques and types to the situation.

Overwhelmed by the amount of data and the task of offering rapid feedback to students, some professors experimented with diversifying the *identity of the assessor.* Self-assessment and peer-assessment were introduced to students in a more vigorous fashion, to deal with the task of mastering the assessment flow. While this is a fruitful solution, if applied correctly, it cannot spread over all types of exams. Students can estimate their success in exams, by having access to the grading system, with details regarding the measured skills and/or knowledge in a given exam, but for graduation exams, for instance, the process is entrusted to an examination committee.

Another element of the assessment that professors may have control over is the timing of the examination interaction. Many examples of the published case studies indicate that the dominant choice was a *synchronous examination*, with instructors doing their best to replicate the familiar exam atmosphere, while ensuring that they share the same medium with students. Access to technology, a fairly good Internet connection and the skill to ensure the flow of the assessment are preconditions for success. An ample debate in pedagogical literature goes towards the manner of organizing the technology-assisted assessment, with a focus on the technological affordances and tools, but also with an eye to the security, fairness, and accuracy of the process. To diminish the concerns about academic ethics a variety of solutions was proposed, among which open book exams seem by far the most interesting, and with the highest degree of implications. Open book exams may revolutionize the assessment type, since students no longer need to rely on memory, but focus, instead, on demonstrating the ability to creatively apply the knowledge to the task at hand. They have to prove concept understanding and skill acquisition, instead of a good memorizing capacity, but challenges to this type of exam are numerous. Students may only reproduce what they find in the resources, without memorizing even the basic information compulsory as guidance towards their future profession. Professors need to be trained in designing and assessing open-book exams and by far these are not simple tasks.

The type of work submitted for assessment is of consequence to the way the activity is organized. Faced with the necessity to ensure access to education and non-discriminatory conditions for students with limited access to technology and/or the Internet, professors embraced to a larger extent *asynchronous exam*, in the form of take-home exams or portfolio-based assessment. These are not merely terminological choices but shifts in the assessment type. Take-home exams are typically unsupervised and open book. Logistically they are simple to organize, the instructor sending the task to students via any medium at hand (e-mail, discussion group, WhatsApp, phone call, etc.). The content of the take-home assessment, however, needs to be meaningful and appropriate for this type of examination. Among major risks, signaled by students, are the work overload (students complained that it increased during the pandemic education), the duration of the exam, and even the complexity of the task.

Emergency remote assessment (ERA) can best work if Boyer's six principles are applied:

- ERA needs to be *educationally purposeful*. While the co-creation of new assessment formats had limited timespans, professors and students needed to negotiate the assessment activities for them to have meaning and to contribute to strengthening teaching and learning. Despite sometimes untested methods of evaluation used to complete the teaching and learning process, an assessment still preserved its's most salient feature: that of accounting for the learning outcomes during a stage or after a course.

- ERA needs to be *open*, in the sense that professors should have the freedom to choose those forms of assessment that are fit for the content of the course and the pedagogical experience of the instructor. While universities may recommend assessment strategies and need to provide the normative frames, especially for end-term, admission and graduation exams, some degrees of freedom should remain with the teachers developing assessment activities and providing their professional expertise.

- ERA needs to be *just*, in the sense that no student should be discriminated because of their lack of technological affordances or skills. The university support needs to go towards ensuring that the learners have the information, means and possibilities to continue their learning voyage throughout the storm of crises and that their accomplishments are properly acknowledged.

- ERA relies on *discipline*, with individuals accepting their responsibilities and working towards the common good. Clear rules, adapted to the situation and brought to the attention of all participants in the educational process, embraced by the academic community, spread over the assessment activities as well.

- ERA needs to be *caring*, in the sense that the well-being of each member is supported and where service to others is encouraged. This feature ensures that teachers continue to feel valued as experts in their field of work, while students enjoy the respect and find support in reducing assessment-related stress.

- Finally, ERA needs to be *celebrative.* Since the foundation of universities, academic life is marked by reiterative rituals [28]. Assessment activities, especially exams are a significant part of academic rituals [12]. Studies show that during the emergency remote assessment activities students missed most, exam-related rituals [12]. Although, some of these, such as verbal interaction with peers before and after the exam could easily be carried into the virtual environment, most students remained encapsulated in their constructed shell that felt like artificial, alienating, although familiar and somewhat supportive, since most of the students were confined to home-staying with their families.

In terms of the elements that need special attention for unfolding the emergency remote assessment, findings in the literature (case studies, surveys, and pedagogical reflections on the matter) show that the following four dimensions need to be considered:

- Technological solutions that facilitate access to the educational process and ensure the support for assessment activities.

- Appropriate pedagogical approaches, that consider the affordances of the newly created learning environment (virtual or otherwise).

- Supporting measures, in the form of norms, regulations and procedures about the exceptionality of the emergency situation and allowing for the accommodation with the adaptive tools and procedures that account for the assessment activities.

- Support structures and provisions ensure the well-being of teachers and learners as well, preventing burnout, technology fatigue, alienation, or disconnectedness.

For the first issue, ERA can benefit largely from the acquisitions of e-learning practices and computer-based assessment [7, 9, 29]. Students' voices, however, warn that while ERA represented a breakthrough in educational practices and they welcome the comfort brought by the use of computers for assessment purposes, the human factor still needs to be present in the appraisal of the results [12]. Students liked that they could use computers or other digital devices during exams and those professors tried to offer feedback on time. However, they also showed that their satisfaction rate depends on the relationship negotiated with the instructor and that they do not fully trust technology to provide an accurate assessment of the learning outcomes, a reaction anticipated also in earlier research [30]. Change in assessment is often unwelcomed [30], but the COVID-19 crisis made it compulsory. Efforts were undertaken to overcome resistance in the face of new forms and in presenting assessment as more than a mechanism for gatekeeping and achievement certification.

In terms of pedagogical approaches, we share the belief that Torrey Trust and Jeromie Whalen voiced in proposing that teachers be trained in emergency remote education as part of their set of professional skills and as a precondition to ensuring the resilience of the educational system in times of future crisis [31, 32]. These authors advance the idea that exploring the difference between emergency, blended teaching, and online teaching "may help scholars and teacher educators identify professional learning topics that can improve teachers' feelings of preparedness for teaching in any situation moving forward", in all the instances about the educational process [32]. Taking one step further, we believe that the experiences of remote teaching and remote assessment should not be forgotten and the return to the "new normal" education needs to preserve the lessons of 2020–2021 in the institutional memory and practices, such as it is recommended by crisis management literature [33]. In reflecting upon the accumulated experiences, teachers and institutions contribute to building resilience, understood as the ability of colleges and universities to prevent, protect against, mitigate, respond to, and recover from the crisis, be it triggered by natural disasters or by man-made disruptive activities. By incorporating the lessons of education during the COVID-19 pandemic into institutional memory and practices, appropriate plans can begin to be formulated on how to steer universities towards being resilient.

Supporting measures were rapidly developed during the pandemic, a synthetic document drafted by the Organization for Economic Co-operation and Development grouping the available resources along with three categories: Curriculum Resources, Professional Development Resources, and tools [34]. These resources were developed by a variety of actors: educational systems, represented by ministries or alliances of universities, by private initiatives, by educational non-governmental organizations, etc. At the micro-level, each institution adopted its' own set of measures to provide support to teachers and/or students, as shown by the numerous cases in the research literature on emergency remote education during the COVID-19 crisis.

Finally, the support measures and provisions ensuring the well-being of teachers and learners ensure the possibility of "building back better" the educational system in the aftermath of the pandemic, as listed among the nine ideas that shape the future of education in the post-pandemic world [35].

## 3. Conclusions

This intellectual journey into the pedagogical, managerial, and political experiences accumulated during the COVID-19 pandemic necessitating the adoption of emergency remote assessment (as part of the emergency remote education) stresses the necessity of researchers, policymakers, and educational practitioners to join forces and find solutions to the unexpected challenges brought by crisis situations. Beyond the immediate *ad hoc* measures aimed at ensuring learning continuity (often referred to as *sudden online* education), higher education institutions need to process the whole string of experiences [36] and extract long-term strategic implications for their return to in-campus learning and their resilience plans.

Throughout its history, the university assessed itself as a learning, adaptive and evolving organization. It follows naturally that the university will use the pandemic lessons in post-event analyses, increasing the knowledge of the organization, in building anticipation of and preparation for future (disruptive) events. The coping phase, manifested at the outbreak of the pandemic in the form of adopting emergency educational solutions was replaced by the adaptation phase, during which acquisitions from other experiences were called upon (mainly from e-learning and technology-assisted education) and, finally, by the transformational phase, during which universities once again prove themselves to be drivers of innovation. Educational systems aim at building sustainable, resilient universities as part of the development of academic life, "continuously influenced by sociocultural, technological, and environmental changes" [37]. In the process, assessment practices need to evolve towards sustainable models, ensuring that appropriate pedagogical resources are activated, that students understand, accept and extract meaning from the assessment activities, that society acknowledges and recognizes the result and those technological affordances are put to use in the process. With each case study, a note from the field, review, or reflection the community of assessment practices enlarges and gains momentum.

Assessment activities, although occurring after a cycle of teaching-learning string, are planned at the initial phase, and incorporated in the curriculum. The specifics of the emergency situations cancel some of the features, if not the entire projection of assessment and new models need to be put in place. The future, resilient university should make room in the curriculum design for sustainable assessment forms, that are less influenced by external factors and allow for a smooth shift from in-campus activities to remote education. Such a sustainable model needs to be not only student-centered, but also co-created with students, to ensure that they understand, accept, and comply with the new provisions in their academic journey. Assessment should gain more visibility in institutional debates and policies, and despite all adverse events it cannot be canceled without risking that the progress of students through the curriculum eludes appraisal instruments. Innovative models of assessment should be encouraged, such as self-assessment, peer assessment, take-home exams, open-book exams, enhancing the responsibility of the learners towards learning, their understanding of the process and their preparation for transitioning from school to work.

## Author details

Mariana Cernicova-Buca
Faculty of Communication Sciences, Politehnica University of Timisoara, Romania

*Address all correspondence to: mariana.cernicova@upt.ro

## References

[1] Boyer EL. Campus Life: In Search of Community. Princeton, NJ: Princeton University Press, (USA); 1990

[2] National Recovery and Resilience Agency. Emergency Planning Handbook, 2nd Ed. Australian Disaster Resilience Knowledge Hub; 2020 Available from: https://knowledge.aidr.org.au/resources/emergency-planning-handbook/

[3] Guide for Developing High-Quality Emergency Operations Plans for Institutions of Higher Education. Washington, DC: U.S. Department of Education; 2013 Available from: https://rems.ed.gov/docs/IHE_Guide_508C.pdf

[4] Petal, D. (2008), Disaster Prevention for Schools Guidance for Education Sector Decision-Makers, Available from: https://www.preventionweb.net/files/7344_DPforSchoolssm.pdf

[5] UNESCO, Education in Emergencies, Available from: https://en.unesco.org/themes/education-emergencies/action

[6] World Health Organization (WHO), Timeline: WHO's COVID-19 response, 2020. Available from: https://www.who.int/emergencies/diseases/novel-coronavirus-2019/interactive-timeline?gclid=EAIaIQobChMIzq335pT58gIVmMx3Ch0ejgLgEAAYASAAEgKblPD_BwE#event-115

[7] Crompton H, Burke D, Jordan K, Wilson SW. Learning with technology during emergencies: A systematic review of K-12 education. British Journal of Educational Technology. 2021;52:1554-1575. DOI: 10.1111/bjet.13114

[8] Inter-agency Network for Education in Emergencies, Available from: https://inee.org/

[9] Ashlee A, Clericetti G, Gladwell J, Mitchell J, Torrance R. Education in emergencies. Rapid evidence review. The EdTech Hub. 2020. DOI: 10.5281/zenodo.4058181

[10] Murphy MPA. COVID-19 and emergency eLearning: Consequences of the securitization of higher education for post-pandemic pedagogy. Contemporary Security Policy. 2020;**41**(3):492-505. DOI: 10.1080/13523260.2020.1761749

[11] Hodges C, Moore S, Lockee B, Trust T, Bond A. The difference between emergency remote teaching and online learning. Educause Review. 2020;**27** Available from: https://er.educause.edu/articles/2020/3/the-difference-between-emergency-remote-teaching-and-online-learning

[12] Cernicova-Buca M, Dragomir G-M. Romanian students' appraisal of the emergency remote assessment due to the COVID-19 pandemic. Sustainability. 2021;**13**(11):6110. DOI: 10.3390/su13116110

[13] Şenel S, Şenel H. Remote assessment in higher education during COVID-19 pandemic. International Journal of Assessment Tools in Education. İzzet KARA, Turkey: Pamukkale University; 2021;**8**:181-199

[14] Whittle C, Tiwari S, Yan S, Williams J. Emergency remote teaching environment: A conceptual framework for responsive online teaching in crises. Information and Learning Sciences. 2020;**121**(5/6):311-319. DOI: 10.1108/ILS-04-2020-0099

[15] UNESCO. (2020a). Exams and assessments in COVID-19 crisis: fairness at the centre, 2020, Available from: https://en.unesco.org/news/exams-and-assessments-covid-19-crisis-fairness-centre [Accessed December 3, 2020]

[16] Fry H, Ketteridge S, Marshall S, editors. A Handbook for Teaching and

Learning in Higher Education Enhancing Academic Practice. New York, London: Routledge; 2009

[17] Secolsky C, Denison DB, editors. Improving Institutional Decision-Making through Educational Measurement, Assessment, and Evaluation. In: Higher Education. Second ed. New York, USA: Routledge; 2017

[18] UNESCO (2014). Education strategy 2014-2021, Available from: https://unesdoc.unesco.org/ark:/48223/pf0000231288

[19] Iosad A, Pauli M, Attewell S. Assessment Rebooted: From Fixes to Foresight. Bristol, UK, Available from: https://repository.jisc.ac.uk/7854/1/assessment-rebooted-report.pdf; 2020 [Accessed: March 1, 2021]

[20] Amzalag M, Shapira N, Dolev N. Two sides of the coin: Lack of academic integrity in exams during the corona pandemic, students' and lecturers' perceptions. Journal of Academic Ethics. Springer; 2021:1-21. DOI: 10.1007/s10805-021-09413-5

[21] Boud D, Solcr R. Sustainable assessment revisited. Assessment & Evaluation in Higher Education. 2016;**41**(3):400-413. DOI: 10.1080/02602938.2015.1018133

[22] Chung S-J, Choi L-J. The development of sustainable assessment during the COVID-19 pandemic: The case of the english language program in South Korea. Sustainability. 2021;**13**(8):4499. DOI: 10.3390/su13084499

[23] United Nations Children's Fund (UNICEF), (2021). Formative learning assessment in contexts of remote educational services in Latin America and the Caribbean: Literature review, guidelines and tools, Available from: https://www.unicef.org/lac/media/20736/file/Formative_Learning_Assesment_LAC.pdf

[24] Gamage KAA, Silva EKD, Gunawardhana N. Online delivery and assessment during COVID-19: Safeguarding academic integrity. Education Sciences. 2020;**10**(11):301. DOI: 10.3390/educsci10110301

[25] Farrell O. From portafoglio to eportfolio: The evolution of portfolio in higher education. Journal of Interactive Media in Education. 2020;(1):19. DOI: 10.5334/jime.574

[26] Zalat MM, Hamed MS, Bolbol SA. The experiences, challenges, and acceptance of e-learning as a tool for teaching during the COVID-19 pandemic among university medical staff. PLoS One. 2021;**16**(3):e0248758. DOI: 10.1371/journal.pone.0248758

[27] Price M, O'Donovan B, Rust C, Carroll J. Assessment standards: A manifesto for change. Brookes eJournal of Learning and Teaching. 2008;**2**(3)

[28] Cernicova-Buca M. Academic rituals and ceremonies in Romanian universities of the 21st century. Conference Proceedings, 4th International Multidisciplinary Scientific Conference on Social Sciences and Arts SGEM. 2017. DOI: 10.5593/sgemsocial2017/41/S16.015

[29] Katz I, Gorin J. Computerising assessment. In: Brown GTL, Harris LR, editors. Handbook of Human and Social Conditions in Assessment. New York, USA: Routledge; 2016

[30] Struyven K, Devesa J. Students' perceptions of novel forms of assessment. In: Brown GTL, Harris LR, editors. Handbook of Human and Social Conditions in Assessment. New York, USA: Routledge; 2016. pp. 129-144

[31] Barbour MK, Labonte R, Kelly K, Hodges C, Moore S, Lockee B, et al.

Understanding Pandemic Pedagogy: Differences between Emergency Remote, Remote, and Online Teaching; State of the Nation. Cobble Hill, BC, Canada: K-12 e-Learning in Canada; 2020

[32] Trust T, Whalen J. Should teachers be trained in emergency remote teaching? lessons learned from the COVID-19 pandemic. Journal of Technology and Teacher Education. 2020;**28**(2):189-199

[33] Bundy J, Pfarrer MD, Short CE, Coombs WT. Crises and crisis management: Integration, interpretation, and research development. Journal of Management. 2017;**43**(6):1661-1692. DOI: 10.1177/0149206316680030

[34] OECD. Supporting-the-Continuation-of-Teaching-and-Learning-During-the-COVID-19-Pandemic. 2020. Available from: https://www.oecd.org/education/Supporting-the-continuation-of-teaching-and-learning-during-the-COVID-19-pandemic.pdf

[35] UNESCO. Education in a post-COVID world: Nine ideas for public action. Paris: UNESCO; 2020b available at https://en.unesco.org/sites/default/files/education_in_a_post-covid_world-nine_ideas_for_public_action.pdf

[36] Amemado D. COVID-19: An unexpected and unusual driver to online education. International Higher Education. 2020;**102**:12-14 [Accessed January 4, 2021]

[37] Bartusevičienė I, Pazaver A, Kitada M. Building a resilient university: ensuring academic continuity—transition from face-to-face to online in the COVID-19 pandemic. WMU Journal of Maritime Affairs. 2021;**20**:151-172. DOI: 10.1007/s13437-021-00239-x

Chapter 6

# Social Distancing Disbanding Learner Groupings: A Case on Language Development

*Bulelwa Makena and Thandiswa Mpiti*

## Abstract

Information sharing is a fundamental aspect in learning an unfamiliar, yet, an additional language, with specific regards to reading comprehension. Language teachers are faced with a task to monitor development, performance, and effectiveness in learner reading proficiencies. This chapter aims to measure if disbanding learner groupings as per the social distancing protocols brought about by COVID-19 restrictions has any impact on language enhancement. Henceforth, there are limited suggestions by literature in relation to disbanding learner groupings, yet improved reading proficiency is one of the crucial language aspects to be mastered for one to be a successful scholar. Nonetheless, this chapter aims to provide teaching strategies applied by English language teachers to necessitate transmitted learning in accordance with information sharing as learners are dependent on one another for language enhancement, thus leading to academic achievement.

**Keywords:** learner groupings, language, social distancing, learner achievement, reading proficiency

## 1. Introduction

For improved academic achievement and acceptable reading proficiency levels, learners need to vigorously engage on varying reading activities. When they work as groups, they tend to learn from one another through collaboration, information sharing, and mentoring each other. There have been identified benefits of working as groups when primary school learners learn an unfamiliar language in the schools studied, this being referred to English language learning [1]. Research reveals that for primary school learners to engage in the form of groups during the processes of language learning and teaching, there are enriched social skills that are acquired, including cooperation and accountability, as such it becomes easy for learners to break down compound tasks into minor and convenient packages [2]. The main benefits of group work when developing language proficiency among learners include cultivated discussions and justifications, let alone contesting learner assumptions, yet the ultimate goal being emerging robust communication skills. This strategy has been observed to curb problems of shyness, lowered self-esteem coupled with self-motivation [3]. As emergent readers, learners in the primary school need daily continued engagement with reading exercises as learning to read has been recently regarded as one of the core educational objectives not for English language learning only, but across all the subjects underpinning the curriculum as there are also texts to be comprehended.

However, in the previously known South African schools' classroom environment prior COVID-19 pandemic era, policy advocated for formation of learner groupings as learning and teaching has to be learner-centered and learner-paced, this being prescribed by the Curriculum and Assessment Policy Statements (CAPS) [4]. English language teachers, through this arrangement, would proudly report on escalating learner achievements that used to be paired up with improved reading proficiency levels. This makes us as authors of this manuscript to acknowledge the importance of group work. To our perception, working as groups when learning a language leads to a more effective and fun collaboration as learners with diverse learning styles and learning abilities are granted an opportunity to engage with others, thereby anticipating the comprehended text from diverse perspectives, yet promoting confidence levels and expanded listening, thinking, speaking, and writing skills. All these are regarded as the core language skills for language learning [5]. For learners to be successful, efficient, and effective scholars, these skills need to be mastered.

## 2. Literature review

Grouping of learners when studying a language has been proved to lead to progress and success in academic achievement [6]. Teamwork is of real importance as learners engaging in this manner were identified to have exhibited better achievement levels when compared with those who preferred to study or learn in a single-handed mode. Henceforth, there is a vital need for English language teachers to be quite conversant that indeed group work has some profits and therefore are expected to apply such strategy during the processes of teaching and learning.

On the other side, social distancing protocols emanating from COVID-19 regulations have resulted in schools being left with no other option than to disband the previously formulated classroom learner groupings [7]. One may ask himself, what then has the current state of the existing new normal put primary school language teachers together with the learners as recipients in the teaching-learning process, as previously been observed by the authors that this cohort of teachers has full confidence for language development when comprehending texts is handled not in an individual perspective, but by learners specifically arranged as groups to interact, engage, thereby learning as peers. Furthermore, learners in the studied schools got intimidated by the abrupt changes in the schooling situation more so that learning English language, being unfamiliar hence not their home language, needs to be nurtured. By so doing, learners would then value own cultural heritages attached to obtaining valued experience in English language [8].

As an operational method to inspire active learning, for communication skills joined mutually with critical thinking, there is a need to encourage group work among learners [9]. On the other side, literature reveals that the current situation across all environments due to the COVID-19 regulations has brought about some negative effects resulting in stress from loss of peer interaction with regard to academic content as learners are no longer denied access to practice the so-called previously known normality of either sitting as groups or as pairs in a classroom setting, as a way of responding to the constraints of social distancing observance [7, 10]. This current state of affairs is declared similar to the period when there was once some disturbance in the schooling mode of behavior. There emerged an influenza first perceived in the United States, then later swiftly blew out across the entire countries of the world. As reported by the public health schools in such communities had to be closed down due to the influenza pandemic [11]. The schooling situation or practices by then were declared to have slightly changed as all inhabitants were expected to give full observance of the prescribed instructions by the then governmental officials.

Furthermore, as learners actively engage in group work, they obtain chances to express own opinions and ideas. As deliberations reach climax within a specific group of learners, critical thinking and robust discussion are also improved [12]. When learners' critical thinking and engagement skills are improved, problem-solving is then enhanced, together with improved communication skills, consequently leading to an enriched cultural awareness [13]. Such improved skills would be eminent as learners would have learnt to listen at others' opinions, then providing feedback. As this entire exercise is carried out, one would notice that learners forming a single group originate from dissimilar linguistic constituencies, different backgrounds, diverse cultures yet with varying learning styles, as such, at their early ages, learners then learn to have respect for each unique individual.

This manuscript is strengthened by Guskey's model of teacher change [14]. A model of teacher change has been used for this investigation pertaining to changes currently championing the education system, as brought about by the COVID-19 etiquettes that need to be observed by all individuals around the country [15]. The framework further portrays ecological changes in consideration of the attitudes and beliefs toward teaching and learning, as is the case in the current schooling situation. Previously, teachers strongly believed that for an operational and functional language development in learners, better results used to be eminent when learners were grouped, yet the current situation has resulted on learner groupings being disbanded.

With respect to the main objective of this chapter, authors opine that for learners to comprehend any text with understanding, there is a dire requirement for a combined practice between the text itself and learners brainstorming as a group. To uplift and motivate this notion, language teachers are therefore anticipated as the ones to constantly allocate reading tasks to learners in the form of groups, irrespective of whether during the normal classroom environment, or for tasks assigned as take-home activities. If English language teachers would embark in this practice, language proficiency among learners would surely be enhanced as perceived by the authors [16]. Teachers therefore are regarded as the core recipients to ensure language enhancement in learners, as suggested by the theory underpinning this manuscript [14]. Innovative reading skills, ease at comprehending with text, and upgraded language skills would then emerge, therefore leading to academic excellence as the greatest percentage of the subjects buttressing the curriculum in the schools investigated are offered in the English medium.

## 3. Methods and materials

For the purposes of this investigation, the authors followed a qualitative approach entrenched by a case study design. This is a research approach applied for generating an in-depth understanding for some compound issues affecting real-life situations. Authors used this type of design in order to have an understanding of recent social distancing trajectories affecting the previous normal running of schools [17]. Truths pertaining human behavior as authors studied the real-world circumstances that unfolded were put together [18]. An inclusive understanding pertaining to teacher perspectives on language development on the view that grouping of learners was no longer a practice, henceforth social distancing code of practice, was followed. For the context of this study, investigation was based on administering semistructured interviews to 10 purposefully selected teachers from three different primary schools in one district of the Eastern Cape Province in South Africa [19, 20]. Authors decided to embark on selecting participants in a purposive manner as this sampling technique allows researchers to rely on own judgment when nominating population members to participate. Henceforth, we decided to identify teachers from the surrounding locations where high COVID-19 death tolls had been reported by statistics [11]. Further than that, purposive sampling was a method that suited us well, hence the limited number of our participants who served as primary data sources by virtue of the case study designed ingraining this investigation. Participants nominated were teachers who offered English language as a medium reinforcing the utmost percentage of subjects enrolled in these particular schools.

As perceived by research, semistructured interviews as a data-collection instrument permitted the authors full engagement with all participants, more so that chances to explore more on crucial emerging themes seemed eminent [21]. Open-ended interview questions revolved around viewpoints of teachers on the subject of learner proficiency reading levels as directed by the abolishing of engaging on reading as groups, despite the previously reported improved readership in learners when such reading exercises used to be tackled in daily learner groupings. Despite the interview schedule containing open-ended questions, authors were at liberty to throw follow-up questions in instances where further clarities were deemed necessary. As a way of observing the current social distancing procedures, as well as avoiding grouping all participants in one common venue, interviews were conducted in a one-on-one fashion. Authors arranged meetings for each single participant at a single time. The interaction or engagements between the authors and participants started in September 2021 and at a later stage got terminated beginning December 2021 as both the interviewers and the interviewees became entangled in the processes of administering examinations in their varying work stations. As the interview schedule was administered, authors took some recordings, which were later replayed again and again. These recordings were taken in a different number of visits and days, for an interval ranging between 15 and 20 minutes for each individual participant. This method helped authors to be able to transcribe all responses from all participants, avoiding not to disregard any single response. Similar or relevant responses were grouped together and thereby coded by the authors as a way of formulating themes [17–22].

## 4. Research results

There are two themes that emerged during data analysis from an argument of findings for this investigation [22]. In consideration of reading proficiency levels, it emerged that reading is affected by disbanded learner groupings due to the COVID-19 pandemic era code of practice. The second finding outlined relates to learner attitudes resulting in feeling isolated from their peers, and yet this is proving to somehow influence language development intertwined with learner achievement.

### 4.1 Proficiency levels in reading

Among the group of participants, one teacher reported own observance on proficiency levels in reading among learners since in the classroom setting, learner groupings had no longer become the talk of the schooling environment: *My greatest worry is that learners in my class previously performed maximally well during the times when I used to group them as per their reading abilities.* On the same view, another participant concurred: *With time, all those who still displayed some difficulties in reading texts would improve through interactions and support made by members in a single group. Learners would later require me as their teacher to allow time to engage in competing as groups as a way to encourage learners to be all in an accepted level with regards to their proficiencies in comprehending with texts.*

### 4.2 Learner attitudes versus isolation

It was divulged that the majority of learners felt isolated from their peers. Henceforth, the current COVID-19 social distancing restrictions pertaining to the seating logic of one learner seated in a stipulated distance away from the other, they no longer had opportunities to either exchange ideas or share information as they used to when seated as groups.

In relation to this encounter, one participant argued that: *Even if those learners who are super gifted than the rest have successfully comprehended with the text within a short space of time, as their teacher I have recently developed reluctance to either pair or group learners according to their reading abilities, with fear of clomping learners together, in case one contaminates the deadly disease from the other.* On that note one participant reported a story that left us so sad, but without any remedy to suggest: *As I came a little bit closer, one by one, to those learners with difficulties to comprehend with the assigned texts, they almost gave me a similar response that they felt so isolated and deserted as groupmates who used to assist them were now seated afar, making it difficult to easily exchange ideas and ask for assistance and mentorship when they came across new, unfamiliar and difficult words.*

## 5. Discussion

Pertaining to reading proficiency levels, a key finding was a noted deterioration in reading progress among learners. Teachers offering English language as a subject debated that motivation within learners as groups no longer exists, actually, it has then been compromised as each learner had to battle or struggle on comprehending the text all alonc, this somchow displaying a sudden lack of collegiality among learners registered for the same subject. This situation was even made worse by the current situation that existed when learners were at their cultural or rather home backgrounds. Learners had reported to respective teachers that isolation also roams in their living environments to such an extent that even if one had a neighbor with whom they are enrolled for the same grade, phase, or subject, parents denied their children access to visit others for purposes of information sharing sessions [23]. As authors of this manuscript, we really feel pity for the cohort of learners experiencing difficulties in comprehending with texts. Actually, this then becomes a call for language teachers to identify alternative strategies that would curb the situation of learners who feel isolated and left alone, as this might lead to implications of increased learner-dropout rate as well as lowered progression levels. On the other side, a reading nation is a wealthy nation, we all need to engage with written texts in order to be an economically balanced country.

To curb the situation, learners need to be motivated so as to be able to adapt in the unfamiliar systems of self-independency. Motivation is known for its importance especially in learning an unfamiliar language, in this instance this being an English language. Motivated learners have since been noted of achieving their goals, while on the other hand those with lack of motivation become victims of not obtaining the intended academic achievement. Nurtured motivation has been identified to lead higher levels of language competence. It therefore lies with English language teachers that as learners are held in situations of no longer vibrantly engaging with group members in the classroom environment, learners be encouraged and driven toward attaining short-term goals such as reading and writing, by so doing, they would improve in language proficiencies. Dissolution of learner groupings is perceived by learners as not supportive toward language learning. With limited collaboration, some learners could undergo stress disorders or related sicknesses [6–10].

Furthermore, as collaborative learning has proved to yield good results, teachers are then advised to let learners learn as either pairs or groups, even if the seating plan makes learners to be scattered from each other [24]. This method of learning collaboratively has been proved by other writers to have some advantages as research argues that in group work learners have an opportunity to learn from each other as they can better unpack some ideas clearer to respective classmates, as compared with how a teacher would have tackled it, this at times resulting from that some learners have an introvert attitude, as such become reluctant to seek assistance from their teachers [25].

From the collected data, it also emerged that the newly designed seating plan for learners to be positioned apart from their peers seemed to have some adverse impacts on learning, and specifically for the purposes of this investigation, isolation led to attitudes of neglect, this having an influence on language development [26]. The current seating plan in the schooling environment is attached with compliance of COVID-19 regulations on social distancing as prescribed by the South African government. Elements of anxiety in learners revolve around logistics encounters with regard to loneliness, discomposure, and loss of peer interaction [27]. To the authors' perspective, these critical aspects are likely to have an influence on academic content and uncertainty in learner progression. Teachers also reported that learners whose comprehension levels were not of the expected average normally raised concerns that the current seating plan causes lots of stress, likely to impact on their development in learning.

On the other side, teachers also reported their concern regarding learner isolation as this might impact on emotional and social learning [28]. Proficiency gaps in reading abilities were noted by language teachers to have erupted ever since the innovations on the classroom seating plans, in so much that isolation even from friends and family in general, have normally resulted into an unhealthy social learning environment. This finding is in line with the views that for a task to be considered as outcomes-based, learners are expected to cultivate some links in between the content learnt and the encompassing learning styles thereof. Moreover, as learners comprehend and intermingle in the target language that is being learnt, there seems to be a crucial need for them to interact and communicate among themselves for easy access to acquire the logistics of the new and the unacquainted language. Engaging in such a strategy is likely to rebuild self-confidence, this leading to improved language proficiency levels [29]. For satisfactory progress, learning in schools needs to be a process administered through social relationships, including oneself, life, as well as collaborating with others through unanimous decision-making [30, 31]. By so doing, the school then becomes a family because of the supportive networking by both teachers and groups of learners. For such networking to be lost, it then really becomes a greatest concern ever. As the authors of this manuscript, we therefore opine for paramount importance that language teachers devise the necessary strategies aimed toward improved language proficiency with revised approaches to help rebuild the lost self-intrinsic inspiration within learners as swept away by isolation logistics.

## 6. Conclusion

The fundamental aim of this chapter was to measure the extent to which terminated learner groupings as a way of responding to the COVID-19 social distancing logistics had any influence on language enhancement. Importance of this investigation is reaffirmed as all the underlying discussions for this article have been proven to be aligned with the model of teacher change [14]. An examination of disbanded learner groupings led to the key finding outlining that indeed group work yields best results in relation to reading proficiency in leaners. From the data analyzed, it has become eminent to note that restricted groupings of learners in the current schooling situation seem to have an effect of redundancy toward a healthy reading culture. As perceived by the authors of this chapter, a nation with restricted or deprived culture of reading is tantamount to a vehicle expected to be in motion, yet fully loaded with a dead engine. Findings of this investigation therefore imply that despite the restrictions to group learners in classroom settings, language teachers are faced with a huge task to motivate the young, yet highlighting to them that with time they need to develop responsive attitudes with that sense of individual drive toward their learning, as the current state of affairs has led to all scholars being held up in the predicament of self-studies, of which no one had ever anticipated. Henceforth, authors recommend that managerial implications of this investigation be vested on the policymakers to redesign functional policies that would act as alternatives into restoring worthwhile sitting plans, yet, rebuilding that sense of inner ambiguity among learners no longer able to collaborate with peers as was in the previously disbanded learner groupings.

## Acknowledgements

First and foremost, let me appreciate and thank the Almighty God for the strength and wisdom. Without His blessings, I doubt if we would have courage to successfully write this manuscript.

To write a book chapter is really hard work than I ever imagined, yet rewarding because as I continue embarking on the process of writing, my research skills coupled with academic writing logistics are sharpened day by day. This chapter encompasses to measure whether disbanding learner groupings as per the social distancing protocols brought about by COVID-19 restrictions has any significant impact on language enhancement.

I would be making a mistake not to acknowledge the amazing obligation that I owe toward researchers who encouraged me on manuscript writing. For this manuscript to be written in completion, an immense amount of work was done and would not have happened without an inspiration by a number of compassionate researchers whom I collaborated with, inclusive of:

Dr. Nomxolisi Mtsi, who was the first person to inspire me on research writing. As I narrated to her that my life situation had its ups and downs, she just told me that there was always a way out for whatever situation experienced. This academic was the one who whispered out loud in my ears that I need to start focusing on research writing. I can assume in me she sensed a hungry academic that needed some inspiration to grow. She went an extra mile to introduce me to Dr. Thandiswa Mpiti, with whom we are in the same field of research: languages. I am so grateful to have networked with such an academic, engaging on research writing, sharing experiences, and stimulating one another.

I cannot turn a blind eye on this one. To Dr. Shakespeare Chiphambo, no matter how the awkward timing would be, he is always eager to read through my drafts and offer whatever form of assistance I require from him in relation to manuscript writing.

I am ceaselessly appreciative to my mentor: Professor Bongani Bantwini, my managers at work: Professor Nolutho Diko and Mrs. Nondwe Mtshatsha. These seasoned academics would always and forever encourage me to make it a priority that I prioritize on manuscript writing to be considered as fully blown in academia. My mentor would always go an extra mile to read through my drafts.

Without proficiencies, collaboration, and support from my colleague at work, Dr. Ntando Elliot Mpahla, the research expertise on manuscript writing, would not have been to this level.

To all the researchers who would preach into my ears that to be regarded as a real academic one has to embark on publishing, thank you so much for inspiring more authors to have courage to convert their ideas to becoming stories. It is because of such inspiring comments that I have obtained some growth opportunities.

For the publication of this manuscript, I wish to extend my sincere gratitude to the Walter Sisulu Research Directorate for offering funding toward our publications. This stimulates and encourages us as researchers to have a maintained zeal toward the project as academic writers.

Writing a chapter about real-life experiences encountered in the workplace during the processes of teaching and learning is indeed a bizarre process, but through the ongoing support of the colleagues in the same field of work, there was continued motivation and inspiration to maintain the passion of bringing all our stories to life.

A very special word of thanks goes to my family. My kids, Yonela, Tina, and Zenazi, for supporting me without complaining even at times when I gave them less attention than they expected. My nephews and nieces, Odwa, Ongeziwe, Lisolethu, Kungawo, Amyoli, and Minathi, for exercising patience when I took longer to assist them with their studies while I was still hooked up in this little piece of writing. Their level of understanding is well applauded. My brother, Campbell, and sisters, Xoliswa and Hombakazi, for always encouraging me in whatever endeavor intending to make my life a better one. My mom, Vuyiswa, who would always and forever urge all her kids to prioritize with engaging in furthering their studies for being successful and prominent citizens. Lastly, my debt goes to my late dad, Erick Vuyisilet, who always dreamt big about the level of education for his children.

Conclusions to this study have been sharpened by contributions of our participants. For the time they excellently dedicated in engaging in this investigation, they are highly acknowledged.

## Appendix A: interview schedule

### Interview Schedule for English First Additional Language Primary School teachers

1. To what extent is social distancing in relation to learner attitudes versus isolation affecting language development?

2. What role does social distancing play with respect to learner groupings on reading proficiency levels?

**Your participation in this regard is of the highest value in this enquiry. Thank You.**

## Author details

Bulelwa Makena* and Thandiswa Mpiti
Walter Sisiulu University, Komani Campus, South Africa

*Address all correspondence to: bmakena@wsu.ac.za

## References

[1] Barkley EF, Cross KP, Major CH. Collaborative Learning Techniques: A Handbook for College Faculty. San Francisco: Jossey-Bass Publishers; 2005. p. 90

[2] Beebe SA, Masterson JT. Communicating in Small Groups. Boston, Massachusetts: Pearson Education Inc; 2020. p. 12

[3] Cooper J. Cooperative learning and college teaching: Tips from the trenches. Teaching Professor. 1990;**4**:1-2. DOI: 10.1177/136548020100400206

[4] DBE Curriculum and Assessment Policy Statements. South African Government; 2011. Available from: https://www.education.gov.za/Curriculum/CurriculumAssessmentPolicyStatements(CAPS).aspx. [Accessed: July 17, 2021]

[5] Astin A. What Matters in College? Four Critical Years Revisited. San Francisco: Jossey-Bass; 1993. p. 75. DOI: 10.2307/1176821

[6] McDonald L. Benefits of Group Work: Classroom Management. 2020. Available from: https://www.teachhub.com/classroom-management/2020/09/benefits-of-group-work/. [Accessed: September 6, 2021]

[7] Hughey D. Lessons Learned-Social Distancing May Impact Student Development. 2020. Available from: https://www.cbs19.tv›education›eyes-on-education. [Accessed: July 9, 2021]

[8] Makena B, Mpahla N. Enhancing English language proficiency through learning styles centered on a perception of migrating from face-to-face to remote online learning culture: A case of a rural South African University. International Journal of Sciences and Research. 2021;**77**(8):33-34. DOI: 10.21506/j.ponte.2021.8.3

[9] Mannix E, Neale MA. What differences make a difference? The promise and reality of diverse teams in organizations. Psychological Science in the Public Interest. 2005;**6**(31-55): 1529-1006

[10] Karasmanaki E, Tsantopoulos G. Impacts of social distancing during COVID-19 pandemic on the daily life of forestry students. Children and Youth Services Review. 2020;**120**(1):1-7

[11] Braunack-Mayer A, Tooher R, Collins JE, Street JM, Marshall H. Understanding the school community's response to school closures during the H1N1 2009 influenza pandemic. BMC Public Health. 2013;**13**:344-349. DOI: 10.1186/1471-2458-13-344

[12] Dano Z. 0,5m Social Distancing Rule at Schools Is Not a Good Idea, but May be Better than Current System. 2021. Available from: https://www.iol.co.za/education/05m-social-distancing-rule-at-schools-is-not-a-good-idea-but-may-be-better-than-current-system-expert-484ee2d9-c966-4554-b824-6c7a7e35abfb. [Accessed: September 1, 2021]

[13] Freeman L, Greenacre L. An examination of socially destructive behaviors in group work. Journal of Marketing Education. 2011;**33**:5-17. DOI: 10.1177/0273475310389150

[14] Guskey TR. Staff development and the process of teacher change. Educational Researcher. 1986;**15**(5):5-12. DOI: 10.3102/0013189X015005005

[15] Cave H. Learning in Extraordinary Times. 2021. Available from: https://bold.experttopicslearning-in-extraordinary. [Accessed: September 11, 2021]

[16] Muchtar N. Intensive and extensive reading in improving teaching reading comprehension. Lingua Pedagogia

Journal of English Teaching Studies. 2019;**1**(2):1-13. DOI: 10.21831/lingped.v1i2.18687

[17] Myers MD. Qualitative Research in Business and Management. 2020. Available from: https://books.google.co.za›books. [Accessed: September 6, 2021]

[18] Denzin NK, Lincoln YS. The SAGE Handbook of Qualitative Research. Los Angeles: Sage; 2018. p. 859

[19] Guest G, Namey E, Taylor J, Eley N, McKenna K. Comparing focus groups and individual interviews: findings from a randomized study. International Journal of Social Research Methodology. 2017;**20**(6):693-708. DOI: 10.1080/13645579.2017.1281601

[20] Brinkman S. Qualitative Interviewing. New York: Oxford University Press; 2013. p. 26

[21] Sweetman D, Badiee M, Creswell W. Use of the transformative framework in mixed methods studies. Journal of Qualitative Inquiry. 2010;**16**(6):441-454. DOI: 10.1177/1077800410364610

[22] Creswell JW. Research Design Qualitative, Quantitative, and Mixed Methods Approaches. Los Angeles: Sage; 2009. p. 168

[23] Maragakis LL. Coronavirus, Social and Physical Distancing and Self-quarantine. 2020. Available from: https://www.hopkinsmedicine.org/health/conditions-anddiseases/coronavirus/coronavirus-social-distancing-and-self-quarantine. [Accessed: August 04, 2021]

[24] Caruso HM, Wooley AW. Harnessing the power of emergent interdependence to promote diverse team collaboration. Diversity and Groups. 2008;**11**:245-266. DOI: 10.1016/S1534-0856%2808%2911011-8

[25] Deardorff J. Gifted Students Benefit from Ability Grouping, Acceleration. 2017. Available from: https://www.sesp.northwestern.edu/news-center/news/2017/01/gifted-students-benefit-from-ability-grouping,-acceleration. [Accessed: July 17, 2021]

[26] Lopez M. Social distance during the COVID-19 pandemic reflects perceived rather than actual risk. International Journal of Environmental Research and Public Health. 2021;**18**(11):5504. DOI: 10.3390/ijerph18115504

[27] Menezes S. The COVID-19 pandemic as an opportunity to weaken environmental protection in Brazil. Biological Conservation. 2021;**255**:2-4. DOI: 10.1016/j.biocon.2021.108994

[28] Kumar A. COVID-19: A Global Transplant Perspective on Successfully Navigating a Pandemic. 2020. Available from: https://timesofindia.indiatimes.com/blogs/indic-positive/social-distancing-and-its-impact-on-kids/. [Accessed: September 06, 2021]

[29] Mpiti T, Makena B, Mpahla NE. Task-based approach in improving the communicative skill of English First Additional Language first-year student teachers. In: Proceedings of 15th International Technology, Education and Development Conference (INTED 21); 08-09 March 2021; Valentia, Spain. pp. 10732-10738

[30] Bates K. How Social Distancing Affects Social Development. 2021. Available from: https://bold.expert/how-social-distancing-affects-social-development/. [Accessed: September 6, 2021]

[31] Burden K, Aubusson P, Brindley S, Schuck S. Changing knowledge, changing technology: Implications for teacher education futures. Journal of Education for Teaching. 2016;**42**:4-16. DOI: 10.1080/02607476.2015.1125432

Chapter 7

# Perspective Chapter: Psychosocial Impact of COVID-19 – Stigma and Xenophobia

*Dogancan Sonmez and Cicek Hocaoglu*

## Abstract

The novel type of coronavirus (COVID-19) pandemic, which affected the whole world and resulted in the death of many people, caused problems in various fields in societies. The effects of the pandemic, especially on health and the economy, have reached important points and studies in these areas have intensified. It is also a known fact that the pandemic causes psychosocial problems in humans. Existing problems have also had negative effects on mental health. Measures, restrictions, and quarantine practices are taken to control the epidemic have caused psychological, social, and economic problems. The spread of the disease and changes in living conditions have led to an increase in negative attitudes among people. The pandemic has also caused discriminatory and stigmatizing attitudes among people. In addition, xenophobic attitudes, defined as fear, hatred, and prejudice against foreigners, have become widespread during the pandemic process. People exposed to stigma and xenophobic attitudes due to the pandemic have experienced social and economic inequalities. It is important to prevent stigmatizing and xenophobic attitudes during the pandemic process in order to ensure social cohesion in society. In this section, the psychosocial effects of stigma and xenophobia associated with COVID-19 will be discussed in light of literature.

**Keywords:** COVID-19, pandemic, stigma, xenophobia, psychosocial impact

## 1. Introduction

The coronavirus disease, which emerged with respiratory symptoms (high fever, cough, shortness of breath) in Wuhan, China's Hubei Province in December 2019, has turned into a worldwide pandemic. The novel coronavirus disease (COVID-19), defined by the World Health Organization (WHO) on January 13, 2020, spread rapidly in 6 continents and hundreds of countries after China, causing many deaths [1]. At the time of preparation for this study (August 23, 2021), approximately 211,730,035 people worldwide were infected and 4,430,697 people died due to COVID-19 [2]. The COVID-19 outbreak, defined as the first pandemic caused by coronaviruses, has caused global concern. The COVID-19 pandemic has brought many challenges. A few of these difficulties are stigma and xenophobia. The stigma associated with COVID-19 has serious implications for the lives of healthcare professionals, patients, and those who have had the disease. This makes a difficult situation, such as the fight against the epidemic, even more difficult. Health workers, infected individuals, and their families are seen as possible sources of infection and are exposed to various discrimination and stigmatization. Not allowing healthcare workers to use public transportation, being asked to vacate their rented houses, being exposed to verbal and physical violence, abandoning the woman with COVID-19 who gave birth by her family, calling the street where the house of a person with COVID-19 is located as a 'corona road' and people avoiding this street are examples of stigma [3]. Epidemics that contain many uncertainties, such as the COVID-19 epidemic, can cause serious social stigma. For example, Russian Jewish immigrants were stigmatized because of the typhus and cholera epidemics in 1892, and Native Americans in the region were stigmatized because of the 1993 hantavirus epidemic in the United States. Also, an epidemic of bubonic plague, the so-called "black death" attributed to rats transported by ship from Hong Kong in the spring of 1900, resulted in discrimination and stigmatization in the San Francisco Chinatown community [4]. Stigmatized persons may give up seeking treatment, people may fear and avoid stigmatized persons, society may be prejudiced against stigmatized persons, and this may turn into verbal or physical violence against stigmatized persons or groups. For fear of being stigmatized and labeled as someone with an infectious disease, many at-risk people may not seek help until symptoms become very severe. In fact, many people may not seek help for treatment at all [5]. The COVID-19 pandemic has created an environment with too many risks for stigma. Xenophobia is a word that means fear and hatred of foreigners [6]. Xenophobia is spreading in many countries during the pandemic and is mostly directed against Asians. Such xenophobic incidents have been reported in countries such as Belgium, Croatia, Finland, France, Germany, Hungary, Italy, the Netherlands, Russia, Ukraine, and the United Kingdom. Cases of xenophobia include verbal attacks and accusations of spreading the virus to the public [7]. In this section, it is aimed to discuss the history of the concepts of stigma and xenophobia, its psychosocial dimension, its relationship with the COVID-19 pandemic, methods of combating risk factors in the light of literature information, and to raise awareness about this situation.

## 2. Definition and theories of stigma

Stigma refers to the situation of being exposed to an accusatory, exclusionary approach and attitude due to the existence of a situation that should be ashamed for a person or group, being different from normal or different from other individuals with any feature. Stigma as a word means a scar, a stain, a sign of shame and humiliation that marks the person [8]. Etymologically, the concept of stigmatization was used for the first time in Ancient Greek with the meanings of hole, puncture, wound, scar, and today it is used in the sense of humiliation and loss of reputation, similar to this definition. Sociologist E. Goffman defined stigma as social rejection resulting from negatively perceived characteristics [9]. According to Goffman, the term stamp goes back to the Greeks who cut or burned the skins of criminals, slaves, and traitors to describe them as tainted or immoral people to be avoided [9]. Stigma is a term that refers to social disapproval, not just a physical marking. Link and Phelan extended Goffman's conceptualization by identifying four attributes of stigma; (1) individual differences are noticed, (2) these differences are perceived negatively by society, (3) the stigmatized group is viewed as an outgroup, (4) the end result is loss of opportunity, power, or status [10].

While explaining the reasons for stigma, 4 terms were used. These are as follows:

a. *Stereotypes:* This concept represents the common general view of societies. It is a concept adopted by the general public. When a "sick person" is mentioned, the person first perceives and evaluates this situation with stereotypes. Some of these definitions share commonalities, but each may also contain unique aspects that may contradict the others. Stereotypes are grouped into positive and negative.

b. *Prejudices:* Prejudices support stereotypes. Different emotional reactions may develop as a result of prejudices and stereotypes. As a result of prejudices, negative emotions such as anger and fear often arise towards patients.

c. *Discrimination:* It is the cognitive and emotional reactions that occur due to certain characteristics of a person or a group as a result of an evaluated situation and are reflected in the behavior. This behavior can be positive or negative. However, the word discrimination is generally understood to mean negative. This behavior is discriminatory and exclusionary. It can also occur as a result of biased behaviors or as a result of an individual with negative stereotypes.

d. *Attitude:* People's perspectives on life is shaped by the society and culture in which they grew up. This perspective also affects the emotional reactions and behaviors of the person to events. These reactions can be sometimes positive and sometimes negative. The perspective formed by the integration of these reactions and the person's worldview is called "attitude" [11].

## 3. Stigma in previous pandemics

Throughout history, human beings have been exposed to dangerous diseases that force them to change their behavior to adapt to new conditions. WHO has defined a pandemic as "the worldwide spread of a new disease". From smallpox of the 19th century to COVID-19 of the 21st century, epidemics and pandemics have always been associated with stigma and serious social consequences [12]. Apart from natural disasters or wars affecting a certain geographical region, infectious diseases affect the whole world and humanity without borders, as we witnessed in the COVID-19 epidemic. To date, there have been 21 pandemics affecting humanity. The most well-known and most severe of these is the plague epidemic that emerged in the fourteenth century. In previous studies, it was reported that the population of the whole world decreased by 1/4 in the plague pandemic and the population of many important cities was completely destroyed [13, 14]. Other major pandemics are Spanish Flu (1918–1920), HIV epidemic, Smallpox in the former Yugoslavia (1972), severe acute respiratory syndrome (SARS) (2003), "Swine Flu" or H1N1/09 (2009), Middle East Respiratory Syndrome (MERS), Ebola (2014–2016), and ZIKA (2015–2016) pandemics. These pandemics have caused many casualties [15]. There are differences between the first known pandemics and more recent pandemics because during the first pandemics the population was independent of each other, that is, isolated. However, in the present times when human mobility has increased, the significant increase in interregional and even intercontinental communication and interaction has changed the course of today's pandemics. On the other hand, the development of transportation and communication in the global arena and increased contact with a different human, animal, and ecosystem populations facilitated the spread of the pandemic [16]. Medical stigma is seen in almost every period of history. Diseases such as leprosy, plague, syphilis, tuberculosis, cancer, AIDS, which affect societies, are the diseases that cause stigmatization [17, 18]. As diseases such as tuberculosis and syphilis became treatable, stigmatizing attitudes towards these diseases decreased over time [19]. Leprosy, which has a history as old as human history and is one of the first stigmatized diseases, was described as an "evil" given to man by God [20]. Those who contracted syphilis in the fifteenth century were condemned by society. Tuberculosis, named in the eighteenth century, was seen as a disease belonging to the lower class. Since the 1900s, with the recognition of cancer types and the increasing number of people receiving this diagnosis, prejudiced behaviors have been made against cancer patients, and discriminatory approaches against cancer patients have continued until the last 20 years. There were comments about AIDS, which emerged in the 1980s and was formerly known as a homosexual disease, as "a punishment given by God to sinners". Along with cancer, tuberculosis, leprosy, syphilis, and epilepsy, AIDS has also become one of the diseases that create stigma [20].

## 4. COVID-19 and stigma

During the pandemic process, people's relationships with each other have changed. Newborn baby visits could not be made, university graduates could not share their graduation moments with their loved ones. Many people were not able to physically meet with their elderly family members. Many people were unable to attend the funerals of their closest relatives and friends, and could not adequately mourn their loss [21]. As a result of all these changes, stigma has been an important problem during the COVID-19 pandemic period. It has been modified through human interactions, social distancing, and other restrictions to limit the spread of the virus. Much more emphasis has been put on health systems, which are often under heavy load, and they have become inadequate. Inadequacies in health systems have led to inequalities among people in accessing health. As a result of health inequalities, the COVID-19 pandemic has rekindled or strengthened sensitive social issues such as stigma, discrimination, and racism [22]. In a qualitative study conducted in Pakistan, participants described their neighbors' hostile attitudes when COVID-19 was detected in their family members. Neighbors asked some people to leave the neighborhood. A person whose spouse had COVID-19 reported that other family members were reluctant to meet with him, even though his spouse's test result was negative. This stigma has even been reported among doctors. A 55-year-old doctor whose wife contracted the coronavirus explained that despite a negative test result and taking protective measures at work, he was treated as if he was a carrier of the infection. People who have been found to have COVID-19 in their relatives have also been exposed to discrimination in the workplace. Some participants felt that the stigma and discrimination they faced in their region were so great. They reported that they had a problem and that they were planning to change their houses [23]. We can say that this group is at high risk of stigmatization since the disease especially affects the population over the age of 65. At the same time, returnees from abroad face stigma [24]. Stigma has become a serious problem for healthcare professionals, especially during the COVID-19 pandemic. During such epidemics of widespread infectious disease, healthcare workers are often stigmatized by people in their own community [3]. During the COVID-19 pandemic, healthcare workers are hailed as "heroes" in the media. However, this does not eliminate the possibility of discriminatory attitudes towards healthcare professionals based on the fear that healthcare professionals are carriers of COVID-19. In a study conducted in the United States and Canada during the COVID-19 pandemic, an online questionnaire about stigmatizing healthcare professionals was administered to 3551 non-healthcare workers. More than a quarter of respondents reported that health workers should be kept separate from their communities and families. More than one-third of respondents reported avoiding healthcare workers for fear of infection. People who stigmatize healthcare workers also tend to avoid other people, avoid pharmacies and supermarkets, and stay at home all the time [25]. In a study conducted in Egypt with 509 physicians, 138 of whom directly care for COVID-19 patients, 159 (31.2%) physicians reported severe COVID-19-related stigma. The overall COVID-19-related stigma score was higher in those working in the quarantine hospital. A significant number of physicians have experienced the stigma associated with COVID-19 [26]. In another study conducted with 529 physicians during the COVID-19 process, approximately one-third (31%) of the participants reported that they were concerned about stigma due to their profession as a healthcare workers. About 13.8% reported that they were worried about avoiding family members due to stigma [27]. Stigma adds an unnecessary burden to healthcare workers' lives and can contribute to healthcare worker burnout [28]. For this reason, protective measures should be taken against stigmatization, especially among healthcare professionals, and more support should be provided to healthcare professionals in this regard. In cases where stigma is high, people may tend to hide the disease as a coping strategy to avoid discrimination. Hiding infections and avoiding testing is a serious problem and can contribute to an increased risk of infection and a decrease in protective behaviors [29]. Additionally, the stigma associated with COVID-19 can become a barrier to control and prevent COVID-19. It is because people with high levels of stigma are less likely to explain their health status and seek treatment [13]. WHO Director-General Dr. As Tedros Adhanom Ghebreyesus stated that "Honestly, stigma is more dangerous than the coronavirus itself" [30]. The stigma associated with infectious diseases is associated with the clinical features of such diseases and socio-cultural factors [31, 32]. For example, hepatitis A survivors rarely suffer from stigma, but hepatitis B and C survivors often experience high levels of stigma due to more serious long-term effects [33]. Because COVID-19 disease is caused by a new virus, it is not clear how widespread or severe stigma is among survivors. The effect of stigma in the future is a matter of curiosity.

## 5. Definition of xenophobia

Xenophobia is literally a compound word formed by two Latin words. It found its semantic equivalent with the combination of the words xénos, which indicates the difference, and phóbos, which means fear and/or horror, and entered the literature in the sense of the individual or society's fear of the foreign and different from themselves. The state of being afraid of strangers, which is mentioned within the scope of the definition of xenophobia, also includes a discriminating, hateful, humiliating, and standardizing hostile attitude towards a different person. In this context, the target audience includes people who are not those from the relevant region, who are not citizens, or who differ in this context [34]. Xenophobia is defined as "attitudes, prejudices, and behaviors that reject, exclude, and often disparage people who are foreign to the society or national identity or who are perceived as a foreign" [35]. In order to understand the concept of xenophobia, it is useful to distinguish it from the concept of racism, which is often confused with each other. While xenophobia expresses a behavior based on the idea that the other is alien to the group; racism explains discrimination based on differences in physical characteristics such as skin color, hair type, and face shape. Racism is also considered the most extreme level of xenophobia [35]. In recent years, migration movements have increased and continue to increase in the world with the expectation of regional conflicts, climate change, security, employment, education, health, and generally higher welfare [36]. While the concept of alien can be considered a universal concept, this is not the case for xenophobia. Xenophobia is an emerging concept: it was first used by Anatole France in 1901 in Monsieur Bergeret a Paris. Situations such as the term anti-Semitism of the Dreyfus affair that shook domestic politics in France at the turn of the twentieth century, and the violent form of nationalism that emerged at the time provided a social and political background for xenophobia [37]. In 1906—the full year of Dreyfus' rehabilitation - xenophobia was first listed in a French dictionary: Nou eau Larousse illustre. In the following years, it was included in the dictionary in many languages, especially in English [38]. The concept of xenophobia came to the fore again in the COVID-19 epidemic and became the subject of research.

## 6. Xenophobia associated with COVID-19

The effects of the pandemic, which has heavily influenced all countries in the world, are felt in many areas socially, economically, politically, and spiritually [39, 40]. Pandemics have historically been linked to political and economic relations, foreign interventions, conflict, and concerns about maintaining social control in society [41]. The COVID-19 pandemic, on the one hand, contributed to the mutual solidarity and support of states, societies, and individuals from different socioeconomic statuses, on the other hand, it also caused widespread fears and concerns that triggered the current culture of distrust and discrimination, especially against immigrants. Due to the pandemic, social and economic inequalities towards immigrants have increased, and immigrants have been discriminated against and stigmatized [42]. Immigrants have been one of the vulnerable groups that have suffered the most during the pandemic [43]. Xenophobia spread like the virus itself, affecting not only those of Chinese descent but also those of any East Asian descent or nationality [44]. The increase in the prevalence of xenophobia causes stigmatization and targeting of various groups in the society and therefore the inability to provide health services appropriately [45]. In order to evaluate xenophobia comprehensively, it is necessary to acknowledge how certain diseases and social conditions fuel fear and discrimination, and that the stigmatization of various groups in society due to the disease is an important challenge for global development [46]. Throughout history, viral diseases have often been associated with the place or regions where outbreaks first occurred. In 2015, WHO issued guidelines to stop this practice and thereby reduce prejudice and xenophobia towards these regions or people of these regions [47]. Despite these guidelines for naming diseases in order to avoid stigmatizing communication, stigmatizing expressions such as "Spanish flu" and "Mexican swine flu" are frequently used. Such stigmatizing statements suggest that there is a relationship between strangers and a particular epidemic, leading to increased fear of strangers [48]. Efforts are ongoing to prevent the use of false and stigmatizing statements. However, as the number of COVID-19 cases increased in the US and around the world in early 2020, terms such as Chinese virus, Kung-Flu, Chinese coronavirus, and Wuhan virus were used for the COVID-19 virus by leaders in the US and some sections of society [49]. Such naming of the virus has led to the legitimization of the negativities towards Asian communities, the disruption of treatment services, and the stigma of these communities. With the study of Reny and Barreto, it has been experimentally proven that linking the pandemic to a social group in this way will activate negative attitudes towards Asian communities [49]. Even the smallest changes in expression styles and communication are reflected in the way socio-cultural structures are presented and perceived. The style and language used in the transmission of information about the virus can contribute greatly to the spread of xenophobia as well as to its prevention. In the current situation, the widespread stigmatization of immigrants with negative expressions causes an increase in xenophobia. It is seen that racist acts against Asians and Asian-Americans have increased in connection with

COVID-19 cases in the USA, and Asian societies have become vulnerable to verbal and physical abuse due to widespread prejudices [45]. Verbal and physical abuse of Asian Americans has been reported at subway stations in Los Angeles and New York [45]. It was reported that 1135 verbal abuse, embarrassment, and physical attacks against Asian Americans took place in the USA in 2 weeks [42]. In another study conducted in Malaysia, it was determined that xenophobia and racism towards Rohingyas increased due to the COVID-19 pandemic. This is supported by reports of increased hate speech against the Rohingya, both on social media and in government discourse [50]. In a study conducted with Asian university students in Poland, it was determined that the COVID-19 pandemic triggered xenophobic attitudes towards students. 61.2% of the students stated that they were exposed to prejudice, and 47.1% stated that these prejudiced attitudes occurred on public transport and on the street. Reactions towards Asian students are keeping away from them, changing seats on the bus, maintaining a safe distance, covering mouth and nose, showing judgmental facial expressions, pointing fingers and speaking in a whisper, spitting, throwing beer bottles, and using offensive language [51]. Another study found that 90% of respondents in China displayed discriminatory attitudes towards people from Hubei province, such as reporting their presence to local authorities, avoiding them, and actively removing them from their communities [52]. There are concerns that verbal and physical attacks on Asians may continue to increase during the pandemic. In hospitals, some patients have been observed verbally abusing Asian service providers and refusing care. Some Asians and Asian-Americans stated that they may not seek help for fear of discrimination, both in public spaces and within the healthcare system. This puts communities at risk. The increase in racist acts against Asian communities, especially due to fear and misinformation, puts these communities at risk in terms of not only their physical health but also their mental health [42].

## 7. Risk factors for stigma and xenophobia associated with COVID-19

There are several risk factors for stigma and xenophobia. One of them is isolation and quarantine practices. Social distancing in the COVID-19 pandemic is an effective way to reduce morbidity and mortality. However, it should be noted that social distancing can increase stigma for affected populations [5]. It has been reported that quarantine, hopelessness, financial losses are associated with social stigma during the COVID-19 process. Quarantined individuals are more likely to be stigmatized and socially rejected. Stigma is a very important issue, especially for involving people who are quarantined. Media reporting is a powerful tool for influencing public opinion and contributed to stigma in previous outbreaks [53]. It is reported in the literature that there may be people who carry the virus asymptomatically in the COVID-19 pandemic. This is another risk factor for stigma and xenophobia. People can see and stigmatize other people as a constant carrier [54]. Those with COVID-19 may be accused of not following stay-at-home directives or not taking appropriate precautions when going out. People can be stigmatized even when they do not have the virus. For example, someone with allergies, congestion, and sneezing may be stigmatized for leaving their home while sick [55]. Another risk factor for stigma is social media. When the COVID-19 outbreak broke out, hate speech about China and Chinese people on social media provoked social stigma. In a study, a search for "china and coronavirus" on Twitter found 3,457,402 tweets about China-related to COVID-19. Hate speech was detected in 25,467 tweets [56]. Another risk factor for stigma is the language used. Researchers are careful when naming the COVID-19 virus to avoid any stigma. Tedros Adhanom Ghebreyesus, the director of the World Health Organization, said he needed to come up with a name that does not refer to a geographical place, an animal, a person, or a group of people, but is also pronounced and related to the disease [57]. This sensitivity suggests that pointing to a certain group will increase stigma even when naming the virus. For example, being able to say a patient with a diagnosis of COVID-19 instead of a patient with COVID can reduce stigma. Words can create a stigma against geographic regions and certain populations and cause prejudice and panic [5]. Pandemics can cause intense stigma in certain populations. For example, during the 2003 SARS epidemic, discrimination against people of Asian descent was widely reported worldwide, affecting the care-seeking behavior and mental health of many people of Asian descent [4]. The African-Americans Policy Forum (AAPF), an advocacy group for Asian Americans in the United States, reported 1500 incidents of discrimination in 45 states between March 19, 2020, and April 24, 2020. These complaints ranged from verbal abuse to physical attacks in public. Most of the complaints were reported as verbal abuse, including children and the elderly [18]. A Chinese group also living in the UK received intense stigmatizing and accusatory Facebook posts [58]. It is necessary to be very careful when giving news about health workers who are at risk of intense stigma. Exposure to dramatic news images of sick and deceased healthcare professionals can cause the viewing public to exaggerate the risk of personal infection and stigmatize healthcare professionals [59]. In the pandemic process, the influence of the media and politicians comes to the fore as two important factors that trigger xenophobic tendencies towards immigrants. Discourses in the media and the way politicians plan and conduct the pandemic process and the expressions they use in this process shape attitudes and perceptions towards immigrants in society [42].

## 8. The economic and psychosocial effects of the stigma and xenophobia associated with COVID-19

With the onset of the COVID-19 pandemic, psychosocial and economic problems began to be experienced all over the world. Some of these problems were related to stigmatizing and xenophobic attitudes. Stigma can lead to disadvantages in many areas of life, including interpersonal relationships, education, and work-life. Such discriminatory attitudes can limit life opportunities, for example, through loss of income, unemployment, reduced access to housing or health care [60]. Individuals who perceive that they are stigmatized may report guilt, self-blame behavior, self-devaluation, self-isolation, low self-esteem, and being ostracized or ignored by others. Stigma is closely related to mental health problems, especially depression. Studies have found strong positive associations between stigma and depression; depression and stigma also have some common symptoms such as guilt, self-blame, and low self-esteem [61]. Reports from various countries show that discriminatory and xenophobic behavior causes food insecurity and the return of immigrants to their home countries [42]. With the rise of xenophobic tendencies in the USA, the demands for Asian Americans to return to their countries have also increased, and this has led to the greater exclusion of Asian Americans in society [62]. Asian Americans face serious problems such as physical assault, verbal abuse, coughing on themselves, being fired from shops and restaurants, discrimination, and vandalism in the workplace [63].

## 9. Groups at risk for stigma and xenophobia associated with COVID-19

People over the age of 65 suffer from the disease more severely due to the effect of other existing medical diseases. With the spread of the coronavirus and growing fear and anxiety, especially among older adults, the issue of coronavirus stigma in older people has become a major social concern. Elderly people are accused of ignoring their own health and public health because they do not comply with protective measures sufficiently [64]. Disregarding their own will, they are the target of more prohibitive measures, and ageism has been exacerbated during this pandemic. The hypothesis that older people are more likely to have COVID-19 leads to the fact that people in the community are less likely to contact with older people. This led to the isolation of the elderly. This stigma can weaken social cohesion in the elderly and lead to social isolation among older adults [65]. In the first days of the epidemic, people living in China, even from all Asian countries, foreigners or foreigners were perceived as a possible threat. Refugees were included in the current risk group. Many names that affect the public, from heads of states to officials, made speeches accusing refugees of spreading the virus; discrimination and hate crimes against Mexicans in the USA, Africans in Italy, and refugee groups in Bosnia, Jordan, Singapore, and Greece took place in the press [66]. Health workers who are in close contact with patients may be excluded, and when people around them see them in shopping, in an apartment, or at home, they may exhibit discriminatory behaviors even when necessary physical distance and adequate precautions are taken. In May 2020, 13 humanitarian organizations such as the World Medical Association, Red Crescent, Red Cross and medical associations made a statement to draw attention to and prevent attacks against healthcare workers during the pandemic. In many different countries, from Mexico to India, healthcare workers are being attacked for fear of transmitting COVID [1]. Burnout is more common in healthcare workers who are faced with stigmatization [67].

## 10. The role of media and information pollution (infodemia) in stigma and xenophobia associated with COVID-19

During the pandemic period, people mostly stayed in touch via social media as part of social isolation measures. However, there is an increase in the number of false information and fake news that can negatively affect the health and life of individuals on social media [68]. WHO director Tedros made a statement as "we are not only fighting a pandemic, we are also fighting an infodemic" when the COVID-19 pandemic started [18]. Infodemia is a word derived from the English words "information" and "pandemic". Infodemia can be defined as the excessive circulation of misinformation. WHO reported that the spread of unrealistic or erroneous information about COVID-19 can cause panic and fear in societies, make it difficult to fight the disease, and increase stigma [69]. The spread of false or false information about COVID-19 can cause panic and fear in communities. It can complicate the fight against the disease as well as increase stigma and xenophobia [70]. One of the most negative consequences of the epidemic is the rise of xenophobia. Media reports can have this effect. The lives of individuals exposed to xenophobia may be adversely affected by this situation [49]. Infodemia is a facilitating factor of the stigma associated with COVID-19 [71]. Infodemia is also a serious problem for vaccination studies. Misinformation about COVID-19 vaccines is a serious threat to both public health and national economic security [72]. The infodemic brought by each epidemic has become one of the most compelling factors at the center of the COVID-19 struggle, with the spread of social media communication networks in the recent period.

## 11. Preventing stigma and xenophobia associated with COVID-19

Stigma and xenophobia are serious problems. Countries that are successful in infection control thanks to methods such as strict screening, patient isolation, contact tracing, and quarantine should also address the risk of stigma and the negative effects that may arise. Disease-related education and provision of quarantine and public health information to the general public can reduce stigma [5]. Applying strategies to reduce stigma in other diseases for COVID-19 may be important to combat stigma. People affected by COVID-19 should be actively involved in the development and implementation of stigma mitigation strategies and interventions. Lack of correct information and misinformation are the main causes of xenophobia and stigma. This should be taken into account in stigma reduction strategies. Information about COVID-19 should be conveyed concisely and in a culturally appropriate manner to the wider population in a variety of local languages, with particular attention to stigmatized communities. Considered a major force in the fight against COVID 19, the media can play a crucial role by not spreading unconfirmed and exaggerated claims that can promote stigma and xenophobia. The media should spread the right information in order to convey hope, unity, and solidarity to large masses. Finally, it is important to involve those who affect society in the fight against stigma, to create public awareness, and to pay attention to cultural characteristics, to combat stigma during the epidemic [73]. In studies, it is recommended that such studies be carried out and educational interventions should be made with professional staff who have leadership characteristics in the society, such as health workers, police and school children, clergy, headmen, journalists, celebrities. Accurately informing the leading professional groups in society is seen as an effective method in alleviating the burden of stigmatization [74].

## 12. Conclusion

In the current pandemic process, we are going through times that we have never experienced before as the whole world. COVID-19 will have devastating consequences on humanity in the short and long term, causing significant sociological, economic, and psychological problems. Stigma and xenophobia is a barrier to medical evaluation, communication, delivering, and receiving necessary care due to fear and is associated with both physical and mental health complications. Healthcare workers who heroically fight the epidemic during this process are especially at risk of stigmatization. Also, various ethnic groups are at risk of xenophobia in epidemics. COVID-19 related stigma needs to be addressed rigorously by professionals and health care providers as well as authorities. Fighting stigma and xenophobia is a vital issue as much as fighting the epidemic. The pandemic will end one day, but the effects of stigma and xenophobia and the effects of the pandemic may continue for many years and cause devastating results. In addition to developing national strategies to prevent stigma and xenophobia, international cooperation is needed. It is necessary to recognize stigma and xenophobia in epidemic periods and to create training and policies to combat these problems. This will lead to a stronger sense of unity, more effective scientific communication, greater adherence to the rules and guidelines set for combating the pandemic, more efficient use of medical means, and ultimately better management of the pandemic as a whole.

## Acknowledgements

I gratefully commemorate all healthcare professionals who lost their lives due to COVID-19.

## Author details

Dogancan Sonmez and Cicek Hocaoglu*
Department of Psychiatry, Medical School, Recep Tayyip Erdogan University, Rize, Turkey

*Address all correspondence to: cicekh@gmail.com

## References

[1] Available from: https://www.who.int/docs/default-source/coronaviruse/situation-reports/20200121-sitrep-1-2019-ncov.pdf/ [Accessed: August 23, 2021]

[2] Available from: https://www.worldometers.info/coronavirus/ [Accessed: August 23, 2021]

[3] Bagcchi S. Stigma during the COVID-19 pandemic. The Lancet Infectious Diseases. 2020;**20**(7):782. DOI: 10.1016/S1473-3099(20)30498-9

[4] Person B, Sy F, Holton K, Govert B, Liang A, Garza B, et al. Fear and stigma: The epidemic within the SARS outbreak. Emerging Infectious Diseases. 2004;**10**(2):358-363. DOI: 10.3201/eid1002.030750

[5] Bruns DP, Kraguljac NV, Bruns TR. COVID-19: Facts, cultural considerations, and risk of stigmatization. Journal of Transcultural Nursing. 2020;**31**(4):326-332. DOI: 10.1177/1043659620917724

[6] Oxford English Dictionary. 2017

[7] Roberto KJ, Johnson AF, Rauhaus BM. Stigmatization and prejudice during the COVID-19 pandemic. Administrative Theory & Praxis. 2020;**42**(3):364-378. DOI: 10.1080/10841806.2020.1782128

[8] Paananen J, Lindholm C, Stevanovic M, Weiste E. Tensions and paradoxes of stigma: Discussing stigma in mental health rehabilitation. International Journal of Environmental Research and Public Health. 2020;**17**(16):5943. DOI: 10.3390/ijerph17165943

[9] Goffman E. Stigma: Notes on the Management of Spoiled Identity - Erving Goffman. Englewood Cliffs, New Jersey: Prentice-Hall; 1963

[10] Link BG, Phelan JC. Conceptualizing stigma. Annual Review of Sociology. 2001;**27**:363-385. DOI: 10.1146/annurev.soc.27.1.363

[11] Corrigan PW. Dont call me nuts: An international perspective on the stigma of mental illness. Tinley Park, IL: Recovery Press; 2001. p. 228-234

[12] Saeed F, Mihan R, Mousavi SZ, Reniers RLEP, Bateni FS, Alikhani R, et al. A narrative review of stigma related to infectious disease outbreaks: What can be learned in the face of the Covid-19 pandemic? Frontiers in Psychiatry. 2020;**11**:565919. DOI: 10.3389/fpsyt.2020.565919

[13] Hocaoglu C. The Impact of COVID-19 Pandemic on Suicidal Behavior. Londra: IntechOpen; 2021. DOI: 10.5772/intechopen.97663

[14] Yang Y, Peng F, Wang R, Guan K, Jiang T, Xu G, et al. The deadly coronaviruses: The 2003 SARS pandemic and the 2020 novel coronavirus epidemic in China. Journal of Autoimmunity. 2020;**109**:102434. DOI: 10.1016/j.jaut.2020.102434

[15] Huremović D. Brief history of pandemics (pandemics throughout history). In: Psychiatry of Pandemics. 2019. p. 7-35. DOI: 10.1007/978-3-030-15346-5_2

[16] Mak IWC, Chu CM, Pan PC, Yiu MGC, Chan VL. Long-term psychiatric morbidities among SARS survivors. General Hospital Psychiatry. 2009;**31**(4):318-326. DOI: 10.1016/j.genhosppsych.2009.03.001

[17] Gary FA. Stigma: Barrier to mental health care among ethnic minorities. Issues in Mental Health Nursing. 2005;**26**(10):979-999. DOI: 10.1080/01612840500280638

[18] Yılmaz Y, Erdogan A, Hocaoglu C. COVID-19 ve Damgalanma. Kocaeli

Medical Journal. 2021;**10**(1):47-55. DOI: 10.5505/ktd.2021.99266

[19] Oran TN, Şenuzun F. Toplumda kırılması gereken bir zincir: HIV/AIDS stigması ve baş etme stratejileri. Uluslararası İnsan Bilimleri Dergisi. 2008;**8**:1-16

[20] Avcil C, Bulut H, Sayar GH. Psikiyatrik Hastalıklar ve Damgalama. Uluslararası İnsan Bilimleri Dergisi. 2016;**2**:175-202. DOI: 10.32739/uskudarsbd.2.2.4

[21] Bitusikova A. COVID-19 and Funeral-by-Zoom. City Life Beyond Times Pandemic. Journal of Urban Ethnography [Internet]. 2020;**10**(4):515. Available from: http://www.anthrojournal-urbanities.com/vol-10-suppl-4-september-2020/

[22] van Dorn A, Cooney RE, Sabin ML. COVID-19 exacerbating inequalities in the US. Lancet. 2020;**395395**(10232):1243-1244. DOI: 10.1016/s0140-6736(20)30893-x

[23] Rizvi Jafree S, Ul Momina A, Naqi SA. Significant other family members and their experiences of COVID-19 in Pakistan: A qualitative study with implications for social policy. Stigma Health. 2020;**5**(4):380-389. DOI: 10.1037/sah0000269

[24] Aacharya RP, Shah A. Ethical dimensions of stigma and discrimination in Nepal during COVID-19 pandemic. Ethics, Medicine, and Public Health. 2020;**14**:100536. DOI: 10.1016/j.jemep.2020.100536

[25] Taylor S, Landry CA, Rachor GS, Paluszek MM, Asmundson GJG. Fear and avoidance of healthcare workers: An important, under-recognized form of stigmatization during the COVID-19 pandemic. Journal of Anxiety Disorders. 2020;**75**:102289. DOI: 10.1016/j.janxdis.2020.102289

[26] Mostafa A, Sabry W, Mostafa NS. COVID-19-related stigmatization among a sample of Egyptian healthcare workers. PLoS One. 2020;**15**(12):e0244172. DOI: 10.1371/journal.pone.0244172

[27] Al Sulais E, Mosli M, Alameel T. The psychological impact of COVID-19 pandemic on physicians in Saudi Arabia: A cross-sectional study. Saudi Journal of Gastroenterology. 2020;**26**(5):249-255. DOI: 10.4103/sjg.SJG_174_20

[28] Lai J, Ma S, Wang Y, Cai Z, Hu J, Wei N, et al. Factors associated with mental health outcomes among health care workers exposed to coronavirus disease 2019. JAMA Network Open. 2020;**3**(3):e203976. DOI: 10.1001/jamanetworkopen.2020.3976

[29] Fischer LS, Mansergh G, Lynch J, Santibanez S. Addressing disease-related stigma during infectious disease outbreaks. Disaster Medicine and Public Health Preparedness. 2019;**13**(5-6):989-994. DOI: 10.1017/dmp.2018.157

[30] Yuan Y, Zhao YJ, Zhang QE, Zhang L, Cheung T, Jackson T, et al. COVID-19-related stigma and its sociodemographic correlates: A comparative study. Globalization and Health. 2021;**17**(54):1-9. DOI: 10.1186/s12992-021-00705-4

[31] Banerjee D. The impact of Covid-19 pandemic on elderly mental health. International Journal of Geriatric Psychiatry. 2020;**35**(12):1466-1467. DOI: 10.1002/gps.5320

[32] Adom D, Mensah JA, Osei M. The psychological distress and mental health disorders from COVID-19 stigmatization in Ghana. Social Sciences & Humanities Open. 2021;**4**(1):100186. DOI: 10.1016/j.ssaho.2021.100186

[33] Cooke GS, Andrieux-Meyer I, Applegate TL, Atun R, Burry JR, Cheinquer H, et al. Lancet

Gastroenterology & Hepatology Commissioners. Accelerating the elimination of viral hepatitis: a Lancet Gastroenterology & Hepatology Commission. Lancet Gastroenterol Hepatol. 2019;**4**(2):13584. DOI: 10.1016/S2468-1253(19)30099-8

[34] Philippas D. Xenophobia [Internet]. Encyclopedia of Quality of Life and Well-Being Research. Dordrecht: Springer;2014.DOI:10.1007/978-94-007-0753-5_3296

[35] Declaration on racism, discrimination, xenophobia and related intolerance against migrants and trafficked persons. Asia-Pacific NGO Meeting for the World Conference. 2001

[36] Crush J, Ramachandran S. Xenophobia, international migration and development. Journal of Human Development and Capabilities. 2010;**11**(2):209-228. DOI: 10.1080/19452821003677327

[37] Villard P. Naissance d'un mot grec en 1900. Anatole France et les xénophobes. Mots. 1984;**8**:191-195. DOI: 10.3406/mots.1984.1147

[38] Wicker HR. Xenophobia. In: International Encyclopedia of the Social & Behavioral Sciences. Pergamon: Elsevier; 2001. pp. 16649-16652

[39] Akat M, Karataş K. Psychological effects of COVID-19 pandemic on society and its reflections on education. Turkish Studies. 2020;**15**:1-13. DOI: 10.7827/TurkishStudies.44336

[40] Banerjee D, Rai M. Social isolation in Covid-19: The impact of loneliness. The International Journal of Social Psychiatry. 2020;**66**:525-527. DOI 10.1177/0020764020922269

[41] Leach M. Echoes of Ebola: Social and political warnings for the COVID-19 response in African settings. 2020. Available from: http://somatosphere.net/forumpost/echoes-of-ebola/ [Accessed: August 25, 2021]

[42] Bozdağ F. COVID-19 Pandemisinin Toplumsal Etkileri: Zenofobik Eğilimler ve Sonuçları. Psikiyatr Guncel Yaklasimlar. Current Approaches in Psychiatry. 2021;**13**(3):537-550. DOI: 10.18863/pgy.822767

[43] He L, Zhou W, He M, Nie X, He J. Openness and COVID-19 induced xenophobia: The roles of trade and migration in sustainable development. PLoS One. 2021;**16**(4):e0249579. DOI: 10.1371/journal.pone.0249579

[44] Coates M. Covid-19 and the rise of racism. BMJ. 2020;**369**:m1384. Published 2020 Apr 6. DOI:10.1136/bmj.m1384

[45] Batasin SJA. Combating xenophobia in the COVID-19 pandemic: The importance of health literacy. Inquiries Journal. 2020;**12**(7):1

[46] Das M. Social construction of stigma and its implicationsobservations from COVID-19. 2020. Available at: SSRN 3599764. DOI: 10.2139/ssrn.3599764

[47] Zeng G, Wang L, Zhang Z. Prejudice and xenophobia in COVID-19 research manuscripts. Nature Human Behaviour. 2020;**4**(9):879. DOI: 10.1038/s41562-020-00948-y

[48] Hoppe T. "Spanish flu": When infectious disease names blur origins and stigmatize those infected. American Journal of Public Health. 2018;**108**(11): 1462-1464. DOI: 10.2105/AJPH.2018.304645

[49] Reny TT, Barreto MA. Xenophobia in the time of pandemic: othering, anti-Asian attitudes, and COVID-19. Polit Groups, Identities. 2020. DOI: 10.1080/21565503.2020.1769693

[50] Mixed Migration Centre. Understanding the impact of COVID-19

on Rohingya and Bangladeshis in Malaysia [Internet]. 2020. Available from: http://www.mixedmigration.org/wp-content/uploads/2020/07/124_covid_snapshot_Asia.pdf [Accessed: August 23, 2021]

[51] Rzymski P, Nowicki M. COVID-19-related prejudice toward Asian medical students: A consequence of SARS-CoV-2 fears in Poland. Journal of Infection and Public Health. 2020;**13**(6):873-876. DOI: 10.1016/j.jiph.2020.04.013

[52] Adalja AA. Coronavirus, COVID-19: WHO names disease caused by novel [Internet]. Healio. 2020. Available from: https://www.healio.com/infectiousdisease/emerging-diseases/news/online/%7B1cca9ae9-7191-498b-9758-637eab141b71%7D/covid-%0A19-who-names-disease-caused-bynovel-coronavirus [Accessed: August 23, 2021]

[53] Brooks SK, Webster RK, Smith LE, Woodland L, Wessely S, Greenberg N, et al. The psychological impact of quarantine and how to reduce it: Rapid review of the evidence. Lancet. 2020; **395**(10227):912-920. DOI: 10.1016/S0140-6736(20)30460-8

[54] Bai Y, Yao L, Wei T, Tian F, Jin DY, Chen L, et al. Presumed asymptomatic carrier transmission of COVID-19. JAMA. 2020;**14**:1406-1407. DOI: 10.1001/jama.2020.2565

[55] Muschick P. Coronavirus and allergies: Don't sneeze-shame [Internet]. THE MORNING CALL. 2020. Available from: https://www.mcall.com/opinion/mc-opicoronavirus-allegies-sneeze-shaming-muschick-%0A20200313-x7s3bvgdxncs5musjofhsjn5qq-story.html [Accessed: August 23, 2021]

[56] Fan L, Yu H, Yin Z. Stigmatization in social media: Documenting and analyzing hate speech for COVID-19 on Twitter. Proceedings of the Association for Information Science and Technology. 2020;**57**(1):e313. DOI: 10.1002/pra2.313

[57] Organization WHO. Coronavirus disease (COVID19) pandemic [Internet]. 2020. Available from: https://www.who.int/emergencies/diseases/novelcoronavirus-2019 [Accessed: August 23, 2021]

[58] Whitehead D. 'You deserve the coronavirus': Chinese people in UK abused over outbreak [Internet]. Sky News. 2020. Available from: https://news.sky.com/story/coronavirus-chinesepeople-face-abuse-in-the-street-over-outbreak-%0A11931779

[59] Taylor S. The Psychology of Pandemics: Preparing for the Next Global Outbreak of Infectious Disease. Newcastle upon Tyne: Cambridge Scholars Publishing; 2019

[60] Dubey S, Biswas P, Ghosh R, Chatterjee S, Dubey MJ, Chatterjee S, et al. Psychosocial impact of COVID-19. Diabetes & Metabolic Syndrome: Clinical Research and Reviews. 2020;**14**(5):779-788. DOI: 10.1016/j.dsx.2020.05.035

[61] Malta M, Rimoin AW, Strathdee SA. The coronavirus 2019-nCoV epidemic: Is hindsight 20/20? EClinicalMedicine. 2020;**3**(20):100289. DOI: 10.1016/j.eclinm.2020.100289

[62] Cheng H-L. Xenophobia and racism against Asian Americans during the COVID-19 pandemic: Mental health implications. Journal of Interdisciplinary Perspectives and Scholarship. 2020;**3**(1):3

[63] Cheah CSL, Wang C, Ren H, Zong X, Cho HS, Xue X. COVID-19 racism and mental health in Chinese American families. Pediatrics. 2020; **146**(5):e2020021816. DOI: 10.1542/peds.2020-021816

[64] Tehrani H. Mental health stigma related to novel coronavirus disease (COVID-19) in older adults. Geriatrics & Gerontology International. 2020; **20**(8):796-797. DOI: 10.1111/ggi.13985

[65] Wu IHC, Bathje GJ, Kalibatseva Z, Sung DH, Leong FTL, Collins-Eaglin J. Stigma, mental health, and counseling service use: A person-centered approach to mental health stigma profiles. Psychological Services. 2017;**14**(4): 490-501. DOI: 10.1037/ser0000165

[66] Vertovec S. Covid-19 and enduring stigma. Max Planck Inst Study Relig Ethn Divers. Munich. 2020

[67] Ramaci T, Barattucci M, Ledda C, Rapisarda V. Social stigma during COVID-19 and its impact on HCWs outcomes. Sustainability. 2020;**12**(9): 3834. DOI: 10.3390/su12093834

[68] Ren SY, Gao RD, Chen YL. Fear can be more harmful than the severe acute respiratory syndrome coronavirus 2 in controlling the corona virus disease 2019 epidemic. World Journal of Clinical Cases. 2020;**8**(4):652-657. DOI: 10.12998/wjcc.v8.i4.652

[69] Organization WHO. Subject in focus: Developing trans-disciplinary science: Infodemiology, the science behind infodemic management [Internet]. Available from: https://www.who.int/docs/defaultsource/coronaviruse/situation-reports/20200707-%0ACOVID-19-sitrep-169.pdf?sfvrsn=c6c69c88_2

[70] Rathore FA, Farooq F. Information overload and infodemic in the COVID-19 pandemic. The Journal of the Pakistan Medical Association. 2020; **70**(5):162-165. DOI: 10.5455/JPMA.38

[71] Ransing R, Ramalho R, de Filippis R, Ojeahere MI, Karaliuniene R, Orsolini L, et al. Infectious disease outbreak related stigma and discrimination during the COVID-19 pandemic: Drivers, facilitators, manifestations, and outcomes across the world. Brain, Behavior, and Immunity. 2020;**89**:555-559. DOI: 10.1016/j.bbi.2020.07.033

[72] Horton R. Offline: Managing the COVID-19 vaccine infodemic. Lancet. 2020;**396**(10261):1474. DOI: 10.1016/S0140-6736(20)32315-1

[73] Peprah P, Gyasi RM. Stigma and COVID-19 crisis: A wake-up call. The International Journal of Health Planning and Management. 2021;**1**:215-218. DOI: 10.1002/hpm.3065

[74] Thornicroft G, Brohan E, Kassam A, Lewis-Holmes E. Reducing stigma and discrimination: Candidate interventions. International Journal of Mental Health Systems. 2008;**2**(1):3. DOI: 10.1186/1752-4458-2-3

Chapter 8

# COVID-19 Sends the Bill: Socially Disadvantaged Workers Suffer the Severest Losses in Earnings

*Tharcisio Leone*


## Abstract

This work uses a nationally representative household survey conducted by phone during the COVID-19 pandemic to estimate the short-term impacts of lockdown measures on employment and income in Brazil. In May 2020, 18 percent of the employed population (around 15.7 million workers) were temporarily absent from their jobs due to the lockdown policies while 56.6 percent of them were no longer earning an income from work. Similar figures were registered in June 2020. This decrease in employment has generated a fall of 18 percent in the average work income and an increase of 0.014 points in the Gini coefficient. The vulnerable among the population have been hit hardest by the pandemic: the average earnings of the lowest income decile decreased from BRL 389.07 to 0 while for the second-lowest a 70.2 percent reduction has been seen (from BRL 878.08 to BRL 262.06). Thanks to the implementation of the COVID-19 Emergency Aid, the Brazilian government has been able to reduce the losses in income for all social classes. Nevertheless, the average income of the first decile is 5 percent lower than the value pre-pandemic while for the second decile the equivalent figure is 15.2 percent.


**Keywords:** COVID-19, lockdown effects, income, employment, emergency aid, Brazil

## 1. Introduction

Since the outbreak of the novel coronavirus disease in China, COVID-19 has profoundly affected the daily routine of the great majority of the global population and plunged the world into a crisis of unprecedented scope [1]. At an early stage herein, the goal was to avoid the overburdening of the health system. Many countries have worked to "flatten the curve", taking such restrictive measures as travel bans, lockdowns, stay-at-home orders, and quarantines—some of them extremely stringent—to reduce the movement of persons, and, consequently, to slow down the spread of the virus [2].

As the pandemic unfolded, Brazil would become a global hotspot. At the time of this writing, the seventh-most populous nation on the planet was then the second-worst-affected country worldwide with more than 18 million confirmed cases and 510 thousand deaths due to COVID-19. Since the confirmation of the first coronavirus case in Brazil on February 26, 2020, the policy responses to combat the spread of the pandemic have been scattered and uncoordinated [3]. The federal and local governments have found themselves in constant disagreement over the lockdown measures necessary to flatten the curve [4]. However, despite the opposition of President Jair Bolsonaro, all twenty-seven Brazilian states would implement between March 13 and 24, 2020, lockdown measures to reduce the circulation of persons and consequently the spread of the virus. In subsequent weeks, the municipalities followed suit, enacting additional legislation to regulate these stay-at-home orders.

Some empirical studies have already been able to confirm that these lockdown policies were successful in increasing social distancing during the pandemic. Leone [5], for example, used geolocation data from nearly sixty million smartphone users in Brazil to show that the population numbers socially distancing grew considerably after the implementation of the lockdown measures. While the share of stay-at-home individuals in the pre-pandemic phase (January and February 2020) was close to 20 percent, this number increased to 50 percent in the first weeks after lockdown policies were introduced. Similar results were also reported for Italy [6], Sweden [7], and the United States [8–10].

It is therefore no surprise that the impacts of the pandemic go way beyond the mortality rate, and the government responses to it will certainly cause turmoil for the economy. Fernandes [11] estimates a decline of 10.4 percent in global gross domestic product under the scenario whereby the lockdowns last until the end of July. In contrast to many European countries who can mitigate at least parts of their lockdowns' economic disruption through welfare states, in developing ones the most vulnerable among the population have tended to be the biggest losers during the pandemic given the lack of social security coverage [12]. A World Bank study concluded that, at the global level, COVID-19 is pushing between 40 and 60 million into extreme poverty [13]. Sumner et al. [14] also used simulation models to quantify the potential short-term economic impact of the lockdown policies, highlighting that in some regions of the world the pandemic could result in poverty levels being reached similar to those recorded 30 years ago. Based on the worst-case scenario—whereby the per capita income decreases 20 percent—the number of people living in poverty could increase by up to 580 million as compared to 2018.

Despite the valuable contribution of all these empirical simulations of the economic costs related to COVID-19, it is high time to abandon the forecasts and start to estimate the real socioeconomic consequences of the pandemic. This is exactly the main contribution of this chapter to the literature. This work will apply real-time measures of work activities and income levels during the pandemic in Brazil to quantify the short-term economic impacts of COVID-19-related social-distancing policies.

Consequently, this chapter contributes to the rapidly growing literature describing the economic impacts of the coronavirus crisis. While similar studies for developed countries have largely flourished over the past year [15–17], empirical evidence for developing countries is still rare in the literature. Therefore, this work will be the first to apply data from the PNAD COVID-19—a (national) representative household survey conducted by phone with 349,306 Brazilian residents during the pandemic—to estimate the negative impact of the lockdown on employment and income levels in Brazil. Overall, the findings suggest that the measures to flatten the curve have led to a reduction in employment and income—with more significant losses occurring for the most vulnerable parts of the Brazilian populace.

## 2. Data and method

This manuscript uses data from PNAD COVID-19, a recent nationally representative longitudinal survey conducted by the IBGE (Brazilian Institute of Geography and Statistics) with 193,662 households (349,306 individuals). The intention behind it is to continuously produce information about the health status and labor-market characteristics of the domestic population during the pandemic (May–November 2020). Data collection was carried out remotely via telephone calls, and drew on the sample of the PNAD-Contínua (Continuous National Household Sample Survey).[1]

To provide information in real time about the pandemic, PNAD COVID-19 adopts a rotating panel scheme of interviews to produce weekly and monthly consolidated data. This means that every week one-quarter of the involved households are interviewed, and the ongoing main descriptive statistics are published immediately. Then, at the end of the month, the data for the whole sample (193,662 households) are consolidated and made available to the public in the form of microdata. Given the panel structure of the survey, the households can be correctly identified across all the months of PNAD COVID-19, and they can be also linked with the data of the Continuous PNAD—thereby providing the relevant information for the period pre-coronavirus.

From the PNAD COVID-19 sample, two main pieces of information related to personal income will be used in this study here. The first variable (C10) refers to the (normal) earnings before lockdown policies were implemented in March 2020, while the latter (C11a) investigates the same type of income during the pandemic itself. In addition, I use the information on the allocation of COVID-19 Emergency Aid (D0051) to estimate the effects of this social scheme on income distribution.

In a first step, the manuscript identifies the economically active population from the sample, which corresponds to employed and unemployed persons aged 15–64. Employed are those individuals who have worked at least one hour during the reference week or who were temporarily absent from their job; unemployed persons meanwhile are those who were not employed but made some specific active effort to find a job in the same reference week. PNAD COVID-19 shows that the lockdown policies have deeply affected job-seeking, since many people were dissuaded from leaving the home or have anticipated that companies would postpone their new hires. For this reason, this chapter assumes as unemployed also those persons who have not looked for a job but wanted to be working during the identified reference week. Finally, this manuscript differentiates between the population employed in the formal and informal labor markets. Informal are those workers with no employment contract registered via the Work and Social Security Card and self-employed persons who do not pay social security contributions (INSS).

## 3. Home office option

In order to reduce the negative labor-market impacts arising from the lockdown measures to flatten the curve, many governments are encouraging their residents to work from home [18]. A recent policy brief of the International Labour Organization indicated that with the pandemic, 59 countries had implemented telework for nonessential publicly employed staff [1]. In Brazil, a phone-interview survey conducted on 03/20/2020 reported that 46 percent of respondents believed that it would indeed be possible to carry out their employment duties via home office [19]. However empirical evidence shows that the chance to work from home is not distributed equally across the population, since many occupations such as

[1] The PNAD COVID-19 database is publicly available on the website of IBGE. See data collection instrument (available here) and microdata files (available here).

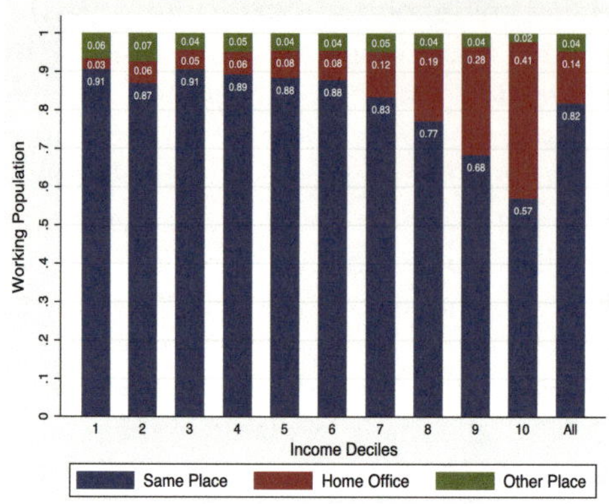


**Figure 1.**
*Workplace during the lockdown. Notes: Income deciles use (normal) personal work income pre-lockdown. Working population refers to individuals aged 15–64 that have worked in the reference week. Percentages are weighted for population size. Workplace in May 2020. Source: Author's own estimates, based on PNAD COVID-19.*

construction workers or street vendors cannot be fulfilled from there [1]. Saltiel [20], for example, found that work-from-home jobs are strong correlated with the educational levels of the workforce; therefore, vulnerable groups are more likely to suffer the negative economic impacts of the coronavirus as their jobs cannot be done from home.

**Figure 1** above examines this hypothesis with the data obtained from the Brazilian case during the month of May 2020.[2] For that, the individuals who have worked in the reference week are sorted according to their (personal) work earnings pre-lockdown and then divided into income deciles.

During the pandemic, 81.9 percent of employees—meaning those who had worked in the reference week—conducted this activity in the same workplace as in the time pre-coronavirus and only 13.5 percent were working from home. However, as predicted in the literature, the chances to work via home office differ greatly according to socioeconomic status. This share is 2.8 percent for the bottom 10 percent of the income distribution, and 40.7 percent for the highest income decile meanwhile.

Looking beyond employment functions can help us to understand this difference across income deciles. PNAD COVID-19 data show that employees with occupations requiring more extensive higher education qualifications were more often found to be working from home during the pandemic. Some 45.4 percent of teachers and 39.6 percent of lawyers, engineers, and journalists were doing home office, while these figures were close to 0 for domestic workers (0.0), doorkeeper (0.2) farmers (0.2), butchers and bakers (0.4).

## 4. Work absenteeism

**Figure 1** was limited to the individuals who continued to work during the pandemic. However, the coronavirus crisis has had also a strong impact on the employment status of workers. **Figure 2** reports the share of the employed

[2] **Figure 3** in Appendix reports the same results for the month of June 2020.

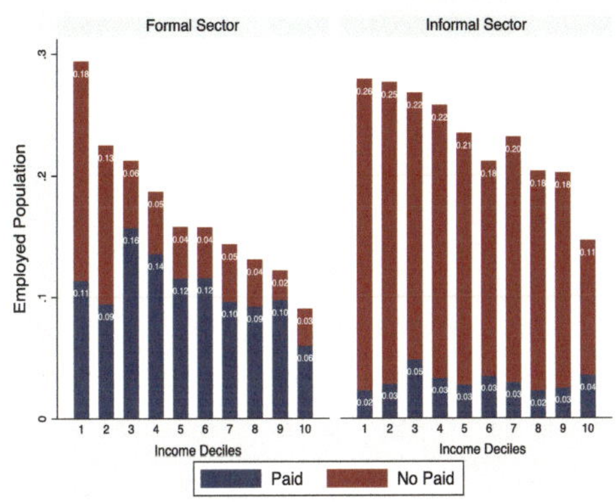


**Figure 2.**
*Temporary work absenteeism due to lockdown. Notes: Income deciles using (normal) personal work income pre-lockdown. Employed population refers to individuals aged 15–64 who worked or were temporarily absent from their jobs in the reference week. Percentages are weighted for population size. Absenteeism related to the month of May 2020. Source: Author's own estimates, based on PNAD COVID-19.*

population who had a job before the lockdown measures but who are in May 2020 temporarily absent from it due to the lockdown policies.[3]

In May 2020, 18.8 percent of the employed population of Brazil—equivalent to 15.7 million workers—were temporarily absent from their job due to social-distancing measures.[4] From this total, 56.9 percent continued to receive (at least one part of) their work earnings, while 43.1 percent had a complete loss of such income. **Figure 2** confirms that vulnerable workers have been hit hardest by the pandemic. The lower the work income, the higher the chance of having become detached from the labor market as a direct result of the lockdown. Informal workers have been especially affected by this trend because they have—independent of their income—a higher chance of being absent from their job, and are more likely to lose all their income in case of work leave. Some 65.5 percent of informal workers who were absent from their job due to the lockdown received no work income in May 2020, compared with a figure of 11.6 percent among the formally employed.

## 5. Impact on income distribution

To highlight the impact of this lockdown-related temporary work absenteeism on income levels, **Table 1** below reports the income distribution in Brazil both before and during the pandemic. Measured are (personal) work incomes for the economically active population aged 15–64, and in the third block (Columns 6 to 7) I add to the investigation the COVID-19 Emergency Aid provided by the Brazilian government to mitigate the economic impact of the lockdown measures.

As shown in the **Table 1**, lockdown increased income inequality within Brazilian society (Gini coefficient rose from 0.467 to 0.481) and reduced the average monthly (work) income of the population by 18 percent (from BRL 2320.18 to BRL 1888.13). It is worth mentioning that all social classes were affected by this income

---

[3] **Figure 4** in Appendix reports the same results for the month of June 2020.

[4] Two further studies show similarly striking results. Silva and Silva [21] found that 18.6 percent of the employed population in Brazil were temporarily absent from their job in Mai 2020 due to the lockdown. Lameiras and Cavalcanti [22] reported a deep fall in this value over time. From 18.7 percent in Mai to 14.2 percent in June and 8.4 percent in July.

| | No lockdown | | | With lockdown | | Lockdown with COVID-19 aid | | Variation in income (%) | |
|---|---|---|---|---|---|---|---|---|---|
| Income | N | Mean | SD | Mean | SD | Mean | SD | A | B |
| Deciles | (1) | (2) | (3) | (4) | (5) | (6) | (7) | (2) to (4) | (2) to (6) |
| 1 | 16,402 | 389.07 | 165.64 | 0.00 | 0.00 | 369.46 | 265.99 | −100.0 | −5.0 |
| 2 | 12,346 | 878.07 | 119.32 | 262.06 | 119.18 | 744.20 | 56.66 | −70.2 | −15.2 |
| 3 | 16,615 | 1044.74 | 1.96 | 649.06 | 118.18 | 995.51 | 62.94 | −37.9 | −4.7 |
| 4 | 13,075 | 1159.40 | 55.43 | 1020.15 | 41.90 | 1149.24 | 54.91 | −12.0 | −0.9 |
| 5 | 16,660 | 1423.94 | 89.75 | 1155.65 | 56.40 | 1408.45 | 88.55 | −18.8 | −1.1 |
| 6 | 5482 | 1624.69 | 49.60 | 1420.43 | 90.48 | 1623.83 | 28.57 | −12.6 | −0.1 |
| 7 | 12,670 | 1940.66 | 88.25 | 1689.03 | 91.58 | 1878.85 | 110.99 | −13.0 | −3.2 |
| 8 | 16,340 | 2614.84 | 325.28 | 2164.81 | 217.58 | 2331.64 | 192.59 | −17.2 | −10.8 |
| 9 | 8012 | 3787.96 | 402.86 | 3290.82 | 446.96 | 3300.09 | 422.25 | −13.1 | −12.9 |
| 10 | 11,247 | 9159.61 | 7220.26 | 8581.21 | 6044.45 | 8412.53 | 5951.34 | −6.3 | −8.2 |
| Total | 128,849 | 2302.18 | 3272.54 | 1888.13 | 2854.72 | 2121.55 | 2797.30 | −18.0 | −7.8 |
| GINI | | 0.467 | | 0.481 | | 0.433 | | | |

*Notes: Calculation using personal income of the economically active population aged 15–64. No lockdown refers to work income before the pandemic. With Lockdown denotes the work income in May 2020. Lockdown with COVID-19 Aid adds to the work income of May 2020 the emergency support of BRL 600 per person paid by the Brazilian government. Values are in BRL, and weighted for population size.*
*Source: Author's own estimates, based on PNAD COVID-19.*

**Table 1.**
*Atleast Income distribution before and during lockdown.*

reduction. However, in relative terms, it is the bottom decile who have suffered the greatest losses. The average income of this group—which was BRL 389.07 in the period pre-lockdown—decreased to 0 in May 2020; in other words, around 8.5 million people have lost their entire work income during the course of the pandemic.

PNAD COVID-19 reports that 68 million Brazilian households (38.7 percent) have benefited from COVID-19 Emergency Aid. Therefore, as shown in **Table 1**, this financial support has helped to mitigate the economic losses induced by lockdown and has made all the income deciles better off than they would otherwise be.

These findings are in line with the conclusions of other studies. Carvalho [23] and Duque [24] confirmed the effectiveness of the COVID-19 Emergency Aid in reducing poverty and neutralizing, at least in part, the income losses caused by the crisis. Pires et al. [25] emphasized the positive impact of the COVID-19 Aid on income inequality, measured by the Gini coefficient. While the lockdown's initial impact generated an increase of 5 percent in the income inequality, the implementation of the emergency cash transfer was responsible for the reduction of the income distribution to a level lower than the pre-pandemic period.

Despite this positive impact of the COVID-19 Emergency Aid, **Table 1** shows that these gains were not evenly distributed the Brazilian society. The deciles in the center of the income distribution (fourth, fifth, and sixth) enjoyed the greatest

[4] Two further studies show similarly striking results. Silva and Silva [21] found that 18.6 percent of the employed population in Brazil were temporarily absent from their job in Mai 2020 due to the lockdown. Lameiras and Cavalcanti [22] reported a deep fall in this value over time. From 18.7 percent in Mai to 14.2 percent in June and 8.4 percent in July.

benefit in relative terms: the (average) income including also the emergency aid of the fourth decile, for example, was only 0.9 percent lower than the value pre-coronavirus. The second income decile has experienced the highest percentage loss of income meanwhile: between earnings and COVID-19 emergency aid, this group had an average income of BRL 744.20 in May 2020, which is 15.2 percent lower than the equivalent figure pre-pandemic (BRL 878.07).

## 6. Conclusion

Using data from a recently published (national) representative phone survey, this chapter has calculated the impact of the COVID-19-related lockdown policies on employment status and income levels in Brazil. Linking the socioeconomic variables of 349,306 individuals across 193,662 households before and during the imposed social-distancing measures (May and June 2020), this manuscript found that home office is a significant option only for the more advantaged sections of society. For the bottom deciles vis-à-vis income distribution, the chance to work from home remains a distant dream.

With the pandemic, 18.8 percent of the employed population in Brazil (around 15.7 million workers) have been temporarily absent from their professional activities and 56.6 percent of them have completely lost their work income. This reduction in employment has generated a fall of 18 percent in the average work income, with more significant losses for the poorest sectors of the population: the average work income of the lowest income decile decreased from BRL 389.07 to 0 and for the second decile the reduction has been 70.2 percent (from BRL 878.08 to BRL 262.06). Informal workers have been doubly economically burdened during the pandemic, since they have a greater probability of being absent from their job, and —if out of work—they are more likely to completely lose their work income.

In addition, this chapter has addressed the importance of state interventions to mitigate the negative impact of social-distancing measures on the socioeconomic environment of the domestic population. The COVID-19 Emergency Aid implemented by the Brazilian (federal) government has compensated—at least in part—for the income losses due to the enforced lockdown policies, increasing the average income from BRL 1888.13 to BRL 2121.55. However, this value is still 7.8 percent lower than the average work income amount pre-coronavirus.

## Conflict of interest

The author declares no conflict of interest.

## Abbreviations

| | |
|---|---|
| BRL | Brazilian Real |
| IBGE | Brazilian Institute of Geography and Statistics |
| INSS | National Institute of Social Security |
| PNAD | National Household Sample Survey |

# Appendix. Figures for June 2020

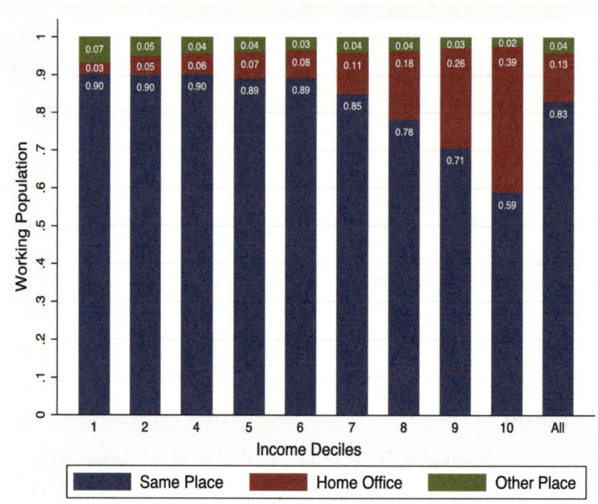


**Figure 3.**
*Workplace during the lockdown. Notes: Income deciles use (normal) personal work income pre-lockdown. Working population refers to individuals aged 15–64 that have worked in the reference week. Percentages are weighted for population size. Workplace in June 2020. Source: Author's own estimates, based on PNAD COVID-19.*

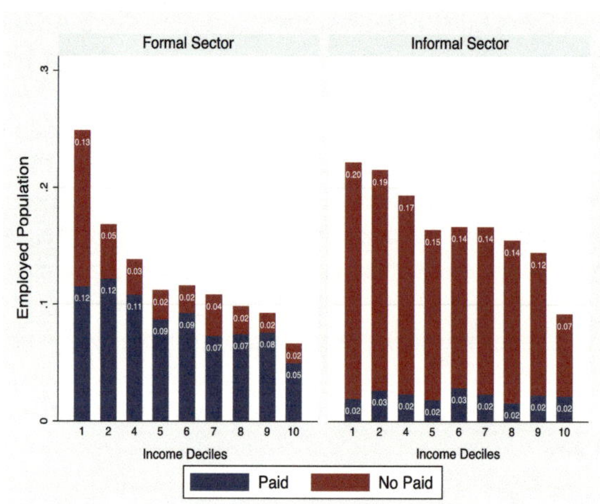


**Figure 4.**
*Temporary work absenteeism due to lockdown. Notes: Income deciles using (normal) personal work income pre-lockdown. Employed population refers to individuals aged 15–64 who worked or were temporarily absent from their jobs in the reference week. Percentages are weighted for population size. Absenteeism related to the month of June 2020. Source: Author's own estimates, based on PNAD COVID-19.*

## Author details

Tharcisio Leone
German Institute for Global and Area Studies (GIGA), Hamburg, Germany

*Address all correspondence to: tharcisio.leone@giga-hamburg.de

## References

[1] Berg J, Bonnet F, Soares S. Working from home: Estimating the worldwide potential. VoxEU CEPR Policy Portal. 2020;**11**. Available from: https://voxeu.org/article/working-home-estimating-worldwide-potential

[2] Nicola M, Alsafi Z, Sohrabi C, Kerwan A, Al-Jabir A, Iosifidis C, et al. The socio-economic implications of the coronavirus pandemic (COVID-19): A review. International Journal of Surgery. 2020;**78**:185-193

[3] Ajzenman N, Tiago C, Da Mata D. Leaders' speech and risky behaviour during a pandemic. VoxEU.org. 2020;**2**. Available from: https://voxeu.org/article/leaders-speech-and-risky-behaviour-during-pandemic

[4] Aquino EM, Silveira IH, Pescarini JM, Aquino R, Souza-Filho JAD, Rocha ADS, et al. Social distancing measures to control the COVID-19 pandemic: Potential impacts and challenges in Brazil. Ciência and Saúde Coletiva. 2020;**25**:2423-2446

[5] Leone T. The harmful effects of denial: When political polarization meets COVID-19 social distancing. Middle Atlantic Review of Latin American Studies. 2021;**4**(3):10-30

[6] Durante R, Guiso L, Gulino G. Civic capital and social distancing: Evidence from italians' response to COVID-19. VoxEU Column. 2020. Available from: https://voxeu.org/article/civic-capital-and-social-distancing

[7] Dahlberg M, Edin PA, Grönqvist E, Lyhagen J, Östh J, Siretskiy A, Toger M. Effects of the COVID-19 pandemic on population mobility under mild policies: Causal evidence from Sweden; 2020. arXiv preprint arXiv:2004.09087

[8] Chiou L, Tucker C. Social Distancing, Internet Access and Inequality. Cambridge, MA: National Bureau of Economic Research; 2020

[9] Farboodi M, Jarosch G, Shimer R. Internal and External Effects of Social Distancing in a Pandemic. Cambridge, MA: National Bureau of Economic Research; 2020

[10] Villas-Boas SB, Sears J, Villas-Boas M, Villas-Boas V. Are We StayingHome to Flatten the Curve? Department of Agricultural and Resource Economics. UC Berkeley: CUDARE Working Papers; 2020

[11] Fernandes N. Economic Effects of Coronavirus Outbreak (COVID-19) on the World Economy (March 22, 2020). IESE Business School Working Paper No. WP-1240-E. Available at SSRN: https://ssrn.com/abstract=3557504

[12] Blofield M, Hoffmann B, Llanos M. Assessing the Political and Social Impact of the COVID-19 Crisis in Latin America. Hamburg, Germany: GIGA Focus Latin America; 2020

[13] Mahler D, Lakner C, Aguilar C, Wu H. The Impact of COVID-19 (Coronavirus) on Global Poverty: Why Sub-Saharan Africa Might be the Region Hardest Hit. Washington, DC: Blog. The World Bank; 2020. p. 20

[14] Sumner, A., Hoy, C., Ortiz-Juarez, E. (2020). Estimates of the impact of COVID-19 on global poverty (No. 2020/43). WIDER working paper

[15] Brynjolfsson E, Horton JJ, Ozimek A, Rock D, Sharma G, TuYe HY. COVID-19 and Remote Work: An Early Look at US Data (No. w27344). Cambridge, MA: National Bureau of Economic Research; 2020

[16] Cameron A. Coronavirus and Homeworking in the UK: April 2020. UK Office of National Statistics (ONS).

2020. Available from: https://www.ons.gov.uk/employmentandlabourmarket/peopleinwork/employmentandemployeetypes/bulletins/coronavirusandhomeworkingintheuk/april2020

[17] Okubo T, Inoue A, Sekijima K. Teleworker performance in the COVID-19 era in Japan. Asian Economic Papers. 2021;**20**(2):175-192

[18] Mongey S, Weinberg A. Characteristics of Workers in Low Work-from-Home and High Personal-Proximity Occupations. Chicago, IL: Becker Friedman Institute for Economic White Paper; 2020

[19] Carta Capital. 54% dos brasileiros dizem que não poderão trabalhar em casa durante quarentena. 2020. Available from: https://www.cartacapital.com.br/sociedade/54-dos-brasileiros-dizem-que-nao-poderao-trabalhar-em-casa-durante-quarentena/ [Accessed: June 14, 2021]

[20] Saltiel F. Who can work from home in developing countries. Covid Economics. 2020;7(2020):104-118

[21] Silva TD, Silva SP. Trabalho, população negra e pandemia: notas sobre os primeiros resultados da PNAD COVID-19. Nota Tãcnica / IPEA. Diest, 46. Brasília. 2020

[22] Lameiras MAP, Cavalcanti MAFDH. PNAD COVID-19: divulgação de 17/7/2020: Principais destaques. Carta Conjunt.(Inst. Pesqui. Econ. Apl.). 2020;**48**:1-5

[23] Carvalho SSD. Os efeitos da pandemia sobre os rendimentos do trabalho e o impacto do auxílio emergencial: os resultados dos microdados da PNAD COVID-19 de junho. Carta Conjunt.(Inst. Pesqui. Econ.). 2020;**48**:1-16

[24] Duque D. Uma avaliação do Auxílio Emergencial: Parte 1. Blog do IBRE. 2020. Available from: https://blogdoibre.fgv. br/posts/uma-avaliacao-do-auxilio-emergencial-parte-1

[25] Pires LN, de Carvalho LB, Rawet EL. Multi-dimensional inequality and COVID-19 in Brazil. Investigación Económica. 2021;**80**(315):33-58

Chapter 9

# Why Knowledge Sharing Increases Well-Being – The Case of Adult Fans of LEGO

*Kei Aoki*

## Abstract

Since 2020, we have faced drastic changes in our lives due to the pandemic. This caused a big paradigm shift in working styles. Parallel careers or multiple jobs are getting more common, and people are ascertaining their own competencies. The utilization of personal knowledge will continue to accelerate and this study sheds light on its societal value; the other side of sharing economy. Aoki (2021) revealed that participation in knowledge sharing has a significant positive impact on contributors' well-being. Those findings are more pertinent as utilization of personal knowledge increases under the ongoing paradigm shift in work style, and the expansion of C-to-C business. However, the reason for the correlation between knowledge sharing and well-being has not been identified. Thus, this study explores this issue by carefully examining knowledge-sharing contributors and their experiences. Finally, this study finds that contributors increased their well-being by deepening their knowledge and experience via competitive co-creation. Furthermore, their concerns shifted towards passing on their knowledge and experience to the next generation. Stakeholders of this study's results are those who utilize personal knowledge. For example, policymakers who wish to shed light on people with hidden potential, managers of knowledge-sharing platforms, such as crowdsourcing, marketing managers who collaborate with consumers, employers who wish to motivate their employees, and so on.

**Keywords:** user innovation, co-creation, social welfare, positive psychology, PERMA

## 1. Introduction

Since 2020, we have faced drastic changes in our lives due to the pandemic. This caused a big paradigm shift in working styles. Parallel careers or multiple jobs are getting more common, and people are ascertaining their own competencies. The utilization of personal knowledge will continue to accelerate and this study sheds light on its societal value.

Aoki [1] revealed that participation in knowledge sharing has a significant positive impact on contributors' well-being. Those findings are more pertinent as utilization of personal knowledge increases under the ongoing paradigm shift in work style, and the expansion of C-to-C business. However, the reason for the correlation between knowledge sharing and well-being has not been identified. This research aims to reveal the relationship between knowledge sharing and well-being.

Due to the growing sharing economy and the large ongoing paradigm shift in work styles caused by the pandemic, people have more opportunities to utilize their personal knowledge than ever before. However, vast amounts of personal knowledge are untapped. For instance, one instantiation of personal knowledge is user innovation, and user innovation research has pointed out the 'market failure' in its diffusion due to a lack of incentives for the innovators [2, 3]. This study contributes to increase knowledge sharing and filling the gap between personal knowledge and society.

### 1.1 User innovation and social welfare

Since von Hippel [4] pointed out that not only manufacturers but also 'users' innovate, user innovation has been studied by various researchers throughout the world. In early research, the term 'users' referred to firms that were supplied products by manufacturers; in other words, user innovation was carried out in the business-to-business community. Over the decades, the importance of individual consumers as user innovators has been articulated (e.g. [5]). In this digital era, the line between a firm and a consumer is becoming blurred, and co-creation between the two has become pervasive.

Some users innovate by themselves and whose innovations occasionally have been commercially successful. Previous studies showed that user innovations increased social welfare because user innovators created financial value from their leisure-time activities [6, 7]. Furthermore, user innovation is distinct from producer innovation in that the former provides benefits from participation, including the use or sale of the output to the innovators themselves [6, 8]. Consequently, user innovation which brings satisfaction to the innovators increases social welfare better than producer innovation.

### 1.2 Diffusion of user innovation

Even if it has a high potential to enhance social welfare, user innovation tends to be restricted to innovators themselves and not diffused. User innovators are likely to choose free information diffusion, rather than paid diffusion, and avoid seeking commercialization on their own or through an existing firm, because it costs more than they would gain. Earlier studies have shown 'market failure' in user innovation diffusion [2, 3]. When valuable innovation remains underground, it is society's loss.

Each user innovation is based on personal needs, which, by nature, are self-centered. Thus, innovation communities play an important role in integrating these isolated individuals [5]. Baldwin et al. [9] revealed that user innovators who commercialized their innovations had participated in innovation communities at an earlier stage and improved their ideas. Earlier research has shown that user communities play an important role in diffusing user innovations and has examined the innovators' motivations to participate in these communities.

People tend to join peer communities (e.g., open-source software communities) to fulfill personal needs. Then, their participation becomes a hobby, and they discover that they are helping other people [10]. In addition to personal needs, feedback from peers and enjoyment were found to be important motivations [11–14]. Feedback in the user community also plays a key role in increasing entrepreneurship [10, 15].

### 1.3 Knowledge sharing and well-being

Diffusion of user innovation is ultimate knowledge sharing and contributors enjoy financial and/or non-financial benefits from sharing. Aoki [1] focused on non-financial benefits and revealed that knowledge sharing increases contributors' well-being.

In terms of psychology, Seligman [16] defined well-being as the ultimate objective of positive psychology. He argued that well-being is sustainable and separate from 'happiness' and suggested the importance of flourishing as a standard to measure well-being. Flourishing consists of five elements, positive emotion, engagement, relationship, meaning, accomplishment, or PERMA for short [16]. Each element represents the following.

- Positive emotion: a subjective feeling of well-being itself
- Engagement: a subjective feeling denoting the extent to which people are absorbed in something
- Relationships with others
- Meaning: the extent how lives are meaningful for themselves
- Accomplishment, the extent how people accomplish something in their lives

Aoki [1] visualized non-financial benefits from knowledge sharing with the measurement of PERMA which was developed by Butler and Kern [17] and have been used to explain the relationship between well-being and a continuous process such as career [18], education [19, 20], and hobby [21]. Although this is an important finding, the cause has not yet been revealed. Thus, this research explores why knowledge sharing increases well-being. In line with Aoki [1], this research follows Seligman's definition of well-being and adopts PERMA to examine the changes in well-being that knowledge sharing contributors' experience.

## 2. Method and data

### 2.1 The case: Adult fan of LEGO

To answer the research question, in-depth interviews with the knowledge-sharing contributors were conducted. The interviewees were sourced from LEGO users who share their original creations. The LEGO Group, one of the world's largest toy manufacturers, was founded in 1932. The brick in its present form was launched in 1958 and has attracted people for over 60 years. LEGO has a lot of adult fans across the world who call themselves AFOL (Adult Fan of LEGO). The LEGO Group has collaborated with these users with novel ideas for decades and much research has revealed the competitive advantages of this collaboration (e.g. [22–26]). Antorini, Muñiz and Askildsen [11] pointed out that the relationship among community members is the strongest motivation for contributors to co-creation with LEGO.

Co-creation among LEGO and its users varies from new product development to programming. Furthermore, users frequently share ideas, some of which are quite new beyond the brand's intention. This research examines how such knowledge sharing affects contributors themselves. This research distinguishes itself from previous research mainly in two aspects. First, this research observes changes in contributors not one specific point but over time. Second, this research shed light to not firms but contributors.

### 2.2 Sample and data

The interview respondents were selected using the following criteria: who share the idea related to LEGO with other people in some form. The interviews reached theoretical saturation with ten respondents. The primary respondent activity was sorted into three groups as follows.

A. Artistic photography of LEGO in scenic environments (n = 4).

B. Designing and creating original crafts with LEGO blocks (n = 4).

C. Programming original LEGO Mindstorms crafts (n = 2).

Their activities were user-generated beyond the firm's original aim. Group A especially, as they go out of their homes with LEGO blocks and/or mini-figures, and enjoy sharing with other people through SNS. These activities were not expected by the firm; however, they have become worldwide trends among LEGO users.

The one-to-one semi-structured interviews covered the beginning of LEGO, current occasion to use, purchase situations, and the relationship with the user community and the firm. The interviews were conducted between September 2020 and February 2021, and each interview lasted 30–120 min (average 59 min).

### 2.3 Analysis

To structurally understand chronological changes in the respondents, the data were analyzed using the Grounded theory approach (GTA) [27]. In line with other marketing research (e.g., [28–30]), this chapter follows the Strauss approach (e.g. [31]). All interviews were transcribed and applied the scheme of open, axial coding converging into theory as follows [32]:

1. breaking down data into manageable analytic pieces.

2. brainstorming with data to arrive at possible meanings and delineate the concepts (open coding).

3. elaborating concepts to form categories (axial coding).

4. integrating categories into a core category and other categories.

5. analyzing data for context.

The data were analyzed (first and second steps) after each interview, and data collecting and analysis were continued until reaching theoretical saturation. The concepts in open coding were based on the actual language respondents used. Then, the concepts were grouped into categories based on theoretical abstracts in axial coding. For analyst triangulation, the coding results were reviewed by the marketing researcher and two of the interview respondents; and the theory was constructed objectively via the reviewers' feedback. Finally, the categories were referred to PERMA [16] to observe the relationship between knowledge sharing and well-being.

## 3. Results

### 3.1 Seven categories extracted from GTA analysis

Through the process of coding, 22 first-order categories were distilled from 67 concepts and consequently converged into the seven second-order categories ending with the two core categories below (**Table 1**). The results are described below for each second-order category.

A. **Formative LEGO experience.** Each respondent had a LEGO experience in their childhood provided by their parents. They habitually played with LEGO and remembered physically clicking blocks, which is the predominant feature of LEGO. As they grew, they stopped playing with LEGO, getting tired of creating with the same blocks. Most respondents were not given enough LEGO blocks, they felt unsatisfied wanting more.

B. **Renewed LEGO experience.** After a while, sometimes more than 10 years later, the respondents rekindled their interest in LEGO for various reasons.

| | First-order categories | Seligman [16] | Second-order categories |
|---|---|---|---|
| 1 | Childhood experiences | | A) Formative LEGO experience |
| 2 | Superiority of LEGO blocks | Positive emotion | |
| 3 | Restart using LEGO | Positive emotion | B) Renewed LEGO experience |
| 4 | Exposed to new playing styles via the internet | Positive emotion | |
| 7 | Absorbed in creating | Engagement | C) Absorption in LEGO |
| 8 | Being an extension of oneself | Engagement | |
| 9 | Huge expenditure | | |
| 5 | Self-recognition of developing creativity | Engagement | D) Satisfaction of intellectual curiosities |
| 6 | Knowledge transformation | Meaning | |
| 10 | Goal representative of ideals | Meaning | E) Goal setting and hardships to reach the achievement |
| 11 | Hurdles to reach achievement | | |
| 12 | Collaboration with peers | Relationship | F) Deepening of knowledge and experiences via competitive co-creation (core category) |
| 13 | Deep communication | Relationship | |
| 14 | Opportunities for feedback | Accomplishment | |
| 15 | Existence of more experienced people | | |
| 16 | Objective judgment of one's own works | Meaning | |
| 17 | Recognition from third parties | Accomplishment | |
| 18 | Collaborative relations with LEGO | Relationship | |
| 19 | Interests and comprehension of brand mission | Meaning | |
| 20 | Social engagement via LEGO | Meaning | G) Passing on knowledge and experience to the next generation (core category) |
| 21 | Awareness of salient issues | Meaning | |
| 22 | Altruism | Meaning | |

**Table 1.**
*GTA results.*

In contrast to their childhood, they purchased LEGO blocks by themselves and found plenty of product lines that were new to them. Furthermore, they enjoyed posting their creations on SNS, a novel experience since their childhood.

> *"When I introduced my creation on YouTube, overseas people visited my channel."*

> *"I posted my creations to Twitter and also saw others' creations. Then, I began communicating with other LEGO users."*

C. **Absorption in LEGO.** When getting back into LEGO, the respondents were first absorbed in creating. Each of them had something to express through LEGO, which they felt was an extension of their body and a method for expression.

> *"When I am deeply moved by something, such as a movie or music, I'd like to express it. LEGO is one option to do so."*

They found themselves spending a lot of time and money as the product lines fired up their enthusiasm for collecting.

> *"I want more of these parts, also those transparent ones, it has become like a collection. I felt it's dangerous, but I really like LEGO."*

D. **Satisfaction of intellectual curiosities.** The respondents experienced the advantages of LEGO which increased their creativity; they could repeat trial and error. The simplicity of combining the blocks provided equal opportunities for competition.

> *"It is not dependent on cutting or pasting, painting or gluing skills, thus it only depends on ideas; how to express them. Even adults and children can compete equally. That's very interesting."*

Moreover, the restrictive regulations of colors and shapes promoted their creativity. The author found that AFOLs usually purchase sets to collect parts necessary for their creations. In other words, they do not follow the official instructions but made original creations using blocks collected from various sources. Furthermore, each respondent is a specialist in a field of their LEGO creations, for example, graphic design or photography. Their LEGO creations inspired them with their specialties, and they recognized this synergy.

> *"While enjoying LEGO, I also enjoy designing!"*

E. **Goal setting and hardships reaching achievements.** Each respondent has a theme and ideal for their creations. They take advantage of their own strengths to pursue originality.

> *"My work affords me opportunities to travel, so I thought I could create my own worldview using Instagram… if I simply do the same as others, my work would remain in obscurity."*

Though they aim to entertain others in addition to their own enjoyment, they face some hardships. First, realizing their ideas is not only fun but quite challenging. Furthermore, all respondents mentioned the high cost of LEGO. Some respondents do not purchase official sets, but individual authentic blocks from overseas through unofficial channels, which needs know-how.

> *"The transactions are all in English. Troubles sometimes happen due to consumer-to-consumer business. It needs experience and know-how. It is difficult for non-fans to understand the proper process and the motivation."*

F. **Deepening of knowledge and experiences via competitive co-creation (core category).** AFOLs collaborate to enhance the quality of their creations and even share information about how to acquire certain blocks. They show their creations and provide feedback to each other, which motivates them and accelerates future creations.

> *"The events are like exhibitions and people bring their creations. We show our best creations, praise each other, and improve ourselves through friendly rivalry."*

Experiencing success in contests or recognizing well-known people in their community enthused the respondents to further create.

Importantly, the LEGO group assists those collaborative relationships. The firm officially recognizes such user communities worldwide as LEGO User Group (LUG). While LUGs contribute to diffusing LEGO, the firm supports its activities. Some respondents belong to LUGs and have indirect collaborative relationships with the firm, whereas some are more directly related to the firm such as by collaborating in new product development.

In summary, AFOLs compete with each other in creating, and such competition increases their motivation. Thus their relationships are co-creative overall. The balance between competition and co-creation enriches the respondents' knowledge and experiences. Furthermore, it broadens their opportunities beyond LEGO creations.

> *"I started to like photos related to LEGO, then decided to major in photography in university. Now I'm interested in cameras and want to make a living shooting photos."*

G. **Passing on knowledge and experience to the next generation (core category).** The respondents eventually received job requests from outside their communities as a result of their LEGO creations. These jobs were not only for additional LEGO creations, but also for writing books about LEGO, lecturing at LEGO schools for children, and so on. The job requests were from both LEGO itself and third parties, from both inside and outside of Japan. Some respondents accepted those jobs as an extension of their hobby, while others did so as a side business. Furthermore, such jobs became the main source of income for some respondents.

> *"Recently, job requests related to LEGO have increased and even become my primary source of income."*

As a hobby or as a source of income, the respondents commonly expanded their fields through LEGO activities and expanded their connection to society.

Moreover, some respondents eagerly passed on their experiences, which was deeply satisfying. Particularly, they were passionate about developing children's creativities and tried to do so by holding events, establishing websites, and so on.

> *"I want children to enjoy creating as I did in my childhood. And I'd like to escalate that exciting feeling within them. That is why I held a LEGO creation contest."*

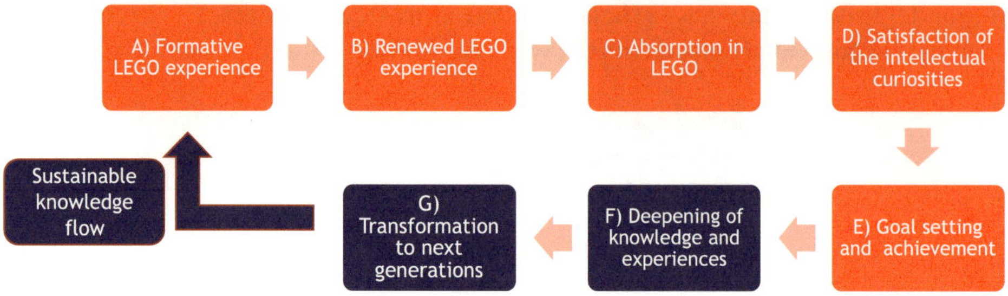


**Figure 1.**
*The flow of knowledge sharing.*

Referring to their beliefs, they tended to be unsatisfied with current product lines and contemporary trends in society which spoils children's creativity.

> *"Children today don't repeat building and destroying. They don't make an airplane from a 'police station' set, but simply purchase an 'airplane' set."*

### 3.2 Matching for the PERMA model

The author finally matched the first-order categories to the PERMA model [16], where appropriate, to observe undergoing changes in the respondents (**Table 1**). The respondents started their experience with a 'positive emotion,' such as fun, then fell into absorption ('engagement'). Then, they recognized the meaning of investing their cultivated knowledge into their creations and their ideals ('meaning'). In the process of achieving their goals, they shared their knowledge with their peers ('relationship') and felt a sense of 'accomplishment' via competition and recognition. Finally, most were motivated to be altruistic (higher level of 'meaning') in the form of knowledge flow to the next generation. Four of the categories do not match PERMA elements but influenced the PERMA outcome. For example, experience in childhood includes unsatisfied feelings but it increases the respondents' absorption in adulthood.

### 3.3 Findings

As a result, it was proven that the flow of knowledge sharing is circular while increasing contributors well-being (**Figure 1**). The respondents had accumulated knowledge and experience with LEGO since their childhood (A). They then found a renewed attraction to LEGO and became reabsorbed in it in their adulthood (B&C). They enjoyed applying their non-LEGO knowledge to their LEGO creations and realizing that it was developing their creativity (D). Sooner after, they each set their own goal which represented their ideal, but there were obstacles (E). To overcome those obstacles, they developed their skills and ideas by collaborating with other users, sometimes competing with them, which resulted in a deepening of their knowledge and experience (F). After reaching their achievements, most respondents were motivated to pass on their experiences to the next generation.

## 4. Conclusions and implications

This study concludes that the reason for knowledge sharing increases contributors well-being is that it further deepens their knowledge and experience. The respondents could further deepen their previously accumulated knowledge and experience with LEGO creation through competitive co-creation with others.

Moreover, regardless of their initial goals, they converged into the broader goal of knowledge flow to the next generation which, importantly, contributes to the realization of sustainability in knowledge development.

This study demonstrates the importance of competitive co-creation with individuals utilizing personal knowledge. This personal knowledge is not necessarily related to their work or major, but rather their outside interests which were accumulated over a longer span. A marriage of diversified ideas could be the resource for innovative ideas.

The COVID-19 pandemic has restricted the flow of people and goods, but owing to the internet, not knowledge. Activation of knowledge sharing increases people's well-being and social welfare.

## Acknowledgements

This work was supported by JSPS Grants-in-Aid for Scientific Research (Grant Number 20K13631).

## Author details

Kei Aoki
Hirao School of Management, Konan University, Japan

*Address all correspondence to: aoki@konan-u.ac.jp

## References

[1] Aoki K. The relationship between well-being and knowledge sharing. Sustainability. 2021;**13**(9):4978

[2] de Jong J, von Hippel E, Gault F, Kuusisto J, Raasch C. Market failure in the diffusion of consumer-developed innovations: Patterns in Finland. Research Policy. 2015;**44**(10):1856-1865

[3] von Hippel E, DeMonaco HJ, de Jong JPJ. Market failure in the diffusion of user innovations: The case of 'Off-Label' innovations by medical clinicians. Science and Public Policy. 2017;**44**(1): 121-131

[4] von Hippel E. The dominant role of users in the scientific instrument innovation process. Research Policy. 1976;**5**(3):212-239

[5] von Hippel E. Democratizing Innovation. Cambridge, MA: MIT Press; 2005

[6] Gambardella A, Raasch C, von Hippel E. The user innovation paradigm: Impacts on markets and welfare. Management Science. 2016;**63**(5):1450-1468

[7] Raasch C, von Hippel E. Amplifying User and Producer Innovation: The Power of Participation Motives. London: Routledge; 2015. pp. 284-309

[8] Hienerth C, von Hippel E, Jensen MB. User community vs. producer innovation development efficiency: A first empirical study. Research Policy. 2014a;**43**(1):190-201

[9] Baldwin C, Hienerth C, Von Hippel E. How user innovations become commercial products: A theoretical investigation and case study. Research Policy. 2006;**35**(9):1291-1313

[10] Shah SK, Tripsas M. The accidental entrepreneur: The emergent and collective process of user entrepreneurship. Strategic Entrepreneurship Journal. 2007;**1**(1-2):123-140

[11] Antorini YM, Muñiz AM Jr, Askildsen T. Collaborating with customer communities: Lessons from the LEGO group. MIT Sloan Management Review. 2012;**53**(3):73-79

[12] Füller J. Refining virtual co-creation from a consumer perspective. California Management Review. 2010;**52**(2):97-122

[13] Janzik L, Raasch C. Online communities in mature markets: Why join, why innovate, why share? International Journal of Innovation Management. 2011;**15**(4):797-836

[14] Ogawa S, Pongtanalert K. Exploring characteristics and motives of consumer innovators: Community innovators vs. independent innovators. Research-Technology Management. 2013;**56**(3): 41-48

[15] Halbinger MA. The role of makerspaces in supporting consumer innovation and diffusion: An empirical analysis. Research Policy. 2018;**47**(10):2028-2036

[16] Seligman MEP. Flourish: A Visionary New Understanding of Happiness and Well-being. New York: Free Press; 2011

[17] Butler J, Kern ML. The PERMA-Profiler: A brief multidimensional measure of flourishing. International Journal of Wellbeing. 2016;**6**(3):1-48

[18] Ascenso S, Perkins R, Williamson A. Resounding meaning: A PERMA wellbeing profile of classical musicians. Frontiers in Psychology. 2018;**9**:1895

[19] Lee J, Krause AE, Davidson JW. The PERMA well-being model and music

facilitation practice: Preliminary documentation for well-being through music provision in Australian schools. Research Studies in Music Education. 2017;**39**(1):73-89

[20] Tansey TN, Smedema S, Umucu E, Iwanaga K, Wu JR, Cardoso EDS, et al. Assessing college life adjustment of students with disabilities: Application of the PERMA framework. Rehabilitation Counseling Bulletin. 2018;**61**(3):131-142

[21] Doyle JP, Filo K, Lock D, Funk DC, McDonald H. Exploring PERMA in spectator sport: Applying positive psychology to examine the individual-level benefits of sport consumption. Sport Management Review. 2016;**19**(5): 506-519

[22] Hienerth C, Lettl C, Keinz P. Synergies among producer firms, lead users, and user communities: The case of the LEGO producer–user ecosystem. Journal of Product Innovation Management. 2014b;**31**(4):848-866

[23] Jensen MB, Hienerth C, Lettl C. Forecasting the commercial attractiveness of user-generated designs using online data: An empirical study within the LEGO user community. Journal of Product Innovation Management. 2014;**31**:75-93

[24] Lauwaert M. Playing outside the box–on LEGO toys and the changing world of construction play. History and Technology. 2008;**24**(3):221-237

[25] Prahalad CK, Ramaswamy V. The Future of Competition: Co-creating Unique Value with Customers. Cambridge, MA: Harvard Business Press; 2004

[26] Schlagwein D, Bjorn-Andersen N. Organizational learning with crowdsourcing: The revelatory case of LEGO. Journal of the Association for Information Systems. 2014;**15**(11):3

[27] Glaser B, Strauss A. The Discovery of Grounded Theory. Chicago: Aldine; 1967

[28] Batra R, Ahuvia A, Bagozzi RP. Brand love. Journal of Marketing. 2012;**76**(2):1-16

[29] Gebhardt GF, Carpenter GS, Sherry JF Jr. Creating a market orientation: A longitudinal, multifirm, grounded analysis of cultural transformation. Journal of Marketing. 2006;**70**(4):37-55

[30] Homburg C, Jozić D, Kuehnl C. Customer experience management: Toward implementing an evolving marketing concept. Journal of the Academy of Marketing Science. 2017;**45**(3):377-401

[31] Strauss AL, Corbin JM. Basics of Qualitative Research: Techniques and Procedures for Developing Grounded Theory. Newbury Park: Sage Publications; 1998

[32] Corbin J, Strauss A. Basics of Qualitative Research: Techniques and Procedures for Developing Grounded Theory. Los Angeles, CA: Sage Publications; 2014

Chapter 10

# Perspective Chapter: Impact of COVID-19 on the Health of Ethnic Minorities in the UK – Salient Features and Recouping Strategies

*Anil Gumber*


## Abstract

COVID-19 has affected selected population groups, professions, and regions much more than others in terms of infection rate, hospital admission rate, and intensive care rate and then premature mortality rate. Globally, the seventh highest deaths due to COVID-19 (>155,000) have been experienced in the UK. The share of Black, Asia, and Ethnic Minorities (BAME) people in the UK is >20% with a high geographical concentration in major cities (London, Birmingham, and Manchester). Government statistics show that Black and Asian people represented disproportionately higher (>3 and 2 times, respectively) than white British in admission to Intensive & Emergency Care Units and resultant deaths due to Coronavirus. This chapter explores underlying reasons for differential impacts on BAME's health and well-being including demographics, socioeconomic condition, health status/long-term conditions (LTCs), diet, and lifestyle. Compared with white British, the BAME people have higher prevalence of LTCs/obesity, lower health literacy, and living and working in most deprivation areas/occupations. These factors are important to plan for short- and long-term impact mitigation strategies to recoup BAME peoples' health and well-being they enjoyed before the Pandemic. Two studies illustrate the Pandemic effect on: BAME access to organ transplants services, and racism experienced at workplace the National Health Services BAME staff.


**Keywords:** pandemic, ethnic minorities, racism, organ transplants, Health & Wellbeing

## 1. Introduction

The Corona virus (COVID-19) was declared a pandemic by the WHO in March 2020. COVID-19 and its subsequent variants (mainly Delta & Omicron) spread exponentially across the World and globally infected over 375 million people with 5.7 million deaths as on 31st January 2022 [1]. COVID-19 has affected some population groups and countries much more than others in terms of infection rate, hospitalisation admissions and discharge, and premature mortality. Globally, the seventh highest deaths due to COVID-19 (>155,000) has been experienced by the

UK; however, in terms of fatality rate per million population the UK ranks at 30th. Both government statistics and media in the UK has pinpointed that the Pandemic has had wider and differential impacts on people from low socio-economic status and those having minority ethnic/cultural background. One in five people in the UK belongs to Black, Asia and Ethnic Minorities (BAME) groups; and they are in majority in London and Birmingham, followed by high concentration in Manchester, Leeds and some other major cities of the England.

According to the report released by the Public Health England on 2nd June 2020 [2], the COVID-19 diagnosis rate, admission to Intensive Care Units and resultant deaths are disproportionately higher among BAME. Age-standardised certified deaths rate due to Coronavirus was more than four times for Black and three times for Asian people when compared with their White British counterparts during the 1st Wave (beginning with 23rd March 2020 Lockdown). There is very limited official release of evidence to explain underlying reasons for such massive differentials in infection, hospitalisation and fatality rates across ethnic and socio-economic groups and resultant health and wellbeing inequalities emerged due to coronavirus pandemic.

This paper explores underlying reasons of differential impacts of COVID-19 on BAME's health and wellbeing. These include demographics, socioeconomic condition, health estate and long-term conditions, as well as diet and lifestyle factors. BAME people have much higher prevalence of long-term conditions/diseases, obesity, low level of health literacy, and living in most deprivation areas and above all working in low-paid occupations. These factors are pivotal in order to plan for short- and long-term impact mitigation strategies as well as to recoup BAME peoples' health and quality of life they enjoyed before the pandemic. The paper also highlights health inequalities for BAME community through two case studies depicting how the Pandemic affected their specialist health services (organ transplants) and how much and type of BAME nursing and allied staff have faced racism whilst working for the National Health Services (NHS) before and during the Pandemic. explores.

## 2. Underlying reasons for differential impact

In fact, due to high infection and spread rate, the coronavirus has not discriminated in terms of providing differential exposure to people with diverse socioeconomic and ethnic/cultural backgrounds. In principle the BAME people are not disproportionately affected because they are BAME in some kind of biological sense, but because of socio-economic and cultural factors which create conditions whereby they are more likely to be exposed to infection and lack the physiological infrastructure to be able to deal with it as effectively as more privileged people. These multiple disadvantageous factors, which triggered and became outrageous when BAME people got exposed to coronavirus, are related at their underlying health issues; lack of physical activity; deprived living conditions; poor hygiene practices; and being engaged in high-risk occupations including low-paid gig sector.

To begin with, the most critical one is the low immunity levels among BAME people to fight against the infection due to unbalanced diet lacking micronutrients, widespread prevalence of anaemia and Vitamin D deficiency prevalence, and predominance of long-term conditions and early onsets of CVD, Type 2 Diabetes and Hypertension (a decade earlier in BAME compared to White British) [3]. COVID-19 affected disproportionately older people and men in the UK [4]; the median age for White British admitted due to coronavirus was above 60 as compared to 55 for BAME people during the 1st Wave. It is found that a majority of BAME people after reaching age 55 milestone, develop a long-term condition (LTC). Among South Asians it was noticed that by age 55 most of them have been on medications for CVD and diabetes for more than 15 years [3]. The high rate of prevalence of LTCs and medications among BAME people, in turn has reduced their immunity levels and thus are unable to fight against infections (most of them even receive every year free winter flu jab from the NHS thus vouching on the prevalence of low level of immunity).

## 2.1 Diet and nutrition

Good nutrition is elemental to improving immunity and with ageing it is pivotal to supplement individual's diet with appropriate magnitude of nutrition. The first line of defence is to choose healthy diet packed with various micronutrients that supports optimal function of the immune system. Based on variety of systematic and evidence-based data, Vitamins: A, C, D, and minerals: Zinc and iron are particularly crucial to boosting immune response [5, 6]. Their details with main contribution, food sources and daily requirement is shown in **Box 1**.

- **Vitamin A**: is an anti-inflammatory because of key role in enhancing immune function and important for epithelial integrity and also crucial for mucosal function. Its main sources are: Animal: Liver, egg yolk, butter, cream, whole milk and cheese; Plant: sweet potato, papaya, melon, apricot, spinach, carrots, pumpkin and red palm oil. It's daily DRIs (Dietary reference intakes), RDA (Recommended dietary allowances), AI (adequate intake), RAE (Retinol activity equivalent) requirements for different population groups are: Infants and young children (AI = 400–500 RAE/day, depending on age); Older children and adolescents (RDA = 600–900 RAE/day, depending on age); Adults (RDA = 700–900 RAE/day, depending on gender); Pregnant (RDA = 750–770 RAE/day) and Lactating women (RDA = 1200–1300 RAE/day).

- **Vitamin C**: increases the production of white blood cells. It protects immunity to fight infections and prevent common cold including allergic symptoms. Its sources are: all citrus fruits, Barbados cherry (acerola), grapefruit, oranges, lemon, limes, guava, goose berries (amla), broccoli, potatoes, tomatoes, cabbage, red amaranth leaves and green peppers. Its daily requirements: Infants and young children (15 mg); Children and adolescents (25-45 mg); Adults (40–60 mg); Pregnant (85 mg) and lactating women (120 mg).

- **Vitamin D**: is thought to be effective to lower the respiratory tract infections and also boost immunity. Its sources are: Eggs, liver, fortified milk, fortified margarines, oily fish and cod liver oil; Sunlight. Its daily requirements: Infants-10 mcg (400 IU); Children and adolescents-15mcg (600 IU); Adults-15 mcg (600 IU) and > 70 age-20 mcg (800 IU); Pregnant-15mcg (600 IU) and lactating women-15mcg (600 IU).

- **Iron:** is a component of haemoglobin, myoglobin and vital in oxygen transfer. Its sources: Animal: Liver meats, egg yolk, shellfish, Plant: dried fruits, whole grain or iron fortified breads and cereals, dark green and leafy vegetables and molasses. Its daily requirements: Infant and young children-7 mg; Children-10 mg; Adolescents-11 mg/day for boys and 15 mg for girls; Adults-8 mg for men, 18 mg for women and 8 mg for menopause; Pregnant- 27 mg and lactating women-9 mg.

- **Zinc:** is essential mineral to boost immunity and prevent depression. Its sources: Animal: oysters, shellfish, dairy and eggs; Plant: Legumes, wheat bran, seeds (black sesame, garden cress seeds, pumpkin seeds). Its daily requirements: Infants and young children-3 mg; Older children and adolescents-5 mg-8 mg; Adults:11 mg for men and 8 mg for women; Pregnant-11 mg and lactating women-12 mg.

**Box 1.**
*Immunity booster vitamins, food sources and daily requirement.*

### 2.2 Physical activity

Daily exercise also boosts immune system and improve physical and mental health wellbeing. WHO recommends regular exercise including brisk walking for adults for at least 30 minutes for five days a week. There is extensive evidence in the UK that physical activity level is low among BAME population with majority of mid-aged do not meet the recommended daily exercise level. NHS health professionals also advice light to moderate intensity exercise daily including Yoga for people suffering from long-term conditions to remain energetic, less stress and manage the condition better. Meditation and breathing exercise especially the *Bhramari* pranayama, a meditative breathing technique, improves immunity, reduces stress, fatigue and also regulates the endocrine glands. Some other breathing techniques are also effective i.e., Pursed lip breathing, diaphragmatic breathing, breath focus technique, lion's breath, alternate nostril breathing, known as *nadi shodhana* pranayama, equal breathing, resonant and coherent breathing and *shitali* breath and deep breathing [7].

### 2.3 Socioeconomic status

The pertinent issue still remains among BAME is their low-income level, poor economic status, employed in low-paid and high risks jobs, and continue to live in poor housing conditions and deprived areas. This in turn directly affects their purchasing power to buy healthy and nutritious food, maintain hygiene and sustaining good health. The level of health literacy among them is low, therefore the key challenge is how to change their food habits, improve their nutrition level and raise their immunity level in order to prepare them against the subsequent waves/variants of the coronavirus and other infectious diseases.

### 2.4 One year with the pandemic

The updated report on the changes in population mental health & wellbeing in England during the COVID-19 pandemic using the UK Household Longitudinal Study showed that mental health deteriorated significantly during the two national lockdown periods [8]. The psychological distress rates increased from 20.8% in 2019 (pre-Covid) to 29.5% in April 2020 (1st Lockdown), then eased at 21.3% by September 2020 and then gone up again to 27.1% in January 2021(2nd Lockdown), then eased at 24.5% in March 2021 end. Mental distress rates were found to be higher among young vs. older adults and women vs. men; During the pandemic period self-reported levels of loneliness were much higher especially during winter lockdown of 2021. Among the young adults who had a pre-existing mental health condition and belonged to lower income group had experienced much worse mental health during the pandemic together with increased alcohol consumption and smoking. Similarly, those with poor physical health reported feeling more socially isolated during the first wave (June-July 2020) than the second (Nov-Dec 2020). It was devastated to observe that the mental health outcomes during the pandemic were found to be worse among minority ethnic groups (BAME) compared to their White counterparts.

According to UCL COVID-19 Social Study the 38 week per week data (starting from 1st Lockdown in 23rd March 2020) showed that both anxiety & depression rates were constantly higher for BAME compared to their White counterparts; the latter group also experienced a faster decline in those rates. It was also noticed that the loneliness rates, Covid stress, Financial stress, thoughts of suicide/self-harm rate were consistently higher for BAME compared to their White counterparts. Finally,

Compare to White community, the life satisfaction rate during the pandemic period was found to be consistently lower for the BAME people. Overall, the deterioration in mental health condition during the pandemic period was higher in BAME, especially among men when compared to White individuals; thus, ethnicity predicts mental health deterioration when interacted with gender [9].

### 2.5 Impact mitigating strategies

Both short- and long-term strategies are thus required to mitigate the devastating impact of COVID on their health and quality of life. These could also be designed according to risk factors and preventable measures including social distancing, maintaining hand hygiene, working remotely and avoiding gathering, clubbing, partying and in groups entertainment. Within BAME community the population is extremely heterogeneous; therefore, any behavioural change strategies need to be contextualised in the six G's framework. The six G's (gender, generation, genes, geography, God/religion, and gaps in resources) in the context of management of diabetes and CVD among BAME through diet and lifestyle behavioural change are discussed in a separate publication [10].

Short-term strategies using social marketing approach are:

- Imparting knowledge through regional language radios and tele-channels through short key messages, expert interviews, talks and discussions on promoting balanced and nutrient diets to raise immunity at the community level.
- Explaining the natural intake of nutrients (through food sources, fresh air, alkaline water and sunlight) to raise levels of Vitamin A, C and D along with Zinc and Iron for adults and children and adolescents.
- Information sheets (possibly in multi-lingual) on promoting these immunities enhancing nutrition to be provided by the organisations and institutions on the basis of their usual/work activities (namely, schools, local government, public and private large employers, charities, places of worships and also through NHS and pharmacies).
- The other critical immunity raising factor is to make people more physically active in accordance with their stamina as well as bring them back into healthy weight threshold. Many successful examples of group walking and gym activities need to be expanded in scope and scale (in order to include BAME people according to their gender and age group).
- It is very important to encourage and introduce indoor activities including Yoga, Meditation and breathing exercises. There are now several mode & medium to teach and deliver these remotely.
- Promote effective vaccine and reduce hesitancy in uptake of COVID vaccines among adults and children from BAME community [11].

Long-term strategies

- Re-emphasise the role of state (Central and local governments) in initiating these preventative strategies at large using the Nobel nudging approach [12].

- To improve health literacy among BAME and people living in deprived area through short courses in colleges which could be delivered remotely or through community centres (this approach has already been used in improving computer and IT skills).

- To promote participation and recruitment of BAME people in new COVID-variants vaccine trials and antibody therapies.

- To regularise and provide greater economic security and employment conditions for people in low-paid, casual and contract jobs particularly to those who are already in the gig-economy.

- Special CPD courses and training programmes for both healthcare professionals and the community on how to manage better specific long-term conditions (such as diabetes, CVD, Asthma, chronic kidney disease, organ transplants recipients, etc.) which get aggravated due to COVID infection.

- Rolling out already successful initiatives to Improve health behaviour in regard to drugs, smoking, and heavy and binge drinking (alcohol intakes).

## 3. Access to organ transplant services during the pandemic

The Pandemic severely affected the UK organ transplant services as the whole NHS (National Health Services) was overwhelmed in treating COVID-19 infected patients in hospitals. In order to treat the heavy influx of COVID patients into respiratory wards and Intensive & Emergency Care Units (ICUs) several speciality hospital services were suspended, and NHS staff and resources were transferred to newly created COVID wards. To ensure the safety of patients transplant centres were also closed during the 1st Lockdown (Mar-Jun 2020) phase and with very limited access during the 2nd Lockdown (Jan-March 2021) period. Our previous study demonstrated that compare to April 2019 there was 73% reduction in deceased donor (DD) transplants and 100% reduction in living donor (LD) in the April 2020 lockdown month; and it was estimated that in the 1st Lockdown quarter 904 fewer transplants were done compared to the pre-pandemic quarter (This shortfall accounted for 16% of waiting list cases) [13].

During the Pandemic period new organ transplants guidelines were implemented with respect to stopping procurement of organs from deceased donors especially those died due to COVID as well as complete suspension of live donor list. This new guideline thus has directly impacted the number of transplant procedures done during the Pandemic affected year 2020–2021. The NHS Blood and Transplant (2021) annual activity report covering the whole Pandemic affected 2020–2021 financial year has reported that due to COVID reason 5307 patients from previous years backlog on transplant lists were temporarily suspended and 4256 new patients were added on the transplant lists during 2020–2021 [14]. Compared to pre-Pandemic 2019–2020 level, 1882 (31%) less patients were newly enrolled on the transplant list with much fewer donors (DD and LD) in 2020–2021. During the Pandemic 2020–2021 number of DD fell by 400 and LD fell by 618 comparted to 2019–2020 (pre-Pandemic year); both together accounted for fall of 1014 (38.4%) donors due to the Pandemic. Consequently 815 (22%) fewer DD transplants were done during 2020–2021. Further, due to temporary suspension of backlog patients on transplant list, their waiting time regrettably got extended further by 12 months and in this process 26% excess deaths occurred whilst waiting for their transplants in the pandemic year (474 vs. 377 in 2019–2020).

The postponement and delay in transplant services have affected the Black, Asian and Minority Ethnic (BAME) patients the most. Compared to 2019–2020, from BAME background 672 (35%) less patients were enrolled; the number of donors fell by 125 (46%) {28 in DD & 97 in LD}; and as a result, 437 (36%) less patients received DD transplants during 2020–2021 [7]. Similarly, 31% excess deaths were recorded for BAME whilst waiting for their transplants in 2020–2021 (169 vs. 100 in 2019–2020). These statistics comparisons (illustrated above and shown in **Table 1**) clearly reflect that BAME patients got affected the most during the Pandemic.

Finally, the Pandemic has impacted the BAME patients unfavourably in terms of waiting time for transplant. For instance, in the pre-Pandemic year the median time to transplant a kidney was 830 days for Asian and 965 days for Black and only 640 days for white patients [13]. Black patients continued to wait almost a year longer for a kidney transplant compared to white patients. Interestingly, 35% of white patients had received their transplant within one year after being listed for a kidney transplant whereas this figure was ironically low at 19% for BAME patients [15]. Thus, due to Pandemic, closer of transplant and suspension of backlog list has resulted in disproportionately extending the wait time for BAME patients; and increased the probability of dyeing whilst waiting for transplant.

## 4. Racism at work during the pandemic

According to the British Medical Association the racism at workplace experienced by BAME staff in the NHS is widespread; however, a surge in such cases during the Pandemic is unfortunate. In our recently concluded online survey of racism cases experienced before and during the Pandemic by the nursing and other healthcare professionals highlights a much wider and deeper problems in such a novel organisation. It is unfortunate to record and report such racism behaviours at the NHS despite several legislations are in place. The online survey conducted during January-May 2021 recorded responses of 308 BAME nurses, midwives and other allied healthcare staff who have faced racism at their workplace any time

| | Pre-Pandemic (2019–2020) | | | Pandemic (2020–21) | | |
|---|---|---|---|---|---|---|
| | All | BAME | BAME per million population | All | BAME | BAME per million population |
| Waiting List | 6040 | 1909 | 28.5 | 4189 | 1237 | 18.5 |
| Total Donors | 2621 | 271 | 4.0 | 1579 | 146 | 2.2 |
| 1. Deceased donors | 1566 | 112 | 1.7 | 1144 | 84 | 1.3 |
| 2. Living donors | 1055 | 159 | 2.4 | 435 | 62 | 0.9 |
| Total Transplants | 4749 | 1204 | 18.0 | 3344 | 767 | 11.4 |
| 1. Deceased donors | 3710 | 1010 | 15.1 | 2903 | 682 | 10.2 |
| 2. Living donors | 1039 | 194 | 2.9 | 441 | 85 | 1.3 |
| Total Deaths while waiting | 377 | 100 | 1.5 | 474 | 169 | 2.5 |

**Table 1.**
*Number of donors, transplants and waiting list in the UK, pre- & during Pandemic Financial Year for BAME & all Ethnicities.*

- Job role (Nurse/Nursing Associate, Midwife, Medical staff, Clinical Support Worker, Allied Health Professional, Social Care Worker, Ancillary staff).
- Employed by (NHS, Agency, Private)
- Type of Care Setting (Hospital, Community, Primary Care, Nursing home/residential, Intermediate care)
- Experience of any forms of racism at work BEFORE the pandemic (Verbal abuse, Physical abuse, Excessive scrutiny/punishment, Prevented from progressing, other harassment, None of these). PROVIDE details of experiences.
- Experience of any forms of racism at work DURING the pandemic (Verbal abuse, Physical abuse, Excessive scrutiny/punishment, Prevented from progressing, other harassment, None of these).
- Treated unfairly regarding any of the following DURING the Pandemic (Distribution of PPE, Physically unsuitable PPE, Working in Covid19 positive environments, Access to risk assessment, Reasonable adjustment following the risk assessment, None of these). Provide details of experiences.
- Ever challenged racist treatment at work (Yes/No). If Yes, were treated fairly (Yes/No).
- Has workplace racism led to any of the followings (Poorer mental health, Took sick leave, Difficult to do job, Left job, None of these)?
- If ever been employed on a work visa, do you believe your immigration status made you more vulnerable to racism and exploitation? (Yes/No/NA).
- Ethnic origin (Black African, Black Caribbean, Black British, Black mixed heritage, Asian Indian, Asian Pakistani, Asian Bangladeshi, Asian Filipino, Asian Other, Asian mixed heritage, Arab, Other –Specify, White British, White Other).
- Age, Gender, Contact email.

**Box 2.**
*Items of information collected in online survey for Nursing & Allied NHS staff.*

during their work-life and including during the on-going Pandemic period [16]. The details of information collected is shown in **Box 2.**

## 4.1 Demographics

Out of 308 BAME respondents, majority of them were working for the NHS (267, 86.7%) and the rest 41 respondents with Non-NHS organisations. Three-fourths of respondents were women and nearly half of the respondents (48.05%) belonged to 31–44 age group which was followed by the middle age group of 45–54 (29.87%). These 308 respondents reported 11 types of ethnic backgrounds which are broadly represent as Black, Asian, and Mixed heritage. The largest number of respondents belonged to Black African (82, 26.62%) which is followed by Asian Indian (45, 14.61%), Black Caribbean (40, 12.99%), Asian Pakistani (39, 12.66%), and Asian Filipino (34, 11.04%). Overall, 165 (53.6%) respondents belonged to Black race. In terms of job role 190 (61.69%) of them were engaged as Nurses or Nursing Associates; the next clustering was of Allied Health Professionals (44, 14.29%). A majority of them were working in a hospital setting (200, 64.94%), which was followed by community setting (71, 23.05%). Out of 308 respondents 140 (45.45%) worked in this country on work permit whereas the remaining 168 (54.55%) did not need the permit.

## 4.2 Types of racism experienced at work

**Table 2** shows the distribution of racism experienced by types at workplace before and during the across seven broad categories of BAME groups. Before the

| Ethnicity | Verbal abuse | Physical abuse | Excessive scrutiny/ punishment | Prevented from progressing | other harassment | None of these | All |
|---|---|---|---|---|---|---|---|
| **Before Pandemic** | | | | | | | |
| Black African | 32 | 2 | 47 | 51 | 30 | 12 | 174 |
| Black Caribbean | 9 | 0 | 23 | 29 | 20 | 5 | 86 |
| Black Other | 12 | 1 | 20 | 20 | 19 | 13 | 85 |
| Asian Indian | 11 | 0 | 12 | 28 | 14 | 8 | 73 |
| Asian Pakistani/ Bangladeshi/Sindhi | 14 | 2 | 15 | 27 | 14 | 13 | 85 |
| Asian Filipino | 14 | 1 | 8 | 15 | 15 | 7 | 60 |
| Asian Other | 6 | 1 | 7 | 16 | 12 | 2 | 44 |
| All BAME (Count) | 98 | 7 | 132 | 186 | 124 | 60 | 607 |
| All BAME (Row%) | 16.14 | 1.15 | 21.75 | 30.64 | 20.43 | 9.88 | 100.0 |
| Black (Count) | 53 | 3 | 90 | 100 | 69 | 30 | 345 |
| Black (Row %) | 15.36 | 0.87 | 26.09 | 28.99 | 20.00 | 8.70 | 100.0 |
| Asian (Count) | 45 | 4 | 42 | 86 | 55 | 30 | 262 |
| Asian (Row %) | 17.18 | 1.53 | 16.03 | 32.82 | 20.99 | 11.45 | 100.0 |
| **During Pandemic** | | | | | | | |
| Black African | 19 | 1 | 31 | 33 | 33 | 23 | 140 |
| Black Caribbean | 3 | 0 | 16 | 12 | 17 | 10 | 58 |
| Black Other | 6 | 2 | 7 | 11 | 12 | 20 | 58 |
| Asian Indian | 5 | 1 | 7 | 16 | 10 | 20 | 59 |
| Asian Pakistani/ Bangladeshi/Sindhi | 8 | 1 | 15 | 14 | 13 | 21 | 72 |
| Asian Filipino | 12 | 1 | 7 | 10 | 15 | 6 | 51 |
| Asian Other | 5 | 1 | 4 | 5 | 11 | 6 | 32 |
| All BAME (Count) | 58 | 7 | 87 | 101 | 111 | 106 | 470 |
| All BAME (Row%) | 12.34 | 1.49 | 18.51 | 21.49 | 23.62 | 22.55 | 100.0 |
| Black (Count) | 28 | 3 | 54 | 56 | 62 | 53 | 256 |
| Black (Row %) | 10.94 | 1.17 | 21.09 | 21.88 | 24.22 | 20.70 | 100.0 |
| Asian (Count) | 30 | 4 | 33 | 45 | 49 | 53 | 214 |
| Asian (Row %) | 14.02 | 1.87 | 15.42 | 21.03 | 22.90 | 24.77 | 100.0 |

**Table 2.**
*Types of racism experienced at work before and during pandemic by BAME groups.*

Pandemic, the main racism type experienced was 'prevented from progressing' which was reported by 186 people. This was followed by 'excessive scrutiny/ punishment' (132), and 'verbal abuse' (98). Compared to Black, a relatively higher proportion of Asian staff reported the main type of racism as 'prevented from progressing' (32.82% vs. 28.99%). The order of importance of next two reasons 'excessive scrutiny/ punishment' and 'verbal abuse' was slightly different between Black and Asian groups; Black staff experienced more 'excessive scrutiny/punishment' whereas Asian staff faced more of 'verbal abuse'.

During the Pandemic, the share of 'other type of harassment' was the highest (111 people) followed by 'none of the listed reasons' (106 people reported). The share of 'prevented from progressing' which was the prominent type before the Pandemic for 186 people was reported by fewer people (101) during the pandemic. Further, 'excessive scrutiny/ punishment' and 'verbal abuse' were reported by 87 and 58 people respectively during the Pandemic. Black people experiencing more of 'excessive scrutiny/punishment' and Asian people facing more of 'verbal abuse' continued during the Pandemic as well. Thus, the important types of racism experienced differed between 'before the Pandemic' and 'during the Pandemic'.

### 4.3 Number of types of racism at workplace

As shown in **Table 2**, 308 respondents mentioned various types of racism at workplace which totalled as 607 before the Pandemic and 470 during the Pandemic. This shows that several of respondents reported more than one type of racism. **Table 3** shows the distribution of 308 respondents by number of types of racism experienced before and during the Pandemic separately for Black and Asian groups. Before the Pandemic, a majority of Asians experienced one (53.15%) or two (20.98%) types of racisms whereas among the Black a relatively higher proportion of them experienced three types (4.24% vs. 14.69%) or 4 types (13.33% vs. 8.39%) of racism. Thus, before the Pandemic Black overall experienced more types of racism compared to the Asian group. The scenario during the Pandemic is bit at a lower intensity as most of the Asians reported only one type of racism and for the Black the portion reporting two types of racism is higher compared to the Asian group (14.55% vs. 9.09%).

| Number of Types of Racism | Black | | Asian | | All BAME | |
|---|---|---|---|---|---|---|
| | Count | % | Count | % | Count | % |
| **Before Pandemic** | | | | | | |
| 0 | 1 | 0.61 | 1 | 0.70 | 2 | 0.65 |
| 1 | 73 | 44.24 | 76 | 53.15 | 149 | 48.38 |
| 2 | 27 | 16.36 | 30 | 20.98 | 57 | 18.51 |
| 3 | 40 | 24.24 | 21 | 14.69 | 61 | 19.81 |
| 4 | 22 | 13.33 | 12 | 8.39 | 34 | 11.04 |
| 5 | 2 | 1.21 | 3 | 2.10 | 5 | 1.62 |
| All | **165** | **100.00** | 143 | **100.00** | 308 | **100.00** |
| **During Pandemic** | | | | | | |
| 0 | 0 | 0.00 | 0 | 0.00 | 0 | 0.00 |
| 1 | 113 | 68.48 | 106 | 74.13 | 219 | 71.10 |
| 2 | 24 | 14.55 | 13 | 9.09 | 37 | 12.01 |
| 3 | 18 | 10.91 | 16 | 11.19 | 34 | 11.04 |
| 4 | 9 | 5.45 | 6 | 4.20 | 15 | 4.87 |
| 5 | 1 | 0.61 | 2 | 1.40 | 3 | 0.97 |
| All | **165** | **100.00** | 143 | **100.00** | 308 | **100.00** |

**Table 3.**
*Count of types of racism at workplace before and during the pandemic.*

| BAME | Respondents | | Before Pandemic | | During Pandemic | |
|---|---|---|---|---|---|---|
| | Count | % | Count | % | Count | % |
| Black African | 82 | 26.62 | 174 | 28.67 | 140 | 29.79 |
| Black Caribbean | 40 | 12.99 | 86 | 14.17 | 58 | 12.34 |
| Black British | 23 | 7.47 | 39 | 6.43 | 30 | 6.38 |
| Black mixed heritage | 20 | 6.49 | 46 | 7.58 | 28 | 5.96 |
| Asian Indian | 45 | 14.61 | 73 | 12.03 | 59 | 12.55 |
| Asian Pakistani | 39 | 12.66 | 71 | 11.70 | 58 | 12.34 |
| Asian Bangladeshi | 5 | 1.62 | 14 | 2.31 | 14 | 2.98 |
| Asian Filipino | 34 | 11.04 | 60 | 9.88 | 51 | 10.85 |
| Asian Other | 12 | 3.90 | 25 | 4.12 | 18 | 3.83 |
| Asian mixed heritage | 2 | 0.65 | 6 | 0.99 | 2 | 0.43 |
| Arab | 6 | 1.95 | 13 | 2.14 | 12 | 2.55 |
| All BAME | 308 | 100.0 | 607 | 100.0 | 470 | 100.0 |
| Black Race | 165 | 53.57 | 345 | 56.84 | 256 | 54.47 |
| Asian Race | 143 | 46.43 | 262 | 43.16 | 214 | 45.53 |

**Table 4.**
*Distribution of racism types at work before and during the pandemic by BAME group.*

**Table 4** shows the distribution of respondents reporting various types of racism experience before and during the pandemic at workplace (607 and 470, respectively) by detailed ethnic groups. The distribution of respondents across 11 categories of BAME group was surprisingly the same as those for the distribution of reporting total types of racism experiences; this implies that quantum of racism experiences was observed across the board by all 11 BAME groups people. Further, there was hardly any difference in the proportion of types of experiences across 11 categories of BAME between "during the Pandemic" vs. "before the Pandemic". Compared to Asian group, the Black group reported lower proportion of types of experiences during the pandemic vis-a-vis before the Pandemic (Black – 54.47% vs. 56.84% and Asian – 45.53% vs. 43.16%).

## 4.4 Covid-kit related unfairly treated cases by types

**Table 5** presents the unfairly Covid-kit related cases by six types. The highest share of the reason was by 'None of the Listed Reason' (30.97%); which was followed by working in 'Covid 19 positive environments' (18.58%), adjustments after risk assessment (17.26%), and access to risk assessment (14.16%). These reasons did not differ much between Black and Asian staff; however, Asian staff relative to Black experienced discrimination in regard to distribution of PPE.

## 4.5 Impact on Health & Wellbeing

The results from the survey clearly highlights that NHS BAME staff had experienced racism both before and during the Pandemic; and several of them had gone through that traumatic experience more than once. The Pandemic period which covered just a span of one year and thus reported a high spurt of work-related and COVID-kit related cases when compared to the whole work-life span before the

| Ethnicity | PPE Distribution | Unsuitable PPE | Covid19 positive environments | Access to risk assessment | Adjustment after risk assessment | None of these | All |
|---|---|---|---|---|---|---|---|
| Black African | 10 | 13 | 27 | 23 | 19 | 38 | 130 |
| Black Caribbean | 5 | 7 | 9 | 8 | 12 | 19 | 60 |
| Black Other | 6 | 2 | 8 | 10 | 11 | 20 | 57 |
| Asian Indian | 7 | 5 | 7 | 4 | 9 | 23 | 55 |
| Asian Pakistani/Bangladeshi/Sindhi | 7 | 7 | 14 | 9 | 13 | 21 | 71 |
| Asian Filipino | 5 | 6 | 15 | 5 | 8 | 9 | 48 |
| Asian Other | 4 | 2 | 4 | 5 | 6 | 10 | 31 |
| All BAME (Count) | 44 | 42 | 84 | 64 | 78 | 140 | 452 |
| All BAME (Row%) | 9.73 | 9.29 | 18.58 | 14.16 | 17.26 | 30.97 | 100.0 |
| Black (Count) | 21 | 22 | 44 | 41 | 42 | 77 | 247 |
| Black (Row %) | 8.50 | 8.91 | 17.81 | 16.60 | 17.00 | 31.17 | 100.0 |
| Asian (Count) | 23 | 20 | 40 | 23 | 36 | 63 | 205 |
| Asian (Row %) | 11.22 | 9.76 | 19.51 | 11.22 | 17.56 | 30.73 | 100.0 |

**Table 5.**
*Distribution of Covid-kit related unfairly treated cases by types.*

Pandemic. More than half of respondents (53%) had experienced unfair treatment in the Pandemic in relation to COVID PPE kit, risk assessment or COVID-ward placement. The experience of racism has severely affected their current or previous placement as well as their health: 59% reported difficulties in doing their job, in 53% cases impacted mental health, and in 36% cases they left the job. Several BAME staff were scared and reluctant to report racism to their superiors/managers. Only about 60% of them reported to the management of which a majority (four-fifths) did not receive a fair response/deal from the management. This clearly reflects that several of BAME nursing and allied staff were deployed to COVID-risk wards and were treated unfairly with respect to both provision of PPE and other safety issues. These instances have affected their health and mental wellbeing and compromised their self-esteem and undermined the confidence to carry-out such a novel healthcare profession for the healthier society.

## 5. Conclusion

COVID-19 has shown widespread impact on social an economic life of people in the UK. The consequences are felt much more on the health and economic livelihood of minority ethnic groups living in the UK. We observed that both Black and Asian background people had experienced much larger COVID-19 and its variants infection rates with greater incidence of hospitalisation and use of Intensive Care Units and resultant high fatality rate when compared to their White counterparts. Men from BAME groups experienced high disability and mortality rates compared to White adults. Even after one-year living in the Pandemic environment both health and mental wellbeing of BAME people continue to remain far below than those of White population; thus, indicating a slow recovery among BAME people when compared with the pre-pandemic levels. Similar slow recovery was noticed in the case of life satisfaction indicator over a year or so. In terms of accessing specialist health services (organ transplants), the Pandemic has pushed up waiting times for transplant for BAME patients and in several cases waiting time has been extended to three years. In this process BAME patients have experienced much higher mortality whilst waiting for their organ transplants when compared to their White counterparts. Finally, a spurt in racism at work for BAME staff in the UK health sector has been noticed during the 12 months of Pandemic period. COVID-19 environment has also contributed enormously towards racism to BAME healthcare staff. Despite working in high risk-Covid wards under difficult time, their health and wellbeing has been affected severely. Unless we cannot adopt and implement zero tolerance racism policy at workplace, the racism against BAME workers cannot be halted. Behind all of these devastating impacts, the real issues lie in the fundamental socio-economic inequalities typically faced by BAME people over several generations caused by the high risks and low-paid employment and inferior living conditions. We will not be able to address the widespread differentials in health outcomes including mortality from COVID-19 until we tackle the disparity in the all-round life opportunities that BAME people have to deal with every day.

## Author details

Anil Gumber
Faculty of Health and Wellbeing, Sheffield Hallam University, UK

*Address all correspondence to: a.gumber@shu.ac.uk

## References

[1] Covid Live – Coronavirus Statistics [Internet]. Available from: https://www.worldometers.info/coronavirus/ [Accessed: 01 January 2022]

[2] Public Health England. Disparities in the Risks and Outcomes from COVID-19. 2020. Available from: https://www.gov.uk/government/publications/covid-19-review-of-disparities-in-risks-and-outcomes [Accessed: 01 January 2022]

[3] Bellary S, O'Hare JP, Raymond NT, Mughal S, Gumber A, et al. Enhanced diabetes care to patients of south Asian ethnic origin (the United Kingdom Asian diabetes study): A cluster randomised controlled trial. Lancet. 2008;**371**(9626):1769-1776

[4] Gumber A, Gumber L. Differential effects of COVID-19 by gender and ethnicity. BMJ Rapid Response. 2020; **369**. https://www.bmj.com/content/369/bmj.m1548/rr-9

[5] Gombart AF, Pierre A, Maggini S. A review of micronutrients and the immune system–working in harmony to reduce the risk of infection. Nutrients. 2020;**12**(1):236

[6] Kathleen Mahan L, Raymond JL. Krause's Food & the Nutrition Care Process. 13th ed. Elsevier Health Sciences. Riverport Lane, St. Louis, Missouri (USA): Saunders; pp. 60-96

[7] Healthline. 10 Breathing Techniques for Stress Relief and More [Internet]. Available from: https://www.healthline.com/health/breathing-exercise [Accessed: 01 January 2022]

[8] COVID-19 mental health and wellbeing surveillance: report by Office for Health Improvement & Disparities (UK) [Internet]. 2021. https://www.gov.uk/government/publications/covid-19-mental-health-and-wellbeing-surveillance-report#full-publication-update-history. [Accessed: 01 January 2022]

[9] Proto E, Quintana-Domeque C. COVID-19 and mental health deterioration among BAME groups in the UK. In: IZA Discussion Paper 13503. Bonn, Germany: Institute of Labour Economics; 2020

[10] Gumber A, Gumber L. Improving prevention, monitoring and Management of Diabetes among ethnic minorities: Contextualising the six G's approach. BMC Research Notes. 2017; **10**(1):774. DOI: 10.1186/s13104-017-3104-9

[11] Gumber A. Hesitancy in uptake of Covid vaccine by certain population groups. BMJ, Rapid Response. 2021;**372**. https://www.bmj.com/content/372/bmj.n513/rr-1

[12] Local Government Association. Changing behaviours in public health: To nudge or to shove? [Internet]. 2013. Available from: https://www.local.gov.uk/sites/default/files/documents/changing-behaviours-publi-e0a.pdf [Accessed: 01 January 2022]

[13] Gumber L, Gumber A. COVID-19 and 'lockdown' in organ transplantation in the UK. Public Health. 2020;**185**: 55-56. DOI: 10.1016/j.puhe.2020.06.017

[14] NHS Blood and Transplant. Organ and Tissue Donation and Transplantation: Activity Report 2020/21 [Internet]. 2021. Available from: https://nhsbtdbe.blob.core.windows.net/umbraco-assets-corp/23461/activity-report-2020-2021.pdf [Accessed: 01 January 2022]

[15] NHS Blood and Transplant. Organ Donation and Transplantation data for Black, Asian, Mixed Race and Minority Ethnic (BAME) communities Report for

2020/2021(1 April 2016 - 31 March 2021) [Internent]. 2021. Available from: https://nhsbtdbe.blob.core.windows.net/umbraco-assets-corp/25529/bame-report-final-2020_2021.pdf [Accessed: 01 January 2022]

[16] Ramamurthy A, Bhanbharo S, Gumber A et al. Nursing Narratives: Racism and the Pandemic. Draft Report submitted to UKRI-Covid Rapid Response Call Project. Sheffield, UK: Sheffield Hallam University; 2022

Chapter 11

# Mental Impact of COVID-19 – Fear, Stress, Anxiety, Depression and Sequels

*Ashwin Parchani, Prasan Kumar Panda and Vijay Krishnan*

## Abstract

Disease pandemics are known to cause mental impact, COVID-19 is not an exception. The ensuing mental health issues are not only restricted to the patients and their relatives/friends but affect the healthcare workers (HCWs) as well. Home isolated/quarantined patients/care takers experience a greater tendency of fear, stress, anxiety, and depression compared to those admitted in the hospital. Similarly, HCWs posted in COVID-19 designated areas of the hospital display higher levels of mental problems in comparison to those posted in non-COVID areas. Furthermore, long COVID-19 syndrome encompasses another large mental impact after 4-12 weeks of acute illness. Several instruments are available to screen for anxiety, fear, stress and depression, including the PSS 10 and DASS 21 questionnaires. These can be used by any HCW and even by educated patients or their care takers with telemedicine guidance from HCW. Treatment is also simple and cognitive behavioral therapy is a major solution and can be markedly practice with tele-consultation. The high degree of uncertainty associated with novel pathogens like COVID-19, both during acute and chronic effects has a profound effect on the mental state of asymptomatic/suspected/confirmed patients, their care takers, friends, as well as HCWs. However, by accepting pandemic with new-normal life of COVID-19 appropriate behaviors, human mankind can overcome these impacts.

**Keywords:** anxiousness, coronavirus, suicide, fearfulness, post-traumatic stress disorder, stress disorder

## 1. Introduction

The development of the coronavirus disease 2019 (COVID-19) epidemic, caused by severe acute respiratory syndrome coronavirus 2 (SARS-CoV-2) infection, triggered a global scenario of socio-economic catastrophe and psychological anguish. Many psychological problems and essential mental health consequences, including stress, anxiety, depression, frustration, uncertainty during the COVID-19 outbreak, emerged progressively.

In response to this dire circumstance, specific public policies were introduced by governments globally. These measures include self-quarantine, isolation, and social distancing. Implementing these policies caused the closure of educational institutes, offices, workplaces, public places, and social gathering restrictions. People were advised to stay at home and follow advice proposed by the WHO to protect



IntechOpen

themselves and others from the spread of COVID- 19. The strict self-quarantine order (lockdown) has kept the entire population in selected jurisdictions in isolation, with a significant impact on people's life [1]. Although social activities have been restricted in most countries, almost all non-essential individual movements were prohibited due to quarantine, while the local hospitals received suddenly thousands of critically ill COVID-19 patients and were forced to implement their emergency protocols.

In this context, the general population and most of the front-line healthcare workers became vulnerable to the emotional impact of COVID-19 infection due to both the pandemic and its consequences worldwide. The modern society, in which everyone can travel and communicate quickly, has seldom been subjected to the present social isolation and constraints associated with feelings of dissatisfaction and uncertainty. This unusual scenario surrounding the COVID-19 epidemic illustrates that people are fundamentally and emotionally unprepared for the negative impacts of biological disasters, which immediately highlight how everyone may be vulnerable and helpless.

There is a constant update about the disease available on news channels and over the Internet, highlighting the number of individuals affected and deaths due to COVID-19. Also, inadequate knowledge and overwhelming news may contribute to fear and anxiety among the public. People at large may experience disappointment, irritability, and boredom under isolation measures [2]. The communication technologies' facilities and transmission of inaccurate or sensational information may increase unacceptable social reactions such as aggression and rage [3].

The psychological reactions to the COVID-19 pandemic may vary from panic behavior or collective hysteria to pervasive feelings of hopelessness and desperation associated with adverse outcomes, including suicidal behavior [4]. Significantly, other health measures may be compromised by abnormally elevated anxiety. According to the social role invested, the security measures adopted in managing the pandemic had different consequences on individuals. Suspected and confirmed COVID-19 cases are likely to experience anxiety, loneliness, depression, denial, insomnia, and fear [5]. Health authorities' strict quarantine policy and mandatory contact tracing policy may lead to social rejection, discrimination, financial loss, and stigmatization. Medical health workers are first-line fighters treating patients with COVID-19. They are a unique subset of exposed individuals as they are equipped with the resources and knowledge to address the dangers imposed by a pandemic. Despite this, they are not impervious to the detrimental impact of the pandemic on their psychological health and behavior. During the challenging times of a pandemic, healthcare workers, the most exposed group, are vulnerable to psychological challenges. Every day, they face a high risk of being infected and are exposed to prolonged and distressing work shifts to meet health requirements. This has placed healthcare workers around the world in an unprecedented situation.

This epidemic, as well as the public health measures put in place to slow it down, has drastically altered people's lifestyles and is believed to pose a threat to their physical and mental health. This significant health catastrophe is impacting numerous countries, with high rates of transmission and death, and extensive outbreaks and mortality are linked to negative mental health consequences.

## 2. Fear

Strasner (1987) defined fear as "an emotional reaction (rational or irrational) to an object (animate or inanimate) or event that is associated with increased risk of danger and also unpleasantness, agitation and a desire to hide, flee or seek protection." Phobia, on the other hand, is characterized by intense, severe, and persistent fear. Such fears lead to persistent efforts to avoid (flee) the source of distress, often by undertaking a number of "safety behaviors". As a new infection with the potential for loss of life, COVID-19 has provoked legitimate fears. However, in a minority of subjects, this has also led to extreme restrictions, which could be characterized as "coronaphobia" [6]. Adequate communication that engenders a realistic appraisal of the risks, along with clear statements of behaviors that can reduce transmission, have been effective to control these fears, while also preventing viral transmission.

### 2.1 Fear among patient population

SARS-CoV2 infected patients experienced a high degree of fear stemming from uncertainity of illness outcome, inability to communicate with family members, lack of complete knowledge of the disease process and the stigma associated with being infected with the virus. Morever, the fear of isolation, discrimination and stigmatization was also noted in this group [7]. Those patients suspected to have SARS-CoV2 infection are also prey to the terror of having the disease, advancement of disease, precariousness of healthcare delivery and quarantine as per government regulations. Besides, even patients suffering from other illnesses displayed features of trepidation of inability to receive proper treatment due to overwhelmed healthcare resources. Patients with chronic diseases like diabetes, TB, and heart failure, for example, were found to avoid seeking medical treatment because they were afraid of contracting the illness from others in a healthcare facility, adding to fear of contagion. The type of chronic disease is a significant predictor of fear with higher levels noted among those diagnosed with autoimmune diseases or receiving immunosuppressants [8].

### 2.2 Fear among HCW population

Despite being the highest risk exposure group, healthcare workers have been found to experience less fear compared to the patient population as well as the general public. In a study conducted in India it was observed that a mere 18.3% healthcare workers reported of fear of contracting the infection. Most healthcare workers displayed concern and fear of transmitting the infection to their families and loved ones, especially to their children and the elderly [9]. Higher levels of fear were present in lab technicians, X-ray technicians and nurses while physicians were found to have the lowest level of fear. A possible explanation of this is that technicians and nurse have more exposure to contracting the illness during sampling, testing and medication of patients [10]. Non-medical healthcare workers were assessed to have lowest fear quotient juxtaposed to medical healthcare workers who are usually in direct contact with SARS-CoV2 infected patients and have a better understanding of the disease and its mortality [11]. Alike patients, healthcare workers are not immune to the fear of social marginalization. Assault on doctors, eviction of resident physicians from their rented houses, and fear of infection from healthcare workers have all been reported [12, 13]. These factors alongwith the shortage of sufficient protective equipment, absence of effective therapy and the virus's high infectivity rate might possibly play a role in their fearfulness of coronavirus pandemic. The presence of fear among HCWs poses a significant threat to their psychological adjustment skills and impede delivery of optimum care to patients.

## 3. Stress

Claude Bernard noted that the maintenance of life is critically dependent on keeping our internal milieu constant in the face of a changing environment. In 1956, Selye coined the term "stress" to represent the effects of anything that seriously threatens homeostasis. The actual or perceived threat to an organism is referred to as the "stressor" and the response to the stressor is called the "stress response." Although stress responses evolved as adaptive processes, Selye observed that severe, prolonged stress responses might lead to tissue damage and disease. During pandemics, the victims and at-risk groups tend to experience stress. As a consequence of the pandemic, even the health professionals who were overworked suffered high level of psychophysical stress. Various tools and questionnaires have been devised to measure stress levels in individuals. The most commonly used are DASS-21 and SAS. Studies have shown that psychological stress can affect the immune system through neuroendocrine pathways [14].

### 3.1 Stress among patient population

The increasing number of confirmed cases, a lack of knowledge of COVID-19, the rapid transmission rate, infection fears, lockdown conditions, difficulties in routine medical treatments, shortages of human resources in hospitals, insufficient psychological preparation, separation from loved ones, financial loss, stigma, loss of freedom, and uncertainty over illness status act as significant stressors for patients. These patients often display features of distress such as feeling nervous, worried in certain situations of panic, tendency to overreact, inability to control things in life, inability to overcome difficulties in daily life, and coping with things. The early months of pandemic had the higher reported prevalence of stress with a significant proportion of individuals reporting being upset due to things happening unexpectedly, inability to overcome difficulties in daily life, and anger at things being outside their control. Among suspected patients, those with history of travel to areas with ongoing community transmission were found to display greater stress [15]. Patients who are kept in isolation and quarantine experience significant levels stress as well [2]. It is expected that individuals may resort to social media during corona-led social distancing for stress relief and with the aim of accessing entertaining content, such as movies, comedies, and communication with family and friends, but frequent media exposure may itself be a source of psychological stress for these patients [16, 17]. Distress and panic during pandemics can propagate and promote misinformation in various ways along with increased digital screen time and unhealthy use of technology. Amid this, there has been a hidden epidemic of "information" that makes COVID-19 stand out as a "digital infodemic" from the earlier outbreaks. Misinformation and fake news are invariable accompaniments to this "information pollution" which can add to existent superior stress levels in the population [18]. Unfortunately, even immunocompromised and chronic disease patients are under tremendous psychological and physical stress in the face of this large-scale infectious public health crisis due to lack of proper healthcare infrastructure and treatment [19–21].

### 3.2 Stress among HCW population

Amid the ongoing unforeseen situation of coronavirus disease 2019 (COVID-19) pandemic, health care workers of multiple disciplines have been predisposed to a considerable amount of stress. A statistically significant association was found between perceived stress and female sex, designation (postgraduate trainees), work hours ≥6 hours/day, COVID-19 positive ward duties and staying with family due to potential risk of transmission to family members [22]. Disturbed sleep time and schedules due to rotational duties exhaust these HCWs both physically and mentally. The physical discomfort and occupational dermatoses associated with the use of PPE have also been shown to be related to greater levels of stress symptoms [23]. Practicing new methods of a discipline different than what he/she has mastered over the years, long hours of working in extreme conditions under PPE kit discomfort, long duty hours with no food/water/urination allowed during the time of duty with PPE, and irritation and physical strain in PPE during the summer season have been constant precipitators of stress among the doctors of all the disciplines working as frontline warriors [22]. With a scarcity of resources and an ever increasing number of patients, life-saving decisions have to be made. Making such decisions amid intense work pressure leads to added stress within emergency departments as well as during after-duty hours [24]. All doctors are susceptible to developing higher stress irrespective of their discipline during the COVID-19 pandemic, and this is further precipitated by their quarantined living conditions [22, 25]. Older HCWs demonstrate a high level of psychological distress, possibly as a result of increased complications of COVID-19 with increasing age and also because older people may have health issues making them more prone to infection with its complications [26]. In conclusion, HCWs are exposed to a protracted source of distress which may exceed their individual coping skills and lead to further chronic psychological problems.

## 4. Anxiety

Anxiety is an emotion characterized by the feeling of tension, worried thoughts and physical changes such as increased heart rate, according to the American psychological association. Since the onset of pandemic, many studies have been conducted to ascertain the prevalence of COVID-19 related anxiety among various sectors of the population. Conventional tools utilized to assess anxiety are:

- Depression, anxiety and stress scale-21 (DASS-21)
- Self-rating anxiety scale (SAS)
- Generalized anxiety disorder scale (GAD-7)
- Chinese version of GAD-7 scale
- Hospital anxiety and depression scale (HADS)

The magnitude of anxiety varies across the country of origin of study, measurement tool used and size of the studied sample.

### 4.1 Anxiety among patient population

Patients suspected or diagnosed with SARS-CoV2 infection experience significant anxiety related to disease and external factors associated with having the infection. Several patient related factors influence the vulnerability to anxiety such as sex, marital status, symptoms and sleep quality, among others [27–30]. There are many patient-related factors associated with anxiety such as:

a. Female gender

b. Older age

c. Divorce/bereavement

d. Married

e. Residing with family

f. Need of oxygen inhalation

g. History of fever

h. Two or more symptoms of infection

i. Suspected/confirmed infection

j. Poor sleep quality

k. Quarantine/isolation

The external factors include spread of misinformation by media, government regulations such as quarantine procedure, lockdown and travel restrictions, and social stigmatization. The current pandemic underlined the vital role played by media in dissemination of information. Ideally, media should ensure that crisis communication helps in dispelling fear and uncertainty, but in the recent pandemic it played a reverse role in spreading anxiety and panic behavior [31–33]. The endless newsfeeds related to COVID-19 infection and death rates considerably increased the adverse psychological outcomes in general population as well as patients. The spread of misleading narratives, provoking controversies and advertisement of unapproved therapies resulted in widespread fear, confusion and panic with serious mental health consequences such as anxiety [34, 35]. Quarantine and isolation of suspected and confirmed cases as per government regulations also led to abnormally increased anxiety. Additional measures like lockdown and travel restrictions also contribute to feeling of uncertainty, perceived lower social support, separation from loved ones, loss of freedom and boredom [2]. Notably, individuals with a previous health disorder experienced worsening of their symptoms due to anxiety.

### 4.2 Anxiety among HCW population

Healthcare workers are directly involved in diagnosis, treatment and care of SARS-CoV2 patients and therefore experience the highest share of mental health issues compared to the other groups in the population. The prevalence of anxiety among healthcare workers is high and has been assessed to be between 23.2% to 30.5% [36, 37]. Several factors have been attributed to cause anxiety in healthcare workers. These include increased workload, inadequate PPE, inadequate isolation precautions, risk of contracting disease, high infectivity and mortality of disease, burnout, lack of clinical experience, young age, chronic health illness and prior history of mental health disorders [31–33]. Socio-demographic variables play a key role in determining the level of anxiety in healthcare workers with higher prevalence among those above the age 40, females, unmarried individuals and presence of offspring [38]. Anxiety in this group manifests as palpitations, tremors, dryness of mouth, feeling scared without any reason and tendency to panic [15]. These symptoms are more prevalent in workers who were assigned duties in COVID designated areas and those who encountered SARS-CoV2 suspected or confirmed patients without adequate protection [5]. Nurses have unfavorable mental health outcomes among the healthcare staff since they usually spend more time caring for patients than any other group of HCWs [11, 36, 39]. The existence of anxiety is associated with reduced performance and fatigue in healthcare workers and impedes optimum healthcare delivery to the population.

## 5. Depression

Depression is one of the five most incapacitating illnesses, and by 2030, it is expected to be one of the major issues in industrialized countries. It's a common reaction to a rapid deterioration in living conditions, which involves isolation and uncertainty. When people are subjected to unpredictable circumstances, they feel helpless and unmotivated, which can lead to sadness [40]. During past epidemic outbreaks (SARS and Ebola), rates of depression in the general population have been reported with a prevalence approaching even 73.10 percent [41]. Past epidemics were more quickly contained, and infection rates were lower despite greater fatality rates, which might explain why depressive symptoms were less common [42]. Furthermore, during the SARS pandemic in Canada, Hawryluck et al. discovered that the length and unpredictability of the lockdown contributed to greater levels of depression [43]. As a result, the present global lockdown measures might explain the increased incidence of depressive symptoms reported during the COVID-19 epidemic. According to a research that looked at 69 million health data from over 62,000 persons diagnosed with COVID-19, 6% of COVID-19 patients suffered mental health problems including sadness and anxiety within three months of diagnosis, compared to 3.4 percent of non-COVID-19 patients [44]. The addition of a psychological burden to an already devastating physical burden affects the prognosis in a number of ways, with long-term consequences. Furthermore, those who are depressed are less likely to seek treatment for physical or mental problems; as a result, depression, like anxiety, can act as a barrier to reasonable medical and mental health interventions during a pandemic.

### 5.1 Depression among patient population

Earlier outbreaks such as SARS and MERS have displayed the presence of depressed mood among those with acute infection [45]. The COVID-19 pandemic is no different. The reported prevalence of depression at 6% in COVID-19 patients is higher to general population [44]. Females are more likely to experience depression than males [46]. According to one study, nearly one-fourth patients had intended to commit suicide or harm oneself [27]. Individuals who were married or underwent a divorce exhibited greater levels of depression than single individuals [27]. This could in part be explained by worries for one's family and grief of separation respectively. Having a family member with confirmed COVID-19, and having two current physical symptoms are independent risk factors for depressive symptoms [28]. Suicide has become a more pressing concern as the pandemic evolved [47]. Those with psychiatric disorders experience worsening symptoms and others are predisposed to develop depression, are all associated with increased suicide risk. Media and other news platforms also affect mental health and psychological behavior [35]. Despite the fact that receiving regular updates on COVID-related health information appears to reduce sadness, it is also claimed that social media exposure is linked to depression and mixed anxiety and depression [48–50]. Unemployment, low social status, a lack of social support, and financial losses are among socioeconomic variables that might contribute to greater incidence of depression [48, 49, 51, 52]. The added impact of quarantine has led to high occurrence of depression and even self-reported suicidal thoughts [29, 53].

### 5.2 Depression among HCW population

The COVID-19 pandemic has significant negative impacts on healthcare workers' psychological health, fostering anxiety, depression, and sleep disturbance. Studies conducted during the SARS have reported a prevalence of depression among the front-line HCWs to be 38.5% [54]. The factors in play causing depression are pretty similar to those contributing to anxiety. Increased workload, burnout, inadequate PPE, the risk of contracting the disease, and the challenge of making difficult moral decisions about care priorities during the pandemic have exposed healthcare workers to severe psychological pressures leading to depression. The high infectivity and mortality rates also contribute to depression among healthcare workers around the world. Furthermore, factors such as a high-risk workplace, a lack of clinical experience, young age, and a history of psychological disorders can contribute to depression among healthcare workers. Working on the front lines was found to be an independent risk factor for poor mental health outcomes across all aspects studied, including the prevalence of depression among HCWs. Between doctors and nurses, the latter have been studied to harbor a greater level of depression [55–57]. This may be partially confounded by the fact that nurses are primarily female but could also be attributed to the fact they may face a greater risk of exposure to COVID-19 patients as they spend more time onwards, provide direct care to patients and are responsible for the collection of sputum for virus detection [55]. Emotional exhaustion, depersonalization, being a nurse, 12- or 24-hour shifts or on-call hours, those who live with people who are at risk, and being very concerned about a possible infection of a family member they do not live with are all positively and significantly related to having depression symptoms [58]. Depression is also significantly higher among HCWs who did not know the latest COVID-19-related research/information. Lack of information may precipitate mental health concerns, and prior studies have suggested that updates and knowledge about COVID-19 may have psychosocial impacts, possibly as they represent an active way of coping and dealing with pandemic-related issues [59, 60]. Research also indicates that healthcare workers who take vacation days experience lower levels of depression [26]. Unfortunately, the COVID-19 pandemic crisis witnessed doctors along with other healthcare workers question their choice of profession, in part due to rising infection rates, unavailability of adequate personal protective equipment and other unexpected pandemic related experiences [60].

## 6. Sequelae

Long COVID is a term used to describe a condition in COVID-19 patients who have symptoms over an extended period [61]. These patients report prolonged, multisystem involvement and significant disability, which can last for more than six months in 93.2% of patients after the acute phase of illness [62]. Musculoskeletal, cardiovascular, gastrointestinal, pulmonary, and neuropsychiatric symptoms are prevalent in >85% of participants. Fatigue, breathing problems and cognitive dysfunction are among the most debilitating symptoms [62]. Such prolonged physical sequelae are associated with and often are a harbinger of psychological sequelae. Multiple studies conducted during previous pandemics also support the development of psychiatric sequelae in survivors. SARS-CoV-1 survivors exhibited posttraumatic stress disorder (PTSD) with an incidence of up to 55%, depression was observed in 39%, pain disorder in 36.4%, panic disorder in 32.5%, and obsessive–compulsive disorder in 15.6% of SARS-CoV-1 survivors [63]. Long term psychiatric complications such as depressed mood, anxiety and insomnia were also reported in 10-20% of patients following SARS and MERS infections [45]. These complications could result from central nervous system involvement of the virus or perhaps a consequence of fear associated with the infection and isolation itself.

Among the psychological sequelae, the most prominent and popular condition is posttraumatic stress disorder [64]. Surviving a critical illness is known to induce PTS symptoms [65]. Data suggests that as many as 43% of COVID-19 patients suffered posttraumatic stress symptoms [66], 'not though true prevalence of PTSD' prevalence. The severity of COVID-19 poses a significant risk factor for PTSD, supported by evidence of higher incidence among ICU patients juxtaposed to non-ICU patients [67, 68]. Even measures of quarantine and isolation, which help to contain the infection from the spread, can have psychological consequences leading to PTSD [2]. Healthcare workers, too, experience significant PTS symptoms. Emotional fatigue, depersonalization, working in a hospital, being highly concerned that someone they live with may become infected, and believing that becoming infected with COVID-19 is very likely are all positively and substantially associated with posttraumatic stress symptoms in the HCW population [56].

Aside from PTSD, COVID-19 infection survivors are more likely to experience depression and anxiety, similar to the acute phase of the disease [64]. The incidence of these disorders is linked to the severity of the disease and the length of hospitalization [69–71]. The baseline systemic inflammation index (SII) is strongly correlated with anxiety and depression [45, 59]. At follow-up, the prevalence of baseline comorbidities, such as mental disorders and female sex, is also linked to depression and anxiety [71, 72]. Although anxiety and depression symptoms generally go away within 1-3 months after infection, their presence increases the risk of developing PTSD later on [61].

## 7. Preventive interventions

### 7.1 Routine screening of patients and their HCWs

Worldwide epidemiological research is urgently needed to evaluate the amount of anxiety, worry, and helplessness and other mental health concerns related to COVID-19. This would aid in developing tailored mental health initiatives (e.g., those who live in villages). Experiences from past pandemics point out the urgent need for screening for mental health problems, monitoring its trend, referral of cases, and providing suitable interventions has to be routine practice during the pandemic period [73, 74]. The target groups of such screening strategies must include COVID-19 infected patients, their high risk contacts, and healthcare workers, as well as those with past history of mental health illnesses. The following questionnaires may be utilized for routine screening:

a. COVID-19 stress scale [75]

b. Perceived Stress Scale modified for COVID-19 (PSS-10-C) [76]

c. COVID-19 Peritraumatic Distress Index (CPDI) [1]

d. Anxiety of COVID Scale (CAS) [77]

e. Fear of COVID-19 Scale (FC-19S) [78]

f. COVID-19 Pandemic Mental Health Questionnaire [79]

The abovementioned questionnaires were newly developed or modified versions of existing mental health screening questionnaires. It is therefore emphasized that the pre-existing validated survey tools such as GAD-65, PSS-10, PHQ-9 and DASS-21 can be also utilized for routine screening purposes and have been validated for the same.

### 7.2 Provision for health services during the pandemic period

- During the pandemic, marginalized groups such as those with chronic health conditions, mental health issues, and the elderly must continue to get health care. Provisions such as telemedicine and clinics independent from COVID-designated facilities should be guaranteed for optimal healthcare delivery in a continuum.

- The mental health and emergency management communities should collaborate to seek, develop, and disseminate evidence-based resources on disaster mental health, mental health triage and referral, unique populations' requirements, and death communication and bereavement support.

- Health care professionals should help patients manage stress and cope (by organizing activities and sticking to routines), introduce patients to social and mental health resources, and encourage them to seek professional mental health help if necessary.

- While most psychological health services can be provided in primary care settings, a few patients will require comprehensive mental health assessment and care, while others might benefit from supportive interventions targeted at enhancing wellbeing and coping such as psychoeducation or cognitive behavioral therapy.

- Patients with suicidal ideation shall necessitate immediate referral, hospitalization, and therapeutic intervention by a psychiatrist.

- Tele-psychiatry services are vital to maintain the continuum of care in the COVID pandemic era. Certain modifications are warranted to enhance the delivery of tele-health services – **video consultations** may be employed for triaging, screening, and providing first consultation services, **home visits** by a locally available nurse/ health care workers/ social workers augmented with video consultations with the psychiatrist, especially in cases of emergencies, and **construction of telemedicine practice guidelines** to enable physicians in better providing healthcare services telephonically.

### 7.3 Support for healthcare workers

- At each institution, teams of expert psychologists should be accessible for healthcare professionals to call at any time, and quick treatment and follow-ups should be given.

DOI: http://dx.doi.org/10.5772/intechopen.102754

- Peer support and group talks should be promoted as well. HCWs must be provided with stress management training.

- During pandemic conditions, vacations from work are required to reduce psychological distress among healthcare professionals, resulting in decreased levels of despair, fear, worry, and stress. Therefore, healthcare professionals are urged to take vacations from work to help them relax, which helps reduce stress.

- In regions where infrastructure is lacking, the government and health authorities must work together to provide PPEs and the essential infrastructure for HCWs to safely administer healthcare to their patients.

- Health-care systems are required to address the stress on individual providers and overall operations by monitoring reactions and performance indicators, modifying assignments and timetables, moderating expectations, and developing effective mechanisms to deliver psychological support as required.

- HCWs should be encouraged to self-monitor their own stress reactions and seek appropriate assistance. Systems must be in place to quickly identify HCWs who require psychological assistance, send them to a professional, and provide access to specialized consultations as well as intervention, if necessary. Setting up of grievance redressal system will be of great use for all the HCWs to raise any issue pertaining to their current work and prompt resolution and solutions can be offered.

- The process of testing, quarantine and re-joining work should be streamlined and communicated to everyone working in the establishment.

- A rotational basis in the work from highly stressful to low stressful duties can be considered.

- Encouragement and establishment of a buddy system with buddies being aware of need for confidentiality and available resources to help the person in distress.

- All HCWs should be encouraged to follow a healthy lifestyle such as having a daily routine, pursuing their hobbies and stress management and relaxation techniques such as yoga and breathing exercises.

### 7.4 Amendments in quarantine and isolation measures

Isolation and quarantine restrict one's activities severely, causing worry and concern over not fulfilling one's professional and familial obligations. While the methods and processes for mental health support and monitoring in quarantine accommodation differ by jurisdiction, there are several critical areas that should be included in national mental health screening, evaluation, and support protocols. These include:

- It is necessary to set up telephonic/digital contact between the patients and their family members.

- Psychological counseling should be offered in quarantine centers.

- Provision of a clear rationale for quarantine and information about protocols
- Prior to departure, throughout travel, upon arrival, and during the quarantine period, accurate and timely information is critical.
- The provision of a structured day with meaningful activities and opportunities for social connection is critical to preserving mental health. From the start, active participation is required, as well as the availability of a variety of individual and group activities from which to pick. COVID-19-compliant group activities must be delivered, if necessary using virtual methods.
- Every person in quarantine should ideally have access to fresh air through windows or a balcony, space to exercise, and healthy and culturally appropriate food options.
- People should be actively and assertively engaged in activities, well-being checks, and information.
- Effective governance necessitates that all providers involved in assisting persons under quarantine have clear lines of communication, information exchange, and complaint handling.

### 7.5 Role of media

COVID-19 news, as previously discussed, has a positive linkage with depression, anxiety, and stress levels. It can be caused by erroneous statistics data and rumors that circulate through the internet. To avoid misleading information and public health statistics, the government and health authorities must offer accurate and up-to-date information. In this context, the research found that having access to current and accurate health information is linked to less stress. Up-to-date and exact data on the number of new and improved cases, available treatment methods, and transmission routes must be used to reduce the illness's psychological and mental health effects. The psychological impact of misinformation/rumor on the mental health of HCWs and the general public might be greatly reduced if a public health information system that is accurate and updated is widely disseminated.

## 8. Conclusions

COVID-19 is linked to a range of psychiatric problems in addition to physical health issues. The spread of the novel coronavirus may have an influence on people's mental health in many communities. Patients with COVID-19 have a significant rate of negative psychological occurrences. Frontline healthcare professionals caring for COVID19 patients have a high rate of stress, anxiety, and depression. As a result, health policymakers should take steps to regulate and prevent mental illnesses among hospital employees. During the COVID-19 epidemic, the mental health of HCWs is a major issue. Psychological interventions that detect and target persons with varying degrees of psychological distress are desperately required.

## Conflict of interest

The authors declare no conflict of interest.

## Notes/thanks/other declarations

None.

## Author details

Ashwin Parchani[1], Prasan Kumar Panda[2]* and Vijay Krishnan[3]

1 Department of Internal Medicine, All India Institute of Medical Sciences (AIIMS), Rishikesh, India

2 Department of Internal Medicine (Infectious Disease Division), All India Institute of Medical Sciences (AIIMS), Rishikesh, India

3 Department of Psychiatry, All India Institute of Medical Sciences (AIIMS), Rishikesh, India

*Address all correspondence to: motherprasanna@rediffmail.com

## References

[1] Qiu J, Shen B, Zhao M, Wang Z, Xie B, Xu Y. A nationwide survey of psychological distress among Chinese people in the COVID-19 epidemic: Implications and policy recommendations. Gen Psychiatry. 2020;**33**(2):e100213

[2] Brooks SK, Webster RK, Smith LE, Woodland L, Wessely S, Greenberg N, et al. The psychological impact of quarantine and how to reduce it: Rapid review of the evidence. The Lancet. 2020;**395**(10227):912-920

[3] Wang Y, McKee M, Torbica A, Stuckler D. Systematic literature review on the spread of health-related misinformation on social media. Social Science & Medicine. 2019;**240**:112552

[4] Serafini G, Parmigiani B, Amerio A, Aguglia A, Sher L, Amore M. The psychological impact of COVID-19 on the mental health in the general population. QJM Int J Med. 2020; **113**(8):531-537

[5] Salari N, Hosseinian-Far A, Jalali R, Vaisi-Raygani A, Rasoulpoor S, Mohammadi M, et al. Prevalence of stress, anxiety, depression among the general population during the COVID-19 pandemic: A systematic review and meta-analysis. Globalization and Health. 2020;**16**(1):57

[6] Asmundson GJG, Taylor S. Coronaphobia: Fear and the 2019-nCoV outbreak. Journal of Anxiety Disorders. 2020;**70**:102196

[7] Abuhammad S, Alzoubi KH, Khabour O. Fear of COVID-19 and stigmatization towards infected people among Jordanian people. International Journal of Clinical Practice. 2021;**75**(4) Apr [cited 2021 Jul 29]. Available from: https://onlinelibrary.wiley.com/doi/10.1111/ijcp.13899

[8] Al-Rahimi JS, Nass NM, Hassoubah SA, Wazqar DY, Alamoudi SA. Levels and predictors of fear and health anxiety during the current outbreak of COVID-19 in immunocompromised and chronic disease patients in Saudi Arabia: A cross-sectional correlational study. Menezes RG, editor. PLoS One. 2021;16(4):e0250554.

[9] Chen Q, Liang M, Li Y, Guo J, Fei D, Wang L, et al. Mental health care for medical staff in China during the COVID-19 outbreak. Lancet Psychiatry. 2020;**7**(4):e15-e16

[10] Shehada AK, Albelbeisi AH, Albelbeisi A, El Bilbeisi AH, El Afifi A. The fear of COVID-19 outbreak among health care professionals in Gaza strip, Palestine. SAGE Open Med. 2021;**9**:205031212110229

[11] Saleem Z, Majeed MM, Rafique S, Siqqiqui Z, Ghandhi D, Tariq H, et al. COVID-19 pandemic fear and anxiety among healthcare professionals in Pakistan [Internet]. In Review. 2020 July [cited 2021 July 29]. Available from: https://www.researchsquare.com/article/rs-37608/v2

[12] Chiara G. NHS doctor kicked out by landlord because of Covid-19 fears. Independent [Internet]. 2020. Available from: https://www.independent.co.uk/news/health/coronavirus-latest-nhs-doctor-evicted-covid-19-oxford-a9425166.html

[13] Datta R. Kolkata landlords evict medical professionals, Resident Doctor's Association steps in. India Today [Internet]. 2020 Mar 25 [cited 2022 Feb 21]; Available from: https://www.indiatoday.in/india/story/bengal-kolkata-landlords-evict-medical-professionals-coronavirus-1659333-2020-03-25

[14] de Punder K, Heim C, Wadhwa PD, Entringer S. Stress and immunosenescence: The role of telomerase. Psychoneuroendocrinology. 2019;**101**:87-100

[15] Parchani A, Vidhya K, Panda PK, Rawat VS, Bahurupi Y, Kalita D, et al. Fear, anxiety, stress, and depression of novel coronavirus (COVID-19) pandemic among patients and their healthcare workers – A descriptive study. Psychology Research and Behavior Management. 2021; **14**:1737-1746

[16] Whiting A, Williams D. Why people use social media: A uses and gratifications approach. Qualitative Market Research: An International Journal. 2013;**16**(4):362-369

[17] Parvin GA, Ahsan R, Rahman MH, Abedin Md A. Novel coronavirus (COVID-19) pandemic: The role of printing Media in Asian Countries. Front Commun. 2020;**26**(5):557593

[18] Banerjee D, Sathyanarayana RT. Psychology of misinformation and the media: Insights from the COVID-19 pandemic. Indian J Soc Psychiatry. 2020;**36**(5):131

[19] Pigozzi E, Tregnago D, Costa L, Insolda J, Turati E, Rimondini M, et al. Psychological impact of Covid-19 pandemic on oncological patients: A survey in northern Italy. Di Gennaro F, editor. PLoS One. 2021;16(3):e0248714.

[20] Liang W, Guan W, Chen R, Wang W, Li J, Xu K, et al. Cancer patients in SARS-CoV-2 infection: A nationwide analysis in China. The Lancet Oncology. 2020;**21**(3):335-337

[21] Ng KYY, Zhou S, Tan SH, Ishak NDB, Goh ZZS, Chua ZY, et al. Understanding the psychological impact of COVID-19 pandemic on patients with cancer, their caregivers, and health Care Workers in Singapore. JCO Glob Oncol. 2020;**6**:1494-1509

[22] Das A, Sil A, Jaiswal S, Rajeev R, Thole A, Jafferany M, et al. A study to evaluate depression and perceived stress among frontline Indian doctors combating the COVID-19 pandemic. Prim Care Companion CNS Disord. [cited 2021 August 16] 2020;**22**(5). Available from: http://www.psychiatrist.com/PCC/article/Pages/covid-19-depression-and-stress-among-frontline-doctors.aspx

[23] Das A, Kumar S, Sil A, Jafferany M. Skin changes attributed to protective measures against COVID -19: A compilation. Dermatologic Therapy. 2020;**33**(4). [cited 2021 Aug 16]. Available from: https://onlinelibrary.wiley.com/doi/10.1111/dth.13796

[24] Koh D, Goh HP. Occupational health responses to COVID-19: What lessons can we learn from SARS? Journal of Occupational Health. 2020;**62**(1). [cited 2021 August 16]. Available from: https://onlinelibrary.wiley.com/doi/10.1002/1348-9585.12128

[25] Podder I, Agarwal K, Datta S. Comparative analysis of perceived stress in dermatologists and other physicians during national lock-down and COVID -19 pandemic with exploration of possible risk factors: A web-based cross-sectional study from eastern India. Dermatologic Therapy. 2020;**33**(4). [cited 2021 August 16]. Available from: https://onlinelibrary.wiley.com/doi/10.1111/dth.13788

[26] Alnazly E, Khraisat OM, Al-Bashaireh AM, Bryant CL. Anxiety, depression, stress, fear and social support during COVID-19 pandemic among Jordanian healthcare workers. Fernández-Alcántara M, editor. PLoS One. 2021;16(3):e0247679

[27] Wang M, Hu C, Zhao Q, Feng R, Wang Q, Cai H, et al. Acute

psychological impact on COVID-19 patients in Hubei: A multicenter observational study. Translational Psychiatry. 2021;**11**(1):133

[28] Dai L-L, Wang X, Jiang T-C, Li P-F, Wang Y, Wu S-J, et al. Anxiety and depressive symptoms among COVID-19 patients in Jianghan Fangcang shelter Hospital in Wuhan, China. Pakpour AH, editor. PLoS One. 2020;15(8):e0238416

[29] Jassim G, Jameel M, Brennan E, Yusuf MA, Hasan N, Alwatani Y. Psychological impact of COVID-19, isolation, and quarantine: A cross-sectional study. Neuropsychiatric Disease and Treatment. 2021; **17**:1413-1421

[30] Kong X, Kong F, Zheng K, Tang M, Chen Y, Zhou J, et al. Effect of psychological–Behavioral intervention on the depression and anxiety of COVID-19 patients. Frontiers in Psychiatry. 2020;**11**:586355

[31] Su Z, McDonnell D, Wen J, Kozak M, Abbas J, Šegalo S, et al. Mental health consequences of COVID-19 media coverage: The need for effective crisis communication practices. Globalization and Health. 2021;**17**(1):4

[32] Gabbiadini A, Baldissarri C, Durante F, Valtorta RR, De Rosa M, Gallucci M. Together apart: The mitigating role of digital communication technologies on negative affect during the COVID-19 outbreak in Italy. Frontiers in Psychology. 2020;**21**(11):554678

[33] Ahmad AR, Murad HR. The impact of social media on panic during the COVID-19 pandemic in Iraqi Kurdistan: Online questionnaire study. Journal of Medical Internet Research. 2020;**22**(5):e19556

[34] Venegas-Vera AV, Colbert GB, Lerma EV. Positive and negative impact of social media in the COVID-19 era. Rev Cardiovasc Med. 30 Dec 2020;21(4):561-564. doi: 10.31083/j.rcm.2020.04.195. PMID: 33388000

[35] Wen J, Aston J, Liu X, Ying T. Effects of misleading media coverage on public health crisis: A case of the 2019 novel coronavirus outbreak in China. Anatolia. 2020;**31**(2):331-336

[36] Pappa S, Ntella V, Giannakas T, Giannakoulis VG, Papoutsi E, Katsaounou P. Prevalence of depression, anxiety, and insomnia among healthcare workers during the COVID-19 pandemic: A systematic review and meta-analysis. Brain, Behavior, and Immunity. 2020;**88**:901-907

[37] Adibi A, Golitaleb M, Farrahi-Ashtiani I, Pirani D, Yousefi K, Jamshidbeigi Y, et al. The prevalence of generalized anxiety disorder among health care workers during the COVID-19 pandemic: A systematic review and meta-analysis. Frontiers in Psychiatry. 2021;**31**(12):658846

[38] Alzaid E, Alsaad S, Alshakhis N, Albagshi D, Albesher R, Aloqaili M. Prevalence of COVID-19-related anxiety among healthcare workers: A cross-sectional study. J Fam Med Prim Care. 2020;**9**(9):4904

[39] Lai J, Ma S, Wang Y, Cai Z, Hu J, Wei N, et al. Factors associated with mental health outcomes among health care workers exposed to coronavirus disease 2019. JAMA Network Open. 2020;**3**(3):e203976

[40] Seligman MEP. Learned helplessness. Annual Review of Medicine. 1972;**23**(1):407-412

[41] Chew Q, Wei K, Vasoo S, Chua H, Sim K. Narrative synthesis of psychological and coping responses towards emerging infectious disease outbreaks in the general population: Practical considerations for the

COVID-19 pandemic. Singapore Medical Journal. 2020;**61**(7):350-356

[42] Huremović D. Social distancing, quarantine, and isolation. In: Huremović D, editor. Psychiatry of Pandemics. Cham: Springer International Publishing; 2019. pp. 85-94. [cited 2021 August 16]. Available from: http://link.springer.com/101007/978-3-030-15346-5_8

[43] Hawryluck L, Gold WL, Robinson S, Pogorski S, Galea S, Styra R. SARS control and psychological effects of quarantine, Toronto, Canada. Emerging Infectious Diseases. 2004;**10**(7):7

[44] Taquet M, Luciano S, Geddes JR, Harrison PJ. Bidirectional associations between COVID-19 and psychiatric disorder: Retrospective cohort studies of 62 354 COVID-19 cases in the USA. Lancet Psychiatry. 2021;**8**(2):130-140

[45] Rogers JP, Chesney E, Oliver D, Pollak TA, McGuire P, Fusar-Poli P, et al. Psychiatric and neuropsychiatric presentations associated with severe coronavirus infections: A systematic review and meta-analysis with comparison to the COVID-19 pandemic. Lancet Psychiatry. 2020;**7**(7): 611-627

[46] Hurissi E, Abu-jabir E, Mohammed A, Mahnashi M, Alharbi S, Alharbi A, et al. Assessment of new-onset depression and anxiety associated with COVID-19. Middle East Curr Psychiatry. 2021;**28**(1):33

[47] Gunnell D, Appleby L, Arensman E, Hawton K, John A, Kapur N, et al. Suicide risk and prevention during the COVID-19 pandemic. Lancet Psychiatry. 2020;**7**(6):468-471

[48] Nguyen HC, Nguyen MH, Do BN, Tran CQ, Nguyen TTP, Pham KM, et al. People with suspected COVID-19 symptoms were more likely depressed and had lower health-related quality of life: The potential benefit of health literacy. Journal of Clinical Medicine. 2020;**9**(4):965

[49] Ni MY, Yang L, Leung CMC, Li N, Yao XI, Wang Y, et al. Mental health, risk factors, and social media use during the COVID-19 epidemic and cordon sanitaire among the community and health professionals in Wuhan, China: Cross-sectional survey. JMIR Ment Health. 2020;**7**(5):e19009

[50] Gao J, Zheng P, Jia Y, Chen H, Mao Y, Chen S, et al. Mental health problems and social media exposure during COVID-19 outbreak. PLoS One. 2020;**15**(4):e0231924

[51] Mazza MG, De Lorenzo R, Conte C, Poletti S, Vai B, Bollettini I, et al. Anxiety and depression in COVID-19 survivors: Role of inflammatory and clinical predictors. Brain, Behavior, and Immunity. 2020;**89**:594-600

[52] Lei L, Huang X, Zhang S, Yang J, Yang L, Xu M. Comparison of prevalence and associated factors of anxiety and depression among people affected by versus people unaffected by quarantine during the COVID-19 epidemic in southwestern China. Med Sci Monit Int Med J Exp Clin Res. 2020;**26**(26):e924609

[53] Wathelet M, Duhem S, Vaiva G, Baubet T, Habran E, Veerapa E, et al. Factors associated with mental health disorders Among University students in France confined during the COVID-19 pandemic. JAMA Network Open. 2020;**3, 10**:e2025591

[54] Su T, Lien T, Yang C, Su Y, Wang J, Tsai S, et al. Prevalence of psychiatric morbidity and psychological adaptation of the nurses in a structured SARS caring unit during outbreak: A prospective and periodic assessment study in Taiwan. Journal of Psychiatric Research. 2007;**41**(1-2):119-130

[55] Liu Z, Han B, Jiang R, Huang Y, Ma C, Wen J, et al. Mental health status of doctors and nurses during COVID-19 epidemic in China. SSRN Electronic. Journal. 2020. [cited 2021 Aug 29] Available from: https://www.ssrn.com/abstract=3551329

[56] Du J, Dong L, Wang T, Yuan C, Fu R, Zhang L, et al. Psychological symptoms among frontline healthcare workers during COVID-19 outbreak in Wuhan. General Hospital Psychiatry. 2020;**67**:144-145

[57] Guo J, Liao L, Wang B, Li X, Guo L, Tong Z, et al. Psychological effects of COVID-19 on hospital staff: A National Cross-Sectional Survey of China mainland. SSRN Electronic Journal. 2020. [cited 2021 Aug 30]. Available from: https://www.ssrn.com/abstract=3550050

[58] Luceño-Moreno L, Talavera-Velasco B, García-Albuerne Y, Martín-García J. Symptoms of posttraumatic stress, anxiety, depression, levels of resilience and burnout in Spanish health personnel during the COVID-19 pandemic. International Journal of Environmental Research and Public Health. 2020;**17**(15):5514

[59] Dubey S, Biswas P, Ghosh R, Chatterjee S, Dubey MJ, Chatterjee S, et al. Psychosocial impact of COVID-19. Diabetes and Metabolic Syndrome: Clinical Research & Reviews. 2020;**14**(5):779-788

[60] Tasnim R, Sujan Md SH, Islam Md S, Ritu AH, Siddique Md AB, Toma TY, et al. Prevalence and correlates of anxiety and depression in frontline healthcare workers treating people with COVID-19 in Bangladesh. BMC Psychiatry. 2021;**21**(1):271

[61] Nabavi N. Long covid: How to define it and how to manage it. BMJ. 2020;370:m3489. doi: 10.1136/bmj.m3489

[62] Davis HE, Assaf GS, McCorkell L, Wei H, Low RJ, Re'em Y, et al. Characterizing long COVID in an international cohort: 7 months of symptoms and their impact. E Clinical Medicine. 2021;38:101019. doi: 10.1016/j.eclinm.2021.101019. Epub 2021 Jul 15. PMID: 34308300

[63] Lam MH-B. Mental morbidities and chronic fatigue in severe acute respiratory syndrome survivors: Long-term follow-up. Archives of Internal Medicine. 2009;**169**(22):2142

[64] Schou TM, Joca S, Wegener G, Bay-Richter C. Psychiatric and neuropsychiatric sequelae of COVID-19 – A systematic review. Brain, Behavior, and Immunity. 2021;97:328-348. doi: 10.1016/j.bbi.2021.07.018. Epub 2021 Jul 30. PMID: 34339806

[65] Sparks SW. Posttraumatic stress syndrome: What is it? Journal of Trauma Nursing. 2018;**25**(1):60-65

[66] Alemanno F, Houdayer E, Parma A, Spina A, Del Forno A, Scatolini A, et al. COVID-19 cognitive deficits after respiratory assistance in the subacute phase: A COVID-rehabilitation unit experience. Di Gennaro F. PLoS One. 2021;16(2):e0246590

[67] Halpin SJ, McIvor C, Whyatt G, Adams A, Harvey O, McLean L, et al. Postdischarge symptoms and rehabilitation needs in survivors of COVID-19 infection: A cross-sectional evaluation. Journal of Medical Virology. 2021;**93**(2):1013-1022

[68] Horn M, Wathelet M, Fovet T, Amad A, Vuotto F, Faure K, et al. Is COVID-19 associated with posttraumatic stress disorder? The Journal of Clinical Psychiatry. 2020;**82**(1). [cited 2021 August 17]. Available from: https://www.psychiatrist.com/JCP/article/Pages/is-covid-19-associated-with-posttraumatic-stress-disorder.aspx

[69] Huang C, Huang L, Wang Y, Li X, Ren L, Gu X, et al. 6-month consequences of COVID-19 in patients discharged from hospital: A cohort study. The Lancet. 2021;**397**(10270): 220-232

[70] Al-Aly Z, Xie Y, Bowe B. High-dimensional characterization of post-acute sequelae of COVID-19. Nature. 2021;**594**(7862):259-264

[71] Mazza MG, Palladini M, De Lorenzo R, Magnaghi C, Poletti S, Furlan R, et al. Persistent psychopathology and neurocognitive impairment in COVID-19 survivors: Effect of inflammatory biomarkers at three-month follow-up. Brain, Behavior, and Immunity. 2021;**94**:138-147

[72] Wong AW, Shah AS, Johnston JC, Carlsten C, Ryerson CJ. Patient-reported outcome measures after COVID-19: A prospective cohort study. The European Respiratory Journal. 2020;**56**(5): 2003276

[73] Duan L, Zhu G. Psychological interventions for people affected by the COVID-19 epidemic. Lancet Psychiatry. 2020;**7**(4):300-302

[74] Ho CS, Chee CY, Ho RC. Mental health strategies to combat the psychological impact of coronavirus disease 2019 (COVID-19) beyond paranoia and panic. Annals of the Academy of Medicine, Singapore. 2020;**49**(3):155-160

[75] Taylor S, Landry CA, Paluszek MM, Fergus TA, McKay D, Asmundson GJG. Development and initial validation of the COVID stress scales. Journal of Anxiety Disorders. 2020;**72**:102232

[76] Pedrozo-Pupo JC, Pedrozo-Cortés MJ, Campo-Arias A. Perceived stress associated with COVID-19 epidemic in Colombia: An online survey. Cad Saúde Pública. 2020;**36**(5):e00090520

[77] Lee SA. Coronavirus anxiety scale: A brief mental health screener for COVID-19 related anxiety. Death Studies. 2020;**44**(7):393-401

[78] Tzur Bitan D, Grossman-Giron A, Bloch Y, Mayer Y, Shiffman N, Mendlovic S. Fear of COVID-19 scale: Psychometric characteristics, reliability and validity in the Israeli population. Psychiatry Research. 2020;**289**:113100

[79] Rek SV, Bühner M, Reinhard MA, Freeman D, Keeser D, Adorjan K, et al. The COVID-19 pandemic mental health questionnaire (CoPaQ): Psychometric evaluation and compliance with countermeasures in psychiatric inpatients and non-clinical individuals. BMC Psychiatry. 2021;**21**(1):426

Chapter 12

# From Face-to-Face to Face-to-Screen: A Correlational Analysis of Psychological Impacts and Perception of Achievement of Ibn Tofail University Students during COVID-19 Times

*Bani Koumachi*


## Abstract

The COVID-19 pandemic, unfolding in early 2020, undoubtedly will bring many additional challenges and new insights as societies come to grips with its social, cultural, and health consequences. This study aimed to verify whether there were significant differences between the aggregate construct of COVID-19 psychological perceived impact factors and the aggregate construct of academic achievement factors during the academic year of 2021. A total of 297 students from the school of Languages, Lettres, and Arts, Ibn Tofail University participated by filling out validated a survey during the months from July to October 2021. Using both descriptive and inferential statistics, the results showed that students' achievement is affected by all the factors composing the bio-ecological environment typically the factors: microsystem and macrosystem. As to the COVID-19 psychological perceived impact factors, it was found a plethora of risk factors affecting the students' life. Moreover, the association between the two constructs has revealed that these are statistically and strongly correlated. From these results, implications for specific guidance were drawn as to the existence of a monotonic relationship between how students felt during COVID-19 times and their bio-ecological environment.


**Keywords:** COVID-19 psychological perceived impact factors, risk factors, students' perception of academic achievement, Ibn Tofail University, school life in Covid 19 pandemic

## 1. Introduction

The COVID-19 pandemic has certainly unprecedently affected all spheres of life including school life. The educational institutions' closure and the necessary gradual move to the online means of instructing inevitably impacted scholastic achievement. Many of these institutions all around the world still grapple with how and when to make informed decisions about when to return to in-person courses.

Studies on how and how much COVID-19 impacted students learning would serve as a backdrop against which balanced decisions about jeopardies associated with the teaching staff and students would be taken.

The COVID-19 pandemic created a state of health emergency and the kingdom has taken drastic measures to prevent its expansion. The Ministry of National Education, Vocational Training, Higher Education, and Scientific Research took decisions to maintain the continuity of school life all along the educational year and decided to stop in-present education in all sectors including higher education levels. Courageous preventive measures were immediately taken and other decisions to adopt online courses and move to distance learning and teaching were also made. Many questions were raised related to teachers' readiness, ability, and aptitude to use information and communication technologies (ICTs), students' availability and ability to be online every time situations call for it, and the abrupt impact that technology could produce while moving from face-to-face to face-to-monitor.

Amidst all this unclarity and uncertainty about how much COVID-19 impacted scholastic achievement, there is growing consensus that this novel virus lockdown closures had negative effects on students' learning. However, the elucidation of this situation comes from the fact that after a year there is ample data in hand to go beyond prophetic measures and begin the testing of this data. Schools have endured the effects and are now after a year can measure the post-COVID-19 pandemic consequences.

For more than 15 years, the Ministry of National Education has introduced the teaching of information and communication technologies (ICTs) for the benefit of university students (ICT module for students of semester 5). A large number of teachers in the school have benefited from continuing training provided within the framework of the strategy of the GENIE program (Generalization of information and communication technologies in education in Morocco) and by the Moroccan-Korean Training Center [1].

For the first time in 2005, the Moroccan government adopted a new ICTs program under the appellation, GENIE, as one way of operationally implementing the national strategy of digitizing the public education sector and enabling students in primary, secondary, and tertiary levels to benefit from four components: infrastructure, teacher training, digital resources, and development of uses. This ICTs' generalization strategy, launched in 2006 and revised in 2009, has set a basis for the equipment of schools with Internet-connected ends with rich digital resources. Encouragement of creation and innovation of these resources as well as support to users was enhanced beside training modules for all stakeholders to guarantee good use and usage. By and large, the main objectives set by the GENIE strategy in 2006 were to convince teachers to accept and to stop resist and to actively involve them in to integrate ICT in their teaching and to contribute to the improvement of the quality of teaching and learning through the use of ICT. However, it is noteworthy to mention here that many teachers did not participate as the training was optional and many of them choose to resist and not to drop in and only some, the motivated, expressed their interest. Some of these were motivated by the awards the ministry granted [1].

The primary focus of this study is to determine whether the students of the faculty of Languages, Lettres, and Arts, Ibn Tofail University suffer psychologically under the influence of the lockdown caused by the COVID-19 pandemic. Using data from hundreds of students, 297 participants, these research questions are set forth for the present study:

1. Is students' perceived scholastic achievement affected by COVID-19 pandemic conditions?

2. What are the impacts of the psychological risk factors on our respondents?

3. Is there any association between the impacts of the psychological risk factors and perception of achievement factors?

The hypotheses emanating from the above research questions are:

1. The students' perceived scholastic achievement is affected by COVID-19 pandemic conditions.

2. The psychological risk factors impact our respondents greatly.

3. The impacts of the psychological risk factors are significantly associated with the perception of achievement factors.

## 2. Review of the literature

The COVID-19 pandemic has caused unprecedentedly considerable repercussions on human life in every aspect and the education sector is no exception to this devastating contagion. Against this backdrop, governments were quick in responding to this devastating contamination as educational institutions halted every aspect of contact and were forced to shift to online classes. This novel virus that was declared a pandemic on March 11, 2020, has spread speedily ravaging peoples' lives and turning them upside down, school life was no exception. The outbreak of this pandemic pushed several if not all scientists to try their best to study its ramifications and effects at various levels, particularly at the educational level.

In this regard, in the educational context, the devastating impacts were also felt [2]. Several concurring factors have converged to make the COVID-19 pandemic a worldwide catastrophe without precedent on school life and hence produced great psychological sufferings [3]. Therefore, there are different types of the risk factors related to COVID-19 psychological perceived impact. Prabhakar, Kapoor, and Mahajan [4]. Stress the fact that the crisis created by the pandemic is cruel to school children as it can lead to stress, mental illnesses, and various psychological problems such as lack of coping skills and even enhanced self-harm behaviors. In the same vein, Handayani & Sri Sumartiningsih [5] claim that like any other pandemic, COVID-19 had diverse effects on different groups with different degrees of impact. University students are a vulnerable group that suffered directly from stress, depression, and anxiety effects due to disruption or cancelation of usual life events like final in-present final exams and/or graduation ceremonies.

Empirically and in a study on stressors, coping strategies, and mental health impacts of COVID-19 in international students studying abroad led by [6], the team discovered that more than 80% of the students had moderate-to-high perceived stress. Exhaustively, in the sample studied, they found that stress related to academics, health, and lack of social support were predictive of higher perceived stress levels and more severe anxiety and depression symptoms. In another study conducted by [7, 8], these scholars have found that the risk impact factors differ according to social groups to which students pertain. Those emanating from financially disadvantaged backgrounds and in developing countries found themselves forced to quit school and give a hand to their breadwinners who already lost their jobs. They also found themselves disadvantaged insofar as the availability of online teaching and learning means and hence cause unwillingness and feeling of bitterness not to pursue their studies online like others where internet connectivity is better.

Extra variables that impacted students' academic achievement, as well as life, can be explained through the learning theories that marked the history of humans as to their learning and environment with particular focus on the bioecological systems theory. The behaviorists with their revolutionizing of our understanding by advancing the principle of operant conditioning trial and error and reinforcement or punishment. Later came the social learning theory by Albert Bandura who elaborated on the behaviorist theory but considered humans as thinking beings who anticipate, punish themselves, and are capable of storing information for later use. The cognitive-developmental theory of the Swiss Linguist Jean Piaget followed strongly later. The theory emphasized the importance of 'constructing' an advanced mode of thinking through a mechanism of combining maturation and experience. Other views of cognitive development along with that of Piaget's were very influential too, the reference here is to Vygotsky's sociocultural and the informative-processing perspectives. The theory adopted here insofar as the academic achievement of our respondents is the Bioecological systems theory by [9].

This persuasive model lays the ground for another deeper understanding of human development in relation to the changing environment and its effects on academic achievement. The system theories postulate that this development is impacted by an interplay between the changing context and the changing environment where one affects the other and where they are joined at the hip units [10]. The complex mutual impacts are seen as a co-acting process between the two parties which are entangled in a dynamic system. According to Bronfenbrenner's perspective, there exist five systems that interact with the individual and many bidirectional or reciprocal impacts are at play as is shown in **Figure 1**.

The first system is the microsystem which is described as the "immediate setting containing that person" [6, p. 514], that is, the direct context in which the person gets in first touch with other people like family, neighbors, and peers. It is the proximal level of context to the individual. The mesosystem is the second layer of the model and is referred to as 'a system of microsystems' through which youth's life is influenced by one or more environments without direct contact with the youth [11]. The macrosystem comprises broad social environments or social beliefs and values that impact the youth incorporating features such as political, religious, and educational values as well as appropriate standards of behavior. The exosystem is described as the system that involves social settings where the individuals

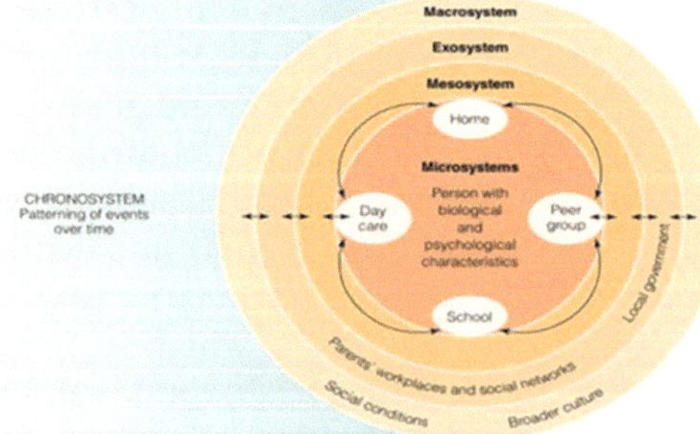


**Figure 1.**
*Bronfenbrenner's ecological model of individual development. (Adopted from Sigelman & Rider [10], p. 114).*

do not interact with but can still influence their development [10]. It shows how distal this system is from the individual, however, decisions taken significantly affect him/her. In addition to the nested series of systems, the chronosystem is the last added system to the model and stipulates that the interplay between the environment and the individual change over time and have different ramifications and schemes [12].

The evolutionary, psychoanalytic, learning, cognitive-developmental, and bioecological systems perspectives capture the complexity of human life with its interplay with the environment be it immediate or distant. However, the bioecological systems theory is more probing as to its complete depiction of the whole human development especially when it comes to academic achievement.

## 3. Method

### 3.1 Research design

In the literature, the selection of a specific type of case study design is guided by the overall study purpose. Our case study, individual learners of the faculty of Languages, Lettres, and Arts, Ibn Tofail University, is to describe and explore [13, 14]. The research design, therefore, adopted is a single explanatory qualitative case study research design with an ex post facto taste to it as the researcher cannot control the independent variable and the influence of COVID-19 pandemic as it already occurred and is impossible to control. The subjects chosen are supposed to possess the characteristics needed for this piece of research, scholastic achievement perception [15]. The use of this type of case study is justified on the ground that the researcher is seeking to answer a question that requires explaining a presumed causal link between two variables, scholastic achievement and COVID-19 pandemic conditions in our case [16]. Moreover, the type of design adopted herein enables the researcher to closely examine the obtained data and explain deeply the complications of the case context.

### 3.2 Participants

A total of 297 students from the school of Languages, Lettres, and Arts, Ibn Tofail University provided their consent to participate in the study and answer the online survey deployed for this purpose. Two hundred and nine participants were able to completely fill in the survey with a response rate of 70.37%. Eighty-eight students did not complete enough items for analysis in the present study, resulting in a final sample of 209 participants.

Conclusions from the outputs of the quantitative survey guarantee most of the time the representativeness of the target group sample; however, in our case, a convenience sampling approach which is considered oftentimes the 'least rigorous technique' is adopted. Even though the researcher targets the most 'easily accessible' respondents, representativeness is guaranteed as the researcher tends to choose easily accessible participants who have experienced the complications of the COVID-19 confinement.

### 3.3 Measures

In the Autumn of 2021, 209 participants were recruited cross-sectionally from a representative and a targeted sample of 297 participants at Ibn Tofail

State University. The obtained cross-sectional data were collected through a web-based questionnaire using representative and convenience sampling to invite students to participate. It was done when most students have become familiar with the coronavirus lockdown and security-related measures were in effect.

Students/participants were asked to respond to questions related to their education following March 2020 school closure. This included asking about which support services they had received (e.g., family counseling, individual counseling, group counseling), engagement with their teacher(s) (e.g., online, in-person, or a mix).

### 3.4 Sample and sampling procedure

The research design of the present study is a single explanatory qualitative case study research design and the population is all the students of the English studies department at the school of Languages, Lettres, and Arts, Ibn Tofail University. A purposive judgment sample is drawn from this population on the ground that the researcher judgmentally selects participants that conform to the criterion of experience with the ramifications of the COVID-19 pandemic, particularly psychological. After the temporary suspension of in-present studies and the shift to online mode starting from March 2020, almost all students were reached out using an online survey, Google Docs, to fill out.

As to recruitment procedure ethics, approval was obtained from a university deanship and facilitated by the fact that the researcher is an insider in the institution. Students from the English studies department were notified through the school Facebook page announcements via directs e-mails enclosing the study link or directing them to the link on the previously mentioned website page. Students started answering the survey, the first days they received it and those who were reluctant were reminded using a reminder email with the survey link. The data collection stage was along a period of approximately a month, from June to July 2021, and was closed on July 31st.

### 3.5 Data analysis

Students' achievement perception is the first co-variable that this study investigated. Therefore, to ascertain the underpinnings of the students' chronosystem nature that reflects academic achievement during the COVID-19 pandemic, Bronfenbrenner's bio-ecological model was adopted. It is a model that contains five layers: the macrosystem, the exosystem, the mesosystem, the chronosystem, and the microsystem. However, for reasons of time and space, the study shall concentrate only on the overall effect resulting in the aggregate effect of the while model. The four levels of this model range from the most personal related to the factors affecting the child in his immediate environment, to the extremist elements of the child's life experience [17].

The data collected from our respondents were fed into the Statistical Package for the Social Sciences (SPSS, Version 22). Measures were taken to ensure that the data gathered were entered correctly and that there are no missing data.

After having completed the preprocessing of the data obtained from the sample chosen, the data screening, checking data for errors, and fixing or removing these errors, took place and were fed into IBM SPSS software, version 22.0 for statistical analysis. A ten-question survey with two sections has been devised and measured on a Likert scale. In order to assure the reliability as well as the adequacy of the sample of the items/questions included in the questionnaire, Cronbach's alpha coefficient along with the Principal Component Analysis with equamax rotation (KMO and Bartlett's Test) were used. The Cronbach's alpha obtained is 0.83, which indicates a high level of internal consistency among the items for our scale with this specific sample. Additionally, the dimensionality of the scale was investigated through the KMO and Bartlett's test. From the results in **Table 1**, the test indicates the data for structure detection is suitable. The Kaiser-Meyer-Olkin Measure of Sampling Adequacy statistic stands at 0.789 and Bartlett's test of sphericity value ($x^2 = 1287.542$; $p \leq 0.005$) is significant indicating that factor analysis or principal component analysis is useful with the data of the sample chosen.

The microsystem is the first level in Bronfenbrenner's theory and contains subcategories such as family, school, peer group, neighborhood, and teachers which are elements in the immediate environment of the child. The individual in this system is influenced by and influences the surrounding. The interactions within microsystems are often very personal and impactful in the sense that if the individual finds a fostering, caring context he/she is positively affected, and if the opposite happens, a negative impact might occur.

As to the mesosystem, it is a system regarding the connections that exists between the components comprised in the microsystem. It is a system that governs the interactions between the immediate environments of the student and epitomizes the type of influences produced-mutual influences. Fundamentally, a mesosystem is a system of microsystems.

If the mesosystem incorporates and typifies the type of influence relationships that exist between the elements composing the microsystem, the exosystem in the ecological systems theory combines other formal and informal social structures that are liable to influence the students from outside his microsystem. Examples of exosystem components include the neighborhood, parent's workplaces, parent's friends, and the mass media. These are contexts where the student gets affected by any external factor, and in our case herein could be COVID-19 pandemic experience.

The macrosystem is the fourth component of Bronfenbrenner's ecological systems theory that focuses on the larger cultural context. The cultural elements of the students as well as other cultures affect how the students/child perceives life. The socioeconomic status, wealth, poverty, region, languages, ideology, and ethnicity are broader factors that underlie the structural fabric of the established cultures the students live in.

Finally, the chronosystem is the fifth level of Bronfenbrenner's ecological systems theory. This system involves all of the patterns of environmental events and transitions throughout the child/student's life. These patterns include the normative life transitions such as school history as well others that occur in parallel and include examples like getting married at an early age or being in charge of a mature man/woman mission like what happens in some African clans.

| | KMO measure of test sampling adequacy | Bartlett's test of sphericity | | |
|---|---|---|---|---|
| **Construct** | | **Chi-square value** | **df** | **Sig. (p)** |
| Questionnaire | 0.789 | 1287.542 | 645 | 0.000 |

**Table 1.**
*KMO and Bartlett's test for the questionnaire.*

## 4. Results

### 4.1 Data processing and analysis

#### *4.1.1 Descriptive statistics*

The first part of the analysis then examines student achievement factors that make up each level of Bronfenbrenner's bio-ecological model. The factors that impact each level are explained and supported by frequencies and percentages.

Microsystem factors (N = 91) accounted for the most frequent response, while the second most frequent response was the macrosystem (N = 72). At third place, came the chronosystem (N = 25), the mesosystem (N = 14) in the fourth place, and the exosystem came last (N = 09).

**Table 2** displays a juxtaposing comparison of the descriptive statistics for the five numeric variables. This allows us to quickly make the following observations about the data: the maximum (83.76) observed here is used to identify a possible outlier or a data-entry error. On assessing the spread of our data by comparing the minimum (53.67) and maximum (83.76), it seems that the spread of the data between the two extremes is compact and is therefore suggestive of the fact that the students' achievement is affected by all the factors composing his/her bio-ecological environment typically the factors: microsystem and macrosystem. This means that the impact is an aggregate of both micro-related to the immediate environment and macro-related to external factors.

The mean as a standard measure of the center of the distribution of the data of this group of participants is (M = 62.761). It is clear from the results in **Table 3** that three factors are above the mean except for exosystem (M = 58.258) and chronosystem (M = 60.123) factors. This adds up to the result of the min and max as the microsystem and the macrosystem factors proved to be effective in determining the nature of the students' achievement during COVID-19 times.

As to the psychological impacts of the COVID-19 pandemic on respondents, a battery of items measuring risk factors coronavirus is used (A survey adapted from [18]). Worth noting here is that the survey contains presumably two sections for the same objective, gauging students' feelings, and perceptions about the COVID-19 pandemic. Thus, regarding the first section of the survey, quantitative segment, and eight survey items based on data gathered from close-ended questions that targeted eight different types of themes, worry, time demands, fear, irritation, sadness, preoccupation, guilt, and stress. These concepts are deemed suitable to provide some guidance on what impacts to measure for the impacts of COVID-19 on college students.

| | N | Min | Max | Max/ Min | Mean | Std. |
|---|---|---|---|---|---|---|
| | Statistic | Statistic | Statistic | Statistic | Statistic | Statistic |
| Microsystem | 201 | 58.98 | 108.54 | 83.76 | 67.876 | 8.753 |
| Mesosystem | 67 | 46.68 | 82.87 | 64.77 | 62.984 | 6.988 |
| Exosystem | 55 | 35.32 | 72.03 | 53.67 | 58.258 | 5.876 |
| Macrosystem | 102 | 52.40 | 101.74 | 77.07 | 64.342 | 7.254 |
| Chronosystem | 72 | 48.91 | 87.67 | 68.29 | 60.123 | 6.789 |
| Valid N (Listwise) | 297 | 48.45 | 90.57 | 69.51 | 62.761 | 7.132 |

**Table 2.**
*Descriptive statistics of the participants COVID-19 psychological perceived impact survey items.*

| Academic Achievement Factors | f | % | Cumulative Percent |
|---|---|---|---|
| Microsystem | 91 | 43.54 | 43.54 |
| Mesosystem | 14 | 06.69 | 50.32 |
| Exosystem | 09 | 04.30 | 54.53 |
| Macrosystem | 72 | 34.44 | 88.04 |
| Chronosystem | 25 | 11.96 | 100.0 |
| Total | 209 | 100.0 | |

**Table 3.**
*Overall descriptive statistics of the questions related to achievement factors as perceived by students.*

Concerning the qualitative segment of the survey, the researcher deemed it appropriate to triangulate results obtained from two diverse data collection instruments by utilizing an open-ended question section that would allow participants to disclose more on the perceived impacts of the phenomenon under study. Also, starting from the conviction that one tool, quantitative measure, is parsimonious in unveiling the broad array of impacts of COVID-19 on students' academic performance, a qualitative side is added to the survey. Two open questions were asked: "List at least three ways among the five presented, microsystem, exosystem, macrosystem, mesosystem, and chronosystem in which COVID-19 pandemic impacted the way you academically performed during the lockdown?"; "which factors, out of the three chosen, do you think affected most your academic achievement?". A word of caution here is that these factors of academic achievement were explained to the participants so that they could decide correctly which system is most affecting.

Qualitative data from the first question of the open-ended responses demonstrated therefore a broad array of impacts caused by COVID-19 lockdown on students' academic achievement. The most common impacts are a decrease in motivation, and even suicidal attempts, feeling of loneliness and isolation, depression, and difficulties to re-socialize with others among others. For example, one of the students commented, "I feel demotivated every day to the extent that I feel hopeless." Another one reacted to the question saying that "I sometimes [felt] depressed and entertained the idea of suicide which hopefully I was able to fight against". "I along with my brothers had the difficulty to get connected to people and even felt that we had become some sort of zombies". These feelings that range from a feeling of mere melancholy to challenges with thoughts of suicide are characteristic of the type of sufferings our respondents were clear about as reflections of parts of their lives during the lethal pandemic. However, a few positive responses were rejected. Some of the respondents reported having the opportunity to sharpen their computer skills; others focused on the idea that they discovered the particularities of online learning and it suited their study skills and even refined others. But the most striking answers were those which expressed liking the experience of being locked and staying away from other people described as intrusive beings.

The quantitative data related to the mean values of the psychological impact survey items are shown in **Table 4**. The seven risk factors used to test for COVID-19 psychological perceived impact were worry, time demand, fear, irritation, sadness, preoccupation, and stress. The first two ones, worry and time demand were measured on a strongly disagree to strongly agree scale and demonstrated the following means ($M = 5.87$and $M = 5.67$, respectively). The two mean values indicate that the respondents scored closely around the mean with substantial feelings of worry and time demand. As to the five remaining risk factors, which were gauged on a different scale, not at all to extremely, three of them: fear, sadness, and stress equal

| Impact | Survey item | Mean/SD | Range |
|---|---|---|---|
| Worry | "I feel worried all the time during COVID-19 pandemic times" | 5.87/1.56 | 1-Strongly disagree to 7- strongly agree |
| Time Demand | "COVID-19 pandemic consumes all my thinking time" | 5.67/1.43 | 1-Strongly disagree to 7- strongly agree |
| Fear | "COVID-19 pandemic makes me feel afraid" | 66.48/25.90 | 0-Not at all to 100- Extremely |
| Irritation | "I feel irritated when I think about my experience with COVID-19" | 55.89/27.87 | 0-Not at all to 100- Extremely |
| Sadness | "How sad do you feel when you think about COVID-19?" | 60.12/26.99 | 0-Not at all to 100- Extremely |
| Preoccupation | "How do you feel when you think about COVID-19?" | 57.81/27.23 | 0-Not at all to 100- Extremely |
| Stress | "How stressed do you feel when you think about COVID-19?" | 62.16/27.01 | 0-Not at all to 100- Extremely |

**Table 4.**
*Descriptive statistics of the participants COVID-19 psychological perceived impact survey items.*

or surpass the main mean value indicating the serious suffering of the respondents with these risks. Furthermore, for the two others, irritation and preoccupation, it seems that they did not score higher than the general average, but the tendency is clearer as to the admittance of undertaking the experience of these risk factors by our respondents even though the impact was not as stronger as the three first ones.

### *4.1.2 Inferential statistics*

The present study investigates the association between risk factors corona virus-related and scholastic/academic achievement factors, a correlational analysis is adopted where each risk factor cluster is equated with a co-variable from the other cluster, academic achievement factors.

Since our correlation that the SPSS statistics generated is not Pearson's correlation, thus, there is no need that our data passes assumption #3 (no outliers) and assumption #4 (normality), it suffices it to satisfy assumption #2 (linear relationship). Therefore, the correlation which is appropriate here is the Spearman Rank Order Correlation coefficient. As could be deciphered from **Table 5**, there is a monotonic relationship between the two variables.

The results of the monotonicity between the two co-variables are presented in a matrix such that, as can be seen above (**Table 5**), the correlations are replicated. Moreover, the table presents Spearman's correlation, its significance value, and the sample size that the calculation was based on. In this example, we can see that Spearman's correlation coefficient, Rho, is 0.697 and this is statistically significant at ($p = 0.000$). That is, the association between the COVID-19 psychological perceived impact factors and academic achievement factors was strong. A positive correlation between them was statistically significant (*Rho* (209) = 0.697, $p = 0.000$). We are allowed therefore to safely conclude that from our two-tailed prediction of the studied relationship, the null hypothesis that there is no association between the two co-variables is rejected in favor of the alternative one which states that the students' perceived scholastic achievement is affected by COVID-19 pandemic conditions.

Consequently, the tendency of the respondents to disclose about the severity of the factors/systems of the bio-ecological environment, mainly microsystem and

| | | | COVID-19 psychological_ perceived_impact_ factors (Aggregate construct) | Academic_ achievement_ factors (Aggregate construct) |
|---|---|---|---|---|
| Spearman's rho | COVID-19 psychological_ perceived_impact_ factors (Aggregate construct) | Correlation Coefficient | 1.000 | 0.697** |
| | | Sig. (2-tailed) | . | 0.000 |
| | | N | 209 | 209 |
| | Academic_ achievement_factors (Aggregate construct) | Correlation Coefficient | 0.697** | 1.000 |
| | | Sig. (2-tailed) | 0.000 | . |
| | | N | 209 | 209 |

***. Correlations significant at the level (2-tailed).*

**Table 5.**
*Correlations between COVID-19 psychological perceived impact factors and academic achievement factors.*

macrosystem, on their academic achievement during COVID-19 times is evocative of the fact that the impact is an accumulation of both micro-related to the immediate environment and macro-related to external factors. With regard to the COVID-19 psychological perceived impact factors, the qualitative and quantitative results have revealed that the respondents went through a tough experience with severe risk factors condemning their academic lives mainly but with different degrees of impact, worry, time demand, fear; irritation, sadness, preoccupation, and stress. It is noteworthy to mention here the impact of other factors as well, such as feelings that range from mere melancholy to challenges with thoughts of suicide, were discovered through open questions. We can conclude here also that the plethora of psychological risk factors categorically impact our respondents' psyches greatly. The previously alternative hypothesis that describes the association between the two co-variables is maintained against the null that states that there is no dependency link between them.

As to the correlation that used Spearman's rho as a popular method for correlating the unvalidated survey instruments or Likert-type survey responses, it was found that there is a strong positive and significant association ($Rho$ (209) = 0.697, $p$ = 0.000) between the COVID-19 psychological perceived impact risk factors and academic achievement factors. Explicitly, it seems that the aggregate construct of COVID-19 psychological perceived impact factors and the aggregate construct of academic achievement factors strongly correlate suggesting that the higher the impact of the coronavirus perceived impact on respondents' lives the stronger it is also on their academic achievement. The monotonic relationship is ascertained between the two co-variables allowing for the researcher to definitely decide on keeping the alternative hypothesis in favor of the null one.

## 5. Discussion

It is worth mentioning here that the findings of the study in relation to the first variable, the COVID-19 psychological perceived impact risk factors are corroborated by other studies mentioned in the literature. For instance, the study conducted by [6] confirms the idea that risk perceptions of Italian respondents concerning health during COVID-19 pandemic time have been recorded to revolve around almost all perceived risks encompassing negative affective states of fear, anger and sadness, anxiety, interpersonal, and psychological risks. Association among perceived stress, depression, and anxiety were found in a study conducted by [19]. Chen and Liu [20] add up to the previous results when they quantified the importance of related risk factors on the level of psychological distress and explored the threshold effect of each risk factor on the level of psychological distress. They found that health risk factors were the greatest contributors in predicting the level of psychological distress, with a relative importance of 42.32% among all influential factors.

With respect to academic achievement factors using Bronfenbrenner's bio-ecological model, the present study revealed a certain taxonomy of effect that situates the microsystem factors which specify the effect of the immediate environment on students' school life. Haleemunnissa et al. [21] substantiate this result when they found that confinement imposed by the COVID-19 pandemic resulted in, especially in conflict-ridden families, augmented symptoms of depression and anxiety. The second in rank was the macrosystem factor that is perceived by our respondents to affect greatly their achievement. The respondents perceive the larger socio-cultural and economic environment to be second in effect as the economic crisis created by the pandemic had its psychological impact and created unease for the respondents. The system ranked third was the chronosystem which is the timeline of change concerning the occurrence of these systems. That is to say the salience of the element of time and history influences and interplay with the individual's life course, the academic achievement in our case particularly [22]. This rank given to the chronosystem is justified on the ground that the family was an immediate context element that impacted much of our respondents' scholastic achievement given the confinement and the break from the other people around. Additionally, it seems that our respondents felt second impacts from factors away from home and that do not need necessarily physical contact, the macro, and the chronosystems. Thus, the transition or change over time in the life situation of the participants indicated by the aggregate effect of both macrosystem and chronosystem is manifested in chronosystem. The mesosystem, where the microsystem elements influence the individual without direct contact with him/her such as the parents' financial situation and workplace difficulties that were indicated by the participants as microsystems that had an impact on their academic achievement as claimed by [23]. As to the exosystem, it is a system that is more distal from the individual's development and this latter does not interact with the social settings. Our respondents ranked it last as they felt the effect distant from them probably considered high the effect that was micro or internal to them in comparison to that one that is external and the exosystem epitomizes this case as shown by [23]. However, and according to [14], significant research has included the proximal ecological levels of the microsystem and mesosystem partially in contrast to our study. Additionally, the effect of the remaining systems is not that effective, the reference here is to the macrosystem, the exosystem, and the chronosystem which our respondents ranked also as levels of less understanding.

## 6. Conclusion

No doubt, COVID-19 pandemic confinement had its impact on every sphere of life and education was no exception [24]. A combination of a bio-ecological perspective focusing on academic achievement factors and COVID-19 psychological perceived impact factors perspective is deemed salient in investigating the association between the two variables. This is crucial to consider as besides the focus of the respondents on the choice of two systems, the microsystem and the macrosystem, to be more influential on their achievement, they chose more frequent COVID-19 psychological perceived impact factors that echoed the literature. What is noteworthy here is the existence of a correlation between the two covariables/constructs proving therefore the monotonicity that proves the scenario in which the increased number of psychological risk factors impact the increased perception of academic achievement factors impact is. These results are evocative of the idea that the respondents were overwhelmed by the COVID-19 experience and this latter had them perceive negative effects on their academic achievement as their psychology has been adversely affected as well.

The study has some limitations. First, the research design was a single explanatory qualitative case study research design with an ex post facto perspective. Thus, the absence of variable control and manipulation might have been less rigorous and experimentation could be more scientifically laborious and is highly likely that it would produce more insightful results. Additionally, basing the study only on perceptions mares also the validity of the results, and an experimental design could make up for this inadequacy. Third, the sample is not representative of all Moroccans as it was difficult to get the sampling frame, and therefore it was impossible to opt for a probabilistic type of sampling procedure. Despite these limitations, however, the study revealed some of the psychological states of the Moroccan students during COVID-19 pandemic times and their perceptions on how influential it was on their academic achievement.

## Author details

Bani Koumachi
Department of English Studies, School of Languages, Lettres, and Arts, Ibn Tofail University, Kénitra, Morocco

*Address all correspondence to: bani.koumachi@uit.ac.ma

## References

[1] How the GENIE Programme from Morocco is doing since receiving. [Internet]. [cited 2021 Nov.4]. Available from: https://en.unesco.org/news/how-genie-programme-morocco-doing-receiving-2017-unesco-ict-education-prize/

[2] Bergan S, Gallagher T, Munck R, Land van't H. Higher education's response to the Covid-19 pandemic: Building a more sustainable and Democratic future. Strasbourg: Council of Europe/Conseil de l'Europe; 2021

[3] Flesia L, Monaro M, Mazza C, Fietta V, Colicino E, Segatto B, et al. Predicting perceived stress related to the Covid-19 outbreak through stable psychological traits and machine learning models. Journal of Clinical Medicine. 2020;**9**(10):3350. DOI: 10.31234/osf.io/yb2h8

[4] Prabhakar H, Kapoor I, Mahajan C. Clinical Synopsis of COVID-19. Springer Nature; 2020

[5] Handayani O, Sri Sumartiningsih N. Proceedings of the 5th International Seminar of Public Health and Education, ISPHE 2020, 22 July 2020, Universitas Negeri Semarang. Semarang, Indonesia; 2020

[6] Lai-kwan AY, Lee L, Wang-ping M, Feng Y, Lai-kwan TT, Ho-ming L, et al. Mental health impacts of the COVID-19 pandemic on International University students, related stressors, and coping strategies. Frontiers in Psychiatry. 2020;**11**:1-13. DOI: 10.3389/fpsyt.2020.584240

[7] Sharma D, Bhaskar S. Addressing the covid-19 burden on medical education and training: The role of telemedicine and tele-education during and beyond the pandemic. Frontiers in Public Health. 2020;**589669**(8):1-14. DOI: 10.3389/fpubh.2020.589669

[8] Bhaskar S, Banach M, Weissert R, Mittoo S, Nurtazina A. Telemedicine during and beyond COVID-19. Frontiers Media SA; 2021;**8**. DOI: 10.3389/fpubh.2020.589669

[9] Bronfenbrenner U. The Ecology of Human Development. Cambridge, Mass: Harvard University Press; 1979

[10] Sigelman CK, Rider EA. Life-Span Human Development. Cengage Learning; 2017

[11] Lerner RM, Schiamberg LB, Anderson PM. Encyclopedia of Human Ecology: Santa Barbara. California: A-H. ABC-CLIO; 2003

[12] Rathus SA. Childhood and Adolescence: Voyages in Development. Cengage Learning; 2016

[13] Stake RE. The Art of Case Study Research. SAGE Publications, Incorporated; 1995

[14] White FA, Hayes BK, Livesey DJ. Developmental Psychology: From infancy to adulthood. Pearson Australia. 2015

[15] Nnadi-Okolo EE. Health Research Design and Methodology. United States of America: CRC Press; 1990

[16] Yin RK. Case Study Research. SAGE Publications, Incorporated; 1994

[17] Hayes N, O'Toole L, Halpenny AM. Introducing Bronfenbrenner. New York: Taylor & Francis; 2017

[18] Browning MHEM, Larson LR, Sharaievska I, Rigolon A, McAnirlin O, Mullenbach L, et al. Psychological impacts from COVID-19 among university students: Risk factors across seven states in the United States. PLoS One. 2021;**16**(1):1-27. DOI: 10.1371/journal.pone.0245327

[19] Li X, Lyu H. Epidemic risk perception, perceived stress, and mental health during COVID-19 pandemic: A moderated mediating model. Frontiers in Psychology. 2021;**11**:1-9. DOI: 10.3389/fpsyg.2020.563741

[20] Chen Y, Liu Y. Which risk factors matter more for psychological distress during the COVID-19 pandemic? An application approach of gradient boosting decision trees. International Journal of Environmental Research and Public Health. 2021;**18**(11):5879. DOI: 10.3390/ijerph18115879

[21] Haleemunnissa S, Didel S, Swami MK, Singh K, Vyas V. Children and COVID19: Understanding impact on the growth trajectory of an evolving generation. Children and Youth Services Review. 2021;**120**:1-30. DOI: 10.1016/j.childyouth.2020.105754

[22] Schell BA, Gillen G, Scaffa M, Cohn ES. Willard and Spackman Occupational Therapy. Philadelphia PA: Lippincott Williams & Wilkins; 2013

[23] Bryan C, Chandan CH. Handbook of Research on Applied Social Psychology in Multiculturalism. Hershey PA, USA: IGI Global; 2021

[24] Lorente LML, Arrabal AA, Pulido-Montes C. The right to education and ICT during COVID-19: An international perspective. Sustainability. 2020;**12**(21):9091. DOI: 10.3390/su12219091

Section 2

# Educational Impacts

Chapter 13

# Perspective Chapter: Impact of COVID-19 on Learning Outcomes of Students

*Dibya Sundar Panda*


## Abstract

Covid-19 pandemic made a paradigm shift in the education scenario across the globe. In an attempt to contain the infection classes were conducted online. Traditional classes and online classes are completely different from the teacher and student perspective but there was no other alternatives. The major domains of teaching and learning are, knowledge, cognitive, interpersonal, communication psychomotor skills. Each domain demands different teaching and assessment methods to achieve the intended learning outcomes. The teaching and assessment methods were modified to a great extent in online teaching. Delivering lectures online can be considered as effective as far as the outcome domain is limited to knowledge but for other domains like cognitive, psychomotor, interpersonal and communication, it is questionable. The various factors affecting in intended learning outcomes are one to one discussion with teacher and peers, adequate prerequisite knowledge, motivation, learning hours and style, active learning, learning interest, attitude of instructor and learner, IT skills. In order to assure the achievement of learning outcomes, careful focus on the identification learning gaps in online teaching has to be done along with implementation of corrective measures to address them.


**Keywords:** learning gap, intended learning outcomes, peers, knowledge, skills

## 1. Introduction

Covid-19 pandemic made a paradigm shift in the education scenario across the globe. In an attempt to contain the infection classes were conducted online. Traditional classes and online classes are completely different from the teacher and student perspective but there was no other alternatives. Commonly used applications for conducting online classes are ZOOM, Google Classroom, Moodle, and Blackboard were instrumental in shifting onsite to online classes as well as e-learning [1]. The COVID -19 pandemic affected the traditional system of education, e-learning was brought in, where the learning is carried out online which can be accessed in any corner of the globe without going to the classroom [2]. However implementing e-learning is a challenge for the learners and educators [3], attempts have been made to embed e-learning through the use of appliances and internet connectivity for seamless conduction of learning process. Delivering lectures online



IntechOpen

can be considered as effective as far as the outcome domain is limited to knowledge but for other domains like cognitive, psychomotor, interpersonal and communication, it is questionable. In the traditional classes the learner has an opportunity to interact with the teacher along with his peers either one to one or in groups. The learner gets an opportunity to learn from his peers. At present education equips the learner with skills and knowledge, to make him employable in the job market. Supervision and observation of the student's activities directly by the teacher plays an important role in enhancing student's ability. Motivation of student is imperative either as a beginner or expert. Learning along with peers, observing their performance and encouragement from the teacher is instrumental in overall achievement of the learning outcomes. This chapter is aimed to give an insight of the possible learning gaps and the contributing factors likely to be encountered in online teaching, effect of online teaching on the intended learning outcomes of learners and ways to address such gaps.

## 2. Learning outcomes

Proclamations describing the knowledge, skills and competence the student should acquire after completion of a lecture, course or program, along with realizing the importance and usefulness of the acquired knowledge and skills.

## 3. Learning domains

The learning outcomes have been categorized into different domains, which are linked to the separate teaching and assessment methods (**Table 1**).

| Domain | Teaching methods during normal condition | Teaching methods during pandemic | Assessment method |
|---|---|---|---|
| Knowledge | Didactic lectures | Didactic lectures | Written and oral test |
| Cognitive | Didactic lectures, Case based learning, Team based learning, Independent learning, Problem based learning | Didactic lectures, Independent learning, Problem based learning online. | Written and oral test, Objective structured examination. |
| Psychomotor | Laboratory demonstration, Clinical onsite training | Online demonstration, Restricted onsite training | Objective structured practical examination. Objective structured clinical examinations |
| Interpersonal skills | Team based learning, Workshops | Online workshops | Objective structured examination. |
| Communication | Journal clubs, Team based learning, Workshops | Online workshops | Objective structured examination. Observations |

**Table 1.**
*Comparison of teaching strategies to achieve the desired outcomes during pandemic with the normal conditions.*

## 4. Factors influencing the intended learning outcomes (ILOs) in online teaching

### 4.1 One to one interaction

Active involvement of students during instructions makes the learning meaningful. In active learning, students apply their minds to get new ideas, crack problems, and use the knowledge they have gained. Doing more instead of mere listening to lectures by the students is followed in active learning process. Interaction in the class only makes it possible for the learners to resolve the assigned problems through logical, systemic and structural thinking process [4, 5]. Online classes do not provide the scope for one two one interaction resulting inability of students to solve the problems in the class. Low level of interaction could be a reason for the decreased student learning outcomes achievement in the Covid-19 pandemic.

It is imperative for the learners to have an understanding and interpretation of definitions and theorems. Learner should acquire the skills to become independent in analyzing and applying statements in problem solving. Learners go through and use the available information [6, 7].

Calculations in kinetics and posology related to proof is not easy to be resolved by students. Cirillo and Herbst have reported that students find it difficult in writing premise and statement for proving in Geometry material [8], along with structuring substantiations, it seems the presence of instructor by the side of students makes the learning easy. In addition, research by Miyazaki, Fujita, Keith [9, 10] also on Geometry material shows that the using of open problems encourages students' understanding of the structure of evidence by providing various assumption relationships with their conclusions. The completion of a proof presented in the Real Analysis book does not provide a clear explanation of the reasoning process, so that students do not understand the analysis of their thinking if there is no interaction in class. This affects student learning outcomes.

### 4.2 Student backgrounds

There are several indicators referring to the learning during the Covid-19 pandemic. The backgrounds factor is related to the grade in the prerequisite course, living in an environment that encourages them to study, living in an area that has wide internet access and well use of IT media. The grade in the prerequisite courses and the learning environment support them to get good learning outcomes [5, 6].

### 4.3 Student's motivation

Indicators on the learning motivation factor are attempting positively to given assignment, acting rationally and preferring to have discussions in studying the courses before starting during conduction of the course [5, 6].

### 4.4 Student's learning style

The indicators of the learning style factor are showing easiness in understanding the material by seeing, reading or writing before the starting of online classes, understanding the material after hearing lecturers' explanations, after discussion with friends, preferring to discussion about the material with their peers. Understanding independently after doing problem solving exercises. Students take help of a wide range of learning resources to understand the course and to have further discussion with the instructor, friends even after the lectures. Unless the instructors and students team up in developing materials for easier understanding, the learning outcomes will be affected [5, 6].

### 4.5 Student's learning hours

For applying Carroll's theory related to learning hours, relatively normal distribution of student's academic performance was noticed by Bloom following non-specific instruction, which resulted in conventional practice of offering same instruction and as a result getting the normal distribution of learning results [11]. Providing enough learning hours to a batch of student, should lead to achievement of the same level of results. According to Bloom learning hour is the time a student dedicates only to school work, instead of the physical sense of time or the natural course of passing time [11, 12]. As said by Yen, there is never a considerable duration of time, which is an abstract that but is ever-present in a student's daily routine [13]. Usually students use their time in various ways, but often have difficulties in learning the concept of time. Considering the impracticability of a student getting the understanding of time by utilizing time, principle related to time concepts can be greatly abstract. Not only it is important to learn the concepts of time on the basis of how daily events are observed, the concept of time is also developed by matching the primacy of events in daily life. As the right understanding of time may not happen eliminating the person's capacity to clench and realize the physical time, also the inner time, the concept of time is established, just like any other concept, in a progressive rather than abrupt manner and matures as one grows older [14]. So, the instructor needs to realize students' progress stages concerning the concept of time, then only he can have a hold on the underscored of teaching materials [13, 15, 16]. The conceptual definition of learning hours has been framed from the literature: having the capacity to clench and realize the physical, as well as inner time, students are inspired by the teacher's instructional attitude that they find satisfying, acquires a correct idea of time and/or aptitude to dedicate extra hours on learning, as per his own or circumstantial needs [14]. There are two sides in the concept of learning hours as proposed by Lai, like: learning hours linked to student's interest and circumstantial interest, the first being an individual's emphasis, driven by own interest, on a basis of prerequisite knowledge combined with emotions, and the subsequent willingness to spend more time on learning eagerly [9]. The second one linked to student's choice to dedicate extra hours on learning based on enthusiasm of teacher related to the delivered lecture. Taking online classes in absence of their peers however may lack the enthusiasm attribute of the teacher and motivation to dedicate more time in reading and understanding affecting the learning outcomes. However in online classes the student has an opportunity to dedicate more time in studying as there will be no preparation or traveling to the institution.

### 4.6 Active learning

There are many reports about studies substantiating the advantages of active learning [17]. Active learning originates from any class activity involving students in doing things and thinking about the things they are doing" [18]. The fundamental thing in active learning is participation of student in activity and engaging them in the learning process. The major difference between active learning and traditional lectures is that, in the former method the student has to do some psychomotor activity in the laboratory or problem solving exercises whereas in the later information is passed from instructor to student [19]. For example, Freeman et al. [20] affirmed that the undergraduate science, engineering, technology and mathematics students receiving active learning in laboratories have performed better than the students receiving traditional classes. In the online classes during pandemic has minimum active learning, may have affected to ILOs achievement to some extent.

### 4.7 Learning interest of students

Curiosity to study a course is one the indicators of the interest factor, in advance devotion to courses ahead of the online lectures schedule, being proactively involved in the courses, availing resources for acquiring an internet package in case of non-availability Wi-Fi, monitor information about lectures on the groups of the learning apps, active involvement in the courses during the online lectures.

Interest is inherent to an individual, it cannot be developed by using external forces. However teacher can play a great role in building interest among the students. According to Li's hypotheses related to importance of interest factor in learning process in a class room, interest should match to the intellectual and emotional need of the student [5].

Based upon psychology, Chang opined that interest can be expressed in two ways, one is person's intrinsic liking to something or someone and the second is the little variation among interest and intention, which are the basis of someone's behavior [6]. According to Chiu although interest is inherent it can be enriched by outer forces [7].

Chen has expressed three types of interest involved in learning. The interest in learning could be personal, which is stable with minimum alterations, circumstantial interest related to emotional condition due to the use of hilarious activities and teaching resources and interest that changes the psychological status that a person shows immense interest in something without getting distracted by surrounding and concentrating on the factor responsible for the ignition of that interest [8].

Her opinion is interest can be developed in a classroom setting to bid important choices to learners by: choosing well-collected teaching resources; choosing variety and animated teaching resources; choosing teaching resource in which the students have prerequisite knowledge; inspiring learners to participate actively; providing necessary quick clues and reminders as needed by the student; using new and varied ideas; and assisting the teacher to become idol by displaying craving and curiosity for the subject he teaches. According to Lai, interest in learning is the choice of the individual, as he chooses one thing over other things may be due to positive impact on his psychological status during the interaction with the situation leading to development of intents of learning [9]. As per the suggested theoretical structure by Krapp, Hidi and Renninger learning interest has two divisions' individual and situational [10]. As pointed by Schraw and Dennison, an individual is independent about a learning assignment which enables him/her to develop strong intentions to participate actively in solo decisions and control-oriented tasks [11]. There are 5 fundamental type of interest like individual, situational, latent, actualized (text and task based) and knowledge [9, 12].

Continuous education can be provided through e-learning but there are not much instructions. As well, providing learning materials was difficult for the instructors [21]. Following the transition of higher educational institutes from traditional teaching to distance online education, there is an advantage of setting flexible e-learning models [22]. Online instruction with quickly created materials has low student engagement, which may lead to low achievement in learning outcomes [23].

There are reports advocating the use of blended teaching (onsite and online) to meet the urgent need in Covid-19 pandemic with an objective to meet the vital educational needs by reducing the student volumes, making best use of the resource persons and technology infrastructure, this could orient the students to become lifelong learners [24].

### 4.8 Learning attitude of the student

The indicators of attitude factors are like, maintaining discipline, applying logics and showing confidence in problem solving exercises, sticking to the course schedule sessions, timely submission of assignment reports [5, 6].

There is a minor dissimilarity among students with high and low level of learning attitude in outcomes on online learning [25]. There is a remarkable positive alignment observed between attitude and teaching efficiency of physical education teachers of elementary school [26]. The best method to attract students attention during teaching is by encouraging competition embedded with novelty, variety and fun among the group [17]. Above method stimulates a feeling of honor and fidelity to the class from the learners as well. Likewise building relation among the parent and teacher, developing partnership providing animated instructional material and demonstrations have proved to develop teacher's skills. In a pleasing and safe study environment encouraging group activities is the best way to activate multidimensional thinking, engagement, strong learning intention and attitude with improved comprehension skills. There is report that a remarkable positive correlation exists in the efficacy of teachers who integrate information technologies in teaching [27].

### 4.9 Instructional attitude of the teacher

In multicultural teaching program, the attitude of teacher is remarkably and positively linked to his teaching efficiency, which functions as an operative tool to assess and improve the efficacy [4]. According to Li instructional attitude of teacher teaching mother tongue has a considerably positive association with his/her sense of self-efficacy [28]. The instructor should encourage online discussion by raising how and why questions to achieve maximum learning outcomes.

### 4.10 Retention of content

Retention is one of the important component of knowledge outcome. Students face the challenge of retaining the course content in online teaching unless the concept is applied in real practice. Frequent formative assessment also helps the student in memorizing the information. Online threaded discussion is another way to retain the contents.

### 4.11 IT skills of student and instructor

The student and instructor need to have the basic skills and knowledge of computer like well aware of technical terms like browses, application software, icons, files, folders, documents etc. Use of keyboards, mouse, basic commands like copy, paste, save, rename, backup delete is essential for seamless learning and teaching. Student and instructor must be well versed with application of software like word, power point, excel. Good knowledge of accessing websites, making online search, creating accounts, creating discussion boards is important in online teaching. Using antivirus tools and basic cyber security aspects is also imperative.

## 5. Conclusion

There are several factors which affects the achievement of learning outcomes. Learning along with the peers in the presence the instructor can influence the behavior, attitude and motivation towards learning ultimately affecting the achievement of the learning outcome. In order to assure the achievement of learning outcomes, careful focus on the identification learning gaps in online teaching has to be done along with implementation of corrective measures to address them. The instructor should always initiate and encourage discussion with the students. Regular planning by the student to have discussion and communication with the instructor is essential to have successful online classes. One to one discussion with teacher and peers helps in understanding the concepts of the subject. Adequate prerequisite knowledge, motivation, learning hours and style, active learning, learning interest, attitude of instructor and learner, IT skills are important determinant of achieving the intended learning outcomes in online teaching.

## Author details

Dibya Sundar Panda
Department of Pharmaceutics, College of Pharmacy, Jouf University, Sakaka, Kingdom of Saudi Arabia

*Address all correspondence to: dibyapanda1974@gmail.com

## References

[1] Stone. Zoom for educators: How to set up virtual classrooms for distance learning. https://getvoip.com/blog/2020/04/08/zoom-for-educators/

[2] Ngampornchai A, Adams J. Students' acceptance and readiness for E-learning in northeastern Thailand. International Journal of Educational Technology in Higher Education. 2016;**13**:34. DOI: 10.1186/s41239-016-0034-x

[3] Kuhad R. We must use modern technology for online education. 2020. https://www.outlookindia.com/newsscroll/wemust-use-mod

[4] Li YN. A Study of the Instructional Attitude and Teaching Efficacy of Elementary School Teachers in Multicultural Education Programs. MA, Taiwan: Department of Social Development, National Pingtung University of Education; 2008

[5] Li CC. John Dewey's Ethics. Taiwan: Sun Yat-Sen Institute for Social Sciences and Philosophy. Academia Sinica; 1981

[6] Chang CH. Educational Psychology: Theories and Practices of the Three Guidelines. Taiwan: Tunghua Book Co; 1996

[7] Chiu LH. Achievement Motivation: Strategies of Theoretical Study and Applications. Taiwan: WINJOIN Book Co; 2007

[8] Chen YZ. An Action Research on Applying Whole-Language Programs to Enhance First- and Second-Graders' Interest in Learning and Reading Comprehension Ability in Chinese Language. Taiwan: National Dong Hwa University, Hualien County; 2008

[9] Lai Q. A Survey of National Taoyuan Senior-High School Students' Interest in Learning Music and Demand for Self-Decision. MA, Taiwan: Department of Music, National Taiwan Normal University; 2010

[10] Krapp A, Hidi S, Renninger KA. Interest, learning and development. In: Renninger KA, Hidi S, Krapp A, editors. The Role of Interest in Learning and Development. Hillsdale, NJ: Erlbaum; 1992. pp. 3-25

[11] Bloom BS. Learning for mastery. U.C.L.A.-C.S.E.I.P. Evaluation Comment. 1968;**1**(2):1-12

[12] Wang CY. Correlations among the Learning-Hours Pattern of on-Line Reading, Interactive Learning and Student's Achievements. MA, Taiwan: Graduate Institute of Information and Computer Education, National Kaohsiung Normal University; 2002

[13] Yan YL. A Research on Learning Achievement of Fifth-Graders in Elementary School Regarding Concept about Time under an on-Line Remedial Teaching Circumstance. MA, Taiwan: Master's Program of Educational Entrepreneurship and Management (in Math Teaching), National University of Tainan; 2005

[14] Piaget. The Development of Thought: Equilibration of Cognitive Structures. New York: Viking; 1969

[15] Chen CY. Elementary-school Children's conception of time and related instructions. Taiwan: A Friend of Teachers. 1992;**33**(3):46-54 152

[16] Tan NC. Exploring children's understanding of measurement from their myths about measurements. Taiwan: Jpurnal of National Taipei Teachers College. 1999;**12**:407-436

[17] Chen BQ. An Action Research on How to Spark Student Interest in Learning about Writing in Native

Language and the Results. MA, Taiwan: In-service Master's Program, Graduate School of Educational Leadership and Development, Fu Jen Catholic University Colleges; 2006

[18] Braxton JM, Milem JF, Sullivan AS. The influence of active learning on the college student departure process: Toward a revision of Tinto's theory. Journal of Higher Education. 2000;**71**:569-590

[19] Prince M. Does active learning work? A review of the research. Journal of Engineering Education. 2004;**93**:223-231

[20] Freeman S, Eddy SL, McDonough M, Smith MK, Okoroafor N, Jordt H, et al. Active learning increases student performance in science, engineering, and mathematics. Proceedings of the National Academy of Sciences USA. 2014;**111**:8410-8415

[21] Allo MDG. Is the online learning good in the midst of Covid-19 pandemic? The case of EFL learners. Jurnal Sinestesia. 2020;**10**(1):1-10

[22] United Nations. Policy Brief: Education During COVID-19 and Beyond. 2020. Available from: https://www.un.org/development/desa/dspd/wp-content/uploads/sites/22/2020/08/sg_policy_brief_covid-19_and_education_august_2020.pdf

[23] Nyer P. &e relative effectiveness of online lecture methods on student test scores in a business course. Open Journal of Business and Management. 2019;**07**(04):1648-1656

[24] Almalnews. 9e Future of Distance Learning in Higher Education after COVID-19. Cairo, Egypt: Egyptian Ministry of Higher Education; 2020 https://almalnews.//المال-آلاف-106-بمشاركة-استق-نتائج-تنشرcom

[25] Gu SM. The Influence of Goal-Setting, Learning Hours and Learning Attitude on Online-Learning Outcomes. MA, Taiwan: Graduate Institute of Information and Computer Education, National Kaohsiung Normal University; 2001

[26] Li MD. Exploring the Relations between the Instructional Attitude of PE Teachers at Elementary Schools and Teaching Efficacy: Taking the Example of Schools in Tainan County/City. MA, Taiwan: Department of Physical 153 Education, National University of Tainan, Taiwan; 2003

[27] Lai JJ. Exploring the Correlations between Junior-High Schools Teachers' Instructional Attitude toward Information Technology-Aided Teaching and Teaching Efficacy: Taking the Example of Schools in Taoyuan. MA, Taiwan: Department of Industrial Education and Technology, National Changhua University of Education; 2007

[28] Li XL. A Study of the Attitude and Sense of Self-Efficacy of Mother Tongue Teachers at Public Kindergartens in Chiayi County/City. MA, Taiwan: Graduate Institute of Early Childhood Education, National Chiayi University; 2009

Chapter 14

# Psychosocial Educational and Economic Impact of COVID-19: Implication for Girl Child Education through Social Studies in Northeast Nigeria

*Adamu Mumini*

## Abstract

The main purpose of this chapter is to examine the psychosocial educational and economic impact of COVID-19 and implication for girl child education through social studies in Northeast Nigeria. COVID-19 pandemic emerged as a global health problem toward the end of 2019. It has presented attendant consequences on human health and the global economy. Families' socioeconomic status cannot afford the psychosocial and educational needs, which later affects the psychological development of children. Psychosocial means the close associations between psychological aspects of the human experience and the wider social experience and then psychosocial education is the term used to refer to awareness regarding unhealthy relationships and maladaptive behaviors among individuals and the families. COVID-19 pandemic affected almost 1.6 billion students across 190 countries of the world, representing 94% of the world's school going children do to school closures, Nigeria is inclusive. A girls' child is biological female offspring from birth to eighteen years of age. This period is made up of infancy, childhood, and early and late adolescence age. As a problems solving and value-laden discipline in it nature, social studies education are school subject that could be used in addressing the challenges of psychosocial and psychological problems caused by COVID-19 to individual's girls' child.

**Keywords:** COVID-19, girl child, psychosocial, educational, social studies

## 1. Introduction

The Coronavirus disease known as COVID-19 emerged in the city of Wuhan, China around the end of 2019 and was declared a worldwide pandemic on 11th of March 2020 by the World Health Organization (WHO). The Coronavirus pandemic has changed the setting, atmosphere, and magnitudes of security threats facing humanity and brought to attention the significance of health security in developing nations. Moreover, there are almost 259,502,031 confirmed cases of COVID-19 and 5,183,003 deaths worldwide, as of 25th November 2021 [1–3].

Pandemics are diseases of very different kinds that exhibit a variety of epidemiologic features. A pandemic is a widespread outbreak of a deadly disease or virus that cuts across boundaries, race, religion, and levels of education, which normally affects health, lives, countries, governments, means of livelihood of individuals, communities, and generally the public [4]. A virus that caused pandemic is called influenza A (HINI) PDM09 also, known as the novel influenza virus. From 1918 to 2020, the world has witnessed a series of pandemics, Spanish influenza occurred in 1918 and it was caused by an H1N1 influenza A virus (IAV) strain. Also, Asian influenza, which occurred in 1957, was caused by an H2N2 IAV draining, similarly Hong Kong flu, a pandemic that occurred in 1968 was caused by an H3N2 IAV strain. In 2003, Canada experienced the outbreak of severe acute respiratory syndrome (SARS), the resurgence of the Ebola pandemic in the mid-millennium in Guinea in 1976 in South Sudan and the Democratic Republic of Congo. From 2009 to 2010, pandemics caused the deaths of 151,700–575,400 worldwide [5–11].

In Nigeria, the first case of COVID-19 pandemic was confirmed in Lagos State on 28 February 2020. It quickly spread to all the 36 States of the federation, including Abuja the federal capital. On 26 March, 2020, the Federal Government of Nigeria announced the lockdown of Lagos and Abuja, and later a national lockdown as a result of widespread of the disease, as part of the effort to contain the spread of coronavirus pandemic [12]. The announcement of lockdown by the governments as one of the global measures for controlling the spread of the ravaging dreaded pandemic has brought about adverse mental health problems, particularly among the girl children in Nigeria. The cases of Coronavirus in Nigeria [13, 14] reported that, as of 29th November, 2021, there were 3862 confirmed cases, 2976 deaths, and 197,143 recovered cases.

Omede and Etumabo in Ref. [15] and Offorma in Ref. [16] describe that "girl children are indeed female children between births to adolescents' age of eighteen (18) years." However, this period is made up of four important stages, that is, infancy, childhood, and early and late adolescence stages of development. Similarly, Fareo and Ateequ in Ref. [17] state that, most societies of the world due to strong religious and cultural beliefs defined a girl child as an undeveloped female person, who would eventually after growing into woman end up marrying, give birth, and take care of the home and the children. Also, girl children are female children between infancy and early adulthood. More so, during this period of development, they are under the custody and supervision of adults who may be their parents or guardians and siblings. The COVID-19 pandemic declared wars against the education of girl children in Nigeria. The education of a girl child is under crisis and threat, particularly those girls that are coming from low-income families.

The number of children not attending formal school system in Nigeria has increased from the initial figure of 10.5 to 13.2 million. The rising figures stipulate that Nigeria has the larger figure of out-of-school children in the world. Inappropriately, the larger percentages are from the northeast region of Adamawa, Borno, and Yobe states where Boko Haram and ISAWP insurgency in the area are responsible factors. Prior to the outbreak of COVID-19 pandemic, violence, child early and forced marriages, lack of schools, inadequate buildings, unsafe environments, limitations in teacher's training, and systematic gender biases impeded girls' participation and learning in formal schooling across Nigeria, the global citizens [18].

Depression means mood disorder. Also, it can be described as feelings of sadness, loss, or anger that interfere with a person's everyday activities. Depression is a common illness worldwide [13], it is estimated that 3.8% of the world population is affected by depression, these categories include 5.0% adults and 5.7% adults older than 60 years. Nearly 280 million people in the world have problems of depression.

"Ravenhills [19] defined psychosocial education to mean, the knowledge given to particular groups of individuals with unhealthy relationship and maladaptive behavior, persons and families." Psychosocial education is relevant to the categories of individuals with psychosocial and psychological problems in order to promote healthy relationships in the individual.

Social Studies education has come to be accepted as [20] "a school subject that should assist students to acquire the basic knowledge, skills, and positive attitudes needed to be responsible citizens and contributing members of society." Also, Mumini and Hussaini in Ref. [21] and Jekayinfa in Ref. [22] discuss that the central focus of Social Studies is man, the physical and social environment (the entirety of men's culture and beyond) is of interest of Social Studies; what man eats, wears, lives, and makes the physical environment conducive for existence are the basis for Social Studies enclosure into to school curriculum." It also deals with man in various perspectives as the scientist, technologist, culture maker historian, politician, and man as being influenced by his culture and conditions of the contemporary world. Therefore, the purpose of this chapter is on psychosocial educational and economic impact of COVID-19: Implication for girl children education through Social Studies. Specifically, the study was to ascertain how psychosocial educational support through Social Studies will impact the girl children with psychosocial problems and how these problems affected their education during the COVID-19 pandemic in Nigeria.

## 2. Conceptual clarifications

### 2.1 COVID-19 pandemic

The 2019 novel Coronavirus disease known as COVID-19 emerged in the city of Wuhan, China around the end of 2019 and was declared a worldwide pandemic on 11th of March 2020 by the World Health Organization (WHO) [23], it defined Coronaviruses as a group of viruses in the family of Coronaviridae that infects both humans and animals. COVID-19 signs and symptoms can range from mild to severe. As a major public health emergency [24], China defines COVID-19 as a category B infectious disease [10]. COVID-19 refers to Coronavirus Disease 2019 and it belongs to the families of SARS-CoV2, Severe Acute Respiratory Syndrome Coronaviruses 2; SARS-CoV, Severe Acute Respiratory Syndrome Coronavirus; and MERS CoV, Middle East Respiratory Syndrome Coronavirus related to H1N1, Hemagglutinin Type 1 and Neuraminidase Type 1, and H5H1 Hemagglutinin Type 5, and Hemagglutinin Type 1 respectively. The signs and symptoms of COVID-19 include respiratory symptoms, fever, shortness of breath, and cough [25].

### 2.2 Lockdown scenario

The primary purpose of lockdown during emergency situation is to crush the outbreak of diseases among peoples, the diseases could be, SARS-CoV2, Acute Respiratory Syndrome Coronaviruses 2, SARS-CoV, Severe Acute Respiratory Syndrome Coronavirus, MERS CoV, Middle East Respiratory Syndrome Coronavirus disease; and the African Ebola disease. During the lockdown period, the anticipated role of the government is to impose a law that would regulate the movement and also enforce people to remain at home for certain period. The lockdown scenario should strictly prohibit large gathering of people in one place, for example, place of religions, markets, schools, hotels, and nightclubs among others [26]. Referring to the opinion of the health experts who have suggested that a complete lockdown is the only measure to stop the exponential infectivity rates of the virus.

In Nigeria, Muhammadu Buhari administration announced the first phase of lockdown on 27th April, 2020, the lockdown period commenced between 4th and 7th May, 2020 for two weeks in the federal capital territories (FCT) Abuja and Lagos [8]. Similarly, the second phase of lockdown was announced on 18th May, 2020 and ended on 1st June, 2020 respectively. More so, two weeks extension of the first phase was further declared, which lasted from 18 May to 1 June 2020. However, the second phase of the gradual easing of the lockdown commenced on 2 June 2020 and lasted for four weeks, which ended on June 29, 2020 as directed by the federal government of Nigeria.

Lockdown has numerous effects. Parvin et al. in Ref. [27] studied on the Psychosocial Anxiety from Lockdown Due to COVID-19 to Income Earner of the Family: An Evidence from Northern Bangladesh. The study attempts to understand the socio-economic crisis and mental stress in managing the family within the limited resources of Bangladesh during the lockdown period. The outcome of the study revealed that lockdown scenario has consequences on men's socioeconomic status and states of psychological development, and it has also attendant health and mental problems, sleeping disorders, reinforcement of hardship on medical system, and inabilities of some families to meet up their obligations, generating short displeasure and confusion in the family.

### 2.3 Psychosocial problems

The lockdown measures posed a terrible effect on the soci0-economic activities of the people in many states of Nigeria [28], including activities such as religious worship, marriage ceremonies, market activities of buying and selling, and movement of goods and services from one state to another or within the state. The COVID-19 pandemic in Nigeria accorded with the security challenges also added salt to the body physique of Nigerians and brought down development indices to all-time low with underdevelopment and unemployment rate currently at 55% with an external debt burden of 79.5 billion dollars [29]. The outbreak of this virus in Nigeria also brought about a decline in the Growth Domestic Product, which was contracted by −2.48; household purchasing power declined, inflation rose to 14.7%, and 40% of the population fell below the poverty line [30].

Unlike other affected countries, the lockdown in Nigeria has not only subjected the already vulnerable households to hunger but also created more tensions, violence, and unfortunate killings of people by either hoodlums who are hungry and resort to attacking neighboring households for food [31]. The socio-economic effect of this pandemic has seriously affected families and well-being in general. On the one hand, it has had undesirable physical and psychological consequences that affect society, families, and individuals [9, 32]. On the other hand, studies indicated that the prevalence rates of depression and general anxiety during the COVID-19 period were higher than the rates before the pandemic [2].

### 2.4 Causes of psychosocial problems among girl children during the COVID-19 pandemic

"School alone cannot meet the basic psychosocial needs of children" [33]. Consequently, students face many circumstances in school and the outcome may lead to psychosocial and health problems rather than for the school to be a source of positive socialization. In this direction, many children in the school experienced an uncaring and unsupportive environment, which can have detrimental consequences on their mental health. The psychosocial aspects of depression are considered with respect to psychological factors (i.e., thinking, personality, and coping style) and social factors (i.e., family, relationships, employment, and life events). Most studies reported negative psychological effects, including post-traumatic stress symptoms, confusion, and anger. Stressors included longer quarantine duration, infection fears, frustration, boredom, inadequate supplies, inadequate information, financial loss, and stigma [9].

However, depression and anxiety levels were higher in households with lower incomes. Furthermore, 55% of parents with a household income of less than £16 k reported feeling "a lot" more anxious compared with 32% of those earning the most [34, 35]. One study found that the rates of mental health symptoms among the Chinese general population during the COVID-19 pandemic were 27.9% for depression and 31.6% for anxiety [36].

### 2.5 Studies on psychosocial problems in relation to COVID-19

However, economist and social psychologist inferred that COVID-19 pandemic, which is a global disease, has destroyed the already bad socio-economic condition of the Nigerians, to these effects, unfamiliar incidences of psychosocial problems were reported [37]. Besides that, worry about infection, specifically among individuals with health conditions related to increased risk for severe COVID-19 such as diabetes mellitus and hypertension, increased social isolation, disruption of social activities, losses of family members and acquaintances to COVID-19-related mortality, and concern about financial instability due to job losses [37].

The paper reviewed five empirical studies related to psychosocial problems and covid-19 pandemic related terms. Studies revealed that there are evidences which created psychosocial problems among the individuals during covid-19 pandemic. Oginni et al. [37] studied depressive and anxiety symptoms and COVID-19-related factors among men and women in Nigeria. The study investigated psychosocial stressors known to be associated with anxiety and depressive symptoms in relation to COVID-19 among the categories of 'heterosexual' and 'non-heterosexual' (comprising 'mostly heterosexual', 'bisexual', 'mostly gay', and 'completely gay') in Nigeria. The findings revealed that, among the categories of respondents studied, female participants were identified with higher depressive and anxiety symptoms significantly. However, COVID-19-related concerns among females such as intimate partner violence and higher worry about infection were identified as the factors that impacted higher levels of psychosocial stressors among women. Also, the study reported mental health disparities in non-heterosexual men compared with heterosexual men in Nigeria. Similarly, the findings indicate that some psychosocial factors related to the COVID-19 pandemic, including worry about infection, disruption due to the pandemic, and isolation during the lockdown, are independently associated with higher depressive and anxiety symptoms.

Banstola [38] and Timalsina et al. [39] investigated the causes of psychosocial problems among school going adolescents in Nepal. The study aimed to find out the factors that are more likely to cause psychosocial problem among adolescents. The findings identified five (5) major factors responsible among the adolescents for psychosocial problems in Nepal, which are as follows: adolescents who were facing abuse from their families, adolescents who do not feel good about their home environment, adolescents not stay with their parents, adolescents from low-income and joint families, and adolescents whose mothers are illiterate and have disrupted marital status of parents. The five categories of school-going children were more likely to develop psychosocial problems. Also, the study can be related to the Nigerian situation during the COVID-19 pandemic.

Lavigne-Cervan et al. [40] studied the consequences of COVID-19 confinement on anxiety, sleep, and executive functions of children and adolescents in Spain. The objectives of the study was to find out whether there consequences of confinement by COVID-19 on anxiety, sleep and executive functioning planning, organization, self-regulation of emotions, flexibility, time management, organization, problem solving, inhibition and containment and motivation of children and adolescents, sex, age, anxiety on the mental health of children and adolescents. The study identified three (3) categories of children of different ages and sexual levels, 9 to 12 age group expresses greater difficulties with anxiety levels while between 13- and 18-year olds express greater sleep disturbances. However, a significant difference between males with intra-sexual executive functioning groups, were also found to have a greater percentage with tendentiously maladjusted problems than their females' counterparts.

Bano and Iqbal [41] studied the cause of psychosocial and emotional problems and the development of psychopathology among university students in Pakistan. The objectives of the study were to identify the psychosocial problems among university students and factors associated with the development of psychopathology. The result of the study found that psychosocial and emotional problems and psychopathology among university students exist.

## 3. Education of a girl child in Nigeria

Education is seen as a process through which an individual is admitted into society by being taught what is worthwhile in order that the individual might play her part well in society. Generally, education involves learners or children; a child is someone who is a young individual between birth and adolescence. The United Nations Convention on the Rights of the Child [42] defines a child as "a human being below the age of 18 years unless under the law applicable to the child." From the social psychological viewpoint, a child is a human being from conception to adolescence. 'The age at which a person ceases to be a child depends on the culture, purpose, and law of the land [43, 44]." More so, Nmaduet al. [45] cited in Murthi et al. [46], "it is a belief that "female education is a powerful mechanism for controlling both mortality and fertility. Recent empirical studies from various social sciences disciplines proved a strong connection between education and demographic change, which confirms that education improves health and reduces fertility." For instance, educated women are much more likely to use dependable family planning approaches, delay marriage and childbearing, and have fewer (and healthier) babies than women without education. However, the scholars affirm that "women with a secondary school education tend to have improved knowledge about health care practices, are less likely to become pregnant at a very young age, tend to have fewer, better-spaced pregnancies, and are more likely to seek antenatal care, postnatal care, and skilled attendance at delivery."

### 3.1 Causes of poor participation of girl children in education in Nigeria

The following are some of the causes of poor participation of girl children in education in Nigeria:-

- **Religious Factor**: According to Crosnoe et al. [47] and Alabi and Alabi [36] "influence of religions of world favored male than a female child. In fact, most religious specialists and leaders are males and this makes for an authoritative image in favor of boys, and it would be a cooperative move if religious leaders of all trusts, beliefs, and denominations were to speak out powerfully in support of the female cause."

- **Health Factor**: Crosnoe et al. [47] state that the general factors related to illiteracy, culture, religion, poverty, and malnutrition have a general effect on the health of school-age children on girls than boys. Boys may get favored feeding, while girls, who are required to carry out domestic responsibilities, are more likely to be undernourished. Even if they go to school, this unfavorableness affects girls' achievement and the retention rate."

- **Socio-Cultural Factor**: "One major factor that hindered the female take up and follow through of educational opportunities, even when these are available, is a near-universal essential cultural bias in favor of males than females [48].

- **Educational Factor**: "It is through that, if you educate one girl, you educate the whole world, therefore, according to Kapur [49], educational factors that affect the participation of females in education are difficulties of accessibility, lack of resources, inadequate infrastructure, and shortage of skilled and competent teachers. However, "within rural areas, the main problem is a shortage of teachers. Parents usually feel hesitant in sending their daughters to schools, when there are not any female teachers [49]."

- **Economic Factor**: "It is believed that good parental economy would boost the education of a girl child. So economic factor is most influential in affecting the participation of girls in education [49]. Finances are imperative areas, especially in higher education. Due to a lack of finances, capable and diligent students are required to give up their aspirations of pursuing higher education. Parents find it difficult to pay for not only the education of their children, but also for making provision of books, stationery, uniforms, clothing, and other materials. Lynn [50] states "The girl child deserved better". Girls are discriminated against in Nigeria in access to educational opportunities, food, and nutrition. Girls carry a heavy burden of farm work and housework. Girls are married off at an early age, which interferes with their education or acquisition of skills needed for survival."

- **Geographical Factor:** Some of the barriers to girl child education in underdeveloped countries according to Brock and Cammish [45] are interconnected with incompleteness of institutional provision (even at lower and middle primary level), which relates directly to difficulties of physical access and adversely affect girls more than boys; there is an overall and profound urban and rural dichotomy that favors towns and cities, especially in respect of secondary school (and especially single sex) provision for girls; patterns of transportation and migration affect the educational provision and take up, again normally disadvantaging females and in some cases, extreme physical difficulties, such as flooding and other hazards act in the same way.

- **Political/Administrative Factor:** Amin [48] cited in Alabi and Alabi [36] are of the opinion that "some countries' educational policies exist in most cases for such developments as universal primary education, equal educational opportunities in terms of gender, and the eradication of gender bias from texts and other materials, the political will to carry these through seems to be weak in the face of severe economic constraint."

### 3.2 Challenges of girl child education in Nigeria

Akhigbe and Koleoso [51] put Nigeria with the highest rate of out-of-school children among the other countries in the year 2013, with less than 50% of girls in schools. Particularly the girls from the northeast region of Nigeria. The Global Coalition to protect education from attack [52] stated that, though attacks have involved the abduction of both school boys and girls, there has been a higher reported number of abduction of school-aged girls and women." In the same vein, GCPEA report indicated that some of the challenges of girl child education in the area include family socioeconomic status and the high rates of poverty, many parents could not afford to send their children to school because of the costs of education, including school fees, uniforms, and textbooks. Furthermore, some parents were resistant to sending their children to formal schools long before the emergence of Boko Haram the Global Coalition to protect education from attack [53].

Also, on the challenges of girl child education "The Global Coalition to protect education from attack [53] quoted Hauwa M., a 16-year-old student of Federal Government College Buni Yadi, Yobe state who witness Boko Haram attack in their respective school in 2014, "*After the attack, I went home. I was too afraid and decided not to go back. I told my parents I would never go back to school. They were also too afraid....Before [the attack], I was so passionate to study and achieve my dream [of being a lawyer]. But now, this experience completely demoralized me....I told my father that I will never go back because of Boko Haram threats and what I saw that night. I cannot go back to face the same thing again.*"

**Table 1** explains the incidences of girl child kidnapped from their school:-.

| S/N | Year | Name Schools | No of Students Abducted | States |
|---|---|---|---|---|
| 1. | 2014 | Government Girls Secondary School Chibok. | 276 | Borno State |
| 2. | 2016 | Government Vocational School, Rijau. | 2 | Niger State |
| 3. | 2016 | State Model College, Igbonla. | 4 | Lagos State |
| 4. | 2018 | Government Girls' Science and Technical College Dapchi. | 110 | Yobe State |
| 5. | 2018 | Maiduguri Capital School. | 2 | Borno State |
| 6. | 2019 | Engravers College, Kakau Daji. | 6 | Kaduna State |
| 7. | 2020 | Good Shepherd Major Seminary, Kakau. | 4 | Kaduna State |
| 8. | 2020 | Prince Academy Secondary School, Damba-Kasaya. | 4 | Kaduna State |
| 9. | 2020 | Government Science Secondary School Kankara. | 344 | Katsina State |
| 10. | 2020 | Dandume Islamiyya School. | 80 | Katsina State |
| 11. | 2020 | Government Science College Kagara. | 42 | Niger State |
| 12. | 2020 | Government Girls Secondary School Jangebe. | 279 | Zamfara State |
| 13. | 2021 | Federal College of Forestry Mechanization Afaka. | 39 | Kaduna State |
| **Total** | | **12** | **1115** | |

*Source: Adamu Mumini et al. 2022 [54].*

**Table 1.**
*Incidents of kidnapping and abduction of school children from school in Nigeria between 2014 and 2021.*

### 3.3 Categories of girl children with psychosocial problems in Nigeria

800,000 persons are reported missing every year, about 2000 missing persons a day [51, 55, 56]. Around 5% of these are under the age of 18. Approximately 400,000 refugee survivors of torture currently live in the United States, a significant portion of which are children [57]. Usually a kidnapped child, after release, often suffer trauma; victims are faced with a whole lot of challenges [58].

### 3.4 Evidence of girl children with psychosocial problems in Nigeria

Psychosocial refers to the importance attached in connection between psychological aspects of the human experience and the wider social experience. Therefore, "Kapur [49] discusses how psychological problems are an integral part of an individual's life. Individuals usually experience psychological problems in one's work, maintaining relationships, health problems, and when they feel overwhelmed due to certain factors, such as, workload, unable to obtain adequate sleep, nutrition, and so forth." However, according to Kapur [49], "When psychological problems, experienced by individuals, are affecting them to a major extent, then it is vital for them to seek solutions. It is good to not that, depression, stress, anxiety, and psychosocial problems are the various psychological problems experienced by individuals' students." Similarly, Omigbodun [59] studied psychosocial issues in children and adolescent psychiatric clinic populations in Nigeria. The study aimed at finding out whether psychosocial stressors and life events existed among 127 children's with psychosocial stressors over the 3 years, and the result of the study revealed that 79 (62.2%) of the 127 new referrals to the clinic had significant psychosocial stressors in the year preceding presentation. However, most of the empirical studies on psychosocial issues in children and adolescents in Nigeria revealed that "the most common psychosocial problems among children and adolescents in Nigeria were problems associated with school adjustment, interpersonal relationships and medical therapy, and perceived depression (Famuyiwa, O O, Matti O O)." Furthermore, study by Omigbodun [59] discovered some of the causes of psychosocial stressors among the children who were referred to psychiatric clinic over the period of 3-year, which are divided into two: the first one are problems associated with lack of primary support, to include: separation from parents to live with relatives, disruption of the family, abandonment by mother, psychiatric illness in a parent, and sexual or physical abuse, occurred in 50 (39.4%) of the subjects. The second causes are problems associated with social environmental factors that occurred in 11 subjects (8.7%), 39 (30.7%) had educational problems, 5 (3.9%) had economic problems, and 15 (11.8%) of the children had "other" psychosocial stressors. More significantly, it is an evidence that more children and adolescents have disruptive behavior disorders and disorders like enuresis, separation anxiety and suicidal behavior, and psychosocial stressors when compared with children with psychotic conditions such as autistic disorder and epilepsy ($chi(2) = 9.6$; $p = 0.048$). More importantly, the study further recommended the importance of the psychosocial diagnostic dimension in routine schedules.

### 3.5 Girl child education and COVID-19 pandemic

The outbreak of COVID-19 pandemic in Nigeria poses a great challenge to the education system in the country's already fragile education system. Obiakor and Adeniran [60] discuss controversial issues of school closure in a very critical moment, and it can have spillover effects on a large number of students in receiving schools. Thus, the consequences of school closure can affect the quality of teaching and learning and academic achievement, particularly for students with special needs or those with learning difficulties that often require more physical attention and guidance from the teachers. Therefore, before the pandemic, there was an estimated total of 10.2 million out-of-school children in Nigeria. About 1.6 billion learners in 190 countries across the world were affected by the pandemic, with 94% of the world's school population impacted by school closures (United Nations *Policy Brief*, The Education Partnership Nigeria (TEP) [61, 62]). The closure of schools has affected 36,400,000 primary and secondary school learners across Nigeria, including those in internally displaced camps.

### 3.6 How psychosocial problems affects girl child education

Psychosocial disorders disrupt the normal functioning of the affected child and the family. Children may lose interest in play and school activities, and relationships with family and friends are usually impaired. The Dakar Framework for Action goal (b) stipulated that all girls child, in difficult circumstances, such as those with Psychological problems or it related terms should have access to complete at least primary education of good quality [63]. Kapur [49] agreed that, psychological problems are an integral part of an individual's life, usually individuals developed and experience psychological problems in one's work, upholding interactions, environmental and health related problems and when individual's feel overwhelmed due to certain factors, such as, workload, inability to obtain adequate sleep, inadequate food and nutrition among others. Child health professionals (CHPs) identified the existence of psychosocial problems among school-aged children, particularly a girls child. One out of ten (20%) adolescents encounter at least one behavioral problem internationally [64]. Half of lifetime mental disorders begin before the age of 14 years, and 75% begin by the age of 24 years [64]. There is a need for early detection of these problems at home and in school especially in preschool [63, 65, 66]. As individuals develop, they usually experience psychological problems in one way or the other, be it in the workplace or in maintaining relationships with loved ones, health problems, and when they feel overwhelmed due to certain factors, such as, workload, unable to obtain adequate sleep, and nutrition [49]. Reijneveld et al. [67] reported the result of study conducted by American Child Health Professionals (CHPs) in Dutch Preventive Child Health Care; confirm that, one or more psychosocial problems were identified in 25% of all children. However, the study further revealed that, 1 in 5 of the identified children with psychosocial problems was referred for further identification and treatment.

## 4. Psychosocial educational

### 4.1 What is psychosocial educational?

Psychosocial is a term used to refer to the active association between psychological aspects of one experiences (including, our feelings, emotions, and behaviors) and our wider social experience (that is, our relationships, family and community networks, social values, and cultural practices), where one influences [68]. Psychosocial education is a terminology of knowledge used to provide to individuals and families to promote awareness regarding unhealthy relationships and maladaptive behaviors. As individuals become aware of such dynamics in their relationships, they can understand the impact and work toward change.

### 4.2 Types of psychosocial problems among girl children

The following are the types of psychosocial problems among girl children [69].

#### *4.2.1 Growing up armed groups*

Child stealing, kidnapping for rape or sexual assault by militant groups exists in Nigeria [70]. The National Center for Missing and Exploited Children states about 800,000 persons are reported missing every year and about 2000 missing persons a day [55]. Around 5% of these are under age 18. United Nations Children's Fund (UNICEF) Nigeria [69] put it that, "Nigeria has vulnerable children who have experienced abduction or forced conscription by non-state armed groups." UNICEF [69] further states that, "children reported having spent crucial periods of their childhood in captivity, in small, hot, enclosed, overcrowded spaces, leading to extreme distress endured over a long duration of time."

#### *4.2.2 The continuance of stressors after release*

UNISEF [69] identified five factors related to stressors after release among the girl child: Separation from family and loss of caregivers, stigma and isolation, prevalence of sexual violence, challenges with attending school and loss of dignity, and child labor.

#### *4.2.3 Prevalence of sexual violence*

Sexual violence means whichever sexual action, and in other words an effort, to attain to acquire sexual act by forcefulness or intimidation. The most vulnerable type of psychosocial problems among Girl Children according to United Nations Children's Fund [69] is sexual violence; the girl child sexual violence is prevalent at the camps and was reported by every girl interviewed for the assessment. Sexual exploitation by volunteers during food and nonfood item distribution was frequently reported during the assessment. The report of the United Nations Children's Fund [69] further cited that, "almost every girl shared that she had been followed by a stranger at the camp more than once. When probed for unsafe spaces, the girls shared that toilet and shower areas were unsafe as there was only a thin metal sheet dividing the male and female showers, with the clothes hung at the same place."

#### *4.2.4 Challenges to attending school*

Boko Haram crisis has extensively expanded the severity of all challenges against formal education in the region, especially the girl child (See 3.2) [53].

#### *4.2.5 Loss of dignity and child labor*

"The volunteers and workers take advantage of girls, seeking sexual favors in exchange for food. If you refuse, they twist it around against your family. And because our parents do not work, we are dependent on aid [69]."

#### *4.2.6 Child marriage*

In northern Nigeria, religion and culture influenced parents to marry their children at the exact age of marriage, of 13 to 14 years for girls and 16 to 17 years for boys. Girls were reportedly at higher risk of child marriage and had little choice-making capacity. Often, adolescent girls were married to middle-aged men as one of the multiple wives [69].

#### *4.2.7 Deteriorating interpersonal and family relationships*

It was observed that interpersonal relationships were poor and reportedly getting worse among families [69].

One girl child who has experienced this in her interpersonal family narrated that, "my mother remarried and has another husband and a new baby. if the baby is crying, she asks me to comfort him. But then she insults me if the baby continues to cry. The mother says "it is because you are not related by blood; you do not have the same father'. And the girl children further add that "I have run away from home before [69]." This is evidence an adolescent girl describing poor family relationships in north-east Nigeria.

### 4.3 Effectiveness of psychosocial support on girl child with psychosocial problems

According to the International Network for Education in Emergencies [68], "Psychosocial support is a process of facilitating resilience within individuals, families and communities." Also, according to United Nations High Commissioner for Refugees Africa [71], Canadian Association for Refugee and Forced Migration Studies (CARFMS) [72], United Nations Children's Fund [69], and Save the Children Nigeria [73], psychosocial support refers to a scale of care and support that influence both the individual and the social environment in which people live and ranges from care and support offered by caregivers, family members, friends, neighbors, teachers, health workers, and community members on a daily basis, and also extends to care and support offered by specialized psychologist and social services."

Psychosocial support offered to individuals, their partners and families to remedy their psychosocial problems can assist people in making informed decisions, coping better with illness, and dealing more effectively with discrimination. It improves the quality of the lives of the affected people [74].

### 4.4 Strategies curb with girl child with psychosocial problems

The World Health Organization [74] developed the following Strategies as a measure to curb psychosocial problems:

- Psychosocial support should be exactly to include in the health policy of all nations as guidelines for the management of psychosocial problems.

- Health institutions should incorporate training support of psychosocial care for all health care trainees and providers into their curriculum.

- All nations should develop guidelines for home care services to include the provision of basic psychosocial care by community volunteers and family caregivers.

- It is vital that training courses for community volunteers should be organized and provided by health care workers.

- Compulsory training in professional disciplines such as counseling, psychology, and psychiatry can be made available at the international level.

- Basic strategies for providing psychosocial support should be developed for specific groups, especially women, youth, men who have sex with men, injecting drug users, and health care providers.

### 4.5 How to use social studies education to address the challenges of psychosocial problems among girl children

Social study is a program of instructions or studies that a society uses to instill in learners the knowledge, skills, attitudes, values, and actions that it considers important concerning the relationships that human beings have with each other [75]. One of the primary aims of teaching Social Studies Education in Nigeria is to inculcate the right type of attitude that is desirable for pupils. To do this effectively, Social Studies teachers, at all levels of education in Nigeria, (nursery, primary, secondary or tertiary), must be conversant and knowledgeable with national values. And this can be derived from the national objectives, some of which are as follows: A free and democratic society; a united, strong, and self-reliant nation; a just and egalitarian society; a great and dynamic economy; and a land of bright and full opportunities for all citizens [76]. Social studies gives students the opportunity to inquire, investigate, discover, discuss, experiment, and acquire experiences to make decisions on social issues and problems, and find solutions to them [17].

## 5. Conclusion

The Dakar Framework for Action goal (b) stipulated that all girls child, in difficult circumstances, such as those with Psychological problems or it related terms should have access to complete at least primary education of good quality. Psychological problems are an essential part of an individual's life. Child health professionals (CHPs) identified that psychosocial problems exist among school-aged children, particularly girl children. One out of ten (20%) adolescents encounter at least one behavioral problem internationally. Therefore, the World Health Organization [74] recommended that "Psychosocial support should be made specifically to include in nations guidelines for the management of psychosocial problem, also compulsory training on the provision of psychosocial support should be incorporated into the curriculum for all health institutions and the health care providers, and guidelines for home care services should be developed to include the provision of basic psychosocial care by community volunteers and family caregivers."

## Author details

Adamu Mumini
Department of Social Studies, School of Secondary Education (Arts and Social Sciences), Umar Suleiman College of Education Gashua, Yobe State, Nigeria

*Address all correspondence to: muminiadamu90@gmail.com

## References

[1] Chukwu O, New Dangers to Girls' Education in Northern Nigeria [Internet]. 2021 [Cited 2021 Sep 20]. Available from www.dio.69i57j69i60.2056j0j7&sourceid=chrome&ie=UTF-8

[2] Meraya AM, Syed MH, Yasmeen A, Mubaraki AA, Kariry HD, Maabouj W, et al. COVID-19 related psychological distress and fears among mothers and pregnant women in Saudi Arabia. Plos one. 2021 Aug 24;**16**(8):e0256597

[3] World Health Organization, Depression [Internet]. 2021 [cited 2021 Sep 20]. Available from https://www.who.int/news-room/fact-sheets/detail/depression

[4] Morens DM, Folkers GK, Fauci AS. What is a pandemic? The Journal of Infectious Diseases [Internet]. 2009;**200**:1018-1021 [Cited 2021 Sep 25]

[5] Jordan D. The Deadliest Flu: The Complete Story of the Discovery and Reconstruction of the 1918 Pandemic Virus. Centers for Disease Control and Prevention, National Center for Immunization and Respiratory Diseases [Internet]. 2019 [Cited 2021 Sep 25] Available from https://www.cdc.gov/flu/pandemic-resources/1918-pandemic-h1n1.html

[6] Glezen WP. Emerging infections: Pandemic influenza. Epidemiology Review. 1996;**18**:64-76. DOI: 10.1093/oxfordjournals.epirev.a017917

[7] Viboud C, Grais RF, Lafont BA, Miller MA, Simonsen L. Multinational impact of the 1968 Hong Kong influenza pandemic: Evidence for a smoldering pandemic. Journal of Infectious Disease. 2005;**192**:233-248. DOI: 10.1086/431150

[8] Ibrahim RL, Kazeem AKB. Implications for the healthcare system in Nigeria. Health Policy and Technology. 2020;**9**:399-404. DOI: 10.1016/j.hlp.2020.09.004

[9] Brooks SK, Webster RK, Smith LE, Woodland L, Wessely S, Greenberg N, et al. The psychological impact of quarantine and how to reduce it: Rapid review of the evidence. The Lancet. 2020;**395**:912-920

[10] Jabeen K, Husnain Haider MB, Haider Z, Hassan A, Ali S. Coronavirus (COVID-19) pandemic: Outbreak, current scenario and impact on human physiology in Pakistan. Global Journal of Clinical Virology. 2021;**6**(1):021-029. DOI: 10.17352/gjcv.000011

[11] Odigbo J, Nnorom K. Global health conundrum: Interrogating the Nigerian state and its containment responses to covid-19 pandemic. Unpublished International conference Book of Abstract: The state, security and development in the COVID-19 era and beyond. 2021

[12] Campbell J. Lagos and Abuja on Lockdown to Stop Coronavirus in Nigeria. 2020. Available from: https://www.cfr.org/blog/lagos-and-abuja-lockdown-stop-coronavirus-nigeria

[13] Institute of Health Metrics and Evaluation, Global Health Data Exchange. 2021. http://ghdx.healthdata.org/gbd-results-tool?params=gbd-api-2019-permalink/d780dffbe8a381b25e1416884959e88b

[14] Nigerian centre for diseases control, Covid-19. From https://covid19.ncdc.gov.ng/ [Retrieved: November 29, 2020]

[15] Omede AA, Etumabo AG. The implications of girl-child education to nation building in the 21st century in Nigeria. Global Journal of Linguistics & Education. 2016;**16**:3 https://globaljournals.org/GJHSS_Volume16/1-The-Implications-of-Girl-Child.pdf

[16] Offorma GC. Girl-child education in Africa in Africa. In: Keynote Address Presented at the Conference of University WOMWNE of Africa. Lagos, Nigeria; 2009. https://www.researchgate.net/profile/GraceOfforma/publication/280554452_girl-child_education_in_africa/links/55b8c2a708aec0e5f43b6bf7/girl-child-education-in-africa.pdf

[17] Fareo DO, Ateequ W. Determinants of girl child education among the nomads in Nigeria. East African Scholars Journal of Psychology and Behavioural Sciences. 2020;**2**(5):138-145

[18] Global citizens. 2018. Nigeria Has World's Largest Number of Out-of-School Children https://www.globalcitizen.org/en/content/un-nigeria-13-million-

[19] Ravenhills PS. Psycho-Social Education. 2020. https://edisoncourt.com/community-forensic-programs/psycho-social-education

[20] Opoh FA, Edinyang SD, Dominic OI. Introduction of social studies education in Nigeria schools: A success or a failure. International Journal of Education and Research. 2014;**2**(4):144-145. https://www.ijern.com/journal/April-2014/13.pdf

[21] Mumini A, Hussaini MA. Upholding religion and national values through social studies in universal basic education curriculum in Nigeria. Nigerian Journal of Social Studies. 2021;**24**(1):47-50. https://www.njss.org.ng/publications/vol_xxiv_1_april_2021/upholding_religion_and_national_values_through_social_studies_in_universal_basic_education.pdf

[22] Jekayinfa AA. The fortunes and challenges of Social studies in Nigeria. In: Being a Lead Paper Presented at the 34th Annual Conference of the SOSAN. Nigeria: University of Lagos; 2018. Retrieved December 26, 2020, from https://www.sosan.org.ng/2018_conference/fortunes_and_challenges _of_social_studies_education_in_nigeria.pdf

[23] The World Health Organization (WHO) Coronaviruses COVID-19 Pandemic. 2021. From https://www.who.int/emergencies/diseases/novel-coronavirus-2019?gclid= [Retrieved: November 29, 2020]

[24] Li D, Zou L, Zhang Z, Zhang P, Zhang J, Fu W, et al. The psychological effect of covid 19 on home-quarantined nursing students in China. Frontiers in Psychiatry. 2021;**12**:652296. DOI: 10.3389/fpsyt.2021.652296

[25] Anifowose OL, Alle OAA, Assessment of the Impact of covid-19 Pandemic and Lockdown Policy on Female Owned Businesses in Akure, Ondo state, Nigeria, West Africa. 2021. From http://www.osogbojournalofmanagement.com/index.php/ojm/article/view/171/140 [Retrieved: November 29, 2020]

[26] Dutta J, Mitra A, Zaman S, Mitra A. Lockdown and beyond: Impact of COVID-19 pandemic on global employment sector with special reference to India. NUJS Journal of Regulatory Studies. Apr 2021;**2**:1-4

[27] Parvin RA, Islam S, Akter MS, Mohammod SS, Hossain B, Rashid SN. Psychosocial anxiety from lockdown due to covid-19 to income earner of the family: An evidence from northern Bangladesh. Sociology Mind. 2021;**11**:65-80. [Retrieved November 29, 2020]. DOI: 10.4236/sm.2021.113006

[28] Atadoga DU, Odalonu BH. The political economy of covid-19 pandemic and the effect of lockdown measures in Nigeria. Unpublished International Conference Book of Abstract: The State, Security and Development in the COVID-19 Era and Beyond. 2021

[29] Amos U, The state and management of internal security challenges in Nigeria in covid-19 era and beyond. Unpublished International Conference Book of Abstract: The State, Security

and Development in the COVID-19 Era and beyond. 2021

[30] Chinonso AA, Odey OT. Rentier state and the covid-19 economic recovery strategy in Nigeria. Unpublished International Conference Book of Abstract: The state, Security and Development in the COVID-19 Era and Beyond. 2021

[31] Amusan L, Agunyai SC. The COVID-19 pandemic and the crisis of lockdowns in Nigeria: The household food security perspective. Africa's Public Service Delivery and Performance Review. 2021;**9**(1):1-19

[32] Liu JJ, Bao Y, Huang X, Shi J, Lu L. Mental health considerations for children quarantined because of COVID-19. The Lancet Child & Adolescent Health. 2020;**4**(5):347-349. DOI: 10.1016/S2352-4642(20)30096-1

[33] Famakinwa TT, Olagunju OE, Akinnawonu CI. A study of psychosocial challenges of public secondary school students in a semi-urban area of Southwest-Nigeria. Journal of Community Medicine and Primary Health Care. 2016;**28**(1):59-64

[34] Saunders B, Hogg S. Babies in Lockdown Listening to Parents to Build Back Better. 2020. Retrieved from https://babiesinlockdown.files.wordpress.com/2020/08/babies-in-lockdown-main-report-final-version-1.pdf

[35] Huang Y, Zhao N. Chinese Mental Health Burden during the COVID-19 Pandemic. Asian journal of psychiatry; Jun 2020;**51**:102052

[36] Alabi T, Alabi OS. Female education: A sociological analysis of girl-child education in Nigeria. International Journal of Educational Policy Research and Review. Jan 2014;**1**(1):006-013

[37] Oginni OA, Oloniniyi IO, Ibigbami O, Ugo V, Amiola A, Ogunbajo A, Esan O, Adelola A, Daropale O, Ebuka W, Mapayi B. Depressive and anxiety symptoms and COVID-19-related factors among men and women in Nigeria. Plos one. 26 Aug 2021;**16**(8):e0256690

[38] Banstola RS. Psychosocial problem among school-going adolescents in Pokhara, western Nepal. Journal of Janapriya Interdisciplinary Studies. 2017;**6**:121-126

[39] Timalsina N, Kafle M, Timalsina R. Psychosocial problems among school going adolescents in Nepal. Psychiatry Journal. 2 Jul 2018;**2018**

[40] Lavigne-Cerván R, Costa-López B, Juárez-Ruiz de Mier R, Real-Fernández M, Sánchez-Muñoz de León M, Navarro-Soria I. Consequences of COVID-19 confinement on anxiety, sleep and executive functions of children and adolescents in Spain. Frontiers in Psychology. 16 Feb 2021;**12**:565516

[41] Bano A, Iqbal N. Psychosocial, emotional problems and development of psychopathology among university students. Clinical and Experimental Psychology. 2018;**4**:201. DOI: 10.4172/2471-2701.1000201

[42] The United Nations Convention on the Rights of the Child: The children's version. https://www.unicef.org/media/60981/file/convention-rights-child-text-child-friendly-version.pdf

[43] Kebede E, Striessnig E, Goujon A. The Relative Importance of women's Education on Fertility Desires in Sub-Saharan Africa: A Multilevel Analysis. Population Studies. 2 Jan 2022;**76**(1):137-156

[44] Mallum JO, Haggai MP, Ajegbu KJU. An Introduction to Child Development. Jos: Deka Publication; 1999

[45] Nmadu G, Avidime S, Oguntunde O, Abdulkarim VDB, Mandara M. Girl child education: Rising

to the challenge. African Journal of Reproductive Health. 2010;**14**(3):108

[46] Murthi M, Guio A, Dreze J. Mortality, Fertility and Gender Bias in India: A District level analysis. 1995. Retrieved from: http://www.histecon.kings.cam.ac.uk/docs/mortal.PDF

[47] Amin ME Social Science research: Conception, Methodology and Analysis. Kampala: Makerere University Press. 2005

[48] Brock C & Cammish N. Factors affecting Female Participation in Education in Seven Developing Countries – Education. 1997. https://core.ac.uk/download/pdf/7052376.pdf

[49] Kapur R. Psychological Problems among Students. 2019. https://www.researchgate.net/publication/334956226_Psychological_Problems_among_Students/link/5d467f67a6fdcc370a79df2d/download

[50] Lynn NG. The Girl Child Deserve Better. 2020. https://ng.opera.news/ng/en/sex-relationship/5b04ce7cf6ba35ba57378087bb28675f

[51] Akhigbe KO, Koleoso ON. Psychological and psychiatric considerations in a kidnapped for-ransom victim: A clinical case study. Journal of Dental and Medical Sciences. 2013;**10**(5):01-05. http://www.iosrjournals.org/iosr-jdms/papers//Vol10-issue5/A01050105.pdf

[52] The Global Coalition Nigeria Has Highest Number of Out-of-School Children in the World https://www.globalcitizen.org/en/content/nigeria-has-largest-number-of-children-out-of-scho/

[53] Global Coalition to Protect Education from Attack. "I will never go back to School" the Impact of Attacks on Education for Nigerian Women and Girls. 2018. https://reliefweb.int/sites/reliefweb.int/files/resources/attacks_on_nigerian_women_and_girls.pdf

[54] Mumini A, Ariya DA, Mariam BA. Social studies: A panacea in managing the menace of kidnapping and abduction of school children in Nigeria. African Journal of Social Studies. 2022;**3**(2):121

[55] Ruwan IIF, Zamani A, Ishaya DS, Audu G, Pailiya V. Assessing the incidences of kidnapping in Kaduna state from 2015-2018: The way forward. Sapientia Global Journal of Arts, Humanities and Development Studies. 25 Sep 2020;**3**(3)

[56] Ford D. Do 800,000 kids vanish every year in the United States? https://leadstories.com/hoax-alert/2020/08/fact-check-800,000-is-not-an-accurate-number-of-kids-who-vanish-every-year-in-the-us.html

[57] Center for the Study of Traumatic Stress The Impact of Kidnapping, Shooting and Torture on Children. nd https://www.cstsonline.org/assets/media/documents/CSTS_impact_kidnapping_shooting_torture_children.pdf

[58] Abamara N. Psychological impact of kidnapping: A Case Study of a Victim in Anambra State Nigeria. 2018. https://www.researchgate.net/publication/327301236_Psychological_Impact_of_Kidnapping_A_case_Study_of_A_Victim_in_Anambra_State_Nigeria

[59] Omigbodun OO. Psychosocial issues in child and adolescent psychiatric clinic population in Nigeria. Social Psychiatry and Psychiatric Epidemiology. 2004;**39**(8):667-672. DOI: 10.1007/s00127-004-0793-x

[60] Obiakor T, Adeniran A. COVID-19: Risk-Control Measures Threaten To Deepen Nigeria's Education Crisis. Centre for the Study of Economies of Africa. 2020. From http://cseaafrica.org/covid-19-risk-controlmeasures-threatens-to-deepen-nigerias-educationcrisis [Retrieved: February, 28, 2021]

[61] United Nations Policy Brief: Education during COVID-19 and

beyond. 2020. From: https://www.un.org/development/desa/dspd/wpcontent/uploads/sites/22/2020/08/sg_policy_brief_covid-19_and_education_august_2020.pdf [Retrieved: February, 28, 2021]

[62] The Education Partnership Nigeria (TEP) Learning in a Pandemic Nigeria's response to Teaching and Learning during the COVID-19 Pandemic https://education.gov.ng/wpcontent/uploads/2020/08/Learning-in-a-Pandemic-Report_TEP-NESG_2020.pdf

[63] What are the Effects of Psychosocial Disorders in Children? https://nursekey.com/psychosocial-problems-in-children-and-families/

[64] Bista B, Thapa P, Sapkota D, Singh SB, Pokharel PK. Psychosocial problems among adolescent students: An exploratory study in the central region of Nepal. Frontiers in Public Health. 2016;**4**:158. DOI: 10.3389/fpubh.2016.00158

[65] International Bureau of Education. Education for All. 2000. http://www.ibe.unesco.org/en/glossary-curriculum-terminology/e/education-all-efa

[66] Calvince O, Odera F. Interventional Measures for the Control of Psychosocial Issues to Promote Academics in Public Secondary Schools in Migori County –Kenya. 2020. http://ijern.com/journal/2020/July-2020/02.pdf

[67] Sijmen A. Reijneveld, Emily Brugman, Frank C. Verhulst, S. Pauline, Verloove-Vanhorick, MD. Identification and management of psychosocial problems among toddlers in Dutch preventive child health care, Archives of Pediatrics & Adolescent Medicine; 2004;**158**(8):811-817. DOI: 10.1001/archpedi.158.8.811

[68] International Network for Education in Emergencies. Psychosocial Support and Social and Emotional Learning for Children and Youth in Emergency Settings. 2016. https://resourcecentre.savethechildren.net/document/inee-background-paper-psychosocial-support-and-social-and-emotional-learning-children-and/

[69] UNICEF Nigeria. Psychosocial Support for Children: A Rapid Needs Assessment in North-East Nigeria. 2019. https://www.unicef.org/nigeria/media/2956/file/PSS%20Assesment%20Report.pdf

[70] Ugwuoke CU. Nigeria and the menace of kidnapping: The way forward. Journal of Research and Production. 2011;**18**(2):1-14

[71] United Nations High Commissioner for Refugees Africa ARC Resource Pack Study Material Foundation Module 7 Psychosocial Support https://www.unhcr.org/protection/children/4c98a5169/arc-resource-pack-study-material-foundation-module-7-psychosocial-support.html

[72] Canadian Association for Refugee and Forced Migration Studies (CARFMS) http://rfmsot.apps01.yorku.ca/glossary-of-terms/mental-health-and-psychosocial-support/

[73] Save the Children, Child Protection Initiative Newsletter. 2011. https://resource-centre-uploads.s3.amazonaws.com/uploads/3746.pdf

[74] World Health Organization. Psychosocial Support for HIV/AID. 2021. https://www.who.int/hiv/topics/psychosocial/support/en/

[75] Kazi KF. The Menace of Social Problems in Nigeria. Jos: Ais Publishers limited; 2016

[76] Gbadamosi TV. Attitude as a correlate of utilization of information communication technology in instructional delivery among social studies teachers in Oyo state. Contemporary Humanities. Nigeria. 2016;**9**:116-127

Chapter 15

# Perspective Chapter: Pedagogical Approaches and Access to Education among Early Childhood Education Learners with Disabilities in Africa during the COVID-19 Pandemic – Review of Available Literature

*Margaret Nampijja, Lillian Ayiro and Ruth Nalugya*


## Abstract

The COVID 19 pandemic suddenly hit the world disrupting access to education especially in Sub-Saharan Africa, threatening the future of millions of learners. This chapter discusses the effects of COVID-19 on early childhood education (ECE) for learners with disabilities in Africa, focusing on three questions: (1) What pedagogical approaches were used to enable access to education among ECE learners with disabilities during the COVID 19 pandemic? (2) How was access to education for ECE learners with disabilities, and what challenges and opportunities were experienced? (3) How can access to quality and equitable learning for ECE learners with disabilities during the crisis be improved? Literature revealed that the pandemic aggravated the hardships in accessing learning programs among learners with disabilities widening the gap between them and their counterparts. Countries resorted to remote and digital pedagogical approaches to enable continuity of learning; however, many did not cater for learners with disabilities. Where disabilities were catered for, the reach and utilization were limited by lack of resources and capacity. Concerted efforts promoting effective inclusive learning are critical for the current and future pandemics. Barriers to provision of equitable education, and long-term effects of COVID 19 on in ECE learners with disabilities should be investigated.


**Keywords:** COVID-19, pedagogical, education, access, learners, children, disabilities

## 1. Introduction

The COVID-19 pandemic rapidly swept through the world's population affecting over 200 million people and causing over 5 million deaths. Clearly, the unprecedented global pandemic has affected every aspect of people's lives [1] resulting in severe disruptions in livelihoods and access to social services for populations across the globe. Sub-Saharan Africa and similar low-income countries were severely hit by the pandemic disrupting the delivery of health, education, and other essential services as these countries were ill-prepared to deal with the effects of such a sudden major disaster [2].

The pandemic resulted in closure of schools in over 188 countries worldwide, affecting the learning, and threatening the future of over 1.5 billion learners, that is, 91% of all learners [3]. In Africa, about 250 million students were affected. Learning completely stopped for most of them, and millions of students were at risk for permanently dropping out of school, adding to the 100 million out-of-school children before the pandemic [4].

In Uganda, for example, during the 2020 wave, to control the rapidly transmissible infection, 51,000 learning institutions were closed between March and October, meaning that approximately 15 million children missed school for half a year. This was shortly followed by a second wave that resulted in a total lockdown and closure of schools from March 2021 for the rest of the year, amounting to almost 2 years of school closure, the longest on record. During the school closures, children not only lost substantial time of their learning, but they were also prone to several risks including abuse, neglect, teenage pregnancy, child labor, mental health disorders, and suicide, among others.

While all learners were affected, children with disabilities are believed to have been disproportionately disadvantaged by the pandemic since they were already grappling with challenges of access to education services due to disability. People with disabilities (PWD) are often overlooked, their capacities underestimated, and their needs given a low priority [5]. It is likely that as a result of COVID-19, preexisting learning challenges for learners with disabilities were complicated while new ones emerged, further widening the gap in access and learning between these learners with disabilities and their normal functioning counterparts. To date, there is little consolidated information on how the pandemic impacted the learning of early childhood education (ECE) learners with disabilities in sub-Saharan Africa, what approaches were used to tackle the challenges, and what lessons can be drawn for future improvement. In this chapter, we examine available evidence on the impact of COVID-19 pandemic on access to education/learning for early learners with disabilities in the context of sub-Saharan Africa, the challenges, and opportunities and possible strategies for bridging the gaps. We focus on three key questions:

1. What pedagogical approaches were used to enable access to education among ECE learners with disabilities during the COVID 19 pandemic?

2. How was access to education for ECE learners with disabilities, and what challenges and opportunities were experienced?

3. How can access to quality and equitable learning for ECE learners with disabilities during the current crisis be improved, and what can we learn for future crises?

Effective planning and institution of appropriate interventions to optimize learning for children with disabilities during the current and future crises will depend on a good understanding of these issues.

## 2. Methods

This chapter is based on review of literature on the topics above that was available between September 2021 and February 2022 when the chapter was written.

We conducted literature review on the subject focusing on the sub-Saharan African context. We retrieved and included peer-reviewed and gray literature that reported on any of the areas listed above.

### 2.1 Literature search

Literature search was guided by the three research questions. Search terms were generated and used in the search across different databases including PUBMED, and Google scholar, and Google search for gray literature including reports, blogs, webinars etc. Key search terms included (COVID-19 OR SARS-VIRUS) AND (disabilities OR "special needs" OR "vulnerable populations") AND (education OR learning OR schooling OR "pedagogical approaches") AND ("early childhood" OR children) AND (Africa OR "sub-Saharan Africa" OR Africa OR "developing countries") AND (barriers OR challenges) AND (access OR opportunities OR support). After the search was completed, the articles were compiled and screened for relevance and eligibility using the titles, abstracts, and/or on full texts. The selected articles were summarized in a table describing the type of literature, source, focus/objectives, geographical representation, and key findings.

### 2.2 Data extraction and synthesis

Full texts of the eligible articles were reviewed by the three reviewers working independently and focusing on our questions of interest, collaborating evidence from the diverse contexts within the continent, and key lessons for policy and practice but also identifying the important evidence gaps for future research, and any emerging perspectives related to our objectives. Based on this extraction approach, a narrative synthesis was used to describe and discuss the information as organized under the different headings below.

## 3. Results

A total of 41 articles including peer-reviewed and gray literature (reports, blogs, and other gray literature) were reviewed and discussed concisely, starting with a flashback on the status of ECE for children with disability before the emergence of COVID-19; followed by the pedagogical approaches that were adopted by educators in response to the pandemic; how ECE learners with disabilities accessed education during the pandemic, the challenges and opportunities they experienced; strategies through which access to quality and equitable learning for ECE learners with disabilities during the crisis can be improved; and a discussion of these perspectives bringing together the different experiences and highlighting key lessons in a local and global perspective and their implications for the current situation and future crises, in terms of policy, service provision, and research. We wind up the chapter with a conclusion highlighting the take-home message and future direction, along with the limitations of the review.

## 4. Early childhood education and learning for children with disabilities before the pandemic

Learners with disabilities include those who have sensory impairments, cognitive differences, physical difficulties, emotional and behavioral difficulties, communication disorders, and those with multiple disabilities [6]. Whereas some learners with disability may follow regular curriculum with adaptation or modification of the pedagogical approaches used, there are those who may need specialized syllabuses and intervention programs to access meaningful education. A majority of learners who follow regular curriculum with modification include children with visual impairment, hearing impairment, physical handicap, mild cerebral palsy, mild learning disabilities, mild autism, mild emotional and behavioral difficulties, communication disorders, and the gifted and talented [7]. They require additional support and care services such as therapy, assistive devices, and technology to access education. Leaners with disabilities who need special syllabus include those with mental handicap, deaf blindness, severe autism, severe cerebral palsy, multiple handicaps, and those with profound disabilities [8]. They learn social, communication, and activities of daily living skills at school [9]. In this chapter, we focus on reviewing literature on the pedagogical methods that were employed to enhance continuity of learning among millions of African children after the schools closed and how they favored or did not favor early childhood education (ECE) learners with disabilities.

Child-centered teaching approaches have been found to effectively enhance learning of children in early childhood education. This is predominantly learning by doing through imitation of teachers and their peers [10]. The approach has also been found to be crucial for learners with disabilities who have various challenges and need extra support [11]. Education for all children in their early years supports their development of social, communication, problem-solving, cognitive, and emotional skills [10]. This also applies to children with disabilities in early childhood education. According to Davis [9], the pedagogical approaches used for effective learning of these foundational skills among children with disabilities include: formulating clear expectations based on learning needs of the child, stimulating learning activities that enhances learners' participation in classroom, use of audio-visual material, real objects, or simulations to make the learning process concrete, break tasks into less complex tasks and build on already acquired skills and knowledge, peer learning, sharing the learning objectives and process with parents so they can help with homework. Other strategies include carrying out every day routines consistently and aiding active learning by use of immediate reward for good behavior, completing work on time, and participating in class activities. In addition, individualized education plans where lessons are modified to meet each learner's needs are also critical for children with disabilities [12]. Much as the approaches to support learning of these children are well articulated, they are often not practiced because of various reasons including lack of teacher skills, resources, and poor attitude of teachers among others [13, 14]. Moreover, children with disabilities are often stigmatized and discriminated against by teachers and pupils, further hindering them from full participation in learning.

Before the era of COVID-19 pandemic, access to education and other services was a major challenge for people with disabilities (PWD) including children in many low- and middle-income settings. There have been increasing efforts toward inclusive education, which recommends that children with special needs are accommodated within the mainstream teaching; however, implementation of this has been slow. Education for people with disability has been characterized by exclusion, stigma, discrimination, non-supportive attitudes of parents and community members, long distance to school, school environments that are not supportive (access, materials, equipment), and limited training for teachers on special needs education, limited involvement in planning and allocation of resources for learners with special needs as well as lack of enforcement and financing of the inclusive education policies [5, 15, 16]. As a result, there was a major gap in education access for children with disabilities in many countries in Africa prior to the pandemic. Clearly, as we will lean from subsequent sections, the pandemic and resulting school closures worsened the challenges for ECE learners with disabilities especially those in LMICs where governments were least prepared to deal with these challenges. In the section that follows, we take a critical look at the pedagogical approaches that were used to support continued learning for ECE learners with disabilities in Africa.

## 5. Pedagogical approaches for learners with disabilities during COVID-19 lockdown in African countries

COVID-19 severely affected education systems across the world [17], and the most affected were learners in pre-primary and primary level who have little experience of learning outside the classrooms, without support of their teachers, and could not be provided with adequate resources for learning at home (EdTech [18]). The situation was more difficult for learners with disabilities living in middle- and low-income African countries who for a long time have struggled to access quality education [7, 17]. Studies indicate that during the period when schools were closed (as a result of the pandemic), over 30% of learners with disabilities in Africa were not able to read by themselves or be read to by their parents [19]. This could have been due to the mismatch between the learners' needs and the pedagogical approaches that were used to support them access education while at home. Learners with disabilities have unique learning styles such as visual, auditory, and kinesthetic styles that require teachers to employ different teaching strategies in the learning process to achieve effective learning. Apart from Benin, Burundi, Cote d'voire, Congo, Ethiopia, Madagascar, Malawi, Niger, and Togo that lacked remote learning readiness, most of the other African countries responded to the school closure due to COVID-19 in innovative ways by offering distance remote learning [20]. The strategies that were used combined high tech and low-cost solutions that included digital teaching and learning approaches as well as the use of paper-based take-home learning materials [21]. These pedagogical approaches were either audio-based where radios were the most common mode of audio learning, or audio-visual based where the television was the most popular form of instruction. A study established that almost all the countries in Middle East and North Africa (MENA) used television programs and print materials to deliver education content while 65% of countries in Eastern and Southern Africa (ESA) and 81% of countries in Western and Central Africa (WCA) used the television to deliver content [17]. The Ubongo Kids, Edu entertainment, and Akili Kids were the most common televised learning programs. It is estimated that over 25 million children across 40 African countries accessed Ubongo TV program that is broadcast in nine African languages including sign language [22]. The assumption of remote learning was that the intervention would meet the educational needs of all children including those in early childhood and with disability, whose schooling had also been disrupted by the pandemic [21]. However, this notion was biased because the learning platforms could not meet the diverse learning styles of children with different abilities in the early years of education. For example, whereas the deaf could benefit from sign language lessons on TV, they could not gain much from the radio lessons. Children with specific learning difficulties as well as those with mental challenges needed some extra individualized support to be able to follow the remote mode lessons.

Learning management systems using digital devices were the other pedagogical approach that was used in some African countries during the COVID-19 school closure to enhance continuity of learning. This included zoom, Google meet as well as WhatsApp and Facebook platforms [7]. Countries such as Kenya and Rwanda partnered with their telecommunication companies to lower cost of access to ICT devices and Internet connectivity alongside developing and implementing digital literacy programs. All these efforts were made to enhance innovative teaching and learning to achieve the child-centered learning. It was assumed that remote learning would meet the educational needs of all children including those in early childhood and with disability; however, this was not the case [21], as revealed by survey in 52 African countries that showed that early childhood and primary level learners could not access or effectively utilize these methods (EdTech [18]). The situation was worse for learners in early years of education with various disabilities. They not only needed support to migrate the digitalized learning but also needed the approaches to be customized to their needs. However, this support was only available in few countries. In Morocco, for example, Internet was used to aid learning. In rural areas, lessons were recorded and broadcast on Moroccan Television. The government through the Ministry of Education took steps to minimize learning loss for children with disabilities particularly the deaf by producing the educational content in sign language. Further, language teachers were recruited and trained on multisensory structured teaching and learning and later were provided with tablets to enable them deliver the content to the children through digital platforms [19]. These approaches may have achieved a certain degree of teaching; however, lack of child-centered pedagogical practices such as free-choice and small group activities, supportive and reciprocal interaction between teachers and children meant that the online approaches could not achieve optimum effectiveness [23].

In Uganda, children with disabilities were to access the learning materials that were provided by the Ministry of Education on radio and television. Home schooling was encouraged by the government, and parents were expected to support their children study using their school text books. Schools also sent learning materials on the phones or in form of printed booklets [24] but as mentioned above, there were no special considerations for children with disabilities. Moreover, as reported by Mbazzi et al. [25], the majority of the parents of children with disabilities in Uganda do not know how best to manage their children's behavior and teach them at the same time.

In Malawi, the National COVID-19 preparedness and response plan was developed to ensure that teaching and learning continued during the lockdowns. Like in other countries, radio and televised lessons were used to reach out to learners at home and communities were mobilized to support home learning for children with disabilities. As revealed by a survey by Singal and colleagues, in addition to radio and TV lessons, learning materials were sent by the Ministry of Education in the form of ordinary print and could not be read by those who have visual impairment. Where Braille materials were provided, parents were unable to help their children read them since they lacked the skills to do so Singal et al. [24]. The survey showed that there were very few cases where parents of children with disabilities received home-based support on therapy, the absence of which must have further affected learning.

In Kenya, during the COVID-19 instigated school closures, distance learning solutions (DLS)/digital learning, also referred to as education technologies (EdTechs) [26], were adopted. The Teachers Service Commission (TSC) developed a teacher training manual through the collaborative efforts of various agencies in the education sector on remote learning. The aim was to engage learners in a variety of online environments using appropriate devices. The Kenya Institute of Curriculum Development (KICD) introduced programs on Edu channel TV and lessons from early childhood level. There was an increase in content on digital sites that was to be accessed by the learners. The television learning programs were supported with sign language interpreter as an adaptation to cater for learners who had hearing difficulties. This must have enriched the approach in terms of inclusivity;

however, as mentioned earlier, delivery of content on television lacked the component of teacher-child interaction that is critical for ECE learners particularly those with special needs.

Moreover, a study indicated that the majority of teachers and parents were not sufficiently familiar with digital technologies that were used to deliver content to the learners at home [23]. Teachers noted that they lacked directions on how to support learners at home while parents indicated that they could not afford internet bundles required to download the learning materials that were sent online. It was reported in some cases that there was no sign language translator for those who had hearing impairments and that the lessons were too fast for those with learning impairments. Moreover, while learning gadgets such as braille and writing material were present at school, they were not provided at home, making home learning for children with visual impairments impossible. In the same way, deaf children were not able to communicate or get interpreter's support at home, making it hard for them to utilize the teaching that was provided on these platforms [27].

In Ghana, the prolonged school closures placed children with disabilities at a risk of dropping out. Like in other countries, distance learning was rolled out by the Ministry of Education using television, mobile devices, and Internet. Remote learning materials were also sent to learners through postal mail. However, using this mode of teaching and learning, children with disabilities were still at risk of being left out [28].

The Zambian government strengthened radio-based learning programs by distributing solar radios and training of teachers to engage with learners through distance learning and radio programs. In Sierra Leone, the government made it a priority to leverage the radio learning programs that had been started even before the pandemic. However, these too did not provide specific support for children with different needs.

Overall, several pedagogical approaches were adopted in the different countries to enable learning continuation during the pandemic. It is imperative to note that ECE learners with disabilities were often not catered for in many of these strategies. Where special facilities were provided to cater for ECE learners with disabilities, they lacked real-time teacher-learner interaction and the additional individualized support that is critical for effective learning for children with different needs. This is because remote learning is more of teacher-directed rather than an interactive learning process that requires face-to-face presence. Effective teaching and learning of children with disabilities in their early years of education require individualized instructional practices tailored to their different educational needs. However, this was not possible since face-to-face engagements were strongly discouraged during the pandemic, putting the learners with special needs at a greater disadvantage than their normal counterparts.

## 6. Access to education, challenges and opportunities experienced by ECE learners with disabilities during the COVID-19 pandemic

Before the first case of COVID-19 was reported in Uganda in March 2020, a new school term for learners at all levels had just begun. In order to prevent the spread of the COVID 19 infection, the Government of Uganda decided to close all education institutions including those for early childhood learning. The closure of education institutions locked about 15 million Ugandan learners at home for a period of 2 years including young learners aged 1–8 years with disabilities. This was one of the longest lockdown of educational institutions globally. With the emergence of the pandemic, access to education for early childhood education (1–8 years) learners with disabilities faced a number of challenges but also some opportunities were experienced.

First of all, the closure of schools led school leaders to shift from physical contact with learners to online-based mode of instruction [29]. This necessitated use of technologies and digital platforms to deliver distance teaching and learning including computers, radios, and television sets to learners and distribution of printed materials to learners in their communities.

Although this development of technologies that could be used for distance learning was a very good innovation to keep learners engaged during the COVID-19 lockdown, it also created challenges to learners with disabilities. For example, the government of Uganda introduced long-distance teaching through the media, especially radio and television. These methods of teaching are not appropriate for young learners with disabilities especially those who are deaf and those who have visual impairments [30–32]. It is obvious that those with hearing impairments or visual impairments will not hear what is being taught on radio and television and will not see what is being taught on television respectively. Therefore, such platforms only benefited learners without disabilities.

Transitioning to a virtual setting required many educators to learn new technologies and skills and caused stress among both teachers and students [33]. However, both the teachers and learners were not given sufficient time to learn the new methods. In addition to moving to online learning platforms during the COVID-19 pandemic, special educators were faced with multiple challenges ranging from equity issues for learners, providing instruction in a virtual environment, and providing special education services as determined by the learner's individual education plan. On equity, we know that the majority of the early childhood learners with disabilities in the Uganda and similar LMICs come from very poor families [34] and who therefore could not afford paying for online classes or teaching did not have televisions or radio sets in their households to access the content. There were attempts by governments to provide radio and television sets to rural communities; however, these were overtaken by other competing national priorities during the crisis.

Since these online and other distance learning technologies have been developed, education providers and the government must use this opportunity to continue developing these technologies to ensure that they remain prepared for other epidemics/and pandemics that may lead to school closure in future. This should also create an opportunity, for training and to continue delivering special education services for students with disabilities.

At a more global level, the UN guidelines for COVID-19 response recommended mainstreaming of disabilities in the planning and provision of any support and services [35–38]. UNICEF provided guidance for staff and partners on supporting the learning of children in areas of school closures, which included making learning accessible to children with disabilities [39]. These also included provision of learning devices/equipment and connectivity, accessibility of instruction, individualized education plans, caregiver involvement, and the Build Back Better strategy among others. However, in many African countries, people with disabilities were neither involved in the development nor provided for during the implementation of COVID-19 response interventions [25], and as explained above, implementation of inclusive education policies was crippled by several systems' challenges that were present before the pandemic.

## 7. How can access to quality and equitable learning for ECE learners with disabilities during the crisis be improved?

Several strategies have been proposed to support education of learners with disabilities in low- and middle-income countries, and this merits consideration by all stakeholders involved in education. General recommendations addressing pre-COVID-19 challenges are re-emphasized since these challenges have not gone away; they have actually become aggravated. At the global level, the Inclusive Education Initiative recommends first, strengthening teachers' capacity (through training) and motivation to manage children with diverse needs and imparting into them the humane aspect for these children; secondly, constantly involving families in the initiatives that support inclusion since families play a critical role in leading and influencing communities and schools to embrace these innovations as well as making the voices of learners and generally PWD be heard at the local level; thirdly, executing inclusion as early as the planning stage of any initiative and at all subsequent stages and reflecting upon key aspects including curriculum, class sizes, teaching, and learning materials during the design and implementation; fourthly, to ensure that the innovations for inclusive education developed for LMICs are based on locally generated evidence and therefore which address local challenges to policy and practice [40].

The UN and UNICEF have provided guidelines to ensure access to education and other services for people with disabilities. In particular, the UNICEF's Build Back Better guideline is based on the fact that many vulnerable children may not have been accessing quality and inclusive learning opportunities pre-COVID-19, and therefore, resumption of schooling presents an opportunity to "build back better" and capitalize on the strategies and resources being put in place during this crisis to increase access and improve learning opportunities for all children. "This includes ensuring that learning spaces are accessible to those experiencing physical disabilities, that all children – in particular girls- can access school safely, that there are gender-segregated latrines to encourage girls' attendance, that schools are equipped for children experiencing learning impairments, that teachers are prepared to teach students of all abilities, and that communities and caregivers/parents are actively engaged and participate in the local education system and are well-informed of how to support their children" [39].

At the country level, several other strategies have been proposed. In Malawi, for example [41], parents proposed that there was need to prioritize continued learning for children with disabilities and for governments to make educational programs accessible for children with disabilities and actually provide the necessary equipment (e.g. TV, radio, parent training) for these children to access the learning. Intermittent physical access to school facilities, e.g., twice a week and permitting children to take scholastic materials home (e.g., books in Braille) as well as regular follow-up and support on home learning by teachers were also proposed by parents.

Providing parents of children with disabilities with the basic skills such a sign language and Braille to enable them to fully support their children's learning at home, as well as financial support (loans) to enable them provide basic needs for their children was proposed. Furthermore, the need to invest in educational digital technological innovations for children with disabilities and developing teacher, parent, and learners' capacity to use them as well as provide the necessary equipment, e.g., phones and computers to the teachers and learners was highlighted [41].

In summary, access and utilization of education services for children with disabilities during the COVID-19 pandemic have been difficult resulting in an escalation of the preexisting challenges and increasing the demands at the family, teacher, and policy levels, for which different stakeholders were not prepared. Concerted support and commitment through the several recommendations including policy improvements, and teacher, student, and learner-centered interventions, and further evidence generation could provide practical solutions to providing inclusive education services during and after the crisis to enable children with disabilities achieve their educational goals.

## 8. Discussion

COVID-19 pandemic has been a challenge for everyone; however, people with disability have experienced greater difficulties. The current chapter aimed at exploring the pedagogical approaches that were adopted to support continued learning for children with disabilities during the COVID-19 pandemic and the challenges experiences as well as key lessons to note.

The findings from the reviewed studies and reports suggest that COVID-19 significantly exacerbated the inequality to access to essential services particularly education for people with disabilities during the lockdown. Parent's reports indicated that they had difficulties including children with disability in livelihood programs, yet they did this with ease to children without disability. The parents reported that the children were lonely further indicating the difficult parents had in socially including these children. Because of the physical, visual, hearing, or cognitive impairments, there is a communication barrier between the children and family members who are normal functioning jeopardizing interaction and socially isolating the child from the rest of the family. This was the case before COVID-19 but which became more evident when children were now spending the whole day at home. Moreover, it appears that parents have limited skills in sign language, let alone more advanced skills such as reading Braille that children with visual impairment need to read.

It is also imperative to note from the reviewed studies that active learning of children with disabilities mainly takes place at school. This finding indicates that parents are less involved in the actual training or learning activities of their children with disability. This could be partly attributed to lack of skills or poor attitude toward disability and education on the part of parents as revealed by the surveys. Furthermore, parents of children with disabilities usually have very low expectations from these children, and this bias down plays their motivation to support their learning in academic and everyday life activities. Consequently, the children have little contact with parents and other family members, and gradually the gap widens and further reducing the opportunity for the parents and siblings to learn how to interact with the child. This family exclusion and inability to support learning became apparent during the pandemic when all children were grounded at home and had to be supported by their parents to continue schooling. Appropriate steps should be taken to promote inclusion at family level through increased awareness and empowering families with skills to supporting learning for their children with different disabilities.

It is clear from the literature that learners with disabilities and their families struggled to access or utilize the education resources provided because they were provided in formats that were not appropriate for them or because the families lacked the necessary skills and technology to support the learner with disability with specialized material. However, in many cases, these resources were not provided at all. This was evidenced in their outcry of lack of contact between children and teachers, and the concern that a lot of the disability support services, e.g. physiotherapy, were school-based. This reveals a gap and a need for a continuum of care and support for learners with disabilities from home to school and within the wider community.

It is also important to note that disability and poverty have a synergistic relationship where disability causes poverty, and poverty aggravates effects of disability, and the two continuously enhance each other if no intervention is introduced [42]. The parents of children with disability decried their challenges in purchasing devices such as Braille machine and books, as well as voice-embedded computers for those with visual impairments to benefit from e-learning that emphasized during lockdown. Because of extreme poverty, these gadgets were not affordable by most parents from low- and middle-income countries. Financial support including cash transfers to families such as those that that were administered in African countries [4] could enable such parent to access these and other needs including electricity, which is needed for the equipment to work.

Notably, remote learning was academic-oriented with an aim of imparting knowledge for the purpose of mastering concepts and recall, whereas education for a majority of children with disability aims at making them self-reliant and emphasize acquisition of social skills, communication skills, and activities of daily living. Practically, learning for children with disability is individualized, targeting the strength of each individual learner. It is therefore implemented using an Individualized Education Plan (IEP) that could not be implemented using remote learning that replaced face-to-face learning as a result of COVID-19 school closure.

Lastly, we aimed to identify potential strategies and recommendations that could be undertaken to improve the status of learning for children with disabilities during the crisis. Our review indicates that parents need to be empowered through training and active engagements in helping their children with disability with home schooling. They need to be taught skills such as sign language, therapies, and Braille, but also be involved in interventions that aimed at bringing about attitudinal change toward disability and education. Furthermore, homes with children with disability need to be made safe against abusers, and children need to be taught how to protect themselves against abusers and where to seek support in case of abuse. Of note, the extreme poverty levels further incapacitated parents from providing the equipment needed for their children's home schooling should be addressed. Indeed, in contexts where families of vulnerable children received cash transfers, it was clear that these had a significant impact on addressing some of the hardships that they were facing during the pandemic. Such financial supports should be considered by governments.

Importantly, there is need for proper disaster preparedness by governments to guard against adverse effects emerging from future eventualities that would necessitate closure of schools. Practically, this will include allocating sufficient budgets to support necessary response programs, but also involving people with disabilities and their families in making policies, in planning and implementation of the interventions. At the global level, funds such as the Marshall investment [4] should be dedicated to supporting children living in vulnerability including those with disabilities and to enable them recover from the adverse effects caused by the pandemic. However, this can only be achieved if there are sufficient data to enable evidence-informed policies, programs, and budgeting, as well as a deliberate commitment by government to support continued learning for children with disabilities in times of crisis. The immense data challenges on key issues were evident in this review and highlight the need for more research to generate local data on specific indicators of the burden of COVID-19 on education access and well-being of children with disabilities and PWD at large in the African context.

## 9. Summary and conclusion

It is evident from the above literature that the COVID-19 pandemic made learning for ECE learners with disabilities in Africa extremely difficult and hence widened the disparities between these children and typically developing children and brought to the forefront the inequity and exclusion that prevail in planning, allocation, and utilization of education resources for people with disabilities. The literature highlights the difficulties in accessing and utilizing disability-specific pedagogical learning opportunities that early learners with disabilities experienced. It must be noted that these issues not only relate to young learners but to all learners with disabilities in Africa and similar LMICs, making the proposed recommendations relevant to a wider population. In line with the Sustainable Development Goal 4 (ensure inclusive and equitable quality education and promote lifelong learning opportunities for all) and leaving no one behind, deliberate efforts should be invested in addressing the gaps and challenges at all levels (system, school, and household) to enable children with disabilities achieve their educational goals. Concerted efforts through policy improvements, political will, and change of attitude of all stakeholders including decision-makers, teachers, and communities to promote inclusion and learner-centered interventions for learners with disabilities are likely to make significant impact in enabling these learners access education during the current and future crises.

Key lessons from this literature are that across Africa, children with disabilities still grapple with difficulty in accessing quality education due to exclusion, stigma, lack of specialized skills among teachers and parents, and weak government enforcement, and low financing, among other causes. COVID-19 clearly aggravated these challenges and brought about new ones, e.g., the lack of physical interaction between learners and educators and widened the gap. Nevertheless, all is not lost, and a lot can be done to improve the status quo.

It is important to recognize the urgent need for building the education system back better, through concerted efforts, at all levels, and combining the preexisting and new approaches to address the access and utilization gap for children with disabilities. Political will in terms of committing more government funds and enforcement into policies and their implementation, effective inclusive planning, capacity building, and skills strengthening as well as utilizing local evidence to develop the interventions are critical for rolling back the challenges affecting learning of children with disabilities in the pre and post COVID-19 era. Of note, contextual and system barriers particularly household poverty, and limited government resources, and the negative community attitude toward PLD in general, which act as substrates, the inequity must be addressed. Furthermore, innovations and technologies must take into account the diverse needs of all learners particularly those with disabilities, and they should be suited to the local context, for them to yield maximum benefit for all learners.

It is apparent that African governments were ill-prepared to deal with the sudden disruptions COVID-19 caused in the education system, and indeed these countries were hard hit. This is an eye opener for governments to invest in disaster preparedness not only for education but for all sectors. Our experience from this review reveals the fact that there is limited information on the impact COVID-19 had on education, how learners navigated the challenges but also to what extent education policies were aligned with inclusion of children with disabilities, and challenges that were encountered. More post-pandemic surveys are recommended to fully understand the impact in order to institute appropriate measures to roll back the effects, but also plan better pedagogical approaches that optimize learning for all learners today and in future crises.

## 9.1 Limitations

The evidence discussed above is based on literature currently available in the African countries on the impact of COVID-19 on education access for learners with disability, including gray literature, which may be subject to reporting bias. The findings are majorly obtained from qualitative self-reported experiences of learners with disabilities or their families and hence a risk for reporting or social desirability bias and subjectivity particularly exaggeration of the difficulties reported with expectation of some kind of support to be provided. To date, there are generally scanty data from the education service providers (teachers) perspective and policy, and hence, a knowledge gap that calls for more research.

## Authors' contribution

MN, LA, and RN contributed to the conceptualization of the idea, generation, and review of the literature; MN led the writing and revision of the chapter; all authors reviewed and edited the final version of the chapter.

## Author details

Margaret Nampijja[1]*, Lillian Ayiro[2] and Ruth Nalugya[3]

1 African Population and Health Research Center, Nairobi, Kenya

2 Maseno University, Kenya

3 Spina Bifida and Hydrocephalus Association of Uganda, Kampala, Uganda

*Address all correspondence to: maggie.nampijja@gmail.com

## References

[1] United Nations Sustainable Development Group. Shared Responsibility, Global Solidarity: Responding To the Socio-Economic Impacts of Covid-19. Nairobi, Kenya, United Nations; 2020

[2] Ozili P. "COVID-19 in Africa: socio-economic impact, policy response and opportunities", International Journal of Sociology and Social Policy. 2022;**42**:177-200. DOI: 10.1108/IJSSP-05-2020-0171

[3] UNESCO. Covid-19 Education: From Disruption to Recovery. UNESCO; 2020

[4] UNICEF. COVID 19: A Catastrophe for Children in Sub-Saharan Africa [Internet]. UNICEF. 2020. Available from: https://www.unicef.org/esa/media/7626/file/COVID-19-A Catastrophe-for-Children-in-SSA.pdf [cited 31 October 2021]

[5] Bannink F, Idro R, Van Hove G. Teachers' and parents' perspectives on inclusive education for children with Spina Bifida in Uganda. Journal of Childhood & Developmental Disorders. 2016;**2**:18

[6] Ndurumo M. Exceptional Children: Development Consequences and Interaction. Nairobi, Kenya: Longman; 1993

[7] McClain Nnlapo C. An Inclusive Response to COVID 19: Education for Children with Disabilities {BLOG}. 2020. Available from: https://www.ukfiet.org/2020/an-inclusive-response-to-covid-19-education-for-children-with-disabilities/

[8] Michael E, Oboegbulem A. Learners with disabilities in an inclusive education setting in Nigeria: Implications for administrators. US-China Education Review. 2013;**3**(5):313-318. Available from: https://files.eric.ed.gov/fulltext/ED543446.pdf

[9] Davis P. Teaching Strategies and Approaches for Pupils with SNE: A Scoping Study Research Report RR516. 2004. Available from: https://dera.ioe.ac.uk/6059/1/RR516.pdf

[10] Andiema NC. Effects of child centered methods on teaching and learning of science activities in pre-schools in Kenya. Journal of Education and Practice. 2016;**7**(27):1-9. Available from: https://files.eric.ed.gov

[11] Pedro A, Mthimunye B, Bust E. How lockdown could affect South Africa's children with special needs. Health24. 2020. https://theconversation.com/how-lockdown-could-affect-south-africas-children-with-special-needs-137127

[12] Kartika A, Suminar D, Tairas M, Hendriani W. Individual Education Program (IEP) paperwork: A narrative review. International Journal of Engineering & Technology. 2018;7:682. DOI: 10.14419/ijet.v7i2.29.13997 Available from: https://www.researchgate.net/publication/326729522_Individual_Education_Program_IEP_Paperwork_A_Narrative_Review

[13] Avramidis E, Norwich B. Teachers' attitude towards integration/inclusion: A review of the literature. European Journal of Special Needs Education. 2002;**17**:129-147

[14] Wanjiru NJ. Teachers knowledge on the implementation of inclusive education in early childhood development centers in Mwea East Sub County, Kirinyaga County, Kenya, [Masters published thesis]. Kenyatta University, Kenya; 2011. Available from: https://ir-library.ku.ac.ke/bitstream/handle/123456789/18124/Teachers%27%20knowledge%20on%20

the%20iplementation...pdf?sequence=1&isAllowed=y

[15] Ajodhia-Andrews A, Frankel E. Inclusive Education in Guyana: A Call for Change. International Journal of Special Education. 2010;**25**(1): 126-144

[16] Soni A, Reyes SM, Lynch P. A review of the factors affecting children with disabilities' successful transition to early childhood care and primary education in sub-Saharan Africa. Journal of Early Childhood Research. 2022;**20**(1):59-79. DOI: 10.1177/1476718X211035428

[17] World Bank. The COVID-19 Pandemic: Shocks to Education and Policy Responses. Washington, DC: World Bank; 2020. https://openknowledge.worldbank.org/handle/10986/33696

[18] EdTech Hub. The Effect of Covid-19 on Education in Africa and its Implications for the Use of Technology: A Survey of the Experience and Opinions of Educators and Technology Specialists. EdTech Hub. 2020. http://www.guninetwork.org/files/the_effect_of_covid-19_on_education_in_africa.pdf

[19] UNICEF. Transforming Education in Africa: An Evidence Based Overview and Recommendation for Long Term Improvements. UNICEF. 2021a. Available from: https://www.unicef.org/media/106686/file/Transforming%20Education%20in%20Africa.pdf

[20] UNICEF Press Release. At Least 200 Million School Children Live in Countries that Remain Unprepared to Deploy Remote Learning in Future Emergency School Closures. 2021. Available from: https://www.unicef.org/eap/press-releases/least-200-million-schoolchildren-live-countries-remain-unprepared-deploy-remote#:~:text=NEW%20YORK%2C%2028%20October%202021

[21] Zacharia S., & Twinomugisha A (2020). Educational Television During Covid-19: How to Start and What to Consider. Available from: https://blogs.worldbank.org/education/educational-television-during-covid-19-how-start-and-what-consider

[22] Ubongo Kids.Org 2020—Kids' Edutainment. 2021. Available from: www.ubongo.org

[23] James Angoye, Irene Mbari-Kirika, O.G.W, Bruce N. Walker, Ph.D. and Martin Kavua. inABLE, MOE & UKAID 2020 Distanced and Disadvantaged: A Study on the Effects of COVID-19 on Education for Learners with Disabilities in Kenya. inABLE. Available from: https://inable.org/wp-content/uploads/2020/11/Main-Report_Distance-and-Disadvantage_a11y_Oct2020.pdf

[24] Singal N, Mbukwa-Ngwira J, Taneja-Johansson S, Lynch P, Chatha G, Umar E. (2021): Impact of Covid-19 on the education of children with disabilities in Malawi: reshaping parental engagement for the future, International Journal of Inclusive Education, DOI: 10.1080/13603116.2021.1965804

[25] Mbazzi FB, Nalugya R, Kawesa E, Nimusiima C, King R, Geert van Hove & Seeley J. (2021) The impact of COVID-19 measures on children with disabilities and their families in Uganda, Disability & Society, DOI: 10.1080/09687599.2020.1867075

[26] Government of Kenya. Kenya Basic Education Covid-19 Emergency Response Plan. Government of Kenya; 2020 Available from: https://www.education.go.ke/images/Kenya_basic_Education_ COVID-19_Emergency_Response_Plan-compressed.pdf

[27] Achieng VO, Ngware MW. Adoption of education technologies for learning during COVID 19 pandemic: The experiences of marginalized and

vulnerable learner populations in Kenya. International Journal of Education. 2021:1-24

[28] UNICEF. Primary and Secondary Impact of Covid 19 Pandemic on Children in Ghana. UNICEF. 2021b. Available from: www.unicef.org/publications

[29] Tumwesige J. Covid-19 Educational Disruption and Response: Rethinking e-Learning in Uganda. Konrad Adnauer Stiftung; 2020; Nairobi, Kenya Paris, France. https://en.unesco.org/news/covid-19-learning-disruption-recovery-snapshot-unescos-work-education-2020

[30] Aljedaani W, Aljedaani M, AlOmar EA, Mkaouer MW, Ludi S, Khalaf YB. I cannot see you—The perspectives of deaf students to online learning during COVID 19 pandemic: Saudi Arabia case study. Education Sciences. 2021;**11**(11):712

[31] Alshawabkeh AA, Woolsey ML, Kharbat FF. Using online information technology for deaf students during COVID 19: A closer look from experience. Heliyon. 2021;7(5):e06915

[32] Gayatri M. The implementation of early childhood education in the time of COVID-19 pandemic: A systematic review. Humanities & Social Sciences Reviews. 2020;**8**(6):46-54

[33] Asri DN, Cahyono BEH. Trisnani RP. Early reading learning for special needs students: Challenges on inclusive primary school during COVID 19 pandemic. Linguistics and Culture Review. 2021;**5**(S1):1062-1074

[34] WHO. WORLD REPORT ON DISABILITY WHO Library Cataloguing-in-Publication Data. 2011 Available from: www.who.int/about/licensing/copyright_form/en/index.html [cited 31 October 2021]

[35] Armitage R, Nellums LB. The COVID-19 response must be disability inclusive. The Lancet Public Health. 2020;**5**(5):e257. DOI: 10.1016/S2468-2667(20)30076-1

[36] Banks LM, Davey C, Shakespeare T, Kuper H. Disability-inclusive responses to COVID-19: Lessons learnt from research on social protection in low- and middle-income countries. World Development. 2020;**137**:105178. DOI: 10.1016/j.worlddev.2020.105178

[37] Kuper H, Banks LM, Bright T, Davey C, Shakespeare T. Disability-inclusive COVID-19 response: What it is, why it is important and what we can learn from the United Kingdom's response. Wellcome Open Research. 2020

[38] Sakellariou D, Malfitano APS, Rotarou ES. Disability inclusiveness of government responses to COVID-19 in South America: A framework analysis study. International Journal for Equity in Health. 2020;**19**:131. DOI: 10.1186/s12939-020-01244-x

[39] UNICEF. All Means All-How to Support Learning for the Most Vulnerable Children in Areas of School Closures A Checklist for UNICEF Staff on Factors to Consider When Planning COVID-19 Education Response 1 [Internet]. 2021c. Available from: https://sites.unicef.org/disabilities/files/All_means_All_-_Equity_and_Inclusion_in_COVID-19_EiE_Response.pdf [cited 31 October 2021]

[40] Singal N. How can we best support the education of children with disabilities in low and middle income countries? (2021). Inclusive Education Initiative July 6, 2021.. Available from: https://www. inclusive-education-initiative.org/index.php/blog/how-can-we-best-support-education-children-disabilities-low-and-middle-income-countries. 2021 [cited 31 October 2021]

[41] Mbukwa-Ngwira J, Johansson ST, Singal UE, Lynch P, Chatha G. Impact of

COVID-19 on the education of children with disabilities in Malawi: Results from a survey with parents. Inclusive Education Initiative [Internet]. Available from: https://www.inclusive-education-initiative.org/blog/impact-covid-19-education-children-disabilities-malawi-results-survey-parents. 2021 [cited 31 October 2021]

[42] Pinilla-Roncancio M. Disability and poverty: Two related conditions. A review of the literature. Revista de la Facultad de Medicina, 2015;**63**:S113-23. doi: http://dx.doi

Chapter 16

# Unveiling the Uncertainty-Revolutionizing Medical Education in COVID-19 Era

*Rabeeya Saeed, Salman Sharif and Faridah Amin*

## Abstract

The beginning of the year 2020 marked the biggest pandemic of the twenty-first century. COVID-19 not only jeopardized the global health care system but also lead to unprecedented effects on every aspect of life. The tragedy evoked by the virus, resulted in disruption of face-to-face learning across the globe. The aftermath of this pandemic on medical education will be enormous and long-lasting. Therefore, it is of utmost importance to identify the challenges and threats facing medical education, both at undergraduate and postgraduate level. Comparative analysis of the innovative models adapted globally in post-COVID era will help countries learn from success stories. Amidst the uncertainty posed by the pandemic, there is a special prospect for medical education. Medical educationist and health policy makers may convert this crisis into opportunity through innovative strategies maximizing the outcome of e-learning. This is the time to relook medical curricula, redesign assessment, focus on standardization of e-learning and upgrade faculty development programs to produce doctors equipped and prepared to serve in the new era.

**Keywords:** COVID-19, medical education, virtual learning, E-learning, training during COVID, undergraduate, postgraduate

## 1. Introduction

The beginning of the year 2020 marked the biggest pandemic of twenty-first century. COVID-19 not only jeopardized the global health care system but also lead to unprecedented effects on every aspect of human life. The tragedy evoked by the virus, resulted in disruption of the face-to-face learning across the globe. Amidst the uncertainty, fear and crisis situation faced by the world the whole learning cycle came to a halt, till the stakeholders proposed innovative strategies of online learning in medical education. Though blended learning was in vogue in pre COVID times, but the sole dependence on online learning in the "New normal" phase has raised questions. Clinical and soft skills teaching is widely accepted to be best taught through physical interaction with patients. Even for undergraduate pre-clinical years, teaching of basic sciences requires performing procedures and demonstration in the skill laboratory, which was also disrupted due to social restriction.

This chapter gives an in-depth understanding of the impact of the COVID-19 pandemic on transforming medical education and the challenges faced by medical education, both at undergraduate and postgraduate level. It also elaborates how



IntechOpen

countries all over the world embraced this challenge, recognized the opportunities and responded to the crisis by ongoing waves and variants of COVID-19. Amidst the uncertainty posed by the pandemic there is still hope. The tremendous opportunity of innovative advancement in technology along with sensible decisions to adopt learning, need to be aligned to survive in the "new normal" world.

## 2. The knee-jerk response to pandemic

The COVID-19 pandemic that has affected almost 221,134,742 people around the world and has claimed 4,574,089 lives, evoked huge fear and uncertainty among people all over the world [1].

The novelty of the situation, uncertainty and limited research on the clinical course of the virus forced policy makers to rush towards difficult decisions. This led to stopping or slowing down academic and nonacademic activities until the world started adopting the best evidence-based recommendations to deal with the catastrophe.

### 2.1 A hiatus in medical education

Soon after official declaration of pandemic by World health organization (WHO), almost 182 countries in the world closed their educational institutions in response to the regulatory bodies' decision on social distancing and lockdown [2, 3]. Medical schools and universities faced dual challenges; first to respond to the clinical and administrative demands, in order to prevent the health care system from collapsing; second was to maintain an effective educational system in order to produce doctors with strong foundation of patient care. In March 2020, the Association of American Medical Colleges (AAMC), released their guidelines for immediate disruption of all clinical rotations till they get further enlightment and preparedness to handle the situation [4]. Italy has faced the worst situation of COVID-19, with almost 4,574,787 cases reported till September 2021 [5]. At the onset of pandemic, their government responded by immediate suspension of all in-campus learning at medical schools [6]. The example of US, UK, Italy and China was followed by developing countries. Though the numbers of cases affected by the virus were comparatively lower in these countries; however, considering the dreadful situation of the developed world, the underprivileged nations were not ready to risk testing their health care system. In India, Pakistan and Bangladesh, all face-to-face educational activities and clinical rotations were suspended after implementation of a nationwide lockdown [7]. The rationale behind these decisions was to conserve the resources including personal protective equipment for front line workers; minimize exposure of health care professionals, protect well-being of students and their families and prevent the already fragile health care system from further declining.

### 2.2 Fast tracking medical graduates into health care system

Uncertainty lead to halting of the education system in early 2020, hence there was an urgent need to develop an alternative system to enhance capacity. With a case fatality rate of 12.6% and total reported fatalities of 17, 600, Italian government responded in the most urgent manner by taking tough decisions regarding Medical education [8]. The 'Cura Italia' decree passed on 17th March 2020, revolutionized the rules of Italian Medical board examination [8]. According to this decree almost 10,000 medical graduates were given license to practice without taking post graduate examination at the end of their practical training. In other words, this change lead to graduates joining the health care system almost nine months earlier than they would otherwise have done in the pre-COVID era. A 10.3% increase in hospital doctors, was anticipated through its implementation to provide services and support departments or intensive care units (ICUs) dedicated to COVID-19 Care [8]. Exemption from medical licensing exam puts an additional bar on the system to evaluate their medical practices, the impact of which is yet to be seen in the coming years.

This practice of introducing young medical graduates in clinical practice, was followed by other countries including US, Ireland and UK, where health care system needed a boost [9].

## 3. Lack of pandemic preparedness: an identified gap in medical education

While pushing fresh medical graduates to enter into health care system may be beneficial to handle the pandemic, the risks needs to be recognized.

Due to uncertainty and the absence of defined roles in this calamity, the role of students varied across different institutions around the world. While some universities did not allow contact with patients, others deployed final year students or fresh graduates as frontline workers in COVID ICUs and emergencies [10, 11]. In a conventional medical education system, the graduates are gradually introduced to clinical practice in a controlled and supervised learning environment. During clinical rotations their work is mostly passive, shadowing consultants during ward rounds, taking history and observation of clinical procedures. This structure creates a stable learning environment, but it does not necessarily prepare students to function with appropriate level of confidence and skills in a system under crisis. A study conducted among medical students in Ireland found that majority of students (75%) were not confident about their skills for working in an emergency setting [12]. Pre-assessment for an elective on disaster preparedness found 70% participants unprepared to work in an emergency however, this number reduced to 11% after training [13].

Inclusion of students in the health care system without necessary preparation or training can be a serious risk for patients, other colleagues and for themselves. This has been explored in various researches in which students did not have sufficient information to make appropriate clinical decisions in their work setting [14].

The presence of such student volunteers or physician assistants can actually overburden the system capacity and compromise quality of patient care. They can act as vector for virus transmission, deplete resources like personal protective equipment and overstrain teaching faculty or clinicians whose resilience was already at stake in this extraordinary situation [15]. However the balance would still be fluctuating between the duality of providing adequate manpower to the health care system and risk of managing the system with unprepared workforce. A careful and ongoing risk benefit analysis as per situation country wise would lead to practical solutions to overcome this challenge.

## 4. Vulnerability of medical students and trainees to mental health problems

Implementation of unaccustomed public health interventions like social distancing and lockdown, fear and stigma due to COVID-19, closures of medical colleges, anxiety from suspension of clinical training and rotations, apprehension about well-being of older relatives and the abrupt switch to the 'New normal' life had a negative impact on psychological health of medical students [16].

The complexity of this challenge is thoroughly evaluated by researchers all over the world. Available evidence suggest that even in pre-COVID times, the mental health of medical students was at a greater risk as compared to the general population [17]. Moreover, graduates and medical students are recognized as vulnerable strata with a high frequency of suicidal ideation and death by suicide. The results of a recent meta-analysis found suicidal ideation to be more prevalent among medical students as compared to qualified doctors [18].

Data from Turkey, Iran, India and European countries like Malta suggest a high prevalence of depression and anxiety in medical students during COVID-19 pandemic [19–23]. However prevalence of anxiety in medical students is found to be similar to pre-pandemic era according to the results of a recent meta-analysis. Sleep deterioration and decreased appetite was commonly reported symptoms [22, 23].

In contrast to stay at home orders, rapid inclusion of recent graduates or final year students in health care system put an additional challenge, the effect of which is yet to be evaluated [24]. Though many students showed great motivation to volunteer their services, however for many the experience was dreadful and altruism alone cannot justify this rapid transition to work. A recent research conducted on post-graduate trainees identified anxiety, stress and feeling of helplessness while working in a pandemic [25]. Moreover, disruption of training caused by cancelation of elective rotations, procedures or teaching sessions by supervising faculty could be strong predictors of evoking uncertainty regarding their future career.

## 5. Impact on postgraduate clinical training

Transition to post graduate medical education has been a real challenge for young graduates in COVID era. The suspension of clinical rotations, cancelation of distant electives, travel restriction in between countries pose a serious challenge for students to explore their areas of interest [25]. Moreover, cancelation of elective procedures and disruption of outpatient clinics resulted in patchy clinical exposure with patients [26]. Adequate clinical exposure to the specialty of interest at undergraduate level is vital for future career selection [27]. Restrictions on clinical rotation reduced students' physical interaction with mentors who could have positively influenced their choice of career [28].

Fewer opportunities and lack of meaningful recommendations due to cancelation of distant rotation may create negative influence on student's morale affecting their progress. This can also make the selection process challenging for program directors relying on less reliable characteristics, such as medical school reputation [29].

### 5.1 Uncertain competence level of postgraduate medical trainees

This evolving setting does not only create more uncertainty among medical students about their future career but also generates doubts among post graduate trainees regarding their competence at the end of a compromised training tenure. As the pendulum of health care shifted towards addressing a crisis situation, limited attention was given to other non COVID health conditions resulting in reduced patient volume in elective clinic setting [30], thus minimizing the necessary exposure required for training.

## 6. Emergence of technology enhanced medical education (TEME)

As the pandemic unfolded, academic leaders came under immense pressure to adapt and bring innovation in curriculum, learning strategies and assessments [31]. Though technology enhanced medical education or the concept of e-learning was not a novel concept even in pre-COVID era [32], however as an immediate response to the national lockdown, the teaching pivot shifted to online delivery. An abrupt transition from face-to-face learning to online pedagogy challenged principles of integrity, fairness and equity in medical education. Yet, considering safety of medical students and faculty as the priority, the new change was unanimously accepted around the world [31, 33].

### 6.1 Medical education with no geographical restriction

During COVID pandemic TEME was adopted as a learning process for both pre-clinical and clinical sciences. With social distancing as a new norm, the concept of traditional class room now seemed like a fairy tale (**Figure 1**).

For basic sciences subject, lectures were delivered through communication softwares like Zoom and Google meet up for synchronous meeting. Online demonstration of procedures was also implemented through virtual labs [35–38].

For discussion on clinical cases and interpretation of diagnostic tests, hybrid models employing asynchronous and synchronous sessions were used [39, 40]. Many schools used to broad cast their study reading material before the flipped class online sessions, making students learn through interactive exercises on virtual patients [41]. Few medical school in Italy utilized video tele-consultation with simulated patients to mimic the clinical experience [6].

### 6.2 Hurdles on the road to innovation

The paradigm shift to virtual learning brought many impediments. The world was not ready for this unprecedented intervention in medical education. Various studies conducted globally identified numerous challenges [6, 42–46] as depicted in **Table 1**. These are particularly exaggerated in developing countries, where barriers including lack of infrastructure, technological resources, financial constraints and

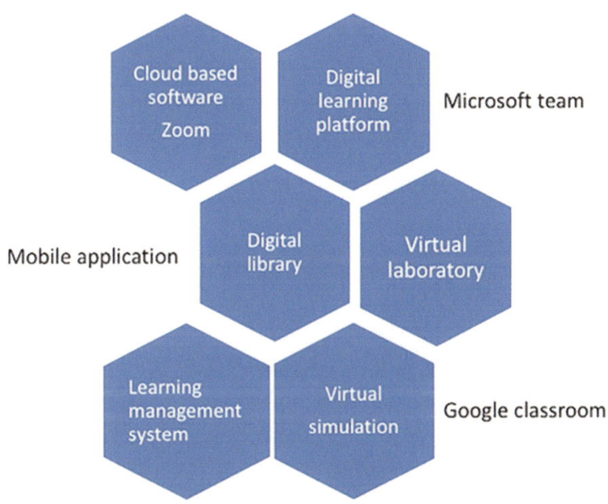


**Figure 1.**
*E-resources used for medical education during COVID-19 pandemic [34].*

| | Factors | Challenges |
|---|---|---|
| 1. | Time management | • Time consuming content preparation<br>• Short notice transition to online pedagogy<br>• Time allocation for learning software |
| 2. | Infrastructure defects and problems | • Internet connectivity issues<br>• Lack of availability of compatible software<br>• Non-availability of hardware resources<br>• Problems with uploading contents<br>• Problems with downloading information |
| 3. | Inadequate student teacher interaction | • Passive participation by students<br>• Compromised clinical teaching due to no patient interaction<br>• Risk of one sided discussion |
| 4. | Noncompliance with virtual class room etiquettes | • Informal attire and attitude of students towards teaching<br>• Disturbance in home environment<br>• Lack of students' commitment to punctuality and attendance<br>• Unfamiliarity with virtual class room rules |
| 5. | Technophobia | • Fear and resistance to use technological tools by experienced and senior teaching faculty and staff |
| 6. | Electronic literacy of teaching faculty | • Teaching faculty with low level of virtual literacy<br>• Need of assistance by the administration for installing and running soft ware |
| 7. | Students adaptability | • Lack of preparedness by students to adapt to this rapid change<br>• Lack of familiarity with software<br>• Doubts regarding effectiveness of online learning model |
| 8. | Lack of human interaction | • Less patient interaction<br>• Lack of social interaction with friends, colleagues and teachers |
| 9. | Ergonomics | • Neck and back problems due to inappropriate posture<br>• Excessive strain on eyes due to prolonged screen time |
| 10. | Formative and summative assessments | • Designing high taxonomy level questions for open book exam<br>• Need to rethink distant mechanisms of individual assessment<br>• Thinking alternative method for OSCE/practical exam |
| 11. | Learning by role modeling | • Lack of interaction with mentors and faculty<br>• Reduce chances of learning professionalism, ethics and communications skills through role models |

**Table 1.**
*Challenges of technology enhanced medical education (TEME) in COVID pandemic [6, 47–49].*

a fragile health care system imposed friction towards smooth transition to a digital system for medical education [7].

### *6.2.1 Challenges faced by medical teachers and staff*

Developing online lectures is more time consuming as compared to face-to-face sessions. Faculty with limited or a complete lack of digital-learning skills, faced immense stress during this rapid transition phase [45, 50].

In their struggle to adapt to the new system, most of the medical faculty overlooked the fact that virtual learning material is different from face-to-face sessions. In the absence of well-established guidelines and standardization procedure for e-learning, the outcome was dubious [47].

#### *6.2.2 Availability of infrastructure for e-learning*

Lack of reliable infrastructure for delivery of online education was one of the widely reported challenges especially in developing countries. Various studies reported lack of compatible software, hardware and internet connectivity issues as major barriers towards e-learning [51].

#### *6.2.3 Lack of social interaction*

The new learning model demanded an unlimited duration of time spent in front of computers. Lack of personal touch and real life interaction may promote a passive learning style, the impact of which is yet to be explored [51]. Online teaching can also compromise one to one interaction with mentors. Yet, it is too early to extrapolate outcomes till we get sufficient evidence.

Various studies reported isolation, stress, lack of concentration and disturbance by domestic affairs as major factors, compromising online learning in home environment [47].

#### *6.2.4 Adaptability by students to new learning environment*

For students of basic sciences, transition to online learning would mean confinement to home. Modifying this new learning environment to make it conducive for e-learning was a real challenge [51].

#### *6.2.5 Dependency of medical education on clinical facilities and clinical educators*

The concept of online learning cannot replace real-time patient interaction and clinical experience which are deeply ingrained, foundation and unique attributes of medical curriculum. Limited (and in some cases none) exposure to clinical teaching raised concerns regarding the competence and skills of final year students, interns and post-graduate trainees who could not get the required clinical experience. Real-life counseling, history taking and examination skills cannot be performed online. Moreover ethics, professionalism and other soft skills are learnt through role modeling for which physical interaction is essential. Though opportunities to provide clinical clerkship through virtual experience were being explored, the idea was not sufficiently imbibed by medical students. In Libya, a study showed 53% of the students expressed their disagreement for this approach.

#### *6.2.6 Virtual assessments*

Just like getting clinical experience online is difficult, assessment of psychomotor and affective domain through clinical examinations or objective structured clinical examination (OSCE) is challenging. Almost 25% medical schools in UK canceled clinical examinations [48]. This lead to a negative impact on preparedness of medical students, as depicted in the survey conducted in UK [52]. While online synchronous and asynchronous methods were widely practiced for teaching and learning, however academic leaders started to brainstorm on the modalities that can be adapted for online assessment. Yet, it is an exhausting task to reinvent assessment modalities, reliable enough to safeguard against the use of unfair means, yet valid enough to produce safe doctors.

## 7. The silver lining in pandemic- success stories

As quoted by Albert Einstein "In the midst of every crises, lies great opportunity". COVID-19 pandemic is not an exception. It has brought immense opportunities for medical educators and leaders to explore innovative strategies and drive advancement into the new model of medical education and training (**Figure 2**).

### 7.1 Revamping medical curricula

This pandemic identified huge gaps in medical education driving rapid modifications in the existing curricula. Some schools realized the importance to expand their courses of community medicine, digital and public health [6]. Schools in Italy, UK, US organized webinars on resilience, self-regulation, disaster preparedness and mental wellbeing [6, 7]. All such efforts would prepare future doctors to develop necessary soft skills and core competence to face the world which was on its knees in response to this disaster.

### 7.2 Rethinking assessments in medical education

#### *7.2.1 Open book examination*

Due to inadequate capacity to organize in-person examinations with social distancing protocols, open book examination (OBE) emerged as an assessment tool in medical education during the pandemic. First successful model of distant online assessment was pioneered by Imperial college of London [53]. Medical students were given 150 scenario based questions with findings from history and examination in which they had to answer regarding diagnosis and management. Randomizing the question order for each student was used as an effective tool to safeguard against cheating. Exposing them to time pressure (approximately 60 seconds per question), minimized chances to search intensively for the answer [54]. OBEs in contrast to conventional examination discourage rote and knowledge recall during assessments. These exams closely mimic actual clinical practice where such information can easily be retrieved from available resources in hospital. OBEs have therefore emerged as a practical assessment modality during the pandemic. As assessment drives learning, this kind of assessment will allow students to study in

| Pre COVID era | Post COVID-19 era |
|---|---|
| Lectures<br>Small group discussion | Online synchronous/asynchronous session<br>Video clips, breakout rooms |
| Basic sciences practical labs(anatomy. Biochemistry) | Online Virtual labs<br>Dividing students into small groups, using PPEs |
| Soft skills and medical humanity | Live online group discussion<br>Video clips |
| Clinical training | Tele medicine with simulated real life patient<br>Short time exposure in wards with PPEs<br>Virtual rounds |

**Figure 2.**
*Transformation of learning strategies in medical education during COVID-19 pandemic [49].*

a way more aligned to real life clinical practice. Written OBE will allow more analytical thinking, evidence based practice and application of knowledge using multiple resources promoting students to be self-directed learners. This type of assessment also minimized anxiety among medical students taking exam while sitting in a home environment [55, 56].

#### *7.2.2 Online proctoring*

Another success story of conducting successful online examination was from a developing country in which they designed an online proctored approach to monitor a group of students at their home by teaching assistants and faculty [57]. The structure of questions and allocation of time were specifically designed in a way to encourage students to utilize their problem solving abilities rather than copy pasting the answers.

#### *7.2.3 Online OSCE, quiz and viva*

Another example of accelerated innovation likely to be introduced soon for final year assessments by Imperial College of London is remote OSCE. This will include history taking of a real or simulated patient through video conferencing and display of examination findings on screen to have a complete clinical picture [53].

#### *7.2.4 Establishing continuum of assessment*

More focus is now being given to develop an assessment process comprising of ongoing formative rather than summative evaluation at the end of academic year. Assignments which need to be submitted within a stipulated time period; e-log books, portfolios, reflective diaries are being considered both for formative and summative assessment [58, 59].

### **7.3 Can clinical posting be done virtually?**

An important aspect of medical education is patient interaction through clinical postings. At the beginning of the pandemic, this was considered non-resolving challenge, since clinical rotations cannot be replaced by distant virtual learning. However with the threat of second, third and fourth wave and emergence of various variants, much has been done to address this issue as well. Imperial College London created an online bank of patient interviews and interactive cases to supplement clinical study. Many university hospitals are piloting the concept of virtual bed-side teaching to avoid overcrowding of clinical areas. Clinicians through the use of specially designed headsets provide feedback to students regarding patient examination findings. However, its feasibility on a larger scale across countries still needs to be explored further [53].

Mayo clinic used the tele-consultation through zoom meetings or video conferences to allow direct patient interaction with students [60]. Such adaptation can be fruitful to cover short term disruption of clinical teaching during peak of COVID waves, however it is hard to believe that it is as effective as learning through physical interaction.

A study conducted in US reported positive feedback of medical students doing clerkship in Emergency Medicine [61]. The students were involved in follow-up care of patients through zoom meetings, conducted under direct supervision of faculty preceptors. They felt more involved and valued the opportunity of engaging with the faculty for critical thinking.

### 7.4 Positive perception of online teaching by medical students

Overall, a positive perception of online learning has been reported by medical students. Some studies show that these remote sessions lead to better attendance as compared to in-person. This could be due to the ease and convenience to access online classes at home, minimizing the traveling time. Another reason could be the close monitoring through digital tracking of the attendance which would otherwise be difficult in large physical sessions. Various studies found online medical education as effective or in some cases more effective than conventional learning [62]. Some of the factors reported in the literature include flexibility and convenience of online teaching, students more in control of their own learning, availability of recorded lectures, opportunities to reflect through the given material and reproducibility of educational material or sessions [3]. Even if they miss face-to-face session they can later catch up by accessing the material online. Nonetheless, students see online teaching complementing rather than complete replacement of medical education, perhaps as part of flipped or blended learning approach.

### 7.5 Empowering teachers for a digital world

With the dynamic circumstances emerging due to the crisis, it is of utmost importance for the faculty to upgrade their digital skills. Special training courses are being organized to empower teaching faculty and staff to use innovative learning and assessment tools in medical education.

A major barrier to adopt innovative methods of teaching was a natural preference and comfort level regarding face-to-face learning. However COVID-19 served as a fuel to drive this transformation, bringing a positive inclination towards e-learning [63].

### 7.6 Road to collaborative and inter-professional learning

With the online education system crossing boundaries of location and geographical constraints, new horizons for collaborative learning are arising. Global conferences, webinars and other asynchronous sessions facilitating a wider group of students, allowing students from different classes, universities or countries to get benefit from subject experts [30]. Moreover, a dire need for inter-professional education (IPE) and collaborative approach has been recognized globally, due to unequal distribution of teaching resources in developed and developing countries. Available evidence suggests that knowledge-sharing among the different professionals can lead to better patient outcomes and effective utilization of health care and learning resources [64]. Tremendous work is already underway and new avenues are being explored to deliver online IPE programs [53, 65].

### 7.7 Development of best practice models

As pedagogy transformed, the impact of different online teaching methodologies were studied and reported. This lead to development of learning models and various frameworks were proposed to structure meaningful online interactions. One such example is the "Community of Inquiry" model which is based on the interplay of teaching, social, and cognitive presence in an online environment, for an effective learning experience [66]. Based on experience, educationists also proposed solutions and recommendations for synchronous virtual learning sessions and strategies to optimize transition from face–to-face to online medical education [67, 68]. Moreover, as online medical education evolved, based on need, prediction models for effectiveness of online clinical clerkship curricula were also developed [69]. The experience and insight of health profession education experts therefore promoted best practices in e-learning, improving the quality of online medical education and clerkship.

## 8. Conclusion

The noise created by COVID-19 pandemic has produced a resonating impact on medical education which will last forever. The urgency and necessity of situation acted as a catalyst, driving a rapid transformation of learning pedagogy; a change that was bound to happen and predicted in pre-COVID era.

The global adversity stimulated academic leaders to relook medical curricula, redesign assessment, standardize e-learning and upgrade faculty development programs, producing doctors ready to serve in the modern era. This is time to convert this crisis into opportunity through innovation, maximizing the outcome of e-learning programs. The term "new normal" has been nailed in the human history making it impossible for medical education to go back to pre-COVID learning strategies. The importance of clinical clerkship, social and physical interaction still pose an ongoing challenge. Though novel teaching and learning strategies complement the conventional curriculum, medical educationists and faculty are skeptical as outcomes may make a life and death difference for the patient. Therefore, a total transformation to virtual environment for the time being seems impossible.

As the world is still recovering from the depredation of COVID-19; many will remember this contagion as a driving spur for revolutionizing medical education that was already on the road to evolution for many years.

## Conflict of interest

The authors declare no conflict of interest.

## Author details

Rabeeya Saeed[1], Salman Sharif[1*] and Faridah Amin[2]

1 Liaquat National Hospital and Medical College, Karachi, Pakistan

2 Indus Hospital and Health Network, Karachi, Pakistan

*Address all correspondence to: sharifsalman73@gmail.com

## References

[1] Sharan A, Groff MW, Dailey AT, Ghogawala Z, Resnick DK, Watters WC 3rd, et al. Guideline update for the performance of fusion procedures for degenerative disease of the lumbar spine. Part 15: Electrophysiological monitoring and lumbar fusion. Journal of Neurosurgery Spine. 2014;**21**(1):102-105

[2] World Health Organization. COVID-19 Public Health Emergency of International Concern (PHEIC) Global research and innovation forum. Available from: https://www.who.int/publications/m/item/covid-19-public-health-emergency-ofinternational-concern-(pheic)-global-research-andinnovation-forum [12 February 2020]

[3] Hayat AA, Keshavarzi MH, Zare S, Bazrafcan L, Rezaee R, Faghihi SA, et al. Challenges and opportunities from the COVID-19 pandemic in medical education: A qualitative study. BMC Medical Education. 2021;**21**(1):1-13

[4] Harries AJ, Lee C, Jones L, Rodriguez RM, Davis JA, Boysen-Osborn M, et al. Effects of the COVID-19 pandemic on medical students: A multicenter quantitative study. BMC Medical Education. 2021;**21**(1):1-8

[5] Sihvonen T, Herno A, Paljarvi L, Airaksinen O, Partanen J, Tapaninaho A. Local denervation atrophy of paraspinal muscles in postoperative failed back syndrome. Spine. 1993;**18**(5):575-581

[6] Consorti F, Kanter SL, Basili S, Ho M-J. A SWOT analysis of Italian medical curricular adaptations to the COVID-19 pandemic: A nationwide survey of medical school leaders. Medical Teacher. 2021;**43**(5):546-553

[7] Ahmed F. COVID-19 pandemic and medical education in India. International Journal of Translational Medical Research and Public Health. 2021;**5**(1):1-3

[8] Lapolla P, Mingoli A. COVID-19 changes medical education in Italy: Will other countries follow?: The fellowship of. Postgraduate Medicine. 2020; **96**(1137):375-376

[9] O'Byrne L, Gavin B, McNicholas F. Medical students and COVID-19: The need for pandemic preparedness. Journal of Medical Ethics. 2020;**46**(9): 623-626

[10] Miller DG, Pierson L, Doernberg S. The role of medical students during the COVID-19 pandemic. Annals of Internal Medicine. 2020;**173**(10):859

[11] Iacobucci G. Covid-19: Medical schools are urged to fast-track final year students. BMJ. 2020;**368**:m1064

[12] Murphy B. COVID-19: how the virus is impacting medical schools. American Medical Association; 2020. Available from: https://www.amaassn.org/deliveringcare/public-health/covid-19-how-virus-impactingmedical-schools [20 February, 2020]

[13] Gouda P, Kirk A, Sweeney AM, O'Donovan D. Attitudes of medical students toward volunteering in emergency situations. Disaster Medicine and Public Health Preparedness. 2020;**14**(3):308-311

[14] Patel VM, Dahl-Grove D. Disaster preparedness medical school elective: Bridging the gap between volunteer eagerness and readiness. Pediatric Emergency Care. 2018;**34**(7):492-496

[15] Mortelmans LJ, De Cauwer HG, Van Dyck E, Monballyu P, Van Giel R, Van Turnhout E. Are Belgian senior medical students ready to deliver basic medical care in case of a H5N1 pandemic? Prehospital and Disaster Medicine. 2009;**24**(5):438-442

[16] Vala NH, Vachhani MV, Sorani AM. Study of anxiety, stress, and depression

level among medical students during COVID-19 pandemic phase in Jamnagar city. National Journal of Physiology, Pharmacy and Pharmacology. 2020;**10**(2):1043-1045

[17] Bergmann C, Muth T, Loerbroks A. Medical students' perceptions of stress due to academic studies and its interrelationships with other domains of life: A qualitative study. Medical Education Online. 2019;**24**(1):1603526

[18] Que J, Shi L, Liu J, Gong Y, Sun Y, Mi W, et al. Prevalence of suicidal thoughts and behaviours among medical professionals: A meta-analysis and systematic review. The Lancet. 2019;**394**:S11

[19] Pandey U, Corbett G, Mohan S, Reagu S, Kumar S, Farrell T, et al. Anxiety, depression and behavioural changes in junior doctors and medical students associated with the coronavirus pandemic: A cross-sectional survey. Journal of Obstetrics and Gynaecology of India. 2020;**71**(1):1-5

[20] Aker S, Mıdık Ö. The views of medical faculty students in Turkey concerning the COVID-19 pandemic. Journal of Community Health. 2020;**45**(4):684-688

[21] Cuschieri S, Calleja AJ. Spotlight on the shift to remote anatomical teaching during Covid-19 pandemic: Perspectives and experiences from the University of Malta. Anatomical Sciences Education. 2020;**13**(6):671-679

[22] Nakhostin-Ansari A, Sherafati A, Aghajani F, Khonji MS, Aghajani R, Shahmansouri N. Depression and anxiety among Iranian medical students during COVID-19 pandemic. Iranian Journal of Psychiatry. 2020;**15**(3):228-235

[23] Torun F, Torun SD. The psychological impact of the COVID-19 pandemic on medical students in Turkey. Pakistan Journal of Medical Sciences. 2020;**36**(6):1355-1359

[24] H S. Final-Year medical students graduate early to fight Covid-19 2020. Available from: https://www.theguardian.com/world/2020/mar/20/final-yearmedical-students-graduate-early-fight-coronavirus-covid-19 [Accessed: 25 April, 2020]

[25] Fodje T, Choo E. Applying for residency in the time of COVID-19. Lancet. 2020;**396**(10264):1718

[26] Elsawy F, Malik RB, Kazi M, Ladan Z. A UK perspective on the effect of the COVID-19 pandemic on medical student career perceptions. Medical Education Online. 2020;**25**(1):1810968

[27] Byrnes YM, Civantos AM, Go BCM, Williams TL, Rajasekaran K. Effect of the COVID-19 pandemic on medical student career perceptions: A national survey study. Medical Education Online. 2020;**25**(1):1798088

[28] Farlow JL, Marchiano EJ, Fischer IP, Moyer JS, Thorne MC, Bohm LA. Addressing the impact of COVID-19 on the residency application process through a virtual subinternship. Otolaryngology and Head and Neck Surgery. 2020;**163**(5):926-928

[29] Abdelhamid K, ElHawary H, Gorgy A, Alexander N. Mentorship resuscitation during the COVID-19 pandemic. AEM Education and Training. 2020;**5**(1):132-134

[30] Shaikh Y, Sharif S, Amin F. The challenges in neurosurgery training in a third world country. World Neurosurgery. 2021;**152**:19-23

[31] Liang ZC, Ooi SBS, Wang W. Pandemics and their impact on medical training: Lessons from Singapore. Academic Medicine. 2020;**95**(9):1359-1361

[32] Torda AJ, Velan G, Perkovic V. The impact of the COVID-19 pandemic on medical education. The Medical Journal of Australia. 2020;**213**(4):188-188.e1

[33] Gallagher TH, Schleyer AM. "We signed up for this!" - student and trainee responses to the Covid-19 pandemic. The New England Journal of Medicine. 2020;**382**(25):e96

[34] Sharif S, Hafiz M. The light at the end of the tunnel: Neurosurgery education during COVID. World Neurosurg. Nov 2021;**155**:196-198

[35] Srinivasan DK. Medical Students' perceptions and an anatomy Teacher's personal experience using an e-learning platform for tutorials during the Covid-19 crisis. Anatomical Sciences Education. 2020;**13**(3):318-319

[36] Pather N, Blyth P, Chapman JA, Dayal MR, Flack N, Fogg QA, et al. Forced disruption of anatomy education in Australia and New Zealand: An acute response to the Covid-19 pandemic. Anatomical Sciences Education. 2020;**13**(3):284-300

[37] Sandhu P, de Wolf M. The impact of COVID-19 on the undergraduate medical curriculum. Medical Education Online. 2020;**25**(1):1764740

[38] Shih KC, Chan CJ, Chen JY, Lai JS. Ophthalmic clinical skills teaching in the time of COVID-19: A crisis and opportunity. Medical Education. 2020;**54**(7):663-664

[39] Ferrel MN, Ryan JJ. The impact of COVID-19 on medical education. Cureus. 2020;**12**(3):e7492

[40] Abi-Rafeh J, Azzi AJ. Emerging role of online virtual teaching resources for medical student education in plastic surgery: COVID-19 pandemic and beyond. Journal of Plastic, Reconstructive & Aesthetic Surgery. 2020;**73**(8): 1575-1592

[41] Dedeilia A, Sotiropoulos MG, Hanrahan JG, Janga D, Dedeilias P, Sideris M. Medical and surgical education challenges and innovations in the COVID-19 era: A systematic review. In Vivo. 2020;**34**(Suppl. 3):1603-1611

[42] Gishen F, Bennett S, Gill D. COVID-19: The impact on our medical students will be far reaching: The BMJ Opinion; 2020. Available from: https://blogs.bmj.com/bmj/2020/04/03/covid-19-the-impact-on-our-medical-students-will-be-far-reaching/ [Accessed: 25 April, 2021]

[43] Rose S. Medical student education in the time of COVID-19. Journal of the American Medical Association. 2020;**323**(21):2131-2132

[44] Sahi PK, Mishra D, Singh T. Medical education amid the COVID-19 pandemic. Indian Pediatrics. 2020;**57**(7):652-657

[45] Longhurst GJ, Stone DM, Dulohery K, Scully D, Campbell T, Smith CF. Strength, Weakness, Opportunity, Threat (SWOT) analysis of the adaptations to anatomical education in the United Kingdom and Republic of Ireland in response to the Covid-19 pandemic. Anatomical Sciences Education. 2020;**13**(3):301-311

[46] Fernandez AA, Shaw GP. Academic leadership in a time of crisis: The coronavirus and COVID-19. Journal of Leadership Studies. 2020;**14**(1):39-45

[47] Gu GF, Zhang HL, He SS, Gu X, Zhang LG, Ding Y, et al. The clinical results of minimally invasive transforaminal lumbar interbody fusion for lumbar spinal stenosis with lumbar instability. Zhonghua wai ke za zhi [Chinese Journal of Surgery]. 2011;**49**(12):1081-1085

[48] Choi B, Jegatheeswaran L. The impact of the COVID-19 pandemic on final year medical students in the United Kingdom: A national survey. BMC Medical Education. 2020;**20**(1):206

[49] Goh P-S, Sandars J. A vision of the use of technology in medical education

after the COVID-19 pandemic. MedEdPublish. 2020;**9**(49):1-16

[50] Binks AP, LeClair RJ, Willey JM, Brenner JM, Pickering JD, Moore JS, et al. Changing medical education, overnight: The curricular response to COVID-19 of nine medical schools. Teaching and Learning in Medicine. 2021;**33**(3):334-342

[51] Gaur U, Majumder MAA, Sa B, Sarkar S, Williams A, Singh K. Challenges and opportunities of preclinical medical education: COVID-19 crisis and beyond. SN Comprehensive Clinical Medicine. 2020;**2**(11):1992-1197

[52] Zagury-Orly I, Durning SJ. Assessing open-book examination in medical education: The time is now. Medical Teacher. 2021;**43**(8):972-973

[53] Tapper JBD, Savage M. Medical students take final exams online for first time, despite student concer. Available from: https://www.theguardian.com/education/2020/mar/22/coronavirus-forces-medical-students-sit-final-exams-online [Accessed: 1 July, 2021]

[54] Broyles IL, Cyr PR, Korsen N. Open book tests: Assessment of academic learning in clerkships. Medical Teacher. 2005;**27**(5):456-462

[55] Stowell JR, Bennett D. Effects of online testing on student exam performance and test anxiety. Journal of Educational Computing Research. 2010;**42**(2):161-171

[56] Baqir SM, Mustansir F. Online medical education and examinations during COVID-19: Perspectives of a teaching associate. Journal of the College of Physicians and Surgeons–Pakistan. 2021;**30**(1):S16-Ss8

[57] Birch E, de Wolf M. A novel approach to medical school examinations during the COVID-19 pandemic. Medical Education Online. 2020;**25**(1):1785680

[58] Sabzwari S. Rethinking assessment in medical education in the time of COVID-19. MedEdPublish. 2020;**9**(80):1-15

[59] Suh GA, Shah AS, Kasten MJ, Virk A, Domonoske CL, Razonable RR. Avoiding a medical education quarantine during the pandemic. 2020;**95**(9):S63-S65

[60] Chandra S, Laoteppitaks C, Mingioni N, Papanagnou D. Zooming-out COVID-19: Virtual clinical experiences in an emergency medicine clerkship. Medical Education. 2020;**54**(12):1182-1183

[61] Ruiz JG, Mintzer MJ, Leipzig RM. The impact of E-learning in medical education. Academic Medicine. 2006;**81**(3):207-212

[62] O'Doherty D, Dromey M, Lougheed J, Hannigan A, Last J, McGrath D. Barriers and solutions to online learning in medical education - an integrative review. BMC Medical Education. 2018;**18**(1):130

[63] Chan LK, Ganotice F, Wong FKY, Lau CS, Bridges SM, Chan CHY, et al. Implementation of an interprofessional team-based learning program involving seven undergraduate health and social care programs from two universities, and students' evaluation of their readiness for interprofessional learning. BMC Medical Education. 2017;**17**(1):1-12

[64] Singh J, Matthees B. Facilitating Interprofessional education in an online environment during the COVID-19 pandemic: A mixed method study. Healthcare (Basel). 2021;**9**(5):567

[65] Kim JW, Myung SJ, Yoon HB, Moon SH, Ryu H, Yim J-J. How medical education survives and evolves during COVID-19: Our experience and future direction. PLoS One. 2020;**15**(12): e0243958

[66] Haras C, Calhoun A, Olson AP, Rosenberg M. Mindful medical

education online. Medical Science Educator. 2021;**31**(2):863-872

[67] Sharp EA, Norman MK, Spagnoletti CL, Miller BG. Optimizing synchronous online teaching sessions: A guide to the "new normal" in medical education. Academic Pediatrics. 2021;**21**(1):11-15

[68] Jiang Z, Wu H, Cheng H, Wang W, Xie AN, Fitzgerald SR. Twelve tips for teaching medical students online under COVID-19. Medical Education Online. 2021;**26**(1):1854066

[69] Kuroda N, Suzuki A, Ozawa K, Nagai N, Okuyama Y, Koshiishi K, et al. Predicting the effectiveness of the online clinical clerkship curriculum: Development of a multivariate prediction model and validation study. PLoS One. 2022;**17**(1):e0263182

Chapter 17

# COVID-19 and the Dynamic Role of Telemedicine

*Grace Koehler, Saadiq F. El-Amin III and Ashim Gupta*


## Abstract

The COVID-19 pandemic brought never before seen changes in the use of telemedicine in healthcare. With a contagious and unfamiliar virus spreading worldwide, patients and physicians began to utilize contactless options of communication like telephone calls and video visits out of necessity. Prior to March 2020, telemedicine was in use, but on a markedly smaller and limited scale. As 2020 progressed, the use of telemedicine rapidly expanded, especially in the United States, presenting both positive aspects like safety and convenience as well as negative aspects like loss of patient physical contact/exam and concern for new socioeconomic inequities. The adaptation of greater telehealth use in primary care specifically appears to hold potential for long term sustainability and use with patients experiencing new ways to interact with the healthcare system. Going forward, addressing such challenges as payment models and quantifying patient long term outcomes are important to the viability of telemedicine. The future of telemedicine will certainly cause dynamic changes in healthcare far outlasting the pandemic, both for patient and provider.


**Keywords:** telehealth, telemedicine, COVID-19, primary care, public health

## 1. Introduction

The World Health Organization announced on March 11, 2020 that the coronavirus 2019 outbreak was a pandemic, sending healthcare systems across the world into overdrive to respond. Millions of infections were occurring worldwide and many health systems were overwhelmed by the volume and in need of a strategy to prevent further infections while still providing healthcare for the ailing [1].

The initial goals for mitigation of the spread of COVID-19 focused on triage. Steps of this triage were as follows: early identification and diagnosis of the virus, isolating the patient, monitoring contacts and quarantining as appropriate. Telemedicine emerged as the perfect tool for contactless triage and suddenly, everyone from clinical administration, nurses, medical assistants, resident doctors and physicians of all specialties were learning to use and exploit its benefits in an effort to slow the spread of COVID-19.

Overrun hospitals then looked to catalyze the implementation of telemedicine for everything from triage of coronavirus symptoms to off site-physician assessment in understaffed intensive care units and finally to the outpatient clinic setting for general health and specialist visits. Due to the acuity of the pandemic, non COVID related patient visits were threatened with disruption of routine care as in-person visits dropped rapidly. Thus, Telemedicine, which will here on be used in this chapter interchangeably with telehealth, became a major focus in the outpatient, clinic setting to address this threat.

This text will focus on the history of telehealth prior to COVID-19, and the initial spike in telemedicine at the onset of the pandemic. The strengths and weaknesses of virtual visits will be outlined, and primary care physician specific considerations will be addressed along with financial and ethical concerns. Finally, deductions regarding the future of telemedicine will be considered.

## 2. Telehealth prior to Covid-19

Telehealth while more recently a "hot topic", has long been discussed both globally and nationally since at least the 1980s. As early as the year 1996, Medicare was paying for rural telehealth visits, but buy in by both physician and patient was extremely poor. In the United States in 2019, only one percent of rural patients had partaken in telemedicine of any form [2, 3].

At times throughout global health history, the use of telehealth would increase for public health crises response such as during a Public Health Emergency of International Concern (PHEIC) for viruses such as Ebola, Zika and severe acute respiratory syndrome (SARC-COV) and Middle East Respiratory Syndrome Coronavirus (MERS-CoV) [1]. Despite these signs of promise of telehealth as a helpful tool, global or national public health guidelines including ethical guidelines never solidified. Perhaps, the technological landscape was not quite right. In contrast, data from 2019, one year prior to COVID-19, showed that 89% of the US population had internet access and 77% were online daily [4].

While telemedicine has historically been on the horizon for several decades, its future value was undecided by both policy makers and patients until recently. The US department of Health and Human Services actually cut the budget of the Hospital Preparedness Program in half in 2018 from what it had been back in 2004. At that time, there had been no trial of a telehealth workforce that could respond rapidly to national emergencies such as a pandemic or a natural disaster. Conversely, also in 2018, the US government expanded telehealth services system wide for the Department of Defense and the Department of Veterans Affairs [5]. As late as January 2020, merely 24% of United States healthcare entities had telehealth programs [3] although their use was only a small percentage of visits.

Before discussing telehealth further, it is vital to define the term because since its use in the 1980s, the definition has expanded to include different modalities. The World Medical Association has refined its definition the past two decades several times and in 2020 defined telehealth as real-time audio and visual communication between providers and patients. Additionally, this recognized definition of telehealth also represented photo and data collection, remote patient monitoring capability, and virtual check in. Other organizations such as the World Health Organization defined telemedicine in 2007 more generally as a delivery of healthcare in which distance plays a role [6]. More recently, the Department of Health and Human Services released a broader definition of telehealth as, the use of electronic information and telecommunication technologies to support long distance clinical health care, patient and professional-related health care education, health administration and public health [7].

## 3. The start of the pandemic and telehealth

Telemedicine has been nothing if not crucial to support the strains put on healthcare since the abrupt onset of the COVID-19 pandemic. As discussed, the surge in the need for telemedicine appeared to occur overnight and healthcare systems including physicians, clinic and hospital staff, and payment systems had to move rapidly in response. Congress passed The Telehealth Services During Certain Emergency Periods Act of 2020 which allowed for a temporary waiving of previous Medicare restrictions surrounding telehealth [8].

Many general practice offices decided to close their physical spaces temporarily to limit staff exposure [9]. In-person office based visits dropped by over 100 million visits in the second quarter of 2020 when compared to the first quarter of 2020 [10]. Leading up to March 2020, less than 10,000 telehealth visits were submitted to the National Health Institute (NHI) in the United States. By the end of that same month, in the midst of the pandemic, more than 400,000 calls were being submitted to the NHI each week [1].

The initial increase in use of telemedicine very clearly pertained to triaging for COVID-19 infections. This served a dual purpose: to mitigate transmission and also to assist in gate-keeping of increasingly overwhelmed emergency departments. Primary care centers quickly adopted these telehealth visits into their practice as the first line of a COVID-triage framework. Symptomatic patients were given a questionnaire by clinical staff and if appropriate, spoke with a physician via telephone or video service. General practitioners would then assess for severity of illness and whether the patient required monitoring, hospital care, or even intensive care [1].

Telemedicine was soon employed to address non-COVID related concerns that were accumulating and unable to be addressed in-person. Initial vital roles of telehealth included blood pressure and cholesterol checks and most notably for increased psychiatric concerns encountered across the United States population in 2020 [10].

## 4. Strengths and weaknesses

As the COVID-19 pandemic continues on and more time passes, multiple benefits of increased telemedicine use have emerged. Working adults, caregivers and frequent travelers who previously were lost to follow up or in need of a timely appointment with their primary care physician may more easily be triaged virtually without missing work. Overall, the time and resources patients have to commit to a telemedicine visit is substantially lower than the time it takes for most patients to drive, park and visit their doctor. Even more importantly, telehealth is associated with decreased financial costs to patients [11].

One analysis of patient's response to a telemedicine visit showed a majority of patients reported being satisfied with their televisit. This analysis also concluded that a majority of patients would choose a televisit over an in-person visit in the future and there was no difference in satisfaction between telephone and video groups [11]. Another strong point for telemedicine is it does not exclude a person from in person services. Telehealth calls or videos can easily be converted to in-person visits as deemed necessary by the physician.

Telemedicine has emerged at seemingly the perfect moment in time as cell phones are more ubiquitous. In the United States especially, telehealth video calls support the technologically saturated culture and provide new opportunities to educate via email, phone call, video, or social media.

A new modality of care will always bring with it various problems and the same has been proven with the increased use of telemedicine. Telehealth visits more often than not do not include lab work, blood pressure or other vital checks, and screening tests as frequently as in-person visits. Patients may not feel like enough was done for them at their visit if there is not in-person physician interaction and/or an intervention of some kind.

Another concern is the barriers created for certain socio-economic populations. An extensive review of telehealth visits across the year 2020 showed that older age was independently associated with decreased telemedicine use as well as decreased video use. Non-English speaking patients are also significantly less likely to complete a telemedicine visit. Patients with Medicaid, of black race, of Latino ethnicity, of female sex or with a lower median income were less engaged with video use as well. Interestingly, patients with increased risk of morbidity had higher rates of telemedicine completion rates [12]. These patients however, may be the population most in need of more regular in-person services.

Studies that support the safety and efficacy of managing multiple chronic conditions via telehealth and what amount and frequency of in-person follow up are necessary for good outcomes have yet to be done. This ambiguity leaves room for a large range of physician judgment calls which has the potential for missing an opportunity for intervention on a condition like uncontrolled blood pressure. Primary physicians will also find it difficult to be certain of patient compliance. In-person medication refill follow-up visits are often a way in primary care medicine to make sure the patient is on track and to check vital signs and draw periodic labs. Patients in the future will still need assessment of their vital signs and labs. A potential negative effect of telemedicine on the patient is that they may end up having to set up a telemedicine visit and then after evaluation have to travel to a lab or office for a lab draw. This could negate the efficiency of a telemedicine visit when in person office visits can provide all of those services under one roof.

A concern of telehealth expansion, especially whilst the pandemic continues to affect in-person interaction is the loss of new patient pickup. Currently, the recommend use of telehealth is for established patients only. Telehealth therefore may encroach on the opportunity for providers to have availability to accept new patients. However, for those patients that are established with a primary care provider, virtual visits have shown promise for similar clinical effectiveness with less patient cost [4].

Overall, the benefits of telemedicine to keep healthcare running especially in the midst of a pandemic outweigh difficulties that must be addressed along the way. As medicine continue to accept and explore the capabilities of phone and video visits, telemedicine will become a way to make medicine a more efficient and meaningful experience for physician and patient.

## 5. Telemedicine and the primary care physician

The most acutely attuned group of providers to the dramatic shifts in virtual care arguably is the primary care physicians. Since March 2020, outpatient primary clinicians, as well as behavioral health care have accommodated the majority of telehealth calls in the country. Understandably, a large proportion of adults initially postponed routine care as many parts of the country went into lockdown in 2020 and primary care clinics temporarily shut down as well. Chronic conditions therefore went unchecked for prolonged periods of time, creating a longer and more uncontrolled list of ailments when patients returned to the care of their doctor [13]. Primary care physicians, also carry a responsibility to educate on the COVID-19 virus itself and promote vaccination with each encounter, including telehealth. This adds another layer of both time and complexity to each visit.

This demand on the primary care physician for change of practice has sparked new utility of telemedicine and continues to create innovative physician-patient experiences. For example, primary care has implemented a wide spectrum of routine telehealth visits now for things such as chronic condition monitoring, medication reconciliations and management, patient counseling, acute visits and triage. A noticeable gap with telemedicine is that it does not appear to offer much practicality for annual preventative exams [10].

Primary care physicians do have their own concerns as well. While providing further reaching care to the population is advantageous, providers are already expressing concerns about an ever revolving door of new tasks expected of them, a potential extension of office hours cutting into their lifestyle, and diminution of the patient-physician relationship. Specifically, there is concern around an already formidable threat to the working doctor: physician burnout. With an ever changing workflow adapting to new COVID-19 policies, physicians now have to or will have to navigate a schedule with both in-person and telehealth visits and the increased risk of schedules running behind. Another concern voiced from seasoned physicians, is that many nuanced non-verbal cues cannot be picked up by the physician during a telemedicine telephone visit. Even telehealth visits using video do not replace the vital role of the physical examination in the completeness of an assessment of a patient. Providers trained to examine the body are now limited by the resolution of a screen to extract clues around disease process.

However, physicians interviewed did report greater convenience overall for their patients which ultimately, could result in better compliance. Other positives reported included more time for counseling and the capability of evaluating patient home environments via video calls [14].

## 6. Ethical concerns and financial strains

The American Medical Association makes clear in their Code of Ethics that telemedicine should occur when there is a pre-existing and real patient-physician relationship with the exception being in emergencies and extenuating circumstances [3]. As the initial shock of the pandemic subsides, it is important to assess the quality of the telehealth services being provided to the general population. There is certainly a risk of COVID-19 education, assessment, and prevention overshadowing the pivotal pillar of medicine: preventative health care. Many primary care physicians are now juggling yet another piece of an already complex puzzle comprised of treating chronic conditions, acute conditions, preventative screening, labs, and immunizations.

Privacy is another ethical concern expressed by patients. Many people cannot secure a private place to talk confidentially to their provider without interruption at home. Patients may not trust a telephone or video visit to be as secure as a face-to-face interaction.

Perhaps an even bigger concern for healthcare as a whole is the compensation models surrounding telemedicine. Historically, payment rules have dampened many health care provider's efforts to implement telemedicine as payment for telemedicine visits did not compete with in-person visits. At the onset of the pandemic, in the spring and summer of 2020, temporary changes in payer rules suddenly allowed reimbursement for providers who administered telemedicine visits equal to in-person visit reimbursement [2]. This benefitted both the healthcare system as an overarching structure to ease the case load burden of the emergency department, but additionally, helped keep many outpatient practices in business. Of note, during this time period, many clinics were not able to have in-person visits at all.

Currently in 2021, further away from the initial shock of the pandemic, the fee-for-service model of payment is causing some physicians to back track on the initial shift toward telemedicine. The pressure from health care systems to move back toward more, if not all, in-person visits stems from the uncertainty of digital service reimbursement. There continues to be too much "red-tape" for some health care providers to remain trusting that virtual visits will financially be at parity with in-person visits. Some experts are pushing for a move toward capitation as the ideal payment model for telemedicine.

At this moment in time, payers are struggling with how to reimburse these multiple new digital options. The question of what will be compensated now extends to telephone visits, video visits, digital monitoring, patient portals and lab and imaging result phone calls and more. Services that once were complimentary with many practices like digital monitoring, may now carry a fee that could deter patients used to a free service. Increased digital modalities will then present new coding and billing challenges as well [15] and with that increased administrative costs. Despite these financial concerns, it is clear that long-term clinic cost could be reduced by keeping telemedicine as a viable part of a practice, but efficiency and payment models will need to catch up.

## 7. The future of telemedicine

As the world shifts to digital communication in every sector and the pandemic continues on, telemedicine appears to be here to stay in a more substantial and meaningful way than prior to the COVID-19 pandemic. Improved internet access and increased access to technologies like smart phones and web cameras should be addressed to ensure widespread adaptation and "buy-in" to telemedicine. Many countries, in fact, do not have the frameworks or the funding in place for public health emergencies much less for telemedicine to thrive long term. To implement telemedicine effectively, there must be adequate access to technology and sufficient technological and business related support. Vital to its success is restructuring the payment model to include systems like capitation. However, a cohort study evaluating Medicare Advantage health maintenance organization (HMO) plan beneficiaries continuously enrolled from the beginning of 2019 through 2020 found that the use of telemedicine increased at a greater rate and overall volume for organizations using value-based payment models versus fee-for-service payment models. This result bolsters the idea that a strong infrastructure may in fact hold more importance for actualization of telemedicine than a stronger reimbursement incentive [16].

Physicians, especially primary physicians and behavioral health care providers need structured guidelines and education on telemedicine technology and its proper use. There is currently a lack of formal training for physicians in telemedicine as well as lack of literature to support this learning [17]. Further, coordination of care amongst primary care office staff to determine the appropriateness of a telehealth visit and the necessity of length of that visit are vital to ensure a physician can incorporate both virtual and in-person visits into the same work day.

Regarding the future of telemedicine and patient experience and compliance, socioeconomic inequities must be addressed. Non-English speaking patients cannot be left behind as telemedicine continues on; translation services are an essential component of a long-lasting telehealth system. Additionally, distinct and innovative user-friendly telehealth for the elderly population and other populations with audio, motor and visual impairments could help connect a large percentage of healthcare consumers to the benefits of telemedicine [12].

## 8. Conclusion

The COVID-19 pandemic shook up all of healthcare and with it sparked a new surge in telemedicine use. Telehealth implementation has protected thousands of healthcare workers and countless patients from excessive and unnecessary virus exposure. Due to its increased use during the pandemic, telemedicine now has been tested by a large population of patients as a supplement or replacement for normal in-person visits. Benefits of having telehealth as an additional way to reach patients appears to outweigh the growing pains that its adaptation presents. Primary care physicians, alongside behavior health care providers, are amongst the top torch bearers of telehealth and must commit to advocating for payer systems that make sense to both a health care practice and their patients.

Ultimately, further quantitative research needs to be carried out to assess the effectiveness of telemedicine's use alongside traditional clinic visits versus only in-person clinic visits to ensure similar long term health outcomes. Currently, retrospective studies, qualitative studies, and meta-analysis studies exist, but very few if any randomized controlled trials were found in the literature review. Other areas of study that need further investigation include comparison of compliance, patient satisfaction, patient cost and provider compensation.

Without a doubt, the realized and potential benefits of telemedicine if imagined correctly, will open new opportunities for physicians to reach previously underserved or unserved populations [18]. While the Covid-19 pandemic has limited traditional health care models, necessity has driven health care systems and policy makers toward innovation that could benefit all consumers while simultaneously protecting vulnerable patient populations from unnecessary risk.

## Conflict of interest

The author declares no conflict of interest.

## Author details

Grace Koehler[1,2], Saadiq F. El-Amin III[3,4,5] and Ashim Gupta[5,6,7]*

1 Northside Gwinnett Family Medicine Residency, Lawrenceville, GA, USA

2 Faculty of Medicine, University of Queensland, Brisbane, QLD, Australia

3 El-Amin Orthopaedic and Sports Medicine Institute, Lawrenceville, GA, USA

4 Regenerative Sports Medicine, Lawrenceville, GA, USA

5 BioIntegrate, Lawrenceville, GA, USA

6 South Texas Orthopedic Research Institute (STORI Inc), Laredo, TX, USA

7 Future Biologics, Lawrenceville, GA, USA

*Address all correspondence to: ashim6786@gmail.com

## References

[1] Ohannessian R, Duong TA, Odone A. Global telemedicine implementation and integration within health systems to fight the COVID-19 pandemic: A call to action. JMIR Public Health and Surveillance. 2020;**6**(2):e18810. DOI: 10.2196/18810

[2] Werner MD, Glied SA. Covid-induced changes in health care delivery-can they last? New England Journal of Medicine. 2021;**385**:868-870. DOI: 10.105/nejmp2110679

[3] Revisiting KB, Ethical HIT. Legal and social issues and evaluation: Telehealth/telemedicine and covid-19. International Journal of Medical Informatics. 2020; **143**:104239. DOI: 10.1016/j.ijmedinf.2020.104239

[4] Donelan K, Barreto EA, Sossong S, Michael C, Estrada JJ, Cohen AB, et al. Patient and clinician experiences with telehealth for patient follow up care. The American Journal of Managed Care. 2019;**25**(1):40-44

[5] Lurie N, Carr BG. The role of telehealth in the medical response to disasters. JAMA Internal Medicine. 2018;**178**(6):745-746. DOI: 10.001/jamainternmed.2018.1314

[6] Doraiswamy S, Abraham A, Mamtani R, Cheema S. Use of telehealth during the COVID-19 pandemic: Scoping review. Journal of Medical Internet Research. 2020;**22**(12):e24087. DOI: 10.2196/24087

[7] Office for the Advancement of Telehealth [Internet]. 2021. Available from: https://www.hrsa.gov/rural-health/telehealth [Accessed: September 2, 2021]

[8] Coronavirus preparedness and response supplemental appropriations act, 2020, HR 6074. Available from: https://www.congress.gov.bill/116th-congress/house-bill/6074 [Accessed: September 1, 2021]

[9] Silver SL, Lewis MN, CJW L. A stepwise transition to telemedicine in response to COVID-19. The Journal of the American Board of Family Medicine. 2021;**34**(Supplement):S152-S161. DOI: 10.3122/ jabfm.2021.S1.200358

[10] Cortez C, Mansour O, Qato DM, Stafford RS, Alexander GC. Changes in short-term, long-term, and preventative care delivery in US Office-based and telemedicine visits during the COVID-10 pandemic. JAMA Health Forum. 2021;**2**(7):e211529. DOI: 10.1001/jamahealthforum.2021.1529

[11] Allen AZ, Zhu D, Shin C, Glassman DT, Abraham N, Watts KL. Patient satisfaction with telephone versus video-televisits: A cross sectional survey of an urban, multiethnic population. Urology. 2021;**156**:110-116. DOI: 10.1016/j.urology.2021.05.096

[12] Eberly LA, Kallan MJ, Julien HM, et al. Patient characteristics associated with telemedicine access for primary and specialty ambulatory care during the COVID-19 pandemic. JAMA NetwOpen. 202;**3**(12):e2031640. DOI: 10.1001/jamanetworkopen.open.2020.31640

[13] Patel SY, Mehrotra A, Huskamp HA, Uscher-Pines L, Ganguli I, Barnett ML. Trends in oupatient care and delivery and telemedicine during the COVID-19 pandemic in the US. JAMA Internal Medicine. 2021;**181**(3):388-391. DOI: 10.1001/jamainternmed.2020.5928

[14] Gomez T, Anaya YB, Anaya SKJ, Tarn DM. A qualitative study of primary care physicians' experience with telemedicine during Covid-19. Journal of American Board of Family Medicine. 2021;**34**(Suppl):S61-S70. DOI: 10.3122/jabfm.2021.S1.200517

[15] Alder-Milstein J, Mehrotra A. Paying for digital health care-problems with the fee-for-service system. New England Journal of Medicine. 2021;**385**:871-873. DOI: 10.1056/nejmp2107879

[16] Powers BW, Drzayich AD, Zhao Y, et al. Associations between primary care payment model and telemedicine use for medicare advantage enrollees during the COVID-19 pandemic. JAMA Health Forum. 2021;**2**(7):e211597. DOI: 10.1001/jamahealthforum.2021.1597

[17] Garattini L, Badinella Martini M, Zanetti M. More room for telemedicine after COVID-19: Lessons for primary care? Eur J Health Econ Marc. 2021;**22**(2):183-186. DOI: 10.1007/s10198-020-01248-y

[18] Bhaskar S, Nurtazina A, Mittoo S, Banach M, Wessiert R. Editorial: Telemedicine during and beyond COVID-19. Frontier Public Health. 2021;**9**:662617. DOI: 10.3389/fpubh.2021.662617

Chapter 18

# Education Equity in Times of Emergency Remote Teaching: The Case of Slovenia

*Alenka Lipovec, Blaž Zmazek and Igor Pesek*

## Abstract

During the COVID -19 situation, it was often warned that emergency remote teaching increases differences among students. Additionally, some empirical results in Slovenia indicate that the situation at schools in Slovenia was very diverse, leading to a violation of the equity principle in education. In this paper, we investigate teaching methods used by teachers in crisis teaching. The database presents 61 diaries of future teachers from the first grade of elementary school to the fourth grade of secondary school. The results show differences between mentor-teachers emergency remote teaching strategies. Differences are also statistically significant according to the educational stages. The results suggest that secondary school teachers have most effectively adopted and integrated different distance learning strategies into their work. On the other hand, some class teachers have not been as successful, probably also due to the students' distinctive characteristics. The primary purpose of this paper is to describe the Razlagamo.si learning environment, which can reduce differences by providing a common educational point for all Slovenian primary and secondary school students. Finally, we give some implications for physical re-engagement at school.

**Keywords:** emergency remote teaching, video explanations, teachers, students, educational stages

## 1. Introduction

The COVID-19 pandemic is a public health and development challenge, but it is also an opportunity. All stakeholders have a responsibility to ensure that we ground our efforts in human rights principles. The right to basic education is one of the fundamental rights; however, it is often violated. During the pandemic, the impact of e-learning becomes significant. In an emergency, many countries closed schools and switched to distance learning.

An absolute human right, education is the bedrock of just, equal, and inclusive societies and a key driver of sustainable development. Because of the disruption of the social contexts in classrooms and schools, students' relationships with peers, teachers, school leaders, and other staff and the familiar settings that support learning have been disrupted. More than 1.2 billion learners worldwide were affected due to school and university closures because of COVID -19. These nationwide closures are impacting over 60% of the world's student population. As a response to the global education crisis, online emergency remote teaching (ERT) has been implemented. ERT should be considered a temporary solution to an immediate problem. ERT is described as a quick shift from the face-to-face or hybrid teaching of instruction to completely digital education due to external factors (COVID-19) and no time for preparation. Since it is prepared to respond to the emergency, its primary aim is not to develop a robust educational ecosystem but temporary access to instruction and instructors to provide support. Therefore, ERT is about delivery modes, methods, and media. The effectiveness of this measure is still under discussion [1]. Teachers should »in these times (and all other times) think about not only the content of their teaching but also the medium they use«. [2].

Despite the best efforts, teaching staff has not previously had to develop the specialist skills required to create and deliver online learning and are required to upskill very quickly, exacerbating the challenge of sustaining the rate of education and level of engagement. In addition, the COVID-19 outbreak exposed a significant variation in educators' readiness to use technology to support learners at a distance. The gap was noticed in the international context [3, 4] and the Slovenian [5].

An Australian study [6] confirms that the impacts are particularly evident in the early years, critical years for learning, and vulnerable students for whom learning loss is challenging to recover or students from culturally and linguistically diverse backgrounds. These losses are often due to families' lack the physical spaces, technology, and other resources to support learning at home. Additionally, many parents and caregivers require the time to support their children's learning. We believe that similar conclusions could be drawn for the Slovenian context.

In this paper, we will focus on providing equal opportunities for students in times of closure of the schools in Covid 19 in Slovenia.

In the following, we first describe the results of the combined qualitative-quantitative study examining teaching practices conducted by Slovenian teachers in the first COVID-19 wave. The research questions in this part were

- which ERT methods were used for teaching mathematics from 1st to 13th year of schooling, and
- do ERT methods differ according to the age of students?

In the discussion section, we describe the Slovenian response to (as results show) a highly diverse situation, the site *www.razlagamo.si*. In conclusion, we offer some tips for re-engagement at schools.

## 2. Methodology

Using a non-experimental causal methodology of pedagogical research, we will investigate teachers' teaching methods during crisis teaching.

The database consists of 61 records from practice diaries submitted by future teachers after two and a half months of condensed pedagogical practice (April, May and June 2020). We have concentrated on the journals for the subject mathematics.

While working from home, the students carried out the practical training in an adapted form so that the instructions for preparing a report/diary were also modified. One of the nine points in their diaries relates to their teacher-mentor emergency remote teaching practices. The students were asked to find out about the teacher's style and working methods.

Their answers were used to determine whether the teachers:

- gave written instructions (by email, in virtual classrooms, etc.),
- used video lectures (their own or from others),
- held video conferences to explain content,
- checked and evaluated knowledge
- solved learning problems expressed by the students etc.

In Slovenia, a self-contained instruction system is applied, where the primary teacher (so-called class teacher) teaches all school subjects until 5th grade (10–11 years old students), including mathematics. We will call this period educational stage I, followed by stage II from 6th to 9th grade, where a subject (mathematics) teacher teaches students. In stage II, teachers are educated as double-subject teachers (e.g., mathematics major and physics major, mathematics-major and history major...). Finally, at stage III (secondary school level), only a single-subject teacher (only mathematics major) is licenced to teach.

The diaries of condensed pedagogical practice submitted by 24th June 2020 were analysed. The diaries were written by students of three programs: 1st cycle program Primary Education (stage I teachers), unified master's study program Subject teacher (stage II teachers) and 2nd cycle program Educational Mathematics (stage III teachers). At the educational stage I 71 students submitted diaries, and 34 (49%) diaries were included in the analysis, as the required information could be derived from them. We analysed 10 (83% of all) diaries at stage II, and at stage III18 (75% of all) diaries were included in the analysis. Thus, in total, 61 diaries were included in the analysis.

The data were analysed using patterns of common reference to relationship issues. With the use of narrative analysis, each dairy entrance was first determined predominant form of teacher-mentor ERT practices. Analysis was done using thematic analysis in six phases: familiarising with the data (transcribing, reading and re-read the data while simultaneously noting initial ideas), generating initial codes (systematic coding of interesting features of the data and collating data according to the codes), searching for themes (collating of the codes into potential themes), reviewing themes (checking of themes against the coded statements and the data as a whole), defining and naming themes (refining each theme and generating clear definitions for each theme), producing the report (providing extracts for each theme to illustrate the participants' accounts and comparing themes and extracts with relevant literature).

## 3. Results

We first present the results of qualitative analysis in **Table 1**. Then, to give voice to participants in the qualitative analysis, we add excerpts from diaries. Finally, the information about the educational stage addressed by a quote is provided in brackets.

In future teachers' diaries, it was usually possible to detect which method was predominant in teacher-mentor teaching. However, most records contained several methods.

In the following, we present the frequency of remote working methods perceived by students during the condensed internship. The results can be found in **Table 2**.

| Theme | Description | Future teachers' diary excerpt |
|---|---|---|
| Written instructions | The mentor-teacher guides the student's learning process with written instructions. The student receives written instructions through various channels (e.g., email, online classroom, MS Teams). The instructions include a more detailed explanation of the content and assignments that the student should fulfil to consolidate knowledge. However, the instructions are in static text format, which rarely contains links to various multimedia and interactive content. | Every Sunday, the mentor-teacher sent new instructions to the students (and parents) by email, which included a written explanation of the material, worksheets, and some pictures. I prepared the material myself, as the students were used to the system. (I)<br>During the internship, the mentor teacher told me that some students are unresponsive and that work via video conferencing is almost impossible. Her teaching style is thus tied to email and resources in the online classroom. (II) |
| Synchronous video conference | The teacher guides the student's learning process with video conferences. Video conferencing follows traditional lesson elements but is adapted for distance learning in specific segments (e.g., shorter time, omitted parts that cannot be taught at a distance, a particular class contract regarding the rules of operation in a virtual environment). | Mentor-teacher had video conferencing with each class three times a week via Zoom. Students were able to ask questions regarding explained content in that and the previous week. (II)<br>The professor told me that her lessons are conducted exclusively through videoconferencing. In the beginning, all students must say hello. Then she teaches new material and shows animations. In the meantime, she also calls students by name to answer questions. It was interesting that no one, neither the students nor the professor, has the cameras on during this videoconference. (III) |
| Asynchronous video explanation | The teacher guides the student's learning process with video conferences. A video explanation is a video that follows the principles of the method of explaining or the Socrates method. In video explanations (VE), the teacher follows a pedagogy that helps students critically reflect on their understanding of a particular issue with guided questions. VEs can additionally use multimedia tools (e.g., videos of natural phenomena), videos of virtual manipulators (e.g., virtual versions of experiments), or screencasting. Usually, a video explanation contains a combination of these elements. | The teacher prepared a video for essential concepts (e.g., fractions), which the students watched independently. She told me that it took 6 hours of work for a five-minute-long video. (III)<br>Pupils learned from videos made by other teachers or videos on the internet. The teacher opted for this method because she did not have the technical skills to make recordings. She told me that she found it very difficult to find suitable recordings in Slovene. (II) |

**Table 1.**
*ERT methods for mathematics.*

All teachers used written instructions. Two-thirds of the teachers used video conferencing when students had problems. The teachers identified the issues in the knowledge tests, the student themselves asked for help, or they were students with perceived learning difficulties. Among diary entries, we find the excerpt below. The quote indicates that not all those in need may have been helped. The names of the students are anonymised.

*The teacher offered to help the students in class and explain the material to them, but none chose to do so. It seems that the students were embarrassed to need further explanations.* (stage I).

| | f | f% |
|---|---|---|
| A (Also) written instructions | 61 | 100 |
| B1 self-designed video explanations | 6 | 10 |
| B2 video lectures designed by another author | 12 | 20 |
| C1 video conferencing to explain the content | 24 | 39 |
| C2 video conferencing to check and evaluate knowledge | 23 | 38 |
| C3 video conferencing to solve learning problems expressed by the students. | 41 | 67 |

**Table 2.**
*Emergency remote teaching practices.*

The lowest percentage is observed in video explanations, where only 11% of teachers prepared their video explanations. Teachers also did not use video explanations from another author. In the following excerpt, the situation is partly explained.

*First, my mentor confided to me her concerns about implementing distance learning. She was worried that her parents would not be able to cope with the learning content. When I offered her to make a video explaining the learning content, she flatly refused, arguing that she knew her class as well as her parents.* (stage II).

The teachers used several methods for emergency remote teaching. Since they combined several different teaching ways, we checked how often a combination of methods occurred. Only written instructions (provided through various channels such as online classrooms, email, social networks) were used by 31% of the teachers. Another 38% of teachers used video conferencing for various purposes in addition to written instructions. Only 31% of teachers used written instructions as well as video conferencing and video explanations. Only three teachers (1%) used written instructions and video conferencing, and asynchronous video explanations.

As used methods ERT depend on the age of the students, **Table 3** shows the data separately by the educational stage. The letter coding used is explained in **Table 2**.

Additional analyses showed that up to 42% of the teachers at stage I used only written instructions. About one-third (30%) of teachers at stage II were using only written instructions, and only 17% of stage III teachers used only this method. At stage II most teachers used video explanations designed by another author (50%) and video conferencing for explanatory purposes (50%). At stage II, teachers used more videoconferencing for knowledge assessment and solving learning difficulties than their colleagues at stage I, but less than stage III teachers.

There are statistically significant differences for all forms of work except for written instructions (A), depending on the educational stage. We have used the Kruskal-Wallis test and obtained the following values for significance: $P_{B1}$ = 0.031,

| | A | | B1 | | B2 | | C1 | | C2 | | C3 | | total | |
|---|---|---|---|---|---|---|---|---|---|---|---|---|---|---|
| stage | f | f% | f | f% | f | f% | f | f% | f | f% | f | f% | f | f% |
| I | 33 | 100 | 0 | 0 | 5 | 15 | 4 | 12 | 3 | 9 | 18 | 55 | 33 | 100 |
| II | 10 | 100 | 2 | 20 | 5 | 50 | 5 | 50 | 4 | 40 | 7 | 70 | 10 | 100 |
| III | 18 | 100 | 4 | 22 | 2 | 11 | 15 | 30 | 16 | 89 | 16 | 89 | 18 | 100 |
| total | 61 | 100 | 6 | 11 | 12 | 21 | 24 | 39 | 23 | 37 | 41 | 66 | 61 | 100 |

**Table 3.**
*ERT methods by educational stages.*

| stage | II | III |
|---|---|---|
| I | B1: 0.048*<br>B2: 0.195<br>C1: 0.099<br>C2: 0.239<br>C3: 1.000 | B1: 1.000<br>B2: 0.035*<br>C1: 0.000*<br>C2: 0.000*<br>C3: 0.040* |
| II | | B1: 0.041*<br>B2: 1.000<br>C1: 0.259<br>C2: 0.034*<br>C3: 0.935 |

**P-value less than 0.05.*

**Table 4.**
*Pairwise comparisons of remote working methods by educational stage.*

$P_{B2}$ = 0.021, $P_{C1}$ = 0.000, $P_{C2}$ = 0.000, $P_{C3}$ = 0.046. We then used the Dunn-Bonferroni post-hoc method. The results of the pairwise comparisons are shown in **Table 4**.

Stage III teachers differ statistically significantly in several areas. For example, **Table 4** shows that they tend to use more strategies typical for distance learning (self-designed video explanations and video conferencing for different purposes).

On the other side of the spectrum are teachers at stage I. Both video explanations and video conferencing are statistically significantly lower than for the teachers at the other two stages.

## 4. Discussion

The results show that ERT methods used by Slovenian teachers were very diverse. Some teachers immediately switched effectively to distance learning. They prepared interactive materials, taught in video conferences, developed innovative ways of giving feedback and adapted lessons according to the specific needs of students. On the other hand, some teachers did not do so well. They needed more time. But there was no time during the pandemic. There was no time to train teachers to work with new ICT tools. There was no time for detailed instructions on how to work. That is why the spirit of solidarity came to life. Those teachers who knew helped colleagues who had not yet found themselves. Unfortunately, this assistance is by nature limited to smaller collectives (e.g., schools). Results suggest that secondary school mathematics teachers were more prone to adopt new ERT ways quickly. Indonesian secondary mathematics teachers faced a great challenge in using e-learning as a tool of instruction during school closures due to the COVID-19 pandemic. Their most significant barriers were at the student level, including student lack of knowledge and skill in e-learning use and their lack of access to devices and internet connection [7]. Similar barriers were also found in the Slovenian situation.

Our results are in line with a broad survey, the results of which were published by the Slovenian National Agency for Education [5]. In the study, more than 2200 Slovenian teachers were interviewed. In the subchapter on the organisation and implementation of distance education using digital technology in several places, secondary school teachers differ statistically significantly from elementary school teachers. However, this study does not provide insight into the differences between elementary school teachers. We believe that our results complement this aspect.

Nevertheless, [5] reports show that teaching was most demanding and stressful for elementary school teachers on the primary school level (educational stage I).

Moreover, they perceived less energy during distance learning than at teaching in the classroom. The most concerning fact is that only 2% of primary level teachers choose video lectures as the direct distance learning mode. The results also show that only around half of the primary teachers combined video lectures in the teaching process by adding written instructions. In addition, most primary level teachers think that they do not have a realistic insight into the achievements of students' goals at a distance. Students on the primary level also responded that they did not receive the teacher's explanations. Results revealed that explanations mainly were given to those students whose teachers have used video lectures or a combination of video lectures with written work instructions.

Based on the described results, we hypothesise that Slovenian learners were not treated according to the equity principle due to a lack of open educational resources (OER). There was an urgent need for an OER environment in the first wave allowing video sharing for all teachers and students. Therefore, a portal Razlagamo.si was established in Slovenia in March 2020 and is intended for mutual assistance in distance learning. The users are both students and (serving or future) teachers. It offers collected interactive materials for all elementary and secondary schools subjects and supports conversations when learners have problems. It was created on the initiative of all three faculties where University Maribor teachers are trained and result from voluntary work. More than 20 university teachers and more than 230 (serving or future) teachers take part. By the end of June 2020, the website's visitor counter registered more than 190,000 hits, about 800 video explanations were produced, and about 350 pupils and students were involved in supportive discussions.

The support point consists of two elements: video explanations and support conversations. Both elements develop understanding, a distinctive feature of *razlagamo.si* compared to other similar material repositories. In the crisis, it has become clear that synchronous teaching (live lectures for all pupils or students at the same time) is not always possible. Therefore, the learner needs also an asynchronous (pre-recorded) explanation. Such video explanation allows him/her to manage his own time independently (e.g., when and how much time he will devote to learning with video explanation). It also allows and individualised material procurement (e.g., repeated playback of individual video sections). For this reason, Razlagamo.si offers video explanations and synchronous communication about problems in a group or one-on-one conversations.

A Video explanation (VE) is an educational video that follows the principles of the method of explaining. The method of explaining or Socrates method has traditionally been one of the most widely used teaching methods. It is also a relatively effective teaching method in various fields [8] and approaches to teaching and learning, including e-learning [9]. Delić and Bećirović [10] define the Socrates method as "pedagogy that helps students critically reflect on their understanding of a particular issue with guided questions". In asynchronous use of this method, the teacher usually lets the students think about the answer for some time after the question is asked and then offers some of the expected (correct or incorrect) answers. The Socrates method used in an asynchronous VE follows similar principles. VE can additionally use multimedia tools (e.g., videos of natural phenomena), videos of virtual manipulators (e.g., virtual versions of experiments) or screencasting. Usually, a VE contains a combination of all the above elements. The VEs are intended for a reversed (flipped) classroom approach [11] based on conceptual teaching. Several studies suggest that flipped learning positively correlates with academic students' achievements in secondary [12] and elementary school [13].

VEs are short films that present the essence of the concept the student is learning interactively. With a VE, we focus the student on the essential elements of knowledge. Besides, the student can expand their knowledge with the help of interactive i-textbooks. VEs are contributed by active teachers from all over Slovenia and by students - future teachers from all three faculties. The added value of the Razlagamo.si lies in covering all compulsory subjects, except Slovenian language, both in elementary and secondary education. VEs have also been prepared for the general baccalaureate. There are also VEs by special education teachers, covering general psychological and unique education aspects such as learning, memory, motivation, etc.

It was shown that additional one-to-one support is necessary to build up high-quality knowledge, especially in mathematical and natural science subjects. The conversations occur in the MS Teams environment and represent asynchronous version of individualised teaching. Also, in supportive conversations, in which the student can find additional explanations, the future teachers' pay special attention to leading the students to solutions with tips and their activity. At the beginning of May 2020, the conversations covered more than 100 elementary and secondary school subjects, including music school topics. The specialised team also offers advice on general learning difficulties. Future teachers stem from different fields, from natural sciences and social sciences to psychologists and pedagogues.

Most VEs are for stage II. STEM fields are strongly dominated, especially mathematics and the highest number of VEs could be found for 12–15-year-old students [14]. Perhaps the STEM area is relatively better suited to teaching with videos. It is also possible that the subject area's specifics do not allow effective teaching without video explanations, or STEM teachers are more inclined to create videos than teachers of other fields. Whatever the reason, the study of videos for mathematics is vital for developing mathematics teaching, especially in the current situation where many schools are forced to work this way. More than a hundred mathematics topics (e.g., linear function, derivatives...) are offered for the entire educational vertical of mathematics, Ves are available in 63 (57%) topics. Mostly in topics that were in schools at the time of the COVID 19 lock-down. The Slovenian joint educational point Razlagamo.si is mainly in line with the recommendations of Chinese researchers [15] on how to ensure quality learning even during the outbreak of pandemic COVID -19. Additionally, it is in line with the system model MEET [16]. MEET is a system-oriented model [17] and provides a systematic model on planning, preparing, and evaluating response in an abrupt emergency as COVID-19 was.

## 5. Conclusions

The presented results will have important implications for student learning and the development of e-resources. We firmly believe that the age of the students is essential when creating video explanations. Unfortunately, research that would provide insight into younger students' characteristics in this area is still in its infancy. However, since it could happen that schools will be forced to address ERT for some time to come, we believe that research in this area is also welcome. While we agree that distance learning is not a good solution for younger students, we recognise that such learning could last for some students. Therefore, we hope that this work will help teachers who decide to implement ERT through video explanation.

We conclude with the following recommendations for the resumption of school operations in autumn 2021, based partly on Brown et al. [6]. First, according to the strategy for physical re-engagement at schools should:

- Recognise that the necessary input from parents to support learning at home goes beyond the physical provision of resources.

- Where full-time reconnection of a significant number is not going to be possible for safety or logistical reasons, plan for a blend of online and physical presence.

- Encourage universal full-time on-site attendance for pre-school to year three.

- Utilise direct and personalised invitations to specific vulnerable school students and their families/carers to see those students attend school and complement this group with invitations to a balanced cohort of students to reduce stigmatisation of specific groups and 'normalise' attendance.

- Invest in targeted and personalised learner engagement for students who are not physically attending and who cannot access online learning, are not engaging in education, or are at risk of disengaging over the short and long term.

- Invest in and support teachers to manage the increased workload of teaching both offline and online by providing additional staffing on a short-term basis: teachers, teacher assistants, and social/youth workers

- Design professional teacher training for skills and expertise in the creation of non-school-based learning strategies, such as high-quality online content, lower technology radio, and television content.

Razlagamo.si was designed as an open educational environment. Several resources commented on the importance of openness [18]. As we can see from the literature, obstacles to e-learning can involve several problems [19]. Technology, access to the internet, and the lack of an e-learning and assessment curriculum and tools for effective student assessment limit what teachers can teach [20]. The motivation for online learning, confidence in e-learning technology, and teachers' attitudes towards online learning influence how and how much a student will learn. All these barriers need to be considered when faced with an event such as a pandemic. Due to the exceptional success of the support point, we decided that the point will remain active after the end of the crisis. The Razlagamo.si model is also useful when only a part of the student population is involved in distance learning.

Future lines of research are two folded. We will try to overcome the language barrier of Razlagamo.si materials. We will upgrade and improve learning materials, translate these materials using advanced machine learning models to English (pivot language), include materials into the Learning management systems (LMS), and explore new models for use in classrooms in an international environment. We are aware of the low acceptance of the technology by teachers, so we will prepare explicit Instructional Principles for distance teaching and learning in cyber-flipped classroom pedagogy and additional instructions for adapting the learning paths in the LMS to the needs of the students.

The second research track will focus on designing a taxonomy of video lectures. The taxonomy of video explanations will be designed to help teachers choose the appropriate video explanation for their students. We will define a list of attributes that quality video lectures should have and categorise features according to several criteria (i.e., pedagogical, technical, needed for machine translation purposes...). We will summarise the various characteristics into several principles. Some principles are going to be more didactically oriented, probably the most important being the principle of interactivity, followed by the principle of generative activity, the principle of dynamic drawing and the principle of seductive details. Among the slightly more technical principles, which are also related to pedagogy, are: the principle of the perspective of the recording, the principle of the teacher's visibility, the principle of the teacher's emotional state, the principle of the gaze guidance, the principle of subtitles and the principle of the live composite of the recording.

Many educational institutions face a fall semester2021 that is either fully or partially online. Razlagamo.si is paving the road to engaging students with the content, providing collaboration, and creating community. The joint educational point will help teachers who prepare materials according to the principles of flipped learning even in a non-crisis situation (e.g., for sick students, student-athletes, students with another status).

## Author details

Alenka Lipovec[1,2]*, Blaž Zmazek[1] and Igor Pesek[1]

1 Faculty for Natural Sciences and Mathematics, University of Maribor, Slovenia

2 Faculty for Education, University of Maribor, Maribor, Slovenia

*Address all correspondence to: alenka.lipovec@um.si

## References

[1] Viner RM, Russel SJ, Croker H, Packer J, Ward J, Sansfield C, Booy R. School closure and management practices during coronavirus outbreaks including COVID-19: A rapid systematic review. The Lancet. Childs & Adolescent Health. 2020;**4**(5):397-404. DOI: 10.1016/S2352-4642(20)30095-X

[2] Coeckelbergh M. The postdigital in pandemic times: A comment on the Covid-19 crisis and its political epistemologies. Postdigital Science and Education. 2020;**2**. DOI: 10.1007/s42438-020-00119-2

[3] Trust T, Whalen J. Should teachers be trained in emergency remote teaching? Lessons learned from the COVID-19 pandemic. Journal of Technology and Teacher Education. 2020;**28**(2):189-199

[4] Armitage R, Nellums L. Considering inequalities in the school closure response to COVID-19. The Lancet Global Health. 2020;**8**(5):e644

[5] Rupnik VT, Preskar S, Silvar B, Zupanc GR, Kregar S, Holcer BA, et al. Analiza izobraževanja na daljavo v času epidemije Covid-19 v Sloveniji. Delno poročilo, julij 2020. Ljubljana: ZRSŠ; 2020. Available from: https://www.zrss.si/digitalnaknjiznica/IzobrazevanjeNaDaljavo/2/ [Accessed: 15 July 2021]

[6] Brown N, Te Riele K, Shelley B, Woodroffe J. Learning at Home during COVID-19: Effects on Vulnerable Young Australians. Independent Rapid Response Report. Hobart: University of Tasmania, Peter Underwood Centre for Educational Attainment; 2020. Available from: https://icponline.org/wp-content/uploads/2020/05/L-at-H-rapidresponsereport-30April2020-updated.pdf [Accessed: 15 July 2021]

[7] Mailizar M, Almanthari Z, Maulina S, Bruce S. Secondary school mathematics teachers' views on e-learning implementation barriers during the COVID-19 pandemic: The case of Indonesia. Eurasia Journal of Mathematics, Science and Technology Education. 2020;**16**(7):1-9. DOI: 10.29333/ejmste/8240

[8] Overholser JC. Guided guided discovery: A clinical strategy derived from the socratic method. International Journal of Cognitive Therapy. 2018;**11**(2):124-139. DOI: 10.1007/s41811-018-0017-x

[9] Liu Y. Using reflections and questioning to engage and challenge online graduate learners in education. Research and Practice in Technology Enhanced Learning. 2019;**14**(3):1-10. DOI: 10.1186/s41039-019-0098-z

[10] Delić H, Bećirović S. Socratic method as an approach to teaching. European Researcher Series A. 2016;**111**(10):511-517

[11] van Alten DC, Phielix C, Janssen J, Kester L. Effects of flipping the classroom on learning outcomes and satisfaction: A meta-analysis. Educational Research Review. 2019;**28**: 1-18. DOI: 10.1016/j.edurev.2019.05.003

[12] Wagner M, Gegenfurtner A, Urhahne D. Effectiveness of the flipped classroom on student achievement in secondary education: A meta-analysis. Zeitschrift für Pädagogische Psychologie. 2020;**35**(1):11-31. DOI: 10.1024/1010-0652/a000274

[13] Zhu G. Is flipping effective? A meta-analysis of the effect of flipped instruction on K-12 students' academic achievement. Educational Technology Research and Development. 2021;**69**:733-761. DOI: 10.1007/s11423-021-09983-6

[14] Pestano PM, Pesek I, Zmazek B, Lipovec A. Video explanations as u

useful digital of education in the COVID 19 situation. Journal of Elementary Education. 2020;**13**(4):395-412. DOI: 10.18690/rei.13.4.395-412.2020

[15] Huang RH, Liu DJ, Tlili A, Yang JF, Wang FF. Handbook on Facilitating Flexible Learning during Educational Disruption: The Chinese Experience in Maintaining Undisrupted Learning in COVID-19 Outbreak. Beijing: Smart Learning Institute of Beijing Normal University; 2020

[16] Lipovec A, Zmazek B, Pesek I. Testing razlagamo.si on models for emergency remote teaching. In: Izzivi in težave sodobne družbe. Rakičan: Ris; 2021

[17] Karalis T. Planning and evaluation during educational disruption: Lessons learned from COVID-19 pandemic for treatment of emergencies in education. European Journal of Education Studies. 2020;**7**(4):125-142. DOI: 10.1024/1010-0652/a000274

[18] Bozkurt A, Sharma RC. Emergency remote teaching in a time of global crisis due to CoronaVirus pandemic. Asian Journal of Distance Education. 2020;**15**(1):i-vi. DOI: 10.5281/zenodo.3778083

[19] Baseer SA. ICT and integration in education: A meta-analysis. Journal of Emerging Technologies and Innovative Research. 2019;**6**(6):117-122

[20] Scherer R, Teo T. Unpacking teachers' intentions to integrate technology: A meta-analysis. Educational Research Review. 2019;**27**:90-109. DOI: 10.1016/j.edurev.2019.03.001

Chapter 19

# Approaches to Teach Cataloguing Modules during Emergencies

*Madireng Monyela*


## Abstract

With reference to COVID-19 pandemic, the study investigated the emergent approaches to teaching and learning cataloguing modules at the institutions of higher learning. Cataloguing modules require face to face interactions between instructors and students for the explanation of concepts. The module involves the practical use of manuals and the application of standards which are skills that students should master. The closure of higher education institutions (HEIs) due to the outbreak of COVID-19 meant that the traditional approach to teach the cataloguing modules was inhibited. Although in some countries and in distance institutions cataloguing modules were already taught online even before the pandemic, their programs were planned as online education was the nature of their business and was not mandated by the pandemic experiences. The face to face institutions had to drastically make changes in their programs in order to continue with their mandates. The chapter explores measures taken by institutions of higher learning in order to continue with teaching and learning amidst COVID-19 pandemic.


**Keywords:** cataloguing education, COVID-19, education, emergency remote teaching, teaching and learning

## 1. Introduction

Cataloguing modules are part of the Library and Information Studies curriculum and has been included in the curriculum since the beginning of the discipline in the late nineteenth century [1]. There are four processes in the cataloguing workflow that completes the cataloguing modules, namely descriptive cataloguing, authority control, subject cataloguing and classification [2]. Descriptive cataloguing according to Lazarinis [3], deals with description of resources, identifying all the metadata that describes the information source in order to improve access of library sources. Authority control on the other hand, facilitates the control and standardization of bibliographic data [4]. Furthermore, subject analysis deals with the creation and representation of subject terms in the catalogue whereas classification deals with the allocation of specific notations that should serve as a shelving device [3]. Teaching all these processes requires the use of cataloguing standards that are recognised internationally and comprised of theory and hands-on.

Generally, cataloguing modules requires face to face interactions between instructors and students due to the practical components which complements theory [2]. Due to the disruptions caused by COVID-19 that among others led to the universities lockdown worldwide, teaching and learning had to be altered to continue with the university mandate and cataloguing modules were not exempted.

UNESCO [5] urged governments all around the world to take measures in order to support teaching and learning to the best possible extent [6]. Rafiu and Nwalo [7] observed that careers in librarianship are incomplete without a deep knowledge of cataloguing modules such as descriptive cataloguing, authority control, subject analysis and classification. Gourkova [8] believes the cataloguing librarians have been the cornerstone of library services for centuries in terms of knowledge organisation. The quality of their education highly influences their ability to effectively deal with the versatile challenges in the demanding field of knowledge management. However, Rafiu and Nwalo [7]; Rafiu [9], Mahlatji et al. [10] reported poor performance of cataloguing students. Elrod [11] opined that many library professionals do not understand cataloguing although it is a core module in several Library and Information Science (LIS) schools. If this is not taken care of, the profession could be in danger because cataloguing is an integral part of the value librarians add to society, without which there could be chaos in the organisation and retrieval of knowledge"

Moreover, Danskin [12], Morgan and Bowden [13] observed that there were fewer cataloguers in the USA and British libraries. In the UK and the USA, the cataloguing component in library education was diminishing and the faculty was aging as indicated by Morgan and Bowden [13]. They further observed that in 2007 it was predicted that 33% of cataloguers in the Library of Congress were to retire in 2010 and there was no evidence that the lost cataloguing posts would be filled or library schools were producing the next generation of cataloguers. Maphopha [14], Bowman [15], Warren [16], Mason [17] and Monyela [18] found few qualified cataloguers in the cataloguing agencies. Therefore, to preserve the cataloguing profession and to upturn cataloguers, cataloguing education should be supported and there should be strategies to teach and learn cataloguing modules beyond the traditional face to face classroom setup during emergencies and unforeseen circumstances to continue equipping students with necessary skills.

## 2. Context and issues

Due to the inequalities existing both within societies and among different countries, UNESCO concerned undertaking all the possible measures to continue with teaching and learning and not only the ones based on ICT (Information and Communication Technologies). The measures could include hi-tech, low tech and no tech solutions [19]. In agreement with their governments, the contact universities around the globe had to change their usual ways of teaching and learning. For example, the University of Patras in Patras, Greece managed to offer all the theoretical-type courses using a system of distance education, based on synchronous education supported by a teleconference software and asynchronous education of a Moodle type platform already available before the COVID crisis [19]. Jandric et al. [20] collected testimonies on teaching in the age of COVID-19. Jandric shared the Call for testimonies on Post Digital Science and Education social network sites and emailed it to the journal's mailing list. His study received 84 testimonies from 19 countries (USA, UK, China, India, Australia, New Zealand, Denmark, Sweden, Croatia, Canada, Spain, Nigeria, Finland, Ireland, Malta, Tanzania, Malaysia, Latvia and South Africa). The respondents from those different countries shared how they carried out teaching and learning during COVID-19. The testimonies around the world indicated that teaching and learning was moved to online using their Learning Management Systems, Zoom, Podcasts, Skype, Teams, video conferencing and other platforms where they could share videos and interact with students in the online space. Some instructors felt that online classes were more focused and tighter than in the face-to-face sessions however some experienced challenges related to lack of proper planning as they had to go online within short notice. Some who believed in facial expression could switch on their cameras while teaching so that they could have the sense of contact with their students, some did not want to switch on their cameras because they did not want students to see their private space, although they believed in facial expressions. However, in Tanzania and Nigeria it was reported that they encountered challenges of internet accessibility and electricity that made it impossible to move to online teaching. In South Africa it was reported that online teaching was adopted however they experienced unstable internet connectivity [20]. Saavedra [21] also suggested that it has been claimed that developed countries are at an advantage in initiating emergency remote teaching but this is not valid for every country.

Hodges et al. [22] differentiated between online instruction and emergency remote teaching, suggesting that the online teaching is mostly deliberate and involves a lot of planning. Remote teaching, on the other hand, is a temporary and abrupt shift to instructional delivery due to crises such as weather, war, or health. Remote teaching is not the same as planned online teaching. Therefore, remote teaching might be carried out differently in different contexts. For example, instruction can be delivered online but might also be provided through podcasts, couriered exercises for students and learners with no or limited access to internet or computers. While planned online teaching is characterized by different teaching modes such as fully online; blended and modes of communication such as synchronous or asynchronous where students could listen to the voice recorder or receive instructions on the email. Remote teaching may actually rely on or avoid technology for instructional purposes [22]. The main purpose behind remote teaching according to Bozkurt and Sharma [23] is to minimize spatial distance to ensure continuity of education, whereas for distance education, it is to minimize transactional and psychological distance to facilitate the continuity of teaching and learning. Bozkurt and Sharma [23] argue that while we are given opportunity to test online pedagogy, we should try to create a climate of empathy and care, and focus on different types of presence, such as teaching, cognitive and social presence and give focus to the students as whole human beings, their backgrounds, emotions, experiences and more importantly, their learning. "Before putting approaches into practice, we have to think about many variables, including target group, age range, technological infrastructure, and social and economic context" ([23], p. 3). Bozkurt et al. [24]; Wetzler [25] observed that, during the COVID-19 epidemic, the entire educational system needed a shift from their normal routines and create educational resources that could be shared among and within educational networks such as open educational resources (OERs) and open educational practices (OEPs). Bozkurt et al. [24] further observed that OERs and OEPs have played a significant role in ensuring the continuity of education even prior COVID. Therefore, stakeholders should also take efforts to reduce social injustice, inequality and inequity in meeting educational needs by producing and encouraging OERs. In the traditional business model such as publishing industry, learning materials like any other materials are copyrighted. During emergency situations, like the COVID-19 crisis, copyrighted learning materials can be an obstacle to delivering educational content since they require permission from or a payment to the copyright holder. Thus, initiatives to raise awareness and incentives as well as policies should be developed to encourage educators and other stakeholders to produce and use OER as a way to sustain OEP [23]. The cataloguing community including cataloguing educators, facilitator and cataloguing librarians should produce peer review OER and upload them online to use during the crises and prepare for the future. According to Jung and Hong [26], OERs are teaching, learning, and research resources that reside in the public domain or have been released under an intellectual property license that permits their free use or re-purposing by others. This includes, course materials, modules, lecture notes, exercises, podcasts, textbooks, videos, tests, assignments, software, full courses any other tools, materials, or techniques used to support access to knowledge. The concept of OER according to Atkins et al. [27] was initiated by the Education Program of the Hewlett Foundation in 2002 as a major component into its strategic plan to use Information Technology to increase access to high-quality educational content. Hewlett program officers were motivated to initiate the component after thoroughly examining learning materials and content for Kindergarten to grade 12 as well as tertiary levels and found poor quality and discrepancies in the content. They also observed that open information resources that were freely available on the internet were of widely varying quality. With rare exception, the available materials neither promoted enhanced learning nor incorporated the latest technological and pedagogical advances. Educational institutions and publishers, lack of quality assurance for the content, and information overload also impeded the educational impact. Therefore, Hewlett Foundation program wanted to catalyse universal access to and use of high-quality academic content on a global scale. The original goal of the OER was to use information technology to help equalize the distribution of high-quality knowledge and educational opportunities for individuals, faculty, and institutions within the United States and throughout the world [27]. On the other hand, Bonk et al. [28] are of the view that since the year 2000, the Massachusetts Institute of Technology (MIT) has been a leader in the use of OER with their Open Course Ware (OCW) program. They gained inspiration and confidence from the free software movement since 1983 and the development of an open content license in 1998. UNESCO [29] coined the term Open Educational Resources at the Forum of Impact of Open Courseware (OCW), and defined OER as the non-commercial study materials adopted by a learning group through the use of information and communication technologies.

Nipa and Kermanshachi [30] observed that, when students are unable to purchase print educational resources because of rising prices or due to the unwillingness to carry heavy physical books, their education is compromised. Therefore, OERs could come handy because they solve these problems by providing free study materials in electronic formats and medium such as text, voice or visual art. To assist the cataloguing education system further, vendors of standards and manuals used in cataloguing such as resource description and access (RDA) should also consider charging library schools less subscription fees of RDA toolkit. The library schools in Africa and other developing countries should also consider to form the consortium to buy cataloguing standards in groups and save on costs especially because those standards are developed in America and subscription charges are based on American Currency United Stated Dollar (USD). Libraries and library schools that have digitised copies of other cataloguing standards such as Dewey Decimal Classification Scheme (DDC) should also share them online. Although the Web Dewey is free for library schools and students, to access it they will need internet connection whereas digitised copies can be used without internet connections. In developing countries, the cataloguing community experience lack of stable internet connectivity. For instance, in Nigeria and Kenya, Ahonsi [31] reported that major cities, libraries, universities and schools as well as other facilities could go for days or weeks without internet connectivity, in that case the cataloguers and library schools and students could not access RDA toolkit because it is accessible through the internet. Teaching and learning will then be affected negatively. Moreover, although there is free scanned full set of DDC edition 20 online, the library schools should share the costs and digitize the latest edition DDC 23 for the students to use while they are learning from home and cannot access the campus to collect the print DDC due to COVID-19 protocols put in place by the institutions of higher learning in order to control the spread of the deadly pandemic. The same should apply to other standards such as Library of Congress Subject Headings, Sears lists of subject headings or any other cataloguing standard used. During this time, it is more important to build support communities. Therefore, all stakeholders such as educators, psychologists, sociologists, therapists, economists, entrepreneurs and others should collaborate to offer better and timely solutions. For example, in some countries like South Africa, the government has initiated different methods such as food parcels to the poor, government temporary grant to the unemployed, and decrease on the repo rate amongst others, to aid the citizens to alleviate poverty and to survive during the pandemic. Vendors should also do the same by supporting higher education with prescribed learning materials such as cataloguing standards in the case of cataloguing education. Bozkurt and Sharma [23] opine that "we should remember, when things go back to normal, people will not remember the educational content delivered, but they will remember how they felt, how we cared for them, and how we supported them." Therefore the education system in general should support students and understand their stress, trauma and uncertainties because, COVID-19 has also affected individuals both emotionally, psychologically, socially and economically. Some students may not have money to buy data even though they have good internet connections. Nevertheless, emergency remote education is about surviving in a time of crisis with all resources available, including offline and/or online [24]. Bali [32] is of the view that, due to the distressing impact of this global crisis, stakeholders such as educators, parents, government ministries should prioritize the issues of care, empathy, emotional and psychological support to all and should not be limited to the classroom setting or only targeted towards students, but also embodied in educational policies and decision-making that impact educators, parents and staff as well.

## 2.1 Different approaches for cataloguing education during emergencies

Bozkurt et al. [24] looked at a global outlook to the interruption of education due to COVID-19 pandemic in a time of uncertainty and crisis using a collective case study design from different countries across the globe. Their study was comprehensive in nature and involved many co-authors and presented a total of 31 cases from 31 countries (China, India, Japan, Philippines, Russia, Saudi Arabia, South Korea, Algeria, Egypt, Ghana, Kenya, Namibia, South Africa, Uganda, France, Greece, Ireland, Romania, Spain, Sweden, the Netherlands, Turkey, the United Kingdom, Australia, Canada, United States of America, Argentina, Brazil, Mexico, Peru and Uruguay). Bozkurt et al. [24]'s findings revealed that while some countries provided multiple entry points such as hi tech, low tech and no tech choices and different paths for learners to follow, some countries with reliable internet connectivity relied heavily on synchronous and asynchronous online technologies. Many countries focussed their efforts on providing digital content or materials, both from Kindergarten to tertiary education levels, particularly those with the existing lecture or content-centric practices. In addition to online technology-centric solutions, some countries also used technologies popular from earlier generations of distance education such as to courier printed materials, lecture notes, activities, exercises, workbook and textbooks to students and also use radio and TV channels to deliver educational contents. These mass communication systems were important in many countries to deal with digital divide and knowledge access issues, and to address concerns that no learners are left behind. Due to the geographical settings in different countries cataloguing instructors should consider sending tutorials to students using Podcast, videos and other materials to support students learning.

Bozkurt et al. [24] are of the view that no single technology is superior to other ones and different technologies, if used purposefully and adequately, can serve well to facilitate education. Bozkurt et al. [24] further found that "online emergency remote education, LMSs such as Moodle, Canvas, Blackboard, Edmodo, Google Classroom, etc., synchronous communication and conferencing tools such as Zoom, Microsoft Teams, Google Meet, Webex, etc. and live broadcasting features of social networking sites such as Facebook Live, Instagram Live, etc. were widely used. In countries, where broadband internet was partly available, or the necessary infrastructure was not available, mobile technologies were used to communicate and deliver educational content. In such cases, it was generally observed that social networking and instant communication tools such as Facebook, WhatsApp, University APP, etc. were used to create communication channels among students, parents, educators, and school administrators. Such an observation implies the importance of freely available tools and further highlights the main ingredients of social learning, that is, communication. In addition to the above technology-centric observations, the change in pedagogy is worth mentioning because, in contrast to the visible impact of the technology, the invisible impact of pedagogies is argued to be deeper and long-term". It is not the first time in contemporary history, learners and parents in the case of primary to high school are given such a great agency and responsibility for their learning. McCracken [33] learned that during the outbreak of Spanish flu pandemic, schools in California was using the telephone, a technology that was only 40 years old at the time as an educational device. Furthermore, Te Kura [34] also learned that during polio epidemic in New Zealand in 1948, which closed all of that country's schools, they opted for traditional correspondence education and used postal services to send lessons to every household, as well as using educational radio to broadcast lessons. Moreover, Barbour et al. [35] reported that during the H1N1 influenza pandemic of 2009, a number of schools in Bolivia experienced high levels of absenteeism, therefore they developed their own virtual classrooms and trained teachers on how to teach in that environment. Again in Hong Kong, Alpert [36] described how online learning helped to facilitate continued access to instruction in 2003 when schools had to close due to the SARS outbreak. In many countries, inflexible curriculum was rejected, willingly and by necessity, its so-called robust assessment and evaluation approaches and, instead, applied approaches based on meaning-making and progress and defined by the values and interests of learners and parents [24]. On the other hand, Barbour et al. [37] are of the view that the rapid approach necessary for emergency remote teaching may diminish the quality of education. A full-course development project can take months when done properly. However the education system did not have enough time to prepare, train facilitators and students, there was a need to "just get it online" as the hard lockdowns had already consumed time when the education sector reopened. There was not much time dedicated to developing a quality course. Online courses created in this way should not be mistaken for long term solutions but accepted as a temporary solution to an immediate problem. Lesson learned from the previous studies is that although many countries resorted to emergency remote teaching, the process has required a huge effort from all participants (teachers, students, parents and administrators), as well as very creative solutions. Apart from technological divide, lack of planning, coordination, communication and management also placed a heavy burden on students, parents and teachers. Therefore, hence cataloguing curriculum is global, the facilitators and students could plan for the future and form blogs and vlogs to share ideas globally by inviting other institutions to participate on the blogs. These platforms may be sustained and used to share ideas and benchmark with other institutions. Series of formal and informal trainings on how to effectively use any available technology should be offered to students. In cases where the physical libraries (academic, public, special) could not open, the government could install the information cubicles that uses renewable energy sources such as solar, wind, hydroelectric and other fossil energy to overcome the challenges of electricity interruption, especially in developing countries where people experience electricity load shedding, unstable network connection and could not afford internet connectivity. These could help to lessen the problems of social divide and inequality in education. Furthermore, Barbour et al. [37] suggests that schools and institutions should conduct research and collect data about the students' needs and experiences during remote learning. The findings will help the education systems to prepare in case the other pandemic could be experienced, rather than to wait and take drastic measures when the pandemic of any nature hits again. The institutions should also set up training plans for students, facilitators and administrators as well as to plan for the allocation of resources such as laptops, electronic devices that are needed to support remote education, they should also plan for digitization projects, to digitize cataloguing standards in the case of cataloguing education, those digitized standards may also be used during normal face to face instruction to avoid carrying "scaring" big books and sharing the books. Anecdotal research revealed that some cataloguing students are intimidated by the big books (LCSH and DDC) in particular, looking at the size of the books they think they may not understand the content in those books and go to class already discouraged and convinced that the modules are difficult. In that case students will have their own electronic copies that they can keep for referral even after they graduated as they do not have to return them at the end of the course for other students to use like with print books. Exchange teaching programs among the institutions could also help when coming to planning for the future. Institutions could learn from each other, some effective strategies such as webinars, blogs, vlogs, etcetera may be sustained and continue to be used even post COVID, that will save costs for transport, booking of venues and food when people need to meet and share ideas. Encourage student's mentors and supplementary instructions among students. Some students are able to cope while some are not. Those who are coping may be encouraged to assist others with activities and assignments. Furthermore, Barbour et al. [37] opined that legislation should be developed to require educational institutions to develop a digital learning framework and policies. Effective evaluation strategies in practical modules such as cataloguing may be applied.

### 2.2 Challenges of cataloguing education during emergencies

Omodan et al. [38] found limited educational resources to be the major challenges of rural institutions in South Africa. Furthermore, the author of this chapter observed that the majority of students enrolled with rural universities in South Africa are from the rural villages that are affected by poverty, do not have much development with regard to infrastructures and ICT. Some areas do not have communication towers due to their remote locations. Omodan [39] also found that "the students that are mostly found in rural institutions are students who are from poor and underprivileged backgrounds. Because of such, they don't have computers or laptops at home, let alone space and a healthy environment." Moreover, Wahab and Tyasari [40] found lack of managerial and professional efficacy toward emergency management in the university system, that could also contravene the postulation of United Nations Office for Disaster Risk Reduction (UNISDR) that advocate for all-inclusive alternative to development to be put in place to mitigate every unforeseen disaster to ensure holistic and sustainable development in rural organisations including university systems. Furthermore, Omodan found that rural universities in South Africa experienced limited educational resources, lack of funds and lack of social and economic viability to sustain technological improvement, shortages of computers, Lack of access to ICT facilities by students from their homes, lack of emergency response strategies, lack of ICT skills from both facilitators and students, network problems. Similarly Ferri et al. [41]; Trust and Whalen [42] found unreliability of internet connections, lack of necessary electronic devices, lack of digital skills, and lack of work physical spaces at home, lack of support from parents and administrators. At the University of Wisconsin–Milwaukee, Miller et al. [43] reported cataloguing student's lack of ICT skills when offering their online courses even though they were running a planned program. Moreover, another anecdotal research at University A in South Africa that offers distance education revealed lack of students ICT skills, unstable internet connection, lack of data, lack of gadgets among other challenges. Once more, another anecdotal research in different face to face universities in South Africa revealed lack of students and staff ICT skills, lack of data, lack of gadgets such as laptops, electricity load shedding, unstable internet connections, and lack of enough cataloguing standards. During face to face instructions students were sharing those standards in class and their residences, it was now difficult for all the students to access the standards as they were geographically spread and learning from their respective homes. The other challenges were no access to RDA and no access to libraries and information centres when moving to remote learning.

## 3. Methodology

This chapter applied the qualitative research approach based on document content analysis extracted from different information sources such as books, journals, databases, conference proceedings, internet and world catalogue. Taylor [44] affirm that the qualitative research approach is significant in addressing contextual studies of this nature. It means literature could be interpreted based on the search of the researcher on key concepts of the chosen topic. The researcher searched the literature using the key concepts of the study such as different approaches to education during emergencies, challenges experienced by the education sector especially the institution of higher learning during emergencies. This was done to have a better understanding of the approaches towards cataloguing education during emergencies. The literature was then interpreted and conclusions were drawn from the results.

## 4. Concluding remarks

Lesson learned from this study is that, although all sectors and institutions of higher learning were affected by the pandemic, there is no one size fits all solution to respond to emergencies and to continue with quality teaching and learning. Some institutions are more vulnerable than the other, therefore schools and institutions of higher learning should learn from each other and create their tailor made programmes to suit their needs. Some may use high tech, low tech or no tech. The Library and Information Science schools should work collectively and share the costs of subscription and digitization of cataloguing standards to afford the students the opportunity to learn from home as previously suggested in this chapter. Concerning the challenges of ICT skills, LIS curriculum should include computer and ICT courses to afford students with skills. Instructors should also go through formal ICT trainings and exchange programmes with other institutions. Furthermore due to other challenges reported in this chapter, the cataloguing instructors may create the podcast and video tutorials that should be accessed by students. Rural universities may also develop learning packages such as printed materials, videos, etcetera and send to students. Supplementary instruction (SI) model should also be imposed in cataloguing education. (SI) "is an academic support model developed by Deanna Martin at the University of Missouri–Kansas City (UMKC) in 1973 that uses peer-assisted study sessions to improve student retention and success within targeted historically difficult courses" ([45], p. 23). On the issue of assessment, different strategies such as portfolios should be imposed. Gaytan and McEwen [46] are of the view that effective assessment techniques associated with online instructions could include projects, portfolios, self-assessments, peer evaluations, and weekly assignments with immediate feedback. Instructors should design activities that promote student interactions and build a sense of community among students and faculty. Boyle et al. [47] opined that online assessment should include development of realistic scenarios for learning, alignment of learning objectives with realistic scenarios, use of software as soon as possible, availability of online mentors as well as SI and tutors. Although the above mentioned studies were carried out long ago, and were imposed in the planned online programs, emergency remote teaching may learn from them. Lau et al. [48] implemented concept mapping assessment in chemistry modules, indicating that concept mapping has a long history of application in science education and professional development. Cataloguing education may also use concept mapping assessment in the computer laboratory using "split lab" as suggested by [48] in order to curb the spread of the virus among the students, where students could practically generate online catalogues on the computer using Senayan Library Management System (SLiMS) a free and open source Library Management System or any other library system. With strong internet connections students can take the assessment remotely.

## Author details

Madireng Monyela
University of Limpopo, South Africa

*Address all correspondence to: jane.monyela@ul.ac.za; madirengm@gmail.com

## References

[1] Snow K, Hoffman GL. What makes an effective cataloging course? A study of the factors that promote learning. Library Resources & Technical Services. 2015;**59**(4):187-199

[2] Monyela M. Cataloguing education in the midst of the coronavirus (COVID-19): The author's perspectives. Library Philosophy and Practice. 2020;**1**:1-11

[3] Lazarinis F. Cataloguing and Classification: An Introduction to AACR2, RDA, DDC, LCC, LCSH and MARC 21 Standards. Amsterdam: Chandos Publishing; 2014

[4] Casalini M. The future of bibliographic services in light of new concepts of authority control. JLIS.it. 2022;**13**(1):107-115

[5] UNESCO. COVID-19 Impact on Education. UNESCO Institute for Statistics Data; 2020. Available from: https://en.unesco.org/covid19/educationresponse

[6] Owusu-Fordjour C, Koomson CK, Hanson D. The impact of covid-19 on learning—The perspective of the Ghanaian student. European Journal of Education Studies. 2020;**7**(3):88-101

[7] Rafiu J, Nwalo KIN. Effect of English Language proficiency on students' performance in cataloguing and classification courses in polytechnic-based library schools in Nigeria. International Journal of Library and Information Science. 2016;**8**(6):54-61

[8] Gourkova H. Education for library cataloguing: International perspectives. Library Management. 2007;**28**(6/7):437-439

[9] Rafiu J. The effect of attitude on student's academic performance in cataloguing and classification course in Nigerian Polytechnics. In: Proceedings of the 2020 The 3rd International Conference on Information Science and System. 2020. pp. 198-203

[10] Mahlatji M, Maphopha K, Dikotla M. Teaching and learning of classification module: Experiences at University of Limpopo (UL). Paper presented at Collaboration, Community in Session S12 – Classification and Indexing. Subject Access: Unlimited Opportunities; IFLA WLIC 2016 – Columbus, OH – Connections; 11-12 August 2016; Columbus, Ohio, USA. 2016

[11] Elrod JM. The case for cataloguing education. The Serial Librarian. 2008;**55**(102):1-10

[12] Danskin A. Tomorrow never knows: The end of cataloguing? IFLA Journal. 2007;**33**(3):205-220

[13] Morgan J, Bawden D. Teaching knowledge organization: Educator, employer and professional association perspectives. Journal of Information Science. 2006;**32**(2):108-115

[14] Maphopha KA. The training of cataloguers in university libraries in South Africa [M.Bibl. thesis]. Department of Information Science; University of Pretoria; 2000. Available from: http://www.netd.ac.za [Accessed: 14 November 2015]

[15] Bowman JH. Education and training for cataloguing and classification in the British Isles. Cataloging & Classification Quarterly. 2006;**41**(3-4):309-333

[16] Warren J. Directors' views of the future of cataloguing in Australia and New Zealand: A survey. Australian Academic & Research Libraries. 2007;**38**(4):239-251

[17] Mason MK. Automation: Has it deprofessionalized the work of

cataloguing librarians?. 2015. Available from: Moyak.com/papers/automating-cataloging.html

[18] Monyela MJ. Cataloguing practices from creation to use: A study of Cape Town Metropolitan Libraries in Western Cape South Africa [PhD thesis]. South Africa: University of Kwa Zulu Natal; 2019

[19] Karalis T, Raikou N. Teaching at the times of COVID-19: Inferences and implications for higher education pedagogy. International Journal of Academic Research in Business and Social Sciences. 2020;**10**(5):479-493

[20] Jandric et al. Teaching in the age of Covid 19: Testimonials. Postdigital Science and Education. 2020;**2**: 106-1230

[21] Saavedra J. Educational challenges and opportunities of the coronavirus (COVID-19) pandemic. World Bank Blogs. 2020. Available from: https://blogs.worldbank.org/education/educational challenges-and-opportunities-COVID-19-pandemic [Accessed: 20 January 2021]

[22] Hodges CB, Moore S, Lockee BB, Trust T, Bond MA. The difference between emergency remote teaching and online learning. 2020. Available from: https://vtechworks.lib.vt.edu/handle/10919/104648 [Accessed: 20 January 2021]

[23] Bozkurt A, Sharma RC. Emergency remote teaching in a time of global crisis due to oronaVirus pandemic. Asian Journal of Distance Education. 2020;**15**(1):i-vi. DOI: 10.5281/zenodo.3778083

[24] Bozkurt A, Jung I, Xiao J, Vladimirschi V, Schuwer R, Egorov G, et al. A global outlook to the interruption of education due to COVID-19 pandemic: Navigating in a time of uncertainty and crisis. Asian Journal of Distance Education. 2020;**15**(1):1-126

[25] Wetzler J. Leveraging OER for COVID-19 response efforts and international partnerships. Creative Commons. 2020. Available from: https://creativecommons.org/2020/06/01/leveraging-oer-for-covid-19-response-efforts-and-long-term-international-partnerships

[26] Jung I, Hong S. Faculty members' instructional priorities for adopting OER. The International Review of Research in Open and Distributed Learning. 2016;**17**(6):28-43

[27] Atkins DE, Brown JS, Hammond AL. A Review of the Open Educational Resources (OER) Movement: Achievements, Challenges, and New Opportunities. Vol. 164. Mountain View: Creative Common; 2007

[28] Bonk CJ, Lee MM, Kou X, Xu S, Sheu FR. Understanding the self-directed online learning preferences, goals, achievements, and challenges of MIT OpenCourseWare subscribers. Educational Technology & Society. 2015;**18**(2):349-365

[29] UNESCO. Forum on the impact of open courseware for higher education in developing countries: Final report. 2002. Available from: CI-2002/CONF.803/CLD.1

[30] Nipa TJ, Kermanshachi S. Assessment of open educational resources (OER) developed in interactive learning environments. Education and Information Technologies. 2020;**25**(4):2521-2547

[31] Ahonsi A. Resource Description and Access (RDA) Handbook for Facilitating the Understanding of RDA Rules by Librarians and Catalogers in English Speaking Countries in Sub-Saharan Africa. Certificate of Advanced Study (CAS) Certificate of Advanced Study.

Urbana: School of Library and Information Science, University of Illinois; 2014

[32] Bali M. Care is not a fad: Care beyond COVID-19. Reflecting Allowed. 2020. Available from: https://blog.mahabali.me/pedagogy/critical-pedagogy/care Is not afad care-beyond—covid-19/

[33] McCracken H. Before Zoom and coronavirus, how the telephone became the 20th century's most successful remote-learning technology for homebound students. The 74. 2020. Available from: https://www.the74million.org/article/how-the-telephone-became-the-20th-centurys-most-successful-remote-learning-technology-for-homebound-students

[34] Te Kura. Who we are: Our history. 2018. Available from: https://www.tekura.school.nz/about-us/who-we-are/our-his

[35] Barbour MK, Brown R, Hasler Waters L, Hoey R, Hunt J, Kennedy K, Ounsworth C, Powell A, Trimm T. Online and blended learning: A survey of policy and practice from K-12 schools around the world. International Association for K-12 Online Learning. 2011. Available from: https://aurora-institute.org/resource/online-and-blended-learning-a-survey-of-policy-and-practice-from-k-12-schools-around-the-world/

[36] Alpert. Online education in Hong Kong. In: Barbour MK, Hasler Waters L, Hunt J, editors. Online and Blended Learning: Case Studies from K-12 Schools Around the World. Vienna, VA: International Association for K-12 Online Learning; 2011. pp. 37-59

[37] Barbour MK, LaBonte R, Hodges C, Moore S, Lockee B, Trust T, Kelly K. Understanding pandemic pedagogy: Differences between emergency remote, remote, and online teaching. State of the Nation: K-12 e-Learning in Canada; 2020. Available from: https://vtechworks.lib.vt.edu/handle/10919/101905

[38] Omodan BI, Tsotetsi CT, Dube B. Decolonising rural-urban dichotomy in South Africa: An asset-based approach. Progressio: South African Journal for Open and Distance Learning Practice. 2019;**41**(1):1-17

[39] Omodan BI. The vindication of decoloniality and the reality of COVID-19 as an emergency of unknown in rural universities. International Journal of Sociology of Education. 2020;**special issue**:1-26

[40] Wahab A, Tyasari R. Entrepreneurial leadership for university leaders: A futuristic approach for Pakistani HEIs. Asia Pacific Management Review. 2020;**25**:54-63

[41] Ferri F, Grifoni P, Guzzo T. Online learning and emergency remote teaching: Opportunities and challenges in emergency situations. Societies. 2020;**10**(4):86

[42] Trust T, Whalen J. Emergency remote teaching with technology during the COVID-19 pandemic: Using the whole teacher lens to examine educator's experiences and insights. Educational Media International. 2021;**28**(2):189-199

[43] Miller SJ, Lee H-L, Olson HA, Smiraglia RP. Online cataloging education at the University of Wisconsin–Milwaukee. Cataloging & Classification Quarterly. 2012;**50**(23):110-126

[44] Taylor B. Qualitative critical methodologies and post-modern influences. In: Taylor B, Kermode S, Roberts K, editors. Research in Nursing and Health Care: Evidence for Practice. 3rd ed. Australia: Nelson; 2007. pp. 236-329

[45] Burmeister SL. Supplemental instruction: An interview with Deanna Martin. Journal of Developmental Education. 1996;**20**(1):22-26

[46] Gaytan J, McEwen BC. Effective online instructional and assessment strategies. The American Journal of Distance Education. 2007;**21**(3):117-132

[47] Boyle SLT, Kolosh K, L'Allier J, Lambrecht J. Thompson NETg's blended-learning model: The next generation of corporate and school-based learning. The Delta Pi Epsilon. 2003;**45**(3):145-161

[48] Lau PN, Chua YT, Teow Y, Xue X. Implementing alternative assessment strategies in chemistry amidst COVID-19: Tensions and reflections. Education Sciences. 2020;**10**(11):323

Chapter 20

# Tensions, Challenges, and Resistance among Academic Mothers during the COVID-19 Pandemic

*Gabriela Rubilar Donoso, Catherine A. LaBrenz and Caterine Galaz Valderrama*

## Abstract

This chapter presents a reflection of the processes through which academic mothers have reconciled work-life balance during the COVID-19 pandemic. Prior research has evidenced gender disparities in academia, with lower proportions of female faculty as rank increases. During the pandemic, academic mothers have encountered intensified productive and reproductive responsibilities. As three academic mothers, we engaged in autobiographical interviews and conducted an analysis of these narratives across diverse points during the COVID-19 pandemic. Three main themes emerged from the analysis: (1) *bodies that produce and reproduce*; (2) *the triple shift of academic mothers;* and (3) *resistance and change.* Implications for research and policy are explored.

**Keywords:** academic mothers, gender disparities, triple shift, COVID-19 pandemic, transformations in academia

## 1. Introduction

This chapter explores the experiences of reconciling work and family life among academic mothers during the COVID-19 pandemic, through an analysis of narratives that we constructed from our own lives. These narratives were constructed through the use of self-interviews, conducted in the context of remote, academic work during the shelter-in-place orders that emerged during the COVID-19 pandemic. Even before the pandemic, women in academia faced tensions between production and reproduction. Traditionally, academic careers have followed a linear trajectory in which productivity is rewarded over time [1, 2]. To be promoted, academics must meet competitive criteria related to research, teaching, and service. These criteria are transnational and have been exacerbated by neoliberal universities [3, 4]. This has led to a colorblind approach to ongoing disparities, in turn maintaining barriers to academic careers among mothering academics [5, 6]. As many of the challenges related to work-life balance have been exacerbated by the COVID-19 pandemic, this chapter explores the narratives of three academic mothers and the tensions and resistance they have displayed since March 2020.

## 2. COVID and transformations in academia across the globe

In the first 3 months of 2020, people across the globe experienced disruptions to their daily routines because of the COVID-19 pandemic and subsequent restrictions. By April 2020, more than 185 countries had closed schools and/or changed to remote-learning, from preschool to higher education [7]. In parallel, remote work became common to comply with shelter-in-place or other sanitary measures to prevent the spread of COVID-19. In academia, remote work was already an option for some research or administrative tasks but expanded greatly as the pandemic worsened.

Nonetheless, these changes were met with resistance from some students and university administration. For example, concerns were raised about issues with internet connectivity. As the pandemic continued, other concerns were raised about a possible gendered impact of COVID-19 on academia [8, 9]. On the one hand, remote work has allowed some advantages such as more flexible schedules and reduction in risk of getting COVID-19. On the other hand, as schools closed and parents became responsible for overseeing their children's remote education, gender inequities became apparent. For example, initial researchers have found that the lack of separation of work and family space has led to challenges setting boundaries and productivity [10, 11]. Furthermore, academic mothers have experienced a triple shift in which they must navigate domestic tasks, work, and childcare [12, 13]. Indeed, multiple studies have found that the proportion of female-authored publications has decreased since the pandemic began [14–16]. Thus, the pandemic has exacerbated already-existing disparities [17], such as tenure and promotion opportunities [18, 19].

One possible explanation for the gendered impact of the pandemic on academics may be due to the lack of separate work spaces. The loss of a separate work space, such as an office, laboratory, or meeting rooms, has affected women academics more than men [20]. In addition to losing the physical space, academics have also missed out on opportunities to build community and collegiality. This has reinforced the notion of individuality and survival and intensified neoliberal practices and policies within academia [21].

Neoliberal practices and policies emerged four decades ago and have led to *academic capitalism* [22]. Through academic capitalism, universities view trajectories through a lens of individualism [23, 24]. Under this lens, academics guide their careers based on standards that require colleagues to compete for limited resources (e.g., awards, grants) [4, 17, 21].

### 2.1 Academia and the gender gap

Researchers across the globe have evidenced a gender gap in academia [4, 25–28]. Robust evidence suggests that female academics publish less, are promoted less, and tend to have more interruptions in their trajectories [29–35]. Indeed, there tends to be a horizontal segregation among disciplines and a vertical segregation in promotion processes [21, 24, 36–38]. In parallel, the dichotomous nature of academic work into teaching-administration or research-publications may also contribute to the gender gap [36].

Academic capitalism, and specifically, competitiveness and individualistic practices, have been observed across national state entities as well. A recent analysis concluded that there was a need to change policies to recognize and value academic trajectories from an anti-sexist lens [39]. At the beginning of an academic career, women may encounter barriers to engage globally as research has found that female academics travel less and may have fewer opportunities to build professional networks. At the mid-career level, women academics tend to have more time dedicated to administration and teaching, which impact the time they can dedicate to research and scholarship. This in turn impacts tenure and promotion opportunities, which often are based heavily on research and scholarship production. At the senior-level, there is a low proportion of women who retire after achieving full professorships or other high-level administrative positions (e.g., deans or provost).

A recent report by the National Agency for Research and Development (ANID) documented gender gaps across doctoral programs and academic careers. In Chile, females are least represented in public universities (around 40%). Across public and private universities and across age groups, male academics hold more academic positions than females. In parallel, for each female-led project that is submitted for federal funding, there are 1.5 male-led projects, a disparity that carries over to awards of funding [40].

In this context, motherhood in academia does not fit or align. By placing the responsibility for work and motherhood on the individual, it is often reported as a barrier to mobility and that can cause delays in academic trajectories of mothers [27, 37].

### 2.2 COVID-19, motherhood, and care

Before the COVID-19 crisis, women constantly faced tensions from horizontal and vertical segregation [41]. Across disciplines, the gender gap has often been conceptualized as a *glass ceiling,* in which there is a barrier that prohibits females access from top positions [37]. The glass ceiling pushes women away from top positions (both prestige-wise and pay-wise) within academia. Difficulties in obtaining top positions may also arise due to ongoing disparities in domestic work and childcare, which continue to fall disproportionately on women, and may impact tenure and promotion trajectories.

The COVID-19 pandemic intensified disadvantages that mothering academics face, while in many ways, it opened up possibilities for their male colleagues. The marketization and neoliberalization of academia create certain metrics of excellence [42]. These metrics have not changed despite the ongoing impact of the pandemic, forcing mothering academics to prioritize the demands of their child(ren) or productivity. The effects of these decisions will have long-term repercussions as research productivity has stagnated and scholarship has decreased.

Notably, mothering academics are pressured by gendered roles that promote *intensive mothering* as well as work productivity and achievement. These gendered norms are different in male academics, from whom society almost exclusively measures success by work productivity and achievement [41]. Even before the pandemic, mothering academics dedicated less time to scientific production, largely due to domestic tasks. This has only been amplified and exacerbated by the COVID-19 pandemic. Therefore, mothering academics have been affected by a triple shift of triple expectations: work excellence at the university, excellence in mothering, and excellence in domestic tasks and chores.

Over time, academic mothers have been subjected to dominant discourse and norms of academic institutions. Among mothering academics, dominant discourse includes intensifying work expectations, gendered demands involving being a "good mother," and a cultural value on individual success and merit. This leads to a polarization between one's public work identity and one's private, invisible family work. Despite these tensions, we also see resistance and solidarity among mothering academics [37].

## 3. Methods

This study used a qualitative approach that allowed for an in-depth and flexible exploration of reconciling tensions among academic mothers during the pandemic [43]. We used a biographical approach so that the academic mothers themselves could guide understanding and interpreting the social conditions they had experienced [44–46].

Using this approach, we explored the lived experiences of three mothering academics during the COVID-19 pandemic. We focused on how they reconciled tensions from the triple shift of work life, childcare, and domestic chores, along with uncertainty from the pandemic. All three mothering academics worked at research-intensive universities that had high expectations for research and scholarship productivity. The autobiographical narratives were constructed as part of an auto-interview [44]. Auto-interviews are a technique that are used in qualitative research; in this study we followed the structure proposed by several experts [44, 47–49] who propose the use of auto-interviews in research to emphasize researcher reflexivity. Often, this technique is used in combination with biographical interviews, and has been used in prior studies [13, 50–52]. In the analysis presented in this chapter, we used fragments from auto-interviews of the three academic mother researchers and analysis of narratives that emerged from the federally-funded FONDECYT project 1,190,257.

The scientificity of this technique is based on the epistemology that guides the research process. The application of the auto-interview is based on the contribution it can make to knowledge of how an individual experienced and perceived a specific event. While this technique has been questioned on occasion, some initial critics such as Bourdieu [53] applied the technique later on, recognizing its value. That being said, we do acknowledge the limitations of auto-interviews, including a more singular, unique focus on an individual process that creates a theoretical-reflexive dialog, instead of generalizable results [54].

Each mothering academic completed three auto-interviews across different phases of the pandemic, and reflected different mothering experiences, family compositions, and academic trajectories. Two of the mothering academics were in Chile, while the third was in the United States. Both Chile and the United States share similar types of government and handled the pandemic response in similar ways: through increasing remote work opportunities and responding with shelter-in-place orders.

From the constructed narratives, we developed processes to reflect and write collaboratively [51, 52, 55] and deconstruct the disruption that COVID-19 has had on our work and family lives. As we constructed our auto-interviews, we were guided by a Feminist lens to consider a critique of emerging gendered roles [56].

## 4. Results: bodies that produce and reproduce

There were three main themes that emerged from the reflection and analysis of auto-interviews: (1) *bodies that produce and reproduce;* (2) *the triple shift in mothering academics*; and (3) *tactics for resistance and change.* All three of the themes reflected experiences of all three academic mothers as they reconciled tensions from disruptions to work, family, and household life during the pandemic. Consistent with other qualitative research, our results were validated through reflection on the research process, saturation of themes, and a triangulation of these auto-interviews with 20 additional interviews that were conducted as part of project FONDECYT 1190257 and an extensive literature review.

### 4.1 Theme 1: bodies that produce and reproduce

The first theme was *bodies that produce and reproduce,* and related to contradicting demands of production and reproduction among mothering academics. The mothering academics reported feeling tension to conform to *intensive mothering* [57] through expectations that they would accompany, educate, and provide stimulation for the children. Even for mothers who work outside of the house, the idealization of the maternal role has resulted in demands to "be prepared for any challenge" [58]. During the pandemic, there were constant domestic and educational responsibilities and, as demonstrated by the following extracts, mothering academics experienced internal tension about their own expectations of their maternal role while also having their private world made public with remote work:

> *"I've had to break many of the rules I had as a mother. Screens, for example, Before, we only allowed them on special occasions or on flights. Now, they have become the best option to entertain M while I work" (Mothering academic of a 3-year-old, USA).*

> *"I've seen how some aspects of my life have been made public, things that before, were considered private. Like my intimate relationships, a move to a new place, even getting new furniture to adapt my home to the new demands of my job" (Mothering academic of two teenagers, Chile).*

On the other hand, all three academic mothers had to meet high research productivity demands, such as multiple publications and presentations. Consistent with prior research [59] the mothers shifted between the need to fulfill productivity demands and their own expectations as a mother. This required them to balance family and work time, as demonstrated by the following quote, in which childcare and household responsibilities acted as a barrier to academic productivity:

> *"Where do you write? When can you write? I've been asking those questions as part of a longitudinal study I am conducting. Today, I must add the following question: 'how have you done it with the pandemic? What have you had to give up?' I'm trying to acknowledge and raise awareness about the juggling act that we academic mothers have had to do to reconcile housework and child care (young or adolescent) with research and scholarship. The urgency of household tasks have caused my research to get delayed or postponed as I wait for better conditions for production" (Mothering academic of two teenagers, Chile).*

> *"I look at some colleagues reading books and writing articles, while I can't even read two pages in a row of anything [...] finally, we started using false documents to be able to move B, so that I could have at least two or three days per week without worrying about him. During these days I tried to make up for late work. Our society assumes that mothers should always be the ones who are with their children more. I feel completely alone" (Mothering academic of a 7-year-old son, Chile).*

When balancing demands related to reproduction and productivity, their bodies were visible affected. The ideal "bodies" that are prioritized in academia tend to connect to the notion of productivity, in which male academics by and large have fewer interruptions or disruptions with their commitment to work [60, 61]. Through a process of embodiment, the academic mothers' bodies have adapted and organized to crisis mode [62]. On the one hand, the three mothers in our study reported feeling *loneliness, exhaustion,* and *stress.* In their cases, their bodies embodied tensions from the productivity demands at all costs, possible as a response to the academic capitalism and neoliberalism present at the universities [63–65]. The demand to finish delayed work, finding time to write, and converting private spaces into spaces for productivity, led to physical problems and embodiment of structural tension.

### 4.2 Theme 2: the triple shift in mothering academics

During the first semester of 2020, confinement policies enacted by governments across the world to try to reduce the spread of COVID-19 led to isolation and disconnectedness. Many mothering academics entered in a cycle of endless tasks that took over their lives. For many, this led to exacerbating the triple shift that included: (i) *work life* with administrative responsibilities, teaching, and research—all virtual; (ii) *family life* with childcare and motherhood, including overseeing child education; and (iii) *domestic life* with chores and actions to convert one's home into one's work place.

For these academic mothers, the pandemic led to an intensification of responsibilities: elimination of any free time, taking over all aspects of their lives. As presented in the following quote, this led some of the mothers to be "on" 24/7 as they always had some duty to fill, whether that be maternal, household, or academic. Furthermore, in the extracts below, we can visualize certain subjections—produced by gendered norms and neoliberal labor—which led to the inability to successfully fulfill all three demands:

> *"Quickly, you realize that you have no free time. That is over. For practically one year, every minute from the time you wake until you go to bed, every day of the week, I was required to accompany my son with his school and homework, to care for him (my son also has a disability that requires additional care), to maintain my household, and to complete my work remotely, which involved administration, research, and teaching. That alone required me to distribute each task or activity at specific times from Monday through Friday. Quickly, I realized that the only free time I had was when I was asleep. Obviously, this led to more stress, less sleep, and anxiety. Constantly feeling like you are not capable or you are not giving one hundred percent in any of these areas: not in your own work, not in your research, not as a mother, not even in household chores" (Mothering academic of a 7-year-old son, Chile).*

> *"It is not just a matter of child care, but rather of coordinating their education that has multiplied during this time. In my work, I also must justify resources, respond to the ongoing financial crisis, or meet external demands. And there is the triple crisis: the academic difficulties that are the base, the transformation of mothering, and reorganizing time that has led to my productivity being diminished after the first third of the pandemic (...) Long work hours that start very early and end at an unpredictable hour. Then it's night, because evening has set in, and without realizing it I'm in front of the computer screen again and promising that this is: 'the last email I'll check, the last evaluation I'll send, the last recommendation that I'll send my students before the new day breaks'" (Mothering academic of two teenagers, Chile).*

On the other hand, these narratives show how the State, by focusing exclusively on a hygienic approach to the pandemic, did not consider how these measures could affect the organization and division of work (both paid and unpaid), or how to promote more equity in the co-responsibility for children. Instead, the state-imposed measures reinforced gendered norms and stereotypes, shifting responsibility instead to mothers. As presented in the following quote, mothers reported feeling drained emotionally, mentally, and physically:

> *"The State has a double presence: It limits our mobility and requires each person to function individually in the middle of a global pandemic, but it also fails to acknowledge the disparate distribution of childcare and household work. It's not that there is an explicit policy, but rather it is doing it implicitly, by reinforcing the idea that mothers are responsible for those areas.....and in parallel, the university demands rhythms of work that do not align with the diverse experiences of the workforce during the pandemic. Obviously, looking at it structurally, the system leaves the responsibility with each individual—in this case, with us as women workers. They say: you have to take care of yourself, engage in self-care, and you will be successfully and achieve excellence. The immediate effect this has on us is obvious: stress, physical exhaustion, mental exhaustion, anxiety, burnout, and anger (Mothering Academic of a 7-year-old son, Chile).*

> *"We get the call from daycare. For the second time since we sent M back to school, they call us to let us know that one of her classmates tested positive for COVID-19. We just adapted to this new normal, and yet another disruption to the routine" (Mothering Academic of a 3-year-old, USA).*

The measures taken by government to curb the pandemic required mothering academics to reorganize their work and develop new strategies to get their work done. Some of these strategies are observed in the following fragments include a more equitable distribution of responsibilities with their partners (among those with partners), contracting external help when possible, or collaborating with other academics to maintain productivity and publications. Through the following narrative, we see how extended family or support is missed, and the disruption in community support and camaraderie:

> *"Our society assumes that mothers should be the ones who are with their children more. I feel extremely alone. I asked my family for help to pay for someone to come and help out, but everyone is scared and no one wants to leave their house (...) I have realized that I am very social and I miss little get togethers and interactions with other people. Perhaps during another era when families were not so nuclear, rather extended, care would have been difference. But how we are currently, I believe that the individualism of this pandemic has been very apparent, more so than solidarity" (Mothering Academic of a 7-year-old son, Chile).*

> *"For now, the semester has finished. My teaching and service responsibilities at the university have been reduced. With my partner we take turns watching M. Once she is asleep, we work late. In contrast to last summer, this time we know it is temporary. In a few more days, daycare will open back up. I will catch up on proposals, articles, and preparing for the upcoming semester. And then, we can go back to our normal schedule" (Mothering Academic of a 3-year-old, USA).*

Strategies to reorganize daily life and responsibilities are described in the following narratives. This takes on a new meaning when coupled with strategies these mothering academics followed to keep up with their academic career, which required them to perform everything at once:

> *"Trying to turn my home into a double work space has been, without a doubt, challenging. I've had to learn to turn off the microphone and camera to respond to scenes in my house where the lines between public and private life have blurred. Three months into the pandemic, I can say that I have found a new way to organize my work, with breaks to prepare food, eat, chat/visit with my children, do some cleaning, and then try to disconnect after hours of online meetings and teaching" (Mothering Academic of two teenagers, Chile).*

Through these processes, mothering academics learned by trial and error, developing strategies over time to accommodate and reconcile the triple shift generated during the pandemic.

### 4.3 Theme 3: tactics for resistance and change

Despite the tensions and challenges faced by the academic mothers, we also were able to see individual and collective tactics for resistance and change. Throughout the pandemic, there has been a focus on individual or family strategies to better cope with stress. For example, several agencies have called for self-care strategies, and families have been tasked with childcare and education.

One tactic that emerged from our auto-interviews was publicly acknowledging discomfort, needs, and problems with the pandemic. The idea of putting the triple shift in the public eye helps raise awareness of the negative impact on careers, creating at the same time coalitions and alliances among peers. Through these tactics, academic mothers retook their space, calling for more inclusion of the family, to generate collective contexts of support. The following narrative focuses on the role of new technology to be able to gather with other academic mothers and organize. Not only for solidarity as they navigate the triple shift, but also to raise a collective critique of governmental practices [66] that have been generated during the pandemic. Furthermore, they can organize and collaborate to demand changes to academia, without risking their own individual careers.

> *"We have created a certain camaraderie among various people who have been aware of this intentional invisibility of the tiple shift imposed on by the governmental policies. Taking advantage of technology, we have opened up spaces to seek solace from the issues of the pandemic, but also to share with one another ways to challenge the pressure and connect with other academics. All of this helps us not stay behind in our own academic careers. This is one small example of how we don't just assume that the invisibility of the triple shift is something that cannot change. These meetings give us an opportunity to consider possible alliances among academic mothers, since we have scarce time to get together in our professional and personal lives" (Mothering Academic of a 7-year-old son, Chile).*

Similarly, resistance can occur in the private sphere. During the pandemic, it has been important (for those who have one) to negotiate daily tasks and responsibilities with a partner. In the following quotes, the academic mothers emphasized strategies they used to change how they performed roles within their families:

> *"With my partner, we begin the negotiations. We open our calendars to compare our scheduled meeting times. We decide which ones we can postpone or miss, and which we could do while watching our three-year-old daughter. Given the confidentiality regulations at institutions of higher education in the USA (FERPA)*

> *and other privacy protections for my students, I try to avoid taking M while I am teaching or attending confidential committee meetings. On his end, my partner avoids attending shorter meetings when he is with M, since the last time he tried she started yelling that he was being "too loud" during his meeting. We try to arrange it so that one of us can pay attention to her, but inevitably we have some overlapping meetings" (Mothering Academic of a 3-year-old, USA).*

> *"Just as there is resistance, there is also adaptation and more subtle tactics like turning off the cameras, mentioning connectivity issues, or equipment problems, to try to adjust paid work and family work. There is a sort of resignification, which leads to new accommodations and in some sense risks in adapting and organizing academic work during the pandemic, which has normalized time and time again inequities in academic work, in child care and domestic chores. I take advantage of the week "of break" that the university gives us, so that I can catch up on all of the work I need to do, with publications, revising articles, and other documents" (Mothering Academic of two teenagers, Chile).*

## 5. Conclusion

This chapter provided a critical reflection of the tension and resistance that have emerged from remote work and conditions during the pandemic for three mothering academics. Their career trajectories have been affected and impacted by the measures the government has taken to contain the pandemic, coupled with gendered norms of household work and childcare, and the demands of productivity imposed by the university. The triple crisis alluded to in this text highlights the tensions and adaptations that these mothers have experienced in the care of their children, household and academic responsibilities, while also confronting gendered notions of motherhood during the pandemic.

As we conclude this chapter, we advocate for additional research to explore how other academic mothers have experienced structural changes in care—both within family systems and beyond. Throughout the pandemic, we have seen evidence of the importance of paid and unpaid work, highlighting the need to value unpaid work in the interior of the family. The COVID-19 crisis has drawn awareness to the need to redistribute responsibilities within the private sphere and convert them into a public problem, with a need for collective responsibility. In summary, more than a "care crisis," there is a need for "policies around care" [67].

The government and universities have not directly observed the care crisis that has intensified during the pandemic. As highlighted by the three narratives in this chapter, research is needed to explore the impact of the COVID-19 pandemic on the academic gender gap. Therefore, it is of upmost importance that we critically review how we view care and its relationship with paid academic work, which often fails to acknowledge other roles or responsibilities individuals may have. Through tactics for resistance, even more subtle ones, we can begin to raise awareness of these inequities and call for collective action for change.

## Acknowledgements

We would like to acknowledge ANID/CONICYT/Fondecyt 1190257, "Estudio longitudinal de trayectorias y transiciones investigativas de trabajadores sociales chilenos", within the Research Group "Diversidad y Genero: abordajes feministas interseccionales" at the Faculty of Social Sciences at the University of Chile.

## Conflict of interest

The authors declare no conflicts of interest.

## Author details

Gabriela Rubilar Donoso[1*], Catherine A. LaBrenz[2] and Caterine Galaz Valderrama[1]

1 Universidad de Chile, Santiago, Chile

2 University of Texas at Arlington, Arlington, USA

*Address all correspondence to: grubilar@uchile.cl

## References

[1] McAlpine L, Amundsen C, Turner G. Identity-trajectory: Reframing early career academic experience. British Educational Research Journal. 2004; **40**(6):952-969. DOI: 10.1002/berj.3123

[2] Wolfinger N, Mason M, Goulden M. Stay in the game: Gender, family formation and alternative trajectories in the academic life course. Social Forces. 2009;**87**(3):1591-1621

[3] Fardella C, Sisto V, Jiménez F. Nosotros los académicos. Narrativas identitarias y autodefinición en la Universidad actual. Universitas Psychologica. 2013;**14**(5):1625-1636. DOI: 10.11144/Javeriana.upsy14-5.nani

[4] Sisto V. Gobernados por los números. El financiamiento como forma de gobierno de las Universidades en Chile. Psicoperspectivas. Individuo y Sociedad. 2017;**16**(3):64-75

[5] Vergés N, Biglia B, Almeda E. Metodologías feministas con tecnologías para la gestión de la información en la enseñanza universitaria. Revista Linhas. 2020;**21**(45):165-182. DOI: 10.5965/1984723821452020165

[6] Sánchez MJA. Las académicas. Profesorado universitario y género. Revista de Educación. 2002;**328**:465-475

[7] Marinoni G, Van't Land H, Jensen T. The Impact of Covid-19 on Higher Education around the World: IAU Flobal Survey Report. 1st ed. Paris, France: International Association of Universities; 2020. p. 50

[8] Fardella C. El teletrabajo académico: Prácticas y vulnerabilidades. Seminario Virtual—Universidad de Valparaíso. 2020. Available from: https://www.youtube.com/watch?v=9v_GCSD9y-M [Accessed: September 28, 2020]

[9] Gutiérrez F. La promesa engañosa de la ley de teletrabajo. Columna de opinión. Ciper Académico. 2020. Available from: https://www.ciperchile.cl/2020/04/17/la-promesa-enganosa-de-la-ley-de-teletrabajo/ [Accessed: September 28, 2020]

[10] Carreri A, Dordoni A. Academic and research work from home during the COVID-19 pandemic in Italy: A gender perspective. Italian Sociological Review. 2020;**10**(3S):821-845. DOI: 10.13136/isr.v10i3S.400

[11] Oleschuk M. Gender equity considerations for tenure and promotion during COVID-19. Canadian Review of Sociology/Revue. 2020;**57**(3):502-515. DOI: 10.1111/cars.12295

[12] Crook S. Parenting during the COVID-19 pandemic of 2020: Academia, labour, and care work. Women's History Review. 2020;**29**(7):1226-1238. DOI: 10.1080/09612025.2020.1807690

[13] Rubilar G, Galaz-Valderrama C, LaBrenz C. Academic and family disruptions during the COVID-19 pandemic: A reflexive from social work. Qualitative Social Work. 2020;**20**:587-594. DOI: 10.1177/1473325020973293

[14] Gabster BP, Van Daalen K, Dhatt R, Barry M. Challenges for the female academic during the COVID-19 pandemic. The Lancet. 2020; **395**(10242):1968-1970. DOI: 10.1016/S0140-6736(20)31412-4

[15] Malisch JL, Harris BN, Sherrer SM, Lewis KA, Shepherd SL, McCarthy PC, et al. Opinion: In the wake of COVID-19, academia needs new solutions to ensure gender equity. PNAS. 2020;**117**(27): 15378-15381. DOI: 10.1073/pnas.2010636117

[16] Minello A, Martucci S, Manzo L. The pandemic and the academic mothers: Present hardships and future

perspectives. European Societies. 2020; **23**(1):S82-S94. DOI: 10.1080/14616696.2020.1809690

[17] Rodriguez C, Tovar E. Discurso de género y emociones en mujeres académicas de alto rendimiento. Social Perspectives. 2009;**11**(1):187-209

[18] Ash A, Carr P, Goldstein R, Friedman R. Compensation and advancement of women in academic medicine: Is there equity? Annals of Internal Medicine. 2004;**141**(3): 205-212. DOI: 10.7326/0003-4819-141-3-200408030-00009

[19] Kaplan SH, Sullivan LM, Dukes KA, Phillips CF, Kelch RP, Schaller JG. Sex differences in academic advancement. Results of a national study of pediatricians. New England Journal of Medicine. 1996;**335**(17):1282-1289. DOI: 10.1056/NEJM199610243351706

[20] Carr R, Lane-Fall M, South E, Brady D, Momplaisir F, Guerra C, et al. Academic careers and the COVID-19 pandemic: Reversing the tide. Science Translational Medicine. 2021;**13**(584). DOI: 10.1126/scitranslmed.abe7189

[21] Ríos N, Mandiola M, Varas A. Haciendo género, haciendo academia: Un análisis feminista de la organización del trabajo académico en Chile. Psicoperspectivas. 2017;**16**(2):114-124. DOI: 10.5027/psicoperspectivas-Vol16-Issue2-fulltext-1041

[22] Slaughter S, Leslie E. Academic Capitalism: Politics, Policies & the Entrepreneurial University. Baltimore, MD: The John Hopkins University Press; 1997. p. 296

[23] Ibarra E. La "nueva universidad" en México: transformaciones recientes y perspectivas. Revista Mexicana de Investigación Educativa. 2002;**7**(14): 75-105

[24] De Armas T, Venegas A. Patriarcado y capitalismo académico: La reproducción de las violencias. In: Del Valle S, editor. Educación no Sexista: Hacia una Real Transformación. Santiago, Chile: Red Chilena Contra la Violencia hacia las Mujeres; 2016. pp. 57-66

[25] Fardella C, Corvalán-Navia A, García-Meneses J, Chiappini F. Ni extranjeras, ni secretarias: discursos de las científicas chilenas sobre el trabajo académico. Pensamiento Educativo. 2021;**58**:1-13. DOI: 10.7764/PEL.58.1.2021.11

[26] Muñoz G, Rubilar G. Social work research in Chile: Tensions and challenges under the 'Knowledge Economy' and managerialist research agendas. British Journal of Social Work. 2020;**51**(7):2839-2856. DOI: 10.1093/bjsw/bcaa132

[27] Simbürger E, Undurraga R. Jerarquías epistemológicas: Formas de invisibilizar el género en las carreras de sociología en Chile. In: Mora C, editor. Desigualdad en Chile: La Continua Relevancia del Género. Santiago, Chile: Ediciones Universidad Alberto Hurtado; 2013. pp. 171-195

[28] Sisto V. Flexibilización laboral de la docencia universitaria y la gestación de la universidad sin órganos. Un análisis desde la subjetividad laboral del docente en condiciones de precariedad. In: CLACSO Consejo Latinoamericano de Ciencias Sociales, editor. Espacio Público y Privatización del Conocimiento. Buenos Aires, Argentina: Estudios sobre políticas universitarias en América Latina; 2005. pp. 523-574

[29] Cruz-Castro L, Sanz-Menéndez L, Aja Valle J. Las trayectorias profesionales y académicas de los profesores de universidad y los investigadores del CSIC. Documento de trabajo 06-08, Unidad de Políticas Comparadas Consejo Superior de Investigaciones Científicas CSIC. 2006. Available from: https://digital.csic.es/bitstream/10261/

1667/1/profesores_universidad_investigadores_csic.pdf [Accessed: December 7, 2021]

[30] Foster S, McMurray J, Linzer M, Leavitt J, Ronsenberg M, Carnes M. Results of a gender-climate and work-environment survey at a Midwestern academic health center. Academic Medicine. 2020;**75**(6):653-660

[31] Marbley AF, Wong A, Pratt C, Jaddo L. Women faculty of color: Voices, gender, and the expression of our multiple identities within academia. Advancing Women in Leadership. 2011;**31**:166-174

[32] Murgia A, Poggio B, editors. Gender and Precarious Research Careers. 1st ed. London: Routledge; 2018. p. 256. DOI: 10.4324/9781315201245

[33] Suárez-Ortega M. Trayectorias y carrera profesional del personal docente e investigador desde un enfoque de género: Estudio de un caso. Revista Iberoamericana para la Investigación y el Desarrollo Educativo. 2015;**12**:1-11

[34] Universidad de Chile. Del biombo a la cátedra: igualdad de oportunidades de género en la Universidad de Chile. 1st ed. Vol. 211. Oficina de Igualdad de Oportunidades de Género; 2014. p. 211

[35] Woodward D. Work-life balancing strategies used by women managers in British 'modern' universities. Equal Opportunities International. 2007;**26**(1):6-17. DOI: 10.1108/02610150710726507

[36] Berrios P. Análisis sobre las profesoras universitarias y desafíos para la profesión académica en Chile. Calidad de la Educación. 2007;**26**:39-53. DOI: 10.31619/caledu.n26.232

[37] Martínez-Labrin S, Bivort-Urrutia B. Procesos de producción de subjetividad de género en el trabajo académico: tiempos y espacios desde cuerpos femeninos. Psicoperspectivas. Individuo y Sociedad. 2014;**13**(1):15-22. DOI: 10.5027/psicoperspectivas-Vol13-Issue1-fulltext-334

[38] Martínez S. Género, subjetividad y trabajo académico. Integración Académica en Psicología. 2015;**3**(8): 47-53

[39] Universidad de Chile. Conversatorio Ser científica en Chile, avances y desafíos, organizado por Dirección de Diversidad y Género, Facultad de Ciencias Físicas y Matemáticas, Universidad de Chile. 2021. Available from: https://www.youtube.com/watch?v=_uPs7G8FAYQ&ab_channel=FCFM-UChileTV [Accessed: December 7, 2021]

[40] ANID. Análisis de participación femenina en convocatorias a financiamiento de la institución 2010-2019, Departamento de estudios y gestión estratégica, ANID, Ministerio de Ciencia, Tecnología, Conocimiento e Innovación. 2020. Available from: https://s3.amazonaws.com/documentos.anid.cl/cti/ReporteDeGenero_2010-2020.pdf [Accessed: December 7, 2021]

[41] Sanhueza L, Fernández C, Montero L. Segregación de género: narrativas de mujeres desde la academia. Revista Polis. 2020;**19**(55):310-334. DOI: 10.32735/s0718-6568/2020-n55-1453

[42] Vizcarra I, Vélez G. Género y éxito científico en la Universidad Autónoma del Estado de México. Estudios Feministas. 2007;**15**(3):581-608

[43] Denzin N, Lincoln Y. Handbook of Qualitative Research. London: Sage; 1994. p. 643

[44] Boufoy-Bastick B. Auto-interviewing, auto-ethnography and critical incident methodology for eliciting a self-conceptualised

worldview. Forum: Qualitative Social Research. 2004;**5**(1):1-16. DOI: 10.17169/fqs-5.1.651

[45] Riessman C. Twists and turns: Narrating my career, Catherine Kohler Riessman. Qualitative Social Work. 2015;**14**(1):10-17. DOI: 10.1177/1473325014522285

[46] Rubilar G. Narratives and biographical approach. Uses, scope, and challenges for interdisciplinary research. Enfermeria, Cuidados Humanizados. 2017;**6**:76-82. DOI: 10.22235/ech.v6iEspecial

[47] Appel M. La entrevista autobiográfica narrativa: Fundamentos teóricos y la praxis mostrada a partir del estudio de caso sobre el cambio cultural de los Otomíes en México. Qualitative. Social Research. 2005;**6**(2):1-35. DOI: 10.17169/fqs-6.2.465

[48] Ellis C, Adams T, Bochner A. Autoethnography: An overview. Forum Qualitative Social Research. 2011;**12**(1):1-14. DOI: 10.2307/23032294

[49] Keightley E, Pickering M, Allet N. The self-interview: A new method in social science research. International Journal of Social Research Methodology. 2012;**15**(6):507-521

[50] Valles M, Baer A. Investigación social cualitativa en España: Pasado, presente y futuro. Un retrato. Forum: Qualitative Social Research. 2015;**6**(3):18. DOI: 10.17169/fqs-6.3.15

[51] Rubilar G. Practices of memory and the construction of research testimonies. A methodological reflection about self-interviewing, testimonies, and social workers' accounts of their research. Forum: Qualitative Social Research. 2015;**16**(3):1-30. DOI: 10.17169/fqs-16.3.2257

[52] Galaz C, Rubilar G. Experiencias profesionales en intervención psicosocial: el ejercicio narrativo como metodología de reflexividad y vigilancia epistemológica. Revista Latinoamericana De Metodología De Las Ciencias Sociales (Relmecs). 2019;**9**(1):1-13. DOI: 10.24215/18537863e050

[53] Bourdieu P. Autoanálisis de un sociólogo. Barcelona: Anagrama; 2006

[54] Piovani J, Muñiz TL. "Condenados a la reflexividad" Apuntes para repensar el proceso de Investigación Social. Buenos Aires: CLACSO; 2018

[55] Cornejo M, Rubilar G, Zapata-Sepulveda P. Researching sensitive topics in sensitive zones: Exploring silences, 'the normal,' and tolerance in Chile. International Journal of Qualitative Methods. 2019;**18**:1-11. DOI: 10.1177/1609406919849355

[56] Biglia B, Bonet i Martí J. La construcción de narrativas como método de investigación psicosocial. Prácticas de escritura compartida. Forum: Qualitative Social Research. 2009;**10**(1):1-24

[57] Medina Bravo P, Figueras-Maz M, Gómez-Puertas L. El ideal de madre en el siglo XXI: La representación de la maternidad en las revistas de familia. Estudios sobre el Mensaje periodístico. 2014;**20**(1):487-504. DOI: 10.5209/rev_ESMP.2014.v20.n1.45244

[58] Arciniega Caceres M, Figueras Maz M. La construcción social de la maternidad a través de los mommy blogs. In Associació Catalana de Sociologia, editor. VII Congres Catala de Sociologia. 2017. pp. 100-103

[59] Leigh J, Bailey R. Reflection, reflective practice and embodied reflective practice. Body, Movement, and Dance in Psychotherapy. 2013;**8**(3):160-171. DOI: 10.1080/17432979.2013.797498

[60] Ahmad S. Family of future in the academy? Review of Educational Research. 2017;**87**(1):204-239. DOI: 10.3102/0034654316631626

[61] Ollilainen M. Ideal bodies at work: Faculty mothers and pregnancy in academia. Gender and Education. 2020;**32**(7):961-976. DOI: 10.1080/09540253.2019.1632808

[62] Coetzee M. Embodied knowledge(s), embodied pedagogies and performance. South African Theatre Journal. 2018;**31**(1):1-4. DOI: 10.1080/10137548.2018.1425527

[63] Cortes Santiago I, Karimi N, Arvelo AZ. Neoliberalism and higher education: A collective autoethnography of Brown women teaching assistants. Gender and Education. 2016;**29**(1):48-65. DOI: 10.1080/09540253.2016.1197383

[64] Marginson S. Dynamics of national and global competition in higher education. Higher Education. 2006;**52**(1):1-39. DOI: 10.1007/sl0734-004-7649-x

[65] Rizvi F. Beyond the social imaginary of 'clash of civilizations'? Educational Philosophy and Theory. 2011;**43**(3):225-235. DOI: 10.1111/j.1469-5812.2009.00593.x

[66] Foucault M. Defender la sociedad. In: Fondo de Cultura económica. 1st ed. Buenos Aires, Argentina: Fondo de Cultura Economica; 2001. p. 209

[67] El RC. cuidado como objeto de políticas públicas inclusivas con enfoque de género. Revista Estado, Gobierno y Gestión Pública. 2017;**30**:15-43

Chapter 21

# Perspective Chapter: Fallout from the Pandemic – A Social and Psychological Description of COVID-19 Related Traumatic Sequelae

*Aishling Collins, Eleanor O'Driscoll and Declan Lyons*

## Abstract

Pandemics are not new phenomena in human history but in a globalised and interconnected planet the differential impact upon each generation may be distinctive. The concept of trauma has been widely discussed over the last 18 months with emphasis on a collective stress and distress but also in respect of those who are vulnerable to psychological adversity because of established prior mental health diagnoses. Much debate has centred on the impact of the pandemic on mental illness, both new and established, and this chapter will examine the utility of interpreting the psychological outcome at individual and societal level through the lens of collective trauma. At risk populations, such as healthcare workers and those recovering from infection will be a special focus of this chapter.

**Keywords:** trauma, stress, healthcare workers, elderly, youth

## 1. Introduction

Arguably the COVID-19 pandemic is the first mass trauma-laden event the world has witnessed since the second World War, and for many people it has been the first collective trauma in living memory. There has been a plethora of discussion about the impact of the pandemic, much of which has focussed on the economic and political fallout and it is no exaggeration to state that global pandemics are heart-breaking biopsychosocial health crises. There has also been debate and speculation about the implications of the pandemic on people's mental health, with many commentators citing increased levels of depression and anxiety [1]. Such psychological adversity has more often than not, been attributed to the social isolation and the heightened levels of stress which people have incurred during the pandemic—not least the fact that all it has taken for so many of our habits to be swept away and their shaky foundations revealed, has been an unseen virus. Less has been spoken about the concept of trauma and the longer-lasting implications which mass trauma can yield in the aftermath of this catastrophe. Trauma has traditionally been perceived as a once-off event albeit one which caused extreme stress and distress to the affected individual, for example road traffic accidents or assaults on one's



IntechOpen

person. Indeed, when one thinks of the term pandemic, "trauma" is perhaps not the first term that springs to mind but the pandemic has not been a brief, once-off incident, confined to a particular geographic area or a discrete population. Rather, it has spanned many months and had no regard for social, geographical or political boundaries. In this chapter the authors will propose that the pandemic has in fact constituted a mass trauma, whereby millions of people have been affected by the same event within a shared time frame, with virtually no corner of the earth escaping completely unscathed. We believe that long after this pandemic has ended and people have returned to their normal ways of life, the psychosocial impact of this mass trauma will have physical and mental health implications for many citizens around the world. In anticipation of the fallout from this trauma, it is paramount to consider how we may start to adapt. In order to do so, we will reflect on previous mass traumas and explore what we know about the long-term sequelae of trauma.

Trauma may be defined as a 'rupture in meaning-making' [2], in that traumatic events can shatter our pre-existing ways of thinking, our belief systems and how we relate to the world around us. When a traumatic event occurs, we are forced to re-evaluate how we view ourselves, others and the world and it is said that a cleft emerges between what we know (our "orienting systems") and the trauma. It can seem as if there are two selves; the one before trauma and the one after the trauma. A new process of meaning-making, where we evaluate our beliefs and sense of self, is required so that we may progress beyond the trauma.

When one considers who has been adversely affected by the pandemic, healthcare workers in the so-called front line against the virus spring to mind first and foremost. There is no doubt that large numbers of healthcare staff were subjected to increased levels of distress amidst the pandemic. Increased caseload numbers, longer working hours, inadequate PPE supplies, fear of contracting and spreading the virus and moral injury are just a few of the challenges faced by those working in the health sector during this time. Couple these challenges with the well-established fact that healthcare professions experience higher levels of work-related stress in comparison to the general population, and we have a perfect storm for a mental health crisis among healthcare professions. We know that a sense of helplessness in the situation increases the likelihood of a stressful experience becoming a traumatic experience. We may argue that healthcare professionals differed somewhat from the general population in that they may not necessarily have felt helpless; they were on the front line, battling the virus in a very tangible "hands on deck" way, as opposed to the many millions who were asked to help by virtue of staying home and staying away from others. We should also keep in mind that trauma is not necessarily proportional to the intensity of the event: it is possible that a person who nursed patients with COVID-19 on a daily basis may feel less traumatised than a person who had no contact whatsoever with patients afflicted by COVID. The key mediator here is resilience, and its role in the processing, or "meaning-making" should not be understated. There is no doubt that an essential element to the healing process will be the nurturing of mental resilience.

## 2. Inherent trauma of death itself

Grief is defined as an internal experience in reaction to the loss of something loved and valued [3]. Though commonly viewed as an emotive or psychological response; grief has numerous manifestations - physical, cognitive, behavioural, social and spiritual. Grief is often referred to as the loss of a person due to death; however, grief involves the concept of loss in general which can also refer to the loss of a job, a relationship or even a role. COVID 19 and its associated impact has caused devastating loss and thus grief in so many aspects of our lives.

Grief is a process and this process often begins prior to loss, it is at times preparatory and anticipatory. Due to the unpredictable course of COVID 19 illness, many deaths were sudden and grossly unexpected. This complicated individuals' grief process and eliminated the preparatory process. The suddenness and abrupt nature of death, after what presented itself as an initial recovery and then rapid deterioration at day 10 or 11 of the illness, prevented the natural acceptance which can be afforded to loved ones when a patient is dying of a more predictable and widely understood illness.

Loss of a loved one is unfortunately a natural, universally experienced life event, and at the same time, among life's most deeply challenging experiences. Although any death of a loved one can be emotionally devastating, unexpected deaths provoke particularly strong responses, given there is less time to prepare for and adapt to the loss [4].

Research has demonstrated that the bereavement period is associated with elevated risk for the onset of a multitude of psychiatric disorders, consistently across the individual's life course and coincident with the experience of the loved one's death [5]. This is demonstrated in clinical practice, where death of a loved one often precipitates an individual's referral presentation to psychiatric services. Feeling vulnerable is an immensely difficult for many people, and there is no greater vulnerability than being faced with the transience of life itself.

The unexpected or sudden death of a loved one is frequently cited as the most severe and potentially traumatic experience in one's life, even among individuals with a high burden of lifetime stressful experiences. Unexpected bereavement is associated with heightened vulnerability for the onset of virtually all commonly-occurring psychiatric disorders.

Irrespective of culture, religion or value system, death is usually followed by a funeral or a mourning service. Such a service provides an outlet for the culturally accepted expression of loss-related emotions and marks a transition in which the certainty of the death is emphasised. It provides a starting point for recovery, processing and adjustment following a bereavement. In an attempt to slow the spread of the COVID 19 virus worldwide, lockdown restrictions were introduced of varying intensity. Significant restrictions on the mourning rituals, such as limits on the number of individuals permitted to attend funerals, has the potential in the author's opinion to hinder the grieving process and deny families the opportunity to express their grief. Bereaved individuals tend to perceive different aspects of the funeral in a positive regard [6]. People do not only respond positively initially but continue to reflect on the funeral with positive regard in the future, even years later. The restrictions on funeral and mourning proceedings and indeed household visits in the initial grief period likely denied individuals this facilitatory event of the support of loved ones and their wider community, and undoubtedly compounded their grief. It remains to be seen what, if any, will be the longer-term impact of such restrictions on those bereaved by COVID-19.

## 3. Trauma of the patients who contracted COVID-19

A person's experience of illness is highly individual and somewhat dictated by the illness-related information they receive. Due to the fact that COVID-19 is a novel virus that is relatively poorly understood, the information available to patients regarding illness trajectory, prognosis and long-term effects is scarce. The lack of information and uncertainty surrounding this illness, may unsurprisingly foster a sense of fear and anxiety in the COVID-infected individual.

A prominent and rather distressing symptom of COVID-19 is dyspnoea or breathlessness. It is widely appreciated that shortness of breath can constitute both a symptom of and precipitant to panic. Anxiety is noted to be an emotional response to breathlessness, but it also increases the perception of breathlessness. There is a strong association between experiencing respiratory symptoms and psychological distress which is further worsened by the uncertainty of disease progression and indeed the exact underlying pathology causing said breathlessness [7].

Uncertainty and the unknown are themes that underpin the global experience of COVID-19. The clinical understanding of the illness is continually evolving and changing in parallel with epidemiological research which is informed by the natural evolution of the pandemic among a human population. Clinicians play an important role in helping their patients to use coping skills for managing the illness, the different phases of infection and residual symptoms. However, clinicians' lack of knowledge about the illness trajectory results in doctors being unable to advise their patients as they would with other disorders or conditions. The impact of this inability of doctors to sufficiently counsel their patients about the disease is likely to be twofold: traumatic for the patient who seeks information about a hitherto unknown illness, and traumatising for the doctor who wants to help, but is limited in the extent to which he or she can do so.

We should also consider that there is exaggerated fear related to infectious illness compared to non-infectious illnesses. Infection possesses unique characteristics that account for this disproportionate degree of fear: it is transmitted rapidly and invisibly; historically, it has accounted for major morbidity and mortality; older forms or strains re-emerge and new forms emerge. By the time the Spanish flu had run its course in 1920, the pandemic had infected over a quarter of the world's population and resulted in some 30 million to 100 million deaths. In comparison to this, the two World Wars are estimated to have killed roughly 77 million combined [8]. Infectious diseases completely consume us: the media and society become enthralled and fascinated, which results in minimal escape for the individual. Infectious illnesses are unique in that the patient is both a victim and a vector; the latter of which may be associated with feelings of guilt and responsibility. Infectious diseases are well documented throughout history and their devastating impact has resulted in more acute deaths than any other pathology [9]. As such, an automatic fear of infection is engraved in our subconscious.

The psychological response to the threat of infection has been well researched with regards to both acute outbreaks such as SARS and more gradually evolving pandemics such as HIV/AIDS. Anxiety extends beyond the physical consequences of infection, to social consequences such as stigmatisation, which, in the case of the current pandemic, manifested itself as anti-Chinese racism which anecdotally have emerged during this pandemic. In the case of an unknown agent such as COVID-19, a complete lack of preparedness on the part of medical authorities and misleading information perpetuated by the media serves to further aggravate pathological psychological responses to illness and infection [9].

## 4. Fear of the unknown/anticipatory fear

COVID-19 proved to be a highly virulent and transmissible infection which has caused panic in individuals and anticipatory anxiety regarding the contraction of infection by this novel virus. Fear is an appropriate and adaptive response in the presence of threat and danger. Fear enables us to engage in safety behaviours in order to mitigate threat and protect ourselves. Fear is also protective and with COVID 19, the threat is uncertain and continuous and as such the fear may

*DOI: http://dx.doi.org/10.5772/intechopen.101499*

become persistent and negatively impact our collective quality of life. The threat from COVID 19 is universal with each individual being at risk. This high personal relevance and has heightened our subjective experience of fear [10].

Uncertainty surrounding a possible future or continuous threat also potentially disrupts one's ability to avoid it or to mitigate its negative impact, and thus results in anticipatory anxiety. Elevated expectations of threat naturally lead to avoidance of situations involving uncertainty and the said threat. However, as the threat from COVID-19 was ubiquitous and present in many aspects of our lives, people were forced to adjust and adapt to living with constant threat. This excessive threat has triggered a response of anticipatory fear. The fear of contracting the virus has led to excessive concern over physiological symptoms, significant stress about personal and occupational loss, increased reassurance- and safety-seeking behaviours, and avoidance of public places and situations, culminating in a marked impairment in our levels of functioning [11].

Epidemic psychology demonstrates that the human brain is pre-wired to thrive on certainty and has a disdain for uncertainty, which represents danger, stability being at the core of humans' schema and derivation of meaning from life [12]. The crisis of COVID-19 disturbs our set system and questions the certainty to which we were habituated. The perplexity surrounding the origin of the virus and the associated and prolonged uncertainties give rise to fear of the unknown, which is becoming a new feature of human existence. This disruption to our stability necessitates and indeed forces us to alter our ways and develop novel coping mechanisms. Paradoxically COVID-19 encapsulates two of our innate fears, fear of uncertainty and fear of death; the latter being life's great certainty. Fear of the unknown appears to be inherent, evolutionarily-derived and a logical reduction of higher order constructs. Fear of the unknown is defensibly a fundamental fear; one which has been immeasurably amplified at a population level by COVID-19 [13]. Perhaps as we journey through this pandemic and learn more about the virus, fear of the unknown may transmute into a fear of the known, the latter of which may prove to be more manageable and less traumatising.

## 5. The impact of COVID-19 on healthcare workers

The analogy of the COVID-19 pandemic as a kind of global war is now very familiar, with the frontline medical staff akin to foot soldiers in the trenches, fighting back against a voracious, viral enemy. Much has been written about the challenges facing healthcare workers in the midst of this pandemic: extended working hours, risk of exposure to the virus, fear of transmitting the virus to family members, insufficient supplies of personal protective equipment, adaptation to new work practices and changing roles, to name but a few. In addition to such practical challenges facing healthcare workers during the pandemic, a vast array of workers has been faced with emotionally fraught, moral and ethical dilemmas. Immeasurable moral injury may have occurred as healthcare workers have been forced to make difficult decisions regarding resource allocation, something which most workers likely never anticipated having to face.

Also worthy of consideration are the feelings of fear and guilt which may arise following infection with the virus. In light of the fact that countless frontline workers contracted the virus in the course of their work, it is plausible that many of these workers grappled with self-blame and a sense of shame about having become infected. Tragically, such feelings, coupled with heavy stress and fear of having contaminated others, are thought to have resulted in the suicides of a number of healthcare workers. Indeed, Reger and colleagues have discussed the possibility of suicide rates increasing across the general population, in the aftermath of the pandemic: they caution that a surge in suicides may occur among people who struggle to cope with the realities of the pandemic [14]. Coupled with the fact that in 2018, the U.S. had its highest age-adjusted suicide rate since 1941, it is not difficult to imagine that the personal and interpersonal struggles presented by the pandemic could exacerbate the situation. It could be argued that frontline working bestows an even higher risk, given the vicarious trauma which many of these workers have sustained.

Notwithstanding these considerations, there is at least some cause for hope: there has been a decrease in suicide rates in the short-term aftermath of previous national disasters, such as the 11th September terrorist attacks [15], although the data on longer-term effects is, admittedly, somewhat mixed. The "pulling-together" effect, wherein members of society have a shared experience of testing times and learn to support each other through their difficulties, is one hypothesis for the downward trend in suicide after national disasters. In addition, a pandemic may give pause for thought and reflection on our mortality, and force us to consider how precious life is, and as a result, possibly make suicide less likely. However, a word of caution: history has taught us that the impact of outbreaks on suicide rates tends to be a negative one. Although there is little data regarding the previous pandemic of Spanish Flu (1918), the general consensus is that suicide rates increased at that time. More recent data following the SARS epidemic showed an increase in the suicide rate of older adults in Hong Kong in 2003, a 31.7% increase from 2002 [16, 17].

The mantra of "we're all in this together" was quickly adopted in order to inspire a sense of community in the fight against the virus. This well-meaning drive to foster a sense of community would chime with Emile Durkenheim's [18] seminal work on the theory of suicide, which postulated that linking suicide almost exclusively with mental illness, and effectively ignoring social connectedness, was inadequate. He linked a rise in suicides at the time to modernity and the associated weakening of family and community bonds, and ultimately asserted that as social integration decreases, people are more likely to die by suicide. In this time of social and physical distancing, it is not difficult to comprehend how people could feel less socially connected and perceive themselves as being more alone than ever before [19], meaning that a rise in suicides is a very real possibility.

On the other hand, a pandemic is not the same as a natural disaster or an act of terror. Although comparative in terms of the mass loss of life and the sense of a loss of control, a pandemic contrasts with manmade or natural disasters in terms of the duration and magnitude of the event; a pandemic is a prolonged crisis, and it is known that prolonged stressors can be especially challenging to adapt to [20]. However, it is not beyond the capabilities of the human condition to overcome unimaginable suffering: Viktor Frankl's account of life and the search for meaning in a Nazi concentration camp springs to mind as a shining example of human courage in the face of difficulty and suffering [21]. This pandemic has given rise to levels of unemployment not seen for decades, and it is widely anticipated to result in a global economic downturn. It is known that rates of suicide tend to increase during periods of recession [22]: it was estimated that a 22.8% increase in suicide occurred in the United States during the Great Depression of 1929–1933 [23]. Similarly, following the Asian economic crisis of 1997–1998, male suicide rates soared by 39% in Japan, 44% in Hong Kong and 45% in South Korea from 1997 to 1998 [24]. More recently, Irish data found that by the end of 2012, the suicide rate for men was 57% higher than if the pre-recession trend had continued [25], while self-harm rates were 31% higher for males and females. Of note, Stuckler [26] found that countries with the most severe economic downturns had the greatest increase in suicides, while countries such as Austria, with strong social support structures and protective labour markets, had a net decrease in deaths by suicide. It remains to be seen what the impact of this economic downturn will be on suicide rates.

We know that, for many of us, our job plays a key role in our identity and sense of self. Consider being dismissed from a job or unexpectedly losing a job: most people would consider either of these events upsetting at best, traumatic at worst, and there is a real risk to mental well-being involved. One study showed that long-term (more than 52 weeks) unemployment was significantly correlated with large negative effects on mental health, with even greater effect sizes observed in minority groups [27]. Having a job fosters self-confidence, and, for many, inspires a sense of purpose. Many healthcare workers will say they entered the field of health in order to help others in a real and meaningful way. If trauma is a rupture in "meaning-making" [2], then the pandemic was perhaps the greatest rupture these healthcare workers will witness in their careers: the way they viewed themselves, the world, and others was overturned by this frightening event which was unprecedented in living memory. The concern is that a gap has now arisen between what these workers knew, or their "orienting systems", and the traumatic event. As we emerge gradually from the pandemic and healthcare workers have some time to reflect on their experiences, some will undoubtedly process events, harness their resilience, and move past the trauma. Others will likely struggle to process the magnitude of what they have experienced amidst the pandemic, and are at risk of developing mental health difficulties.

In attempting to plan adequately for the increased need for mental health supports for healthcare workers in the aftermath of this pandemic, we should regard it as inevitable that an increase in mental health needs will arise. We need only look to the outcomes for healthcare workers who have worked through previous, smaller outbreaks. One study [28] found that more than three-quarters of healthcare workers who cared for patients during the SARS outbreak reported experiencing mental health difficulties, such as sleep disturbance, anxiety and low mood. Various authors have lamented the paucity of training in mental health care delivery for healthcare professionals in the context of working in a pandemic [29]. Others have argued that it is imperative that healthcare managers take steps to protect the mental health of their staff and to correctly identify those who suffer psychological injury as a result of the pandemic [30].

Regarding the psychological sequelae to trauma, it is widely accepted that a lack of post-trauma social support and exposure to stressors during recovery constitute the two risk factors which confer the highest risk in terms of long-term mental health status [30]. On a positive note, we know that healthcare managers can play an instrumental role influencing the experience of workers, in that they can foster a supportive environment for workers and take steps to reduce workplace stressors following the acute crisis period. Once again, history has taught us that supportive managers can have a powerful effect on the mental well-being of their staff, as demonstrated in research from previous outbreaks [31].

Greenberg discusses six elements, based on the best evidence available, which are necessary in the protection of healthcare workers' mental health [30]. Firstly, it is felt that healthcare workers should be thanked, because resilience is thought to be nurtured through an appropriate acknowledgement of the difficult work carried out by frontline workers. Greenberg suggests that potential psychological and emotional issues should be acknowledged and information should be forthcoming as regards support options which are available to healthcare workers. Secondly, it is advised that healthcare workers who are absent from work be actively followed up by managers. Given that avoidance is a cardinal symptom of traumatic stress, this may manifest as being absent from work. Healthcare managers should engage with workers who have unplanned absences from work, in order to ascertain if the workers are experiencing mental health difficulties and to facilitate signposting to appropriate support services. Thirdly, the case is made for "return to normal work" interviews, as healthcare workers journey from crisis roles back to the "new normal". Such meetings should facilitate a supportive conversation regarding mental health needs, and should be conducted by managers who are experienced in and comfortable with speaking about mental health needs. Research in trauma-exposed occupations has demonstrated that workplace mental health training of managers can reduce employee sick leave [32].

In addition, Greenberg argues that healthcare managers ought to be particularly cognisant of the potential mental health needs of healthcare workers who belong to high-risk groups, including black, Asian and ethnic minority people, as well as junior or inexperienced staff [30]. The identification of ongoing stressors, such as bereavement, is of paramount importance. There is also a need for special focus on those healthcare workers who have taken on roles and responsibilities beyond their usual role, e.g. workers who were redeployed to novel roles.

The UK National Institute for Health and Care Excellence endorses the active monitoring of anyone who has experiences a potentially traumatic event, especially those who are already considered to be at increased risk of mental health difficulties. In the aftermath of the 2005 London bombings, Brewin and colleagues demonstrated that proactively reaching out to people about their mental health can result in an increased take-up of mental health care [33].

Healthcare workers being able to make sense of and derive meaning from their traumatic pandemic experiences is the final piece in the puzzle of protecting their mental health. It is widely believed that it is not events per se have the most significant impact on our coping, but rather how we think about, interpret and perceive events and ascribe them a meaning [20]. Healthcare managers should strive to assist workers in developing a meaningful narrative of their experiences, one that does not apportion blame to the self or others for the distressing challenges they faced amidst the pandemic. Schwartz rounds and Balint groups are two methods by which healthcare workers may process the trauma they have experienced and foster a sense a purpose. After all, oft-quoted in the words of the Friedrich Nietzsche, "he who has a why to live for can bear almost any how".

## 6. Older people and COVID-19

During the COVID-19 pandemic, older adults have been considered a high-risk group. As such, they became a focus of government guidelines and regulations concerning their day-to-day living, which has undoubtedly impacted significantly on their quality of life. Although COVID-19 is a physical health crisis, within it lies the core precipitating factors for a mental health crisis [34]. It has been suggested that the measures taken by government in relation to social distancing and isolation or 'cocooning', especially targeting groups at risk including older adults, can result in social isolation and indeed loneliness. The latter variables are known to decrease psychological well-being and increase the risk for depression and cognitive dysfunction [35].

COVID-19 has disproportionately affected older people all over the world with utterly devastating consequences. An analysis of confirmed deaths by the Central Statistics Office in Ireland has shown that COVID-19 has had the greatest impact on people aged 65 or over. This age group accounted for almost 92% of confirmed deaths between 11th March to 15th May 2020, while similar trends have been observed in other countries.

People aged 70 and over were instructed to stay indoors, avoid all social visits from friends and family, and largely avoid outdoor exercise – activities that are vital to everyday routine and indeed quality of life. Social interaction, physical activity and behavioural activation are heavily encouraged for older people to ensure psychological and physical well-being and suddenly this was curtailed in many societies with no knowledge or certainty of time frame as to when these restrictions would be lifted and a sense of normality could return. Older adults with regular social interaction demonstrate greater psychological well-being and life satisfaction [35]. The pandemic robbed older adults of this opportunity and, consequently, perpetuated the loneliness and social isolation which older adults often experience and feel.

Socioemotional selectivity theory, a life-span theory of motivation which maintains that age differences in goals results from shrinking time horizons, is an area of interest when considering the importance of social connections in older adults. It proposes that older adults use their social network as a buffer against negative experiences [36]. Earlier in life, physical and mental health are strongly interconnected; however, as we age this association is weakened [36]. As physical health declines, subjective well-being is maintained which may be conceived as 'a paradox of aging'. Older adults place emphasis on emotional well-being and their relationships as a maintaining factor in this.

Not only does meaningful social interaction affect emotional and mental well-being, it impacts on physical health and a lack thereof can precipitate a decline in emotional, mental and physical well-being. Psychologists, sociologists, and epidemiologists have contributed significantly to our understanding of how social processes influence physiological processes, going some way towards explaining the link between social interaction and health. Supportive interactions with other individuals benefit immune, endocrine, and cardiovascular functions and reduce allostatic load, which essentially reflects stress on the body due to chronically overstimulated physiological systems engaged in stress responses [36].

Though necessary and understandable, the restrictions and social isolation enforced on vulnerable at-risk groups such as older adults, may further enhance their vulnerabilities by removing their social connections and their associated benefits. Social connections foster cumulative advantages for older adults over time. The direct impact of COVID-19 and the high mortality rate due to physical illness and complications is apparent but what will be the secondary impact on both physical and mental health? This a serious public health concern.

It is easy to presume that as adults age and they experience bereavements, they become somewhat accustomed to it due possibly to habituation and the expectation that we will continue to experience bereavements as we age. However, research has demonstrated that this is not the case [37]. The grieving process of the elderly is not inherently different to that of any other age group and elderly people will require the type of support and assistance afforded to younger persons during times of grieving. Grieving experiences of the elderly is rarely discussed and explored and this is an emerging area of interest [38]. It is, as yet, unclear what the long-term effects of COVID-related bereavements will be on the older generation, the group who likely experienced the greatest number of COVID-related bereavements.

As a group, older adults have been the victims of the majority of deaths due to COVID-19, while also enduring the strictest restrictions vis-à-vis enforced social Isolation. Recent evidence demonstrates the overall death rate from covid-19 has been estimated at 0.66%, rising sharply to 7.8% in people aged over 80 and declining to 0.0016% in children aged 9 and under [39]. Older adults know that they are more vulnerable to death and disability due to COVID-19 than their younger counterparts and that the treatments for COVID-19 are currently rather limited [40].

Older adults have lost loved ones and have not been afforded the opportunity to grieve with support. Moreover, older adults experience anticipatory anxiety and fear of contracting COVID-19 as through public messaging they are all too aware of the possible eventualities should they contract the virus. This anxiety related to fear of death was termed thanatophobia by Sigmund Freud in 1915 in his seminal essays titled: *Thoughts for the Time on War and Death*. Freud believed this to be related to one's unconscious belief in one's own immortality. Death anxiety is a universal and inherent phenomenon, which affects all humans to varying degrees. For the elderly, their fears are based in the actual process of dying and how they will experience dying, rather than death itself where there is thought to be some level of acceptance as regards the transience of life and the inevitability of death [38] This fear is enhanced by COVID-19 as the illness trajectory of the virus is uncertain and unpredictable, with some individuals recovering after a mild illness and others losing their lives rather suddenly after contracting the virus.

On a practical level, this pandemic has upset the lives of older adults in immeasurable ways, given their reliance on external supports. Due to physiological effects of ageing, worsening mobility and the presence of chronic illnesses, many older adults rely on home help, carers and community services for their activities of daily living [41]. Many such services were either reduced or suspended during the peaks of the pandemic. These support services experienced new, substantial challenges in order to maintain services while keeping clients and aides safe from COVID-19 [42]. This disproportionately affects elderly individuals, whose sole social contact may be outside of the home, such as day care venues, community centres, and places of worship. Those who lack close family or friends, and rely on the support of voluntary services or social care, were placed at additional risk of social isolation, as these people may already be lonely, isolated, or secluded. Unfortunately, older adults are anecdotally less accustomed to and involved in the online world of social media and communications. Older adults have experienced difficulties with telecommunications; telephone interaction has not been favourable given the hearing impairment of some older and challenges in engaging individuals and building rapport [43]. Online technologies and resources could be harnessed to provide social support networks and promote future inclusivity for older adults [44].

The traumatic effects of COVID 19 on older adults have been acute, chronic and considerably complex. Older people are the age cohort most at risk of severe physical illness and death. They have been faced with the trauma of death and dying, including vicarious trauma experienced due to the death of their loved ones. They have been under the most severe of restrictions, while services and supports on which they heavily rely have been reduced and suspended.

At the outset of this pandemic, older people and those with pre-established medical conditions were felt to be the most vulnerable to infection with COVID-19. Communal care settings were especially blighted with high disease and mortality rates. The physical and psychological deconditioning and disengagement due to the pandemic and its associated fear will be hard to counteract in this age group. Older people have the least available time of any to recover despite their inherent resilience and life experience. The needs of older adults, and the consequences if these needs are not met, should be strongly considered in public health recommendations and service provision. The negative psychological and social aftermath of the COVID-19 pandemic is playing out and will continually unfold and older people may once again be over-represented in terms of its' detrimental impact.

## 7. Young people and COVID-19

Young people may have escaped the pandemic relatively unscathed in terms of serious physical health sequelae of COVID-19, given that they were substantially less likely to be afflicted by severe illness, but the same cannot assumed regarding young people's social and emotional well-being. Children are more sensitive (e.g. to news reports on TV) and may develop a view of the world that it is a terrifying place to be. They may witness their parents struggling to cope, and this could reinforce their view of the world as a frightening place. In the longer term, this can colour or cloud the lens through which they view the world. The babies born during the pandemic experienced a lack of socialisation- have they missed critical periods of social and emotional development?

It is well established that adolescence is a stage of life wherein there is a heightened need for peer interaction, and emphasis is placed on social stimuli [45]. The severity and gravity of the COVID-19 situation forced many countries to implement strict public health measures such as physical distancing, self-isolation, school closures, and suspension of most sporting and other recreational activities, resulting in unprecedented levels of social disconnection by effectively precluding young people from engaging in face-to-face contact outside the realm of their own household or social bubble. Many young people missed out on life events which typically punctuate the adolescent and young adult periods of the life span, the so-called "coming of age" events such as school-leaving examinations and graduation ceremonies. Others embarked on their third level educations in a radically-changed educational environment, where online teaching prevailed in lieu of in-person lectures, and students were required to stay at home rather than move into their campus accommodation.

It is not yet known what longer-term social and emotional effects the pandemic may herald for our young people. It may be the case that social deprivation and physical isolation from peers will have a lasting impact on the psyche of young people: research has demonstrated that peer acceptance and peer influence are of paramount importance during adolescence. Indeed, animal studies have even demonstrated that social isolation and deprivation in adolescence can give rise to unique effects on brain and behaviour, in comparison to other stages in the lifespan. In highlighting the power of social networks, Jain [46] explains that irrespective of the particular type of trauma a person experiences, early social supports for the person in the aftermath of the trauma can actually prevent the onset of PTSD. Furthermore, for those who develop PTSD, a supportive social network can be instrumental in the healing process. Jain [46] stresses that early optimisation of social support in the wake of traumatic events is now considered excellent treatment. In addition, the person's perception of the support they receive from others is thought to be of utmost importance in terms of protection against developing PTSD.

On the other hand, it may transpire that the trend towards digital platforms of interaction, such as social media, may bestow some level of protection for young people against feelings of social isolation and thereby result in a less damaging effect to their mental well-being. Jain [46] examines the impact of social media technology during times of natural disaster and asks if such technology can be harnessed to bolster the social networks of post-disaster survivors. For example, in 2010, survivors of the Haitian earthquake turned to social media to tell their stories, which in turn rallied the response of the mainstream media to the disaster. Similarly, online communities were established in the wake of hurricane Katrina, providing support for survivors and a space to help process the trauma they had experienced. Of course, there are drawbacks to social media: trolling, misinformation and privacy concerns, to name just a few. It should also be noted that social media technology is not universally accessible: people of lower socioeconomic status are less likely to have the means to access smart phones, tablets, or similar devices. The tragedy is that it is those of lower socioeconomic means who are more likely to be adversely affected by disasters, such as this pandemic, and therefore are perhaps the most needy of support in our society.

A number of rapid cross-sectional surveys have suggested an increased prevalence of anxiety and depression amidst the pandemic, as well as lower levels of well-being. However, Kwong et al. [47] issue a word of caution regarding such rapid surveying of a population: information relating to the participants' pre-pandemic mental health and potential confounding factors, is lacking, thus preventing a comprehensive assessment of whether adverse mental health outcomes arise in those with pre-existing mental health difficulties, or whether those with no previous psychiatric history develop mental health difficulties which are attributable to the pandemic. In an effort to remedy this situation, Kwong and colleagues [47] aimed to quantify the prevalence of depression, anxiety and mental well-being prior to and during the COVID-19 pandemic. Data were compiled from the Avon Longitudinal Study of Parents and Children [ALSPAC] and Generation Scotland cohort. Results showed that the prevalence of depression during the pandemic was similar to pre-pandemic prevalence in the ALSPAC index generation (mean age of 28 years), while the rates of anxiety had increased almost twofold, i.e. 24% in comparison to the pre-pandemic level of 13%. The authors identified young people, women, people with pre-existing mental or physical health difficulties, and those experiencing socioeconomic adversity, as at-risk groups for developing depression and/or anxiety amidst the pandemic, even when controlling for pre-pandemic anxiety and depression. Similar results were found by O'Connor et al. [48], in a study of just over three thousand people, which found that while levels of depression did not change significantly, suicidal ideation increased over time, and anxiety decreased following an initial spike. Subgroup analyses demonstrated that young people (aged 18–29 years), in addition to women, people from socially disadvantaged backgrounds and people with pre-existing mental health difficulties, had worse mental health outcomes during the pandemic. The authors cited the growing rates of suicidal ideation across waves of the pandemic, particularly in young adults, as cause for concern. It is possible that anxiety arises in response to an ongoing threat and sense of uncertainty, whereas the sense of global community and the "all in this together" attitude may bestow some protection against negative self-talk, self-blame and depressive guilt.

In a 2021 survey conducted by a U.K.-based charity for youth mental health, Stem4, it was found that three in five young people reported experiencing mental health difficulties such as anxiety and low mood. The same organisation witnessed an increase of over 1000% in views of its online resources page (which offers advice on matters such as coping skills for anxiety) during the lockdown period, in comparison to pre-lockdown [49]. In a recent Irish qualitative study [50] examining presentations to the paediatric emergency department, clinicians reported that there was an increase in demand for psychological supports for young people during the pandemic. The authors found that overall, the pandemic and the resultant public health restrictions have had a negative impact on the psychosocial well-being of young people. They found that the difficulty in accessing primary care and community services exacerbated the struggle of young people in need of support. There were anecdotal reports that presentations with self-harm had increased and the reduced access to out-patient child and adolescent mental health teams was cited as a possible contributing factor in this regard. The strife of children with neurodevelopmental disabilities was also highlighted: the authors highlighted that in the absence of a structured daily routine and support services such as specialist schools, some children with autism spectrum disorder struggled significantly, culminating in some being brought to the emergency department by their parents, who were struggling to cope with the escalation in their child's challenging behaviour. There is the additional concern that the closure of schools and other community services equated to the loss of safety nets for vulnerable children, who might have otherwise been referred to appropriate support services. Once again, the long-term consequences, if any, of these pandemic-induced challenges are to be elucidated. Perhaps the best course of action at this point would be to implement adequate services for young people as we emerge from the pandemic, with a focus on those services which were insufficiently resourced during the pandemic, such as community-based mental health services.

Finally, there is the question of intergenerational trauma. Although in its infancy, the study of epigenetics seeks to establish if children of traumatised parents have an increased risk of developing similar difficulties to their parents. It is thought that PTSD may alter gene expression in a trauma survivor, and these alterations could then be passed on to the survivor's progeny at a cellular level it being speculated that such epigenetic alterations are passed to the child by "intergenerational transmission" by way of adversely affecting the parents' sperm or egg quality, or by negatively affecting the mother while she is pregnant. Yehuda et al. [51] examined the epigenetics of PTSD by assessing the effect of trauma exposure on the salivary cortisol levels of pregnant women. They found lower cortisol levels in women who were pregnant when they evacuated the World Trade Centre during the 11th September attacks, and this result was replicated in their one-year-old children. In comparison to women who did not develop PTSD in the wake of the terrorist attack, lower cortisol levels were found in mothers who developed PTSD and their infants, with mothers in the third trimester displaying the lowest cortisol levels. It is hypothesised that traumatic stress may alter the expression of an enzyme in the placenta, which in turn, modifies cortisol into an inactive metabolite. Other research has found that pregnant women with PTSD are at increased risk for impaired uterine blood flow, low birth weight babies and prematurity. It has been argued [46] that in-utero exposure to trauma can have adverse effects on the developing foctus. When we consider some of the obstacles which pregnant women faced during this pandemic: hospital visitor restrictions, fear of contracting the illness and uncertainty about vaccination, it is not difficult to imagine how stressful pregnancy was. Only time will tell if the distress and trauma experienced by many expectant mothers during this pandemic has been passed on to their "COVID babies".

## 8. Conclusion

With potentially swathes of people reporting subjective psychological trauma and stress as a direct consequence of the pandemic, the knock-on effects on mental health services and on primary remain to be seen. Will there be an increased demand for supports in the longer term and how will these increased needs be met? Cullen and colleagues [52] issue a word of caution when considering how we ought to address mental health in the aftermath of the pandemic: "we neglect mental health at our peril and to our long-term detriment". That said, resilience factors may offset some of the adverse effects of the pandemic and these may be determined by individual personality traits and proactive coping styles. It is also obvious that psychological stress does not invariably become disorder. The challenge is for governments to adapt the wider environment and societal structures to support resilience and learn from less successful strategies including inadequate, mixed or inconsistent messaging to assist in preparedness for future health crises.

Finally, we should be eternally mindful of the danger of forgetting. When trauma is not discussed, not processed, and perhaps actively forgotten, healing for some is hindered and probably prevented, yet excessive reflection may also potentially be re-traumatising for others. Arguably a sense of complacency and lack of preparedness for future global pandemics would constitute the worst legacy of COVID-19. There is a danger that we will banish the pandemic to the depths of our subconscious, and ignore the need to actively process what has happened to our world and its citizens over the past 2 years. We know that the last pandemic incurred such a fate, with relatively little having been written about it in one hundred years since it ended. We need to consider what steps we may take to facilitate processing the trauma, in the hope that we can eventually learn from it and move past it. As mentioned previously, it has been recommended that frontline workers be formally thanked for their work during the pandemic, that their emotional and psychological wellbeing be preserved, burnout prevented and that their learning and experience be retained to ensure future responsiveness by health systems. We would suggest that a wider societal approach to actively remember the pandemic and those who lost their lives as a result, such as national and international days of remembrance, should be actively considered, lest we forget and fail to derive meaning from what we have been through during the course of this pandemic.

## Conflict of interest

The authors declare no conflict of interest.

## Author details

Aishling Collins*, Eleanor O'Driscoll* and Declan Lyons
St Patrick's Mental Health Services, Dublin, Ireland

*Address all correspondence to: collinae@tcd.ie; odriscel@tcd.ie

## References

[1] Salari N, Hosseinian-Far A, Jalali R, Vaisi-Raygani A, Rasoulpoor S, Mohammadi M, et al. Prevalence of stress, anxiety, depression among the general population during the COVID-19 pandemic: A systematic review and meta-analysis. Globalization and Health. 2020;**16**(1):1-1

[2] Prideaux E. How to heal the 'mass trauma' of Covid-19. [online] 2021. Bbc.com. Available at: https://www.bbc.com/future/article/20210203-after-the-covid-19-pandemic-how-will-we-heal [Accessed: 5 September 2021]

[3] Näppä U, Lundgren AB, Axelsson B. The effect of bereavement groups on grief, anxiety, and depression-A controlled, prospective intervention study. BMC Palliative Care. 2016; **15**(1):1-8

[4] Afolabi O. Death, Grief and Family Dynamics: The Impact of Family Member's Death and Delayed Grief Resolution on the Family System. 2 May 2014:1-13. Available at SSRN 2826483

[5] Keyes KM, Pratt C, Galea S, McLaughlin KA, Koenen KC, Shear MK. The burden of loss: Unexpected death of a loved one and psychiatric disorders across the life course in a national study. American Journal of Psychiatry. 2014;**171**(8):864-871

[6] Mitima-Verloop HB, Mooren TT, Boelen PA. Facilitating grief: An exploration of the function of funerals and rituals in relation to grief reactions. Death Studies. 2019;**11**:1-1

[7] Leander M, Lampa E, Rask-Andersen A, Franklin K, Gislason T, Oudin A, et al. Impact of anxiety and depression on respiratory symptoms. Respiratory Medicine. 2014;**108**(11):1594-1600

[8] Bloom DE, Cadarette D. Infectious disease threats in the twenty-first century: Strengthening the global response. Frontiers in Immunology. 2019;**10**:549

[9] Pappas G, Kiriaze IJ, Giannakis P, Falagas ME. Psychosocial consequences of infectious diseases. Clinical Microbiology and Infection. 2009; **15**(8):743-747

[10] Mertens G, Gerritsen L, Duijndam S, Salemink E, Engelhard IM. Fear of the coronavirus (COVID-19): Predictors in an online study conducted in March 2020. Journal of Anxiety Disorders. 2020;**74**:102258

[11] Wong LP, Alias H. Temporal changes in psychobehavioural responses during the early phase of the COVID-19 pandemic in Malaysia. Journal of Behavioral Medicine. 2021;**44**(1):18-28

[12] Arora A, Jha AK, Alat P, Das SS. Understanding coronaphobia. Asian Journal of Psychiatry. 2020;**54**:102384

[13] Carleton RN. Fear of the unknown: One fear to rule them all? Journal of Anxiety Disorders. 2016;**41**:5-21

[14] Reger MA, Stanley IH, Joiner TE. Suicide mortality and coronavirus disease 2019—A perfect storm? JAMA Psychiatry. 2020;**77**(11):1093-1094

[15] Salib E. Effect of 11 September 2001 on suicide and homicide in England and Wales. The British Journal of Psychiatry. 2003;**183**(3):207-212

[16] Cheung YT, Chau PH, Yip PS. A revisit on older adults suicides and Severe Acute Respiratory Syndrome (SARS) epidemic in Hong Kong. International Journal of Geriatric Psychiatry: A Journal of the Psychiatry of Late Life and Allied Sciences. 2008; **23**(12):1231-1238

[17] Yip PS, Liu KY, Law CK, Law YW. Social and economic burden of suicides

in Hong Kong SAR: A year of life lost perspective. Crisis. 2005;**26**(4):156-159

[18] Durkheim E. Suicide: A Study in Sociology. London: Routledge; 2005

[19] Rokach A. The Psychological Journey to and from Loneliness: Development, Causes, and Effects of Social and Emotional Isolation. London: Academic Press; 2019

[20] Miller ED. The COVID-19 pandemic crisis: The loss and trauma event of our time. Journal of Loss and Trauma. 2020;**25**(6-7):560-572

[21] Frankl VE. Man's Search for Meaning. New York: Simon and Schuster; 1985

[22] Mann JJ, Apter A, Bertolote J, Beautrais A, Currier D, Haas A, et al. Suicide prevention strategies: A systematic review. JAMA. 2005; **294**(16):2064-2074

[23] Luo F, Florence CS, Quispe-Agnoli M, Ouyand L, Crosby AE. Impact of business cycles on US suicide rates, 1928-2007. American Journal of Public Health. 2011; **101**:1139-1146

[24] Chang SS, Gunnell D, Sterne JA, Lu TH, Cheng AT. Was the economic crisis 1997-1998 responsible for rising suicide rates in East/Southeast Asia? A time–trend analysis for Japan, Hong Kong, South Korea, Taiwan, Singapore and Thailand. Social Science & Medicine. 2009;**68**(7):1322-1331

[25] Corcoran P, Griffin E, Arensman E, Fitzgerald AP, Perry IJ. Impact of the economic recession and subsequent austerity on suicide and self-harm in Ireland: An interrupted time series analysis. International Journal of Epidemiology. 2015;**44**(3):969-977

[26] Stuckler D, Basu S, Suhrcke M, Coutts A, McKee M. The public health effect of economic crises and alternative policy responses in Europe: An empirical analysis. The Lancet. 2009; **374**(9686):315-323

[27] Exploring the link between unemployment and mental health outcomes [Internet]. Available from: https://www.apa.org. 2021. [cited: 6 December 2021]. Available from: https://www.apa.org/pi/ses/resources/indicator/2012/04/unemployment

[28] Chong MY, Wang WC, Hsieh WC, Lee CY, Chiu NM, Yeh WC, et al. Psychological impact of severe acute respiratory syndrome on health workers in a tertiary hospital. The British Journal of Psychiatry. 2004;**185**(2):127-133

[29] Xiang YT, Yang Y, Li W, Zhang L, Zhang Q, Cheung T, et al. Timely mental health care for the 2019 novel coronavirus outbreak is urgently needed. The Lancet Psychiatry. 2020;**7**(3):228-229

[30] Greenberg N. Mental health of health-care workers in the COVID-19 era. Nature Reviews Nephrology. 2020;**16**(8):425-426

[31] Brooks SK, Dunn R, Amlôt R, Rubin GJ, Greenberg N. A systematic, thematic review of social and occupational factors associated with psychological outcomes in healthcare employees during an infectious disease outbreak. Journal of Occupational and Environmental Medicine. 2018;**60**(3):248-257

[32] Milligan-Saville JS, Tan L, Gayed A, Barnes C, Madan I, Dobson M, et al. Workplace mental health training for managers and its effect on sick leave in employees: A cluster randomised controlled trial. The Lancet Psychiatry. 2017;**4**(11):850-858

[33] Brewin CR, Fuchkan N, Huntley Z, Robertson M, Thompson M, Scragg P, et al. Outreach and screening following the

2005 London bombings: Usage and outcomes. Psychological Medicine. 2010;**40**(12):2049-2057

[34] De Pue S, Gillebert C, Dierckx E, Vanderhasselt MA, De Raedt R, Van den Bussche E. The impact of the COVID-19 pandemic on wellbeing and cognitive functioning of older adults. Scientific Reports. 2021;**11**(1):1-1

[35] Nezlek JB, Richardson DS, Green LR, Schatten-Jones EC. Psychological well-being and day-to-day social interaction among older adults. Personal Relationships. 2002;**9**(1):57-71

[36] Löckenhoff CE, Carstensen LL. Socioemotional selectivity theory, aging, and health: The increasingly delicate balance between regulating emotions and making tough choices. Journal of Personality. 2004;**72**(6): 1395-1424

[37] Lekalakala-Mokgele E. Death and dying: Elderly persons' experiences of grief over the loss of family members. South African Family Practice. 2018;**60**(5):151-154

[38] Sinoff G. Thanatophobia (death anxiety) in the elderly: The problem of the child's inability to assess their own parent's death anxiety state. Frontiers in Medicine. 2017;**4**:11

[39] Mahase E. Covid-19: Death rate is 0.66% and increases with age, study estimates. BMJ: British Medical Journal (Online). 1 Apr 2020;369

[40] Mistry SK, Ali AM, Akther F, Yadav UN, Harris MF. Exploring fear of COVID-19 and its correlates among older adults in Bangladesh. Globalization and Health. 2021;**17**(1): 1-9

[41] Smith ML, Bergeron CD, Riggle SD, Meng L, Towne SD Jr, Ahn S, et al. Self-care difficulties and reliance on support among vulnerable middle-aged and older adults with chronic conditions: A cross-sectional study. Maturitas. 2017;**104**:1-10

[42] Sama SR, Quinn MM, Galligan CJ, Karlsson ND, Gore RJ, Kriebel D, et al. Impacts of the COVID-19 pandemic on home health and home care agency managers, clients, and aides: A cross-sectional survey, March to June, 2020. Home Health Care Management & Practice. 2021;**33**(2):125-129

[43] Liu J, Ji B, Lou Y. Impact of the COVID-19 pandemic on community services for homebound older adults in New York City. Health & Social Care in the community. 2021:1-11

[44] Armitage R, Nellums LB. COVID-19 and the consequences of isolating the elderly. The Lancet Public Health. 2020;**5**(5):e256. 1-1

[45] Orben A, Tomova L, Blakemore SJ. The effects of social deprivation on adolescent development and mental health. The Lancet Child & Adolescent Health. 2020;**4**(8):634-640

[46] Jain S. The Unspeakable Mind: Stories of Trauma and Healing from the Frontlines of PTSD Science. New York: Harper Collins; 7 May 2019

[47] Kwong AS, Pearson RM, Adams MJ, Northstone K, Tilling K, Smith D, et al. Mental health before and during the COVID-19 pandemic in two longitudinal UK population cohorts. The British Journal of Psychiatry. 2021;**218**(6):334-343

[48] O'Connor R, Wetherall K, Cleare S, McClelland H, Melson A, Niedzwiedz C, et al. Mental health and well-being during the COVID-19 pandemic: Longitudinal analyses of adults in the UK COVID-19 Mental Health & Wellbeing study. The British Journal of Psychiatry. 2020;**218**(6):326-333

[49] Guest Article: Youth Mental Health Day by stem4 — The Consultation

Institute [Internet]. The Consultation Institute. 2021. [cited: 6 December 2021]. Available from: https://www.consultationinstitute.org/consultation-news/guest-article-youth-mental-health-day-by-stem4/

[50] Conlon C, McDonnell T, Barrett M, Cummins F, Deasy C, Hensey C, et al. The impact of the COVID-19 pandemic on child health and the provision of Care in Paediatric Emergency Departments: A qualitative study of frontline emergency care staff. BMC Health Services Research. 2021;**21**(1):1-1

[51] Yehuda R, Bierer LM. The relevance of epigenetics to PTSD: Implications for the DSM5. Journal of Traumatic Stress. 2009;**22**:427-434

[52] Cullen W, Gulati G, Kelly BD. Mental health in the COVID-19 pandemic. QJM: An International Journal of Medicine. 2020;**113**(5): 311-312

Chapter 22

# Perspective Chapter: Transforming Continuing Medical Education in the COVID-19

*Nikos Christo Secchi Nicolás and Ángel de Jesús Gómez Alarcón*

## Abstract

Medical education is not immune from the heartaches produced by abrupt contemporary changes in our world, such as the COVID-19 pandemic. Unexpectedly, and on very short notice, people can no longer teach or learn alongside other people. The impact on the heart of the educational processes of the health professions is unprecedented. The key concerns of yesterday, such as the need to enhance bedside learning or to enhance the experience of students in the clinical setting, in the clinical workplace, have a different meaning. Medical educators can leverage technology to enhance medical education at both undergraduate and graduate levels. Although the most recent initiatives, such as remote transmissions, have been introduced for a long time, traditional classes, lectures, and face-to-face didactic tutorials continue to be the most important cornerstone of medical education both in our country and abroad. The COVID-19 pandemic has posed challenges in medical education globally. Each society has responded according to its possibilities and needs to take advantage of this situation as a learning opportunity, continue with education, and incorporate students as health workers in the countries where it was necessary.

**Keywords:** continuing medical education, COVID-19, pandemic, teachers, videoconferencing, information and communication technologies

## 1. Introduction

Health science educators were living times of discussion about competency-based education, how this influenced curriculum design, teaching methodologies, and the role of teachers. The beginning of the decade took us in time when medical schools and colleges are incorporating an early approach to the field of practice and have increased the proportion of learning in practice settings. We never assumed a scenario like this. The COVID-19 pandemic is a situation not intended neither for health, nor for the economy, nor medical education. Everything will undoubtedly change during this period. There may be new, moderate forms of quarantine, but the world will certainly not be the same when the pandemic passes.

Medical education is not immune to the heartaches produced by abrupt contemporary changes in our world, such as the COVID-19 pandemic. Unexpectedly, and on very short notice, people can no longer teach or learn alongside other people. The impact on the heart of the educational processes of the health professions is unprecedented. Suddenly, the status quo of undergraduate or graduate medical education has been called into question, perhaps for the better. The key concerns of yesterday, such as the need to improve patient bedside learning or to enhance the experience of students in the clinical setting, in the clinical workplace, have a different meaning.

## 2. Continuing medical education during and after the pandemic

The arrival of the COVID-19 pandemic caused medical schools and faculties to interrupt their activities abruptly, recovering institutional capacities and making evident the strengths and weaknesses of each educational institution. The response in the undergraduate courses consisted in the migration of classes to virtual media, and the attendance of students to hospitals was interrupted to prevent them from being infected and could spread the virus in the communities.

In the case of students who were in undergraduate boarding school or in residencies, these were suspended and clinical rotations were replaced by the review of clinical cases by digital means. In graduate school, the resident physicians stayed in the hospitals and carried out a certain degree of theoretical activities and review of clinical cases on the Internet. Residents located in COVID hospitals suspended their scheduled clinical rotations and focused on responding to the pandemic by disrupting academic activities.

However, in contrast to the aforesaid, distance education remains rudimentary in supporting holistic professional learning. With the suspension of internships in colleges, medical educators must be creative in offering meaningful alternatives. Although virtual patients are not universally available and teaching practical procedures online is not yet feasible, clinical teachers can take advantage of the changes that are available in healthcare to adapt to COVID-19 crises. Additionally, COVID-19 can lead to unavailability of clinicians to teach as a result of the intense clinical workload generated by the disease. We may not be equipped with the tools to respond effectively [1].

The first response of most of the institutions in the world is to increase the use of "e-learning", especially online educational platforms and videoconferences. Strategies had already been imposed, more as support systems for face-to-face courses than as real online education. For initial or preclinical cycles, this may be a good answer, but questions immediately arise for which we still do not have an answer regarding the development of professional skills [2]. On the other hand, it highlights the differences in internet accessibility, either due to availability of equipment, connectivity, or the high consumption of data when it is done from mobile devices, which challenge equity in student access. The positive view of these processes is to reflect on how many of our usual face-to-face theoretical classes could be permanently replaced by this modality, accelerating the incorporation of methodologies such as flipped class or team-based learning.

Medical schools and colleges faced the challenge of maintaining their functioning and helping to respond to the pandemic. To this end, the following activities were developed, all of them supported by information and communication technologies (ICT) [3]:

- Maintain the undergraduate training processes: Because undergraduate students had to leave hospitals, training had to be migrated to ICT to assume totally a digital education.

- Preserve postgraduate training: Resident doctors remained in hospitals and many cases were reassigned to COVID areas, regardless of the specialty they were studying. Academic activities were maintained in most cases virtually.

- Strengthen continuing education: Medical schools and faculties implemented courses, webinars, and seminars to update physicians on preventive actions and the management of COVID-19 patients.

- Support the institutional management and coordination of telework: With closed institutions and with teachers and students located in different places, the coordination of activities and the organization of telework became decisive to develop synergistic actions between teachers and students and to maintain communication with the population.

- Promote access to scientific literature and information on COVID-19, and share it with governments, the health sector, and the general public, to guide evidence-based actions, help to reduce public distress, and avoid false news.

- Maintain communication and coordination with national and foreign experts, to keep abreast of the latest advances and set up collaboration networks.

- Generate research projects related to COVID-19: both local and participation in international multicenter studies.

- Establish advisory groups for governments: through interdisciplinary teams of experts made up of epidemiologists, infectologists, mathematicians, biostatistics, computer scientists, georeference experts, sociologists, and others.

- Provide remote medical assistance: through the installation of telephone assistance centers, telemedicine, and virtual hospitals.

- Organize volunteer student brigades, to strengthen health institutions with the care of non-COVID patients and facilitate the continuity of medical care.

- Take care of the physical and mental health of teachers, students, and workers: The faculties and schools implemented actions to assist their community, maintaining regular contact, establishing support units, and developing protocols for action in mental health.

- Produce medical equipment and personal protective equipment, supported by other university entities and businessmen, personal protective equipment was produced and some ventilators were even developed.

- Return to classrooms and clinical practices: A large part of the present effort is directed to organizing the return to face-to-face activities, preparing manuals with standards that include the use of masks, hand hygiene, and maintaining the minimum distance between people, or aspects such as ventilation.

Medical educators can leverage technology to enhance medical education at both undergraduate and graduate levels. Although the most recent initiatives, such as remote transmissions, have been introduced for a long time, traditional classes, lectures, and face-to-face didactic tutorials continue to be the most important cornerstone of medical education both in our country and abroad. In the case of the epidemic, we are experiencing and given the highly infectious nature of COVID-19, but as in most emerging infections in recent years, face-to-face interactions in large groups are sources of spread and transmission diseases and therefore should be avoided.

To avoid this, technology, for example, video conferencing and e-learning platforms, can be used to deliver them remotely *via* handheld devices and PCs. Faculty, residents, and medical students can initiate sessions at designated moments for them. In addition to lectures, teleconferencing is also being used to demonstrate medical procedures and surgical techniques. In this way, a centralized teaching is carried out, even without the need to hold lectures or face-to-face talks. This is also a good opportunity to encourage medical students and residents to use online resources to facilitate their individual learning. In particular, in specialty residency programs with significant procedural weight, remote training through educational videos or online webinars can be integrated into these residency or training programs [4].

Some technological learning tools are also sure to become massive shortly. It will occur in both undergraduate and graduate degrees. Interactive whiteboards, connected to a computer, will be used even more. There the teachers write, project images or videos, and transmit them in real-time to distant places [5]:

1. Perfecting medical visualizations with 3D images will allow you to learn anatomy or diagnostic imaging.

2. On the other hand, thanks to the use of virtual microscopes, even more about human cells and tissues will be taught.

3. The use of mobile phones or electronic tablets for educational purposes will also increase. These devices will allow—thanks to the download of applications—among other things to receive tutoring for a certain exam.

4. The virtual will allow immersive and augmented reality experiences that will include hospitals, inpatient rooms, or patients. There are already designs that simulate real clinical scenarios, where students assume the professional role, take a medical history, propose diagnoses, and indicate treatments.

Faculties can then set up programs and hold online meetings to continue these types of discussions that further help students and residents consolidate their learning. Courses in subjects such as communication skills, medical ethics, and even clinical or statistical research can also be arranged through these online modalities for medical students or residents. There are already numerous experiences in this regard.

Some countries have shown concern regarding the development of some courses during this pandemic; such is the case of anatomy due to the disposition to cremate the bodies to prevent the spread of the virus, a situation that limits the obtaining of corpses for the development of classes [6]. Furthermore, although virtualization is a viable alternative for many universities, not all have the logistical facilities to implement it. On the other hand, although some contents of the clinical courses can be virtualized, the skills necessary for medical performance—such as performing the physical exam—can only be adequately learned with the patient and virtual adaptations are unsustainable over time; for this reason, some faculties considered it necessary to delay the start of this type of course until the end of the pandemic. While it is true there are many advantages in the virtualization process of courses, it is clear that some universities have and will have limitations to make this process concrete [7].

Advantages and limitations in the virtualization process of undergraduate medicine courses are as follows:

- Advantages

  - Reduces the possibility that students in clinical courses will get sick from COVID-19.

- Reduces the possibility of contaminating patients and health personnel if they are asymptomatic carriers of the disease.

- Avoid the use of personal protective equipment on non-essential personnel in hospitals.

- It allows continuing with academic activities.

- Facilitates the timely review of academic material, ensuring the delivery of updated evidence-based content to students.

- It promotes digital learning in the new generations better adapted for it.

- Limitations

    - Not all universities have a digital platform to teach virtual courses.

    - Not all teachers have the ability to build adequate virtual content.

    - Requires a strong sense of self-motivation and good time management skills on the part of students and teachers.

    - The saturation of care work of doctors who are teachers will not allow them to dedicate themselves to virtual class-work.

    - It is not possible to virtualize all the contents of the clinical courses and some non-clinical ones (such as anatomy and the like).

    - Not all students can have access to a laptop, tablet, or smartphone for their classes.

    - Not everyone has an adequate internet or electricity connection; for example, if they are undergraduate students in rural areas.

    - Limits the collaborative learning experience.

    - Limits the presentation experience with live interaction.

    - Limits real-time feedback from face-to-face classes.

    - Unethical behaviors may occur more frequently (e.g., cheating during virtual evaluations).

But there is an unavoidable aspect that puts the development of competencies and their evaluation in tension. The presence of the student in the clinical environment is essential in medical teaching to acquire these skills. Presence that must be supervised requires close contact between teacher and students. The appearance of the coronavirus pandemic, highly contagious, in which the student can be a vector of infection, or can become infected, added to the dramatic change in the care model and the practices of health institutions, makes it necessary to recreate new forms of education combining technology and educational strategies to cushion the impact of the pandemic on the entire education process and continue in some creative way our way of teaching. On the other hand, the student's displays of commitment and enthusiasm that lead to their participation in volunteering should be evaluated in light of the risks involved, if it brings them into contact with potential patients [8].

But medical education is not just about imparting specific knowledge and skills in a particular domain. A highly qualified surgeon or an experienced physician is not necessarily a good physician. In addition to domain-specific knowledge, holistic non-cognitive attributes such as teamwork, empathy, initiative, and compassion are important qualities to convey to medical students and residents. The participation of these medical students and residents as collaborators, the former, and physicians increasingly involved, the latter, to try to alleviate this crisis is something important not only for that purpose but for their general education as physicians. In this sense, we are not inventing anything new, there are antecedents. In 2003, during the height of the SARS outbreak in Singapore, medical students were asked to help with temperature checks [9].

With the COVID-19 crisis, residents of all medical and surgical specialties in very different locations have also been selected to take shifts on the frontline, where they have assisted with the detection of suspected cases in emergencies and elsewhere. In addition to alleviating labor shortages where labor was scarce, this has helped foster camaraderie among residents as part of the medical community, prompting them to feel like part of the teams fighting this pandemic. This, according to very different testimonies, the residents have been taught important lessons about courage, empathy, and teamwork [2]. It has also provided the opportunity for many residents to review their general medical skills, since in many cases many of them, who belonged to highly technical or specialized specialties, have had to care for patients with this infection. This is a great step in their training and development as medical professionals with more holistic perspectives.

In response to the lack of clinical practice, the first alternative seems to be to alter the academic calendar by postponing the practical load and increasing the clinical reasoning activities at this stage, or the elective activities related to the pandemic. Some institutions incorporate the use of virtual cases, surgical videos, and participation in telemedicine. We must also think creatively, how to maintain contact with virtual and real patients, as well as develop new forms of evaluation. This requires clear indications for students and supervisors because the electronic interface modifies the possibilities of giving feedback and modifies the observed competencies. Nor should we lose contact with the human aspects of pandemics, as literature and film can contribute as triggers for this understanding [10].

The COVID-19 pandemic has posed challenges in medical education globally. Each society has responded according to its possibilities and needs to take advantage of this situation as a learning opportunity, continue with education, and incorporate students as health workers in the countries where it was necessary. A crisis such as the COVID-19 pandemic involves making great efforts to carry out contingency plans that minimize disruptions or profound changes that occur in educational programs.

Many university professors who went through this situation agree that preclinical subjects have been taught, overcoming some inconveniences and without being prepared for such a hasty decision. For others, after this pandemic and forced "natural experiment" something may no longer be strange. Why not think about a preclinical cycle entirely online for future doctors. With users located in various parts of the world, even endowed with the ability to find the best teachers or courses thanks to one click. Exchanging face-to-face classes of 1 hour, for sequences of short videos or podcasts of no more than 15 minutes [11].

However, technology can and should be harnessed to allow students and residents to learn from these experiences and gain extra training in skills such as clinical communication and medical ethics. Beyond the knowledge of a particular domain, the participation of medical students and residents in the clinical tasks that a pandemic like the one we are experiencing can be beneficial to develop another perspective on medicine and what clinical practice means and what it means. Time about what is expected of them as physicians. This type of crisis should be used to improve or instill non-cognitive holistic aspects such as leadership and adaptability. As medical educators, we can and must meet the challenge of continuing to teach even in times of crisis.

Before the outbreak of the SARS-COV-2 virus, online medical education had acquired some evolutionary features. She used to dealing with healthcare professionals who were geographically isolated and distant but connected through virtual communication. He provided solutions to hundreds of them immersed in demanding work hours, and with little flexibility in the agenda. It was based on collective learning, online collaboration, proactivity, and self-directed training [12].

Online had dispensed with the presence of educational leaders and managed to optimize interaction with them from a distance. It had generated between the participants an exchange—both synchronous and asynchronous—through chats, forums, or emails. COVID-19 has done nothing but selects those cited features of virtual education. Also, during these months, he has polished virtual-friendly technological educational tools. But it should not be repaired only in this present. It should be noted that the future seems to have changed a bit as well. Even the most skeptical no longer conceives the future of medical education, as something in total separates from technology and online.

In general terms, the educational emergency caused by the epidemic made evident the high frequency that the expository technique or oral presentation has in the educational activity by the teacher, who by not having the students in physical presence, perceived a lack of control and authority. In the same way, the student, under the same system, felt free and without directivity, which generated anxiety and anguish in not feeling his physical presence and having his direct surveillance; the teacher's immediate action was to commission homework, homework, and more homework, and the students were overwhelmed and disappointed by not receiving feedback.

Online education requires a differential planning of education with physical presence; the conjunction of a team of experts in various disciplinary areas is desirable, such as pedagogues, educational psychologists, software specialists, interactive, and graphic designers, among others, with which the online educational experience is highly meaningful for students [12].

The characteristics of teaching in virtuality include the following: the management of non-face-to-face asynchronous or synchronous educational organizations, transversal (multi or transdisciplinary) and holistic; student-centered, characterized by being flexible, cooperative, personalized, and interactive; the teacher will be a facilitator, who must be more collaborative than lonely, encourage/promote participation, recognize/accept the fact that they no longer have possession, with organizational skills, open to experimentation, and with the ability/ability to modify.

The use of ICT in teachers ranges from the resistance of its use to its formal use in education, with relative or little use for play, recreation, or social networks, while students use them little as an educational tool and their focus is on the play, entertainment, and especially on social networks. The previous dichotomy leads us to think in three moments about the knowledge, attitudes, and practice of ICT: appropriation, use, and access to ICT [13].

1. Appropriation: There is a difference in conceptualization and use between natives and digital immigrants; the former have grown and have developed

as a priority the playful and recreational aspect of digital technologies, especially social networks; in the case of the educational aspect, the job that is done consists of recovering the information, generally without discriminating the objective sources or of scientific certainty, and carries out its work by copying and pasting. The latter, digital immigrant teachers, can discriminate from sources, but their technological management often leaves much to be desired. Both require training, but not the same training, students to consume relevant information for their training and teachers train and train in the use of technology to strengthen the teaching-learning process.

2. Use: It has to do with knowing the potentialities that it offers in its scope of action, such as contributing to the development of other thinking skills (problem-solving) other than communicative ability. To develop these skills, critical thinking must be forged in the student that allows him to discriminate information on the network, evaluate it, verify its veracity, and be able to build new learning, because when thinking critically, arguments are accepted or rejected that later can be applied in different fields of knowledge, that is, establish a dialog between the student and the information that allows him to assess and abstract the arguments of use to the student, take a position before them, pose questions and answers to his personal and intellectual searches, solve problematic situations of his daily life, apply new knowledge to your life, and seek the improvement of the world around you. Thinking and interpreting in technology entail the creation of new educational scenarios.

3. Access: Two elements are inherent to access to ICT, one is inherent to the institution and the other to the student. ICTs are resources, tools, and programs that are used to process, manage, and share information through technological supports such as computers, laptops, cell phones, that is, hardware and software. The institution must provide resources and reliable means, of easy access and availability for teachers and students, but it must be ensured that the student has the appropriate resources for their distance education.

Face-to-face and virtual education are not the same, for us to be successful in virtual education we cannot directly apply what we do in physical presence and what is applied online, nor can it be replicated in a face-to-face class, each one has its methodologies and materials to make them work properly. So you have to adapt and redesign; in the virtual environment, people compete for attention, time, and space on the screen; in addition, students have greater control over the content and how they work with it and must take responsibility and practice autonomy, reflection, and reasoning.

Educational institutions must have robust, adequate, and sufficient technology, both intangible resources such as servers, computers, printers, and intangibles, such as platforms that allow them to carry out administrative, school, and teaching process management—learning. The platforms must have some characteristics such as centralization and automation, flexibility, interactivity, standardization, scalability, functionality, usability, ubiquity, and integration.

Educational institutions, in general, must carry out a process of technological reconversion that allows them to sustain the processes adjacent to the use of ICT. Thus, educational institutions should be supported by broadening their horizons to an institutional philosophy that considers ICT as fundamental elements in educational work, having financial sustainability that allows them to maintain high costs, recondition, and maintain the academic infrastructure for the good development of educational processes, in addition, with a teaching staff prone to change. The reconversion must also be carried out in administrative, pedagogical, and institutional management. The training processes in virtual learning environments are essential for the success in the training of students [14].

## 3. Conclusion

The migration from virtual to classroom education is essential in medical education. It is not a substitute for clinical practice, face to face with the real patient; however, hybrid or mixed strategies and curricular redesigns should be sought in the immediate and mediate future of the training of the medical professional. Among the fundamental elements are not improvising, but planning in hybrid or mixed options; consider the differences between face-to-face and virtual education; managers must be involved in the transformation; carry out adequate and pertinent teacher training about ICT in daily didactic and pedagogical activity. Acquire the relevant technological equipment for migration, including servers, Internet capacity, and diagnosis of the needs of teachers and students to carry out the migration properly.

Students are comfortable with technology-based solutions to support learning and assessment, and with peer communication tools. Pandemic circumstances have pushed teachers to acquire skills in using online resources to teach and meet students like never before. Now, we lack patients and a professional care environment. A lot of work is needed to ensure the privacy of participants, compliance with data protection regulations, quality, inclusion and fairness, support for students and teachers, among other key issues. They can be resolved effectively through intra- and inter-institutional cooperation, preferably on an international scale. The COVID-19 emergency will eventually end. By then, the whole concept and system of medical education will have been reinvented, having served as an *in vivo* experiment. For now, universities and health institutions need to collaborate and promote new forms of distance professional education experiences. COVID-19 will have made us all more aware and interested in participating in this process.

As of this quarantine, every one of the universities, certain policies were generally adopted that were applied throughout the country: Face-to-face classes became virtual; universities have had to offer platforms to include their students and to be able to have classes online. This requires a smartphone that can connect to the respective platform with Internet paid for by the student, or laptop computers or iPad's, owned by the student. In the hospitals where I work (General Hospital of Zone No. 36 of the IMSS and General Hospital of Minatitlán) that are public, residents have all the means such as Internet to carry out their academic care work.

We use ICT a lot, whether for conferences *via* webinars, distance classes, and even on-call delivery. This is because some are rotating in other hospitals. In Internal Medicine, the visit pass, the interaction with the patient and with teachers and colleagues, can never be replaced by the Internet or other digital media. There will be greater and faster access to information through smartphones and computers, but human contact will always be necessary, to be equal to or better than the graduates of the "traditional" programs of medicine depending on the use given to them by each individual.

The new insurance doctors will be different from "the old ones." The simple fact of living in confinement due to the pandemic, implying that they suddenly cut their studies, has made them approach learning issues in different ways. New doctors have to face a "new normal" that we may not know what it will be like once we try to return to the life we had every day. Telemedicine is undoubtedly a tool that has accelerated its use and it seems that it will continue in various ways. They will have to get used to teaching and learning in new formats, but at this point, the fact of reaching the comprehensive review of a patient live and in-person should be landed (see Section 4).

## 4. Complementary information

1. Alemán Bermúdez IJ, Vera León E, Patiño Torres MJ. COVID-19 and medical education: Virtuality from the perspective of the teacher and the student of higher education. Internal Medicine, Medical Education and Community 2020;36(3):116–123

2. UNAM School of Medicine. Post-COVID-19 medical education [Video Archive]. Available from: https://www.youtube.com/watch?v=WsytNWRtOdA [Accessed: 21 April 2021]

3. UNAM School of Medicine. Challenges of medical education in times of COVID-19: Institutional decisions in the face of the pandemic [Video Archive]. Available from: https://www.youtube.com/watch?v=RGhn-fW2424 [Accessed: 1 September 2020]

4. TecSalud. Best practices in medical education in time of COVID-19 [Video File]. Available from: https://www.youtube.com/watch?v=olaDLOBaf7U [Accessed: 7 July 2020]

5. National Academy of Medical Education. Medical education, from face-to-face to virtual in times of contingency [Video Archive]. Available from: https://www.youtube.com/watch?v=hmmCBSLCNvI [Accessed: 4 June 2020]

## Author details

Nikos Christo Secchi Nicolás[1*] and Ángel de Jesús Gómez Alarcón[2]

1 President of the College of Internal Medicine of Mexico A.C. Board of Directors 2021, Minatitlán, Veracruz, México

2 Sub-Investigator of the Center for Medical Research and Specialized Care, Minatitlán, Veracruz, México

*Address all correspondence to: drsecchi@hotmail.com

## References

[1] León Bórquez R, Valdez García J. Problems of medical education in Latin America with emphasis on Mexico in the context of the current crisis. In: Medical Education in a World in Crisis. Mexico City: Mexican Association of Schools and Faculties of Medicine, A.C; 2021. pp. 103-122

[2] Margolis A. Trends in distance continuing medical education. Research in Evaluation. 2013;**2**(1):50-54

[3] Crocker Sagastume RC, Esperón Hernández RI, et al. Medical Education in a World in Crisis. Mexico: Mexican Association of Schools and Faculties of Medicine, A.C. (AMFEM); 2021

[4] Herrera-Añazco P, Toro-Huamanchumo CJ. Medical education during the COVID-19 pandemic: Global initiatives for undergraduate, internship, and medical residency. Acta Médica Peruana. 2020;**37**(2): 169-175

[5] Núñez-Cortés JM. Medical education during the Covid-19 crisis. Elsevier Public Health Emergency Collection. 2020;**21**(3):157

[6] Vergara de la Rosa E, Vergara Tam R, Alvarez Vargas M, Camacho Saavedra L, Galvez Olortegui J. Distance medical education in times of COVID-19. Higher Medical Education. 2020;**34**(2):1-6

[7] Reynés-Manzur JN, Vázquez-Rivera M, Velázquez-Challa S, Kuri-Ayala S, Cravioto-Quintana P, Galván-Castillo F, et al. Learning management in times of COVID-19. Acta Pediátrica de México. 2020;**41**(Suppl 1):S137-S143

[8] Idrovo AJ. First lessons from the COVID-19 pandemic to Colombian medical education. Health UIS. 2020;**52**(2):87-88

[9] Costa MJ, Carvalho-Filho M. A new era for medical education after COVID-19. Medical Education Foundation. 2020;**23**(2):55-57

[10] Díaz Quiñones JA, Valdés Gómez ML. The COVID 19 pandemic and its implications in the conception, design and didactic instrumentation of Cuban higher medical education. MediSur. 2020;**18**(3):1-12

[11] Muñoz Cano JM, Maldonado Zalazar TNJ. Technological resources and the reconfiguration of medical education. Emerging Trends in Education. 2021;**3**(6):1-30

[12] Núñez-Cortés JM, Reussi R, García Dieguez M, Falasco S. COVID-19 and medical education, a look to the future. Ibero-American Forum of Medical Education (FIAEM). Elsevier Medical Education. 2020;**21**(4):251-258

[13] Santos-Peyret A, Durón RM, Sebastián-Díaz MA, Crail-Meléndez D, Gómez-Ventura S, Briceño-González E, et al. Digital health tools to bridge the epilepsy care gap before, during and after the COVID-19 pandemic. Journal of Neurology. 2020;**70**:323-328

[14] Sánchez-Duque JA. Medical education in pandemic time: The case of coronavirus disease 2019 (COVID-19). Educación Médica. 2020;**21**(4):259-260

Chapter 23

# A Doctor's Training in COVID Era

*Jiwesh Kumar, Priyanka Choudhary, Kishor Kunal, Anita Singh, Ravi Prakash and Prabha Pandey*

## Abstract

Doctors have severely been impacted by COVID19 not only by overburden but also by a shift in training programmes. With objective to identify the impact of COVID19 on the present training programme of doctors and delineate the possible future impact and find ways to reduce it, a literature review was carried on. Various impacts and adaptations were found. These could be different for different individuals, specialities, and regions based on available resources and the direct impact of COVID19. Although long-term effects are yet to be seen, it has raised several brows, especially questioning the traditional way of training and competency of individuals trained in specialities. We recommend a hybrid model—a mixture of virtual and real training and assessment—for medical education even in the post-COVID era to reap the benefits of both.

**Keywords:** trainee, resident, impact, medical education, psychological, COVID19

## 1. Introduction

When it comes to saving lives, looking throughout the pandemic, this is dignified sacrifice that each doctor made to look after the ill with uncertainty of disease course, limited supplies of protection gear, working overtime and holding not just onto the duties as a doctor but also a member of family and responsibilities towards non-medico friends and acquaintances. But, rather than seeing all doctors from a single profession, we shall see them as cluster of different specializations in progress. Doctors have severely been impacted by COVID19 not only by overburden but also by a shift in training programmes [1–3].

The aspect of training and duties in COVID19 has been rightly dealt by Cate et al. but at the same time, it is also important to see how trainees perceive the impact of pandemic on their training [4]. Johnson and Blitzer noted how the shift in duties is observed by residents as decrement in competency development. Similar reports were made by Upadhyay et al. [5, 6]. In addition to this, the training also got affected by redeployment, overburdening and secondary traumatic stress disorders [2, 3, 7]. Identifying the root cause and mapping the response can help deal with psychological impact on trainees [8]. Let us look at the impact on training and different adaptive modalities used for the continuation of medical education.

## 2. Methodology

### 2.1 Objectives

i. To identify the impact of COVID19 on present training programme of doctors.

ii. To delineate the possible future impact and find ways to reduce it.

### 2.2 Data acquisition

Literature was reviewed from PubMed and Google Scholar to find out articles describing the impact of COVID19 on training of health care workers. A search was also carried out to find the possible ways to deal with the problem.

### 2.3 Data analysis

The compilation of effects was studied and a way was formulated to better understand the impact. The impact was categorically studied in three stages viz., general impact on training and associated adaptation, the difference of impact in different regions of the world and difference of the impact on different specialities.

## 3. Results and discussion

### 3.1 Impact on training and adaptation

Cate et al. questioned the competence of medical education from three levels- micro, meso and macro levels. Micro-level is from the individual's perspective, the meso level is from institution's perspective and the macro level is from regulatory and societal system's perspective. These perspectives ask several questions that need to be answered. From a micro level, one can ask whether applicants' attributes associated with adaptability and willingness to work in uncertain circumstances be assessed in medical school selection processes? Or, should a level of altruism or courage be expected? From a meso level, there are questions regarding training and emergency deployment like should training be considered over after a fixed duration of time or should it be based on skill set acquired? Should the institute maintain an inventory of skill sets of their employees so that in times of need they can be quickly reassembled? When talking about the perspectives of the administration or society, it is a big question whether the emergency licensing to practice given during the time of crisis is valid after the pandemic and if not, was it ethical to do so in times of crisis? Again, what are the reciprocal obligations of local, state, and federal authorities when requesting redeployment of health care workers, such as adequate infection control policies, sufficient personal protective equipment, training opportunities, and reward structures [4]. It becomes rather imperative to question the competency of training in the pandemic. If eligibility for passing an undergraduate examination was considered to be after a set amount of years—say 5–6 years in majority of countries, will the loss of 2 years to a pandemic affect the eligibility? This becomes more evident when talking of post-graduate examination where the training period can be as less as 3 years.

Dedeilia et al. pointed out the challenges in medical and surgical education during the COVID19 era and stated that all aspects of medical education have been severely impacted. The biggest impact seemed to be on medical students who learned through being part of teams. To avoid unnecessary exposure, they were the first to be removed from these teams. Reducing the time of patient contact has also limited bedside learning opportunities. Surgical trainees are even more affected due to the closure of intake of elective cases and diversion of their posting towards COVID19 wards. Also, the introduction of weekly rotation to limit exposure and ensure backup has limited the time a resident spends in hospital. The de-specialization and redeployment of residents in departments with greater demand for healthcare personnel may address urgent service

Needs but disrupts residency education plans [9]. Another aspect of medical training is by learning through seniors. In usual rounds usually, the junior-most would take a first-round followed by seniors and consultants so a patient would be seen at least 3 times and the chances of missing something would decline, this also helped the juniors to find out what they missed in patient care through continuous scrutiny and surveillance. This part of medical training was hampered and it can lead to gross consequences like learning subpar levels of patient care.

Deployment of technology has made it easy to quickly adapt to changing scenarios however, at times they may not be at par with the conventional techniques of learning and teaching. The conferences have turned to virtual conferences and seminars have gone online too. Case discussions are being done with virtual cases with or without simulation. Online learning has replaced nearly all the aspects of conventional learning except where an assistant is required by specialized personnel like in major surgeries. Group viewing has been proposed by Porpiglia et al. as a more interactive and motivating exercise with additional comments from experts [10]. Dedelia et al. proposed online picture diagnosis quizzes in image-centric specialities like radiology or dermatology, however, this can be used in other clinical specialities too where spot diagnosis of entities can be used to teach differentials and for assessment purposes. Image-based learning is always considered more influential than conventional lectures the reason why bedside clinics have still not lost their importance in clinical teaching [9].

Social media too played an important role in case discussions and 'tweetorials' [10]. Tweetorials refer to clinical tutorials in a series of tweets providing links to educational materials. Telemedicine, which was established as a connecting link between non-emergency patients and doctors too played an important role in training. These were sometimes aided with video conferencing for a better understand ing of patients' problems. This was a new learning experience for residents as it led to faster adaptations to technology which might replace the traditional hospital and OPD management in future. Though it was time-consuming for both patients and doctors, it safeguarded against unnecessary exposure and highlighted the significance of conservative management in various diseases.

The highest level of technology helped to create simulations, virtual reality and 3D learning. All these are different technologies aimed to create a real experience for learning. While simulations help to understand and practice medical techniques in a non-human environment and are ethically superior to learning over a human, it is quite expensive to be available at all facilities and for all techniques. Virtual learning has a similar problem but can be very useful on a lower scale such as case presentations which may not require superior technology. 3D technology is being specially used in learning anatomy.

Even though it is difficult to achieve the training levels that are expected conventionally, these rapid adaptations have rebuilt the confidence in a fraternity that any crisis cannot subdue the confidence of humanity. These have not only helped in training but also in assessment. Other than online tests, simulation and virtual cases are aimed to assess objectively. Whether these objective assessments are superior to conventional subjective assessment is still controversial, but it has opened the doors for more transparent and streamlined assessments, especially in those institutes that still use traditional methods of assessments. Also, one shall look at the impact of training based on the resources available. This became evident as different regions of the world felt the same impact differently as adaptability and patient load differed.

### 3.2 Regional impacts

Edigin et al. reviewed the impact of COVID19 on postgraduate medical trainees in the US. They observed that a reduction in non-COVID inpatients can markedly reduce the clinical skills of a postgraduate trainee as there will be less to practice physical examination and do inpatient procedures. They also reported that some centres had to waiver the minimum inpatient procedures required for completion of 3rd internal medicine programs which can affect the proficiency of a trainee in these procedures and can also theoretically lower their confidence while handling such patients. They argued that the period of postgraduate training is short and a shift from learning special skills to providing COVID care or having off (to reduce unnecessary exposure) can reduce the learning and this paradigm shift if prolonged can affect the quality of their training. Other than learning basic skills when the patient volume is considerably high, another advantage is to see a typical presentation of common cases or a typical presentation of uncommon cases. This will also reduce and they might not have exposure to many presentations thus limiting their thought process while making decisions later on in their practice. Though this may not severely impact their practice or skill development this may affect their clinical acuity, especially when handling these cases. They also noted another problem in which some of the international medical graduates (IMGs) could not enter the US due to COVID thus reducing the workforce required which will have to be compensated by already overburdened available workforce [11].

Liang et al. studied the effect of pandemic on medical training in Singapore. They reported similar problems as their counterparts from USA and UK [11–13]. Yuen and Xle reporting on impact on UK trainees suggested three aspects that a trainee can focus on: facilitation of clinical skills supplemented by simulations and virtual reality technologies; preparation for professional examinations and reflection on self for improvement and introspection. While patient care cannot be jeopardized, taking stress for missing out on clinical opportunities in wake of COVID19 crisis is not going to help both in terms of a resident's efficacy to deliver services and mental health [13].

Sahi et al. while addressing the impact on medical education gave a list of available tools and resources for the continuation of medical education. They also proposed that medical education focus on research and development around various aspects of COVID like the development of indigenous PPE along with online assessment and training of both undergraduate and postgraduate medical education. They also argued for development of new ways for training of next generation of health professionals under the guidance of regulatory bodies or faculties [14]. Odedra et al., in a study on Canadian radiology, trainees showed stress levels of high-extreme in nearly 13.5% which according to them was because radiology is a non-patient-facing speciality. The redeployment rate was very less with only 1% redeployed outside radiology and nearly 5% within radiology. They also showed that transfer to online teaching programmes helped to retain their residency teaching programmes [15]. This also points to the fact that different specialities felt the impact differently.

### 3.3 Impact based on specialities

Agarwal et al., in their article on training in neurology showed the adaptation in times of COVID19 in teaching and training programs. The live sessions were transformed into virtual learning. They noted that online availability of lectures and teaching sessions have made them more readily available, leading to improvement in attendance of residents, fellows and faculty. They also addressed the problem of residents not being able to present their work at national conference by deviating their research to focus on COVID19 and related neurological effects. Focusing on this aspect, not only helped to keep on their academic research but served as a contribution towards rapidly understanding the disease in a better way. However, loss in terms of ambulatory rotations in neuro-oncology, neuro-ophthalmology, vascular neurology, neuroimmunology, epilepsy, neuromuscular medicine, headache/Botox clinic, neuro-rehabilitation, etc were on hold which would definitely reduce the exposure to a variety of cases and presentations [16].

Bambakidis and Tomei in a study on the impact of COVID19 on neurosurgery training reported that with halting of elective cases and in-person conferences the training was affected for at least one-third of the academic year in 2020 which might have doubled with the second wave of COVID-19 in 2021. Also, the conversion of clinic visits to telemedicine has restricted the exposure of residents to outpatient cases. Rotating weekly to reduce exposure has limited the residents and staff by 50% thus effectively reducing the training period. With curbing of all non-essential cases such as unruptured aneurysm surgery, spine surgery, benign tumours and other less urgent cases from elective surgery, has reduced the resident's exposure to these cases. They also reported a shift to virtual teaching programs for residents [17].

Crosby and Sharma reported on otorhinolaryngology training in COVID19 and pointed out that a national didactic curriculum along with the implementation of a research curriculum at institute level helped to regain the track of training where in-person training was not possible during the crisis. They also noted that faculty, chairs and program directors should be considerate about the impact of the pandemic on residents' psychology and shall give them ample time and space to acclimatize with the environment. Also, the increased role in the management of complications like mucormycosis towards the end of the second wave of pandemic has led to an increased workload among the residents with its own psychological impact [18]. Training in specialities such as otorhinolaryngology and ophthalmology where patients are needed to be examined in proximity are theoretically affected the most as usually their elective surgeries tend to restart late along with physical OPDs.

DeFilippis et al. detailed various challenges and potential adaptations in learning of cardiovascular fellows during the crisis. They noticed similar challenges in training and advocated for simulation training, virtual learning and inclusion of fellows in post-COVID19-related cardiovascular research. They also used 'Stump the Professor' sessions for case-based learning [19].

Upadhyay et al. reported the severe impact of COVID19 on orthopaedic training programmes. 88% reported a decrease in surgical exposure, 57% reported a decrease in teaching time and 72% were redeployed to areas outside orthopaedics. Around 70% considered that their decreased exposure to speciality patients will hamper their training and passing of their final exams. With a wide variety of virtual sessions being conducted across countries, 89% faced difficulty in choosing one and nearly 96% of residents felt stress, the majority for loss of surgical exposure and fear of contracting COVID. Dissertations to be submitted for partial fulfillment of master's degree were also affected due to very low inpatient intakes and nearly nil patients in physical OPD. Also, social distancing has resulted in the abandoning of group studies thus leaving online resources and tools as the only source of learning [5].

Ehrlrich et al. observed how the use of virtual learning can help surgical trainees. They also showed that a change in training program where the pandemic time can be utilized for non-surgical rotations which are planned later in the course can minimize the loss of the surgical training time for medical graduates. To annihilate the effect of decreased operating room (OR) time of a surgical trainee, online courses provided by ACS can be used in addition to virtual learning programmes and simulation devices like gaining basic surgical skills. They can also review laproscopic skills and ultrasound techniques through interactive modules. Also, the time spared due to less travelling can be used to get the steam off from burnouts and be utilized for self-care. Another method proposed by them was to divide the workforce into two groups where one focused on clinical care and the other was kept backup focused on academics. This can help mitigate the effects of loss of training time due to pandemic [20].

Gaur et al. noted similar problems for preclinical training. Since preclinical teaching is often done through lectures, these were not as much affected as clinical bedside teaching and adapted better to the conversion of teaching model to 'online'. They showed how the transformation is not too bad. Newer methods became popular like open-book examination by the Imperial College of London. They also reported studies showing higher interaction satisfaction with online learning in medical field [21]. Sklar noted in his paper on the effect of COVID19 on health professional education, that a lot of flaws in medical education which have been thought of great importance in traditional training like in-person attendance for lectures, standardized content tests for recertification of practising clinicians and clerkship for medical students has been thrown out in this crisis from training and helped to see out-of-box in this context. The author also stressed the shift from bioscientific model of health in curriculum towards inclusion of behavioural, social and environmental factors that influence health [22].

### 3.4 Far-sighted indirect consequences

There are two far-sighted indirect consequences which may not directly impact the medical training but need a mention to complete the chapter. One is the decrement of empathy in trainees towards patient. Use of masks by both patient and doctor, social distancing while history taking and use of equipments rather than physical examination in patient care has been practised during the pandemic. Lack of tactile stimulation by not touching the patient and inability to get to know the patient from close proximity (not being able to identify or relate to patients due to the use of masks and caps leading to decrement of visual stimulation) can reduce the empathy in trainees or those taking care of patients. Second the increasing mortality among residents and medicos while serving COVID19 patients has made parents and students both think twice before pursuing the profession. This can also demoralize some sharp minds to take up the profession reducing the quality of trainee world will produce in upcoming years.

## 4. Conclusion

COVID19 has severely impacted the training of medical graduates and post-graduates. The shift to online learning has helped in continuing medical education but also raised a question for traditional methods of teaching as to whether they shall be followed blindly or scrutinized based on available technology. It has also helped include technology inside medical teaching especially in preclinical teaching and for transparent and standardized assessment purposes. However, the loss of surgical time for trainees cannot be compensated for, resorting to simulation and virtual reality training wherever possible can help improve competency.

Virtual case discussions and teachings shall be promoted where patient contact needs to be reduced. We recommend a hybrid model- a mixture of virtual and real training and assessment- for medical education even in post-COVID era to reap the benefits of both. Institutes, where simulations and virtual reality teaching are not possible due to limited resources, shall at least try other modalities of online teaching so that trainees shall not feel left out from rest of the world. In excess of this, the mental impacts of COVID19 on doctors should also be looked for and appropriate actions should be taken. Better preparedness for the next impact with the development of ample resources to backup shall diminish the harsh impacts on medical training in future.

## Conflict of interest

The authors declare no conflict of interest.

## Author details

Jiwesh Kumar[1*], Priyanka Choudhary[2], Kishor Kunal[3], Anita Singh[4], Ravi Prakash[5] and Prabha Pandey[6]

1 RIMS, Ranchi, India

2 Department of Plant Pathology, BHU, Varanasi, India

3 Department of Orthopaedics, AIIMS, Jodhpur, India

4 Department of Anesthesia, Medanta, Gurugram, India

5 Govt of Bihar, India

6 DKTE, Kolhapur, Maharashtra, India

*Address all correspondence to: jjiwesh@gmail.com

## References

[1] Alsoufi A, Alsuyihili A, Msherghi A, et al. Impact of the COVID-19 pandemic on medical education: Medical students' knowledge, attitudes, and practices regarding electronic learning. PLoS One. 2020;**15**:e0242905

[2] Aughterson H, McKinlay AR, Fancourt D, et al. Psychosocial impact on frontline health and social care professionals in the UK during the COVID-19 pandemic: a qualitative interview study. BMJ Open. 2021;**11**:e047353. DOI: 10.1136/bmjopen-2020-047353

[3] Dong F, Liu H, Yang M, Lu C, Dai N, Zhang Y, et al. Immediate psychosocial impact on healthcare workers during COVID-19 Pandemic in China: A systematic review and meta-analysis. Frontiers in Psychology. 2021;**12**:645460

[4] ten Cate O, Schultz K, Frank JR, Hennus MP, Ross S, Schumacher DJ, et al. Questioning medical competence: Should the Covid-19 crisis affect the goals of medical education? Medical Teacher. 2021;**43**:817-823

[5] Upadhyaya GK, Jain VK, Iyengar KP, Patralekh MK, Vaish A. Impact of COVID-19 on post-graduate orthopaedic training in Delhi-NCR. Journal of Clinical Orthopaedics and Trauma. 2020;**11**:S687-S695

[6] Johnson WR, Blitzer D. Residents' perspectives on graduate medical education during the COVID-19 pandemic and beyond. MedEdPublish. 2020 Apr 27;**9**(77):77. DOI: 10.15694/mep.2020.000077.1

[7] Orrù G, Marzetti F, Conversano C, Vagheggini G, Miccoli M, Ciacchini R, et al. Secondary traumatic stress and burnout in healthcare workers during COVID-19 outbreak. International Journal of Environmental Research and Public Health. 2021;**18**:337

[8] Kunal K. Third eye model: A hypothesis to span the diversities of psychiatry and normalcy. Neuropsychiatry. London. 2019;**9**:2397-2418

[9] Dedeilia A, Sotiropoulos MG, Hanrahan JG, Janga D, Dedeilias P, Sideris M. Medical and surgical education challenges and innovations in the COVID-19 era: A systematic review. In Vivo. 2020;**34**:1603-1611

[10] Porpiglia F, Checcucci E, Amparore D, Verri P, Campi R, Claps F, et al. Slowdown of urology residents' learning curve during the COVID-19 emergency. BJU International. 2020;**125**:E15

[11] Edigin E, Eseaton PO, Shaka H, Ojemolon PE, Asemota IR, Akuna E. Impact of COVID-19 pandemic on medical postgraduate training in the United States. Medical Education Online. 2020;**25**:1774318

[12] Liang ZC, Ooi SBS, Wang W. Pandemics and their impact on medical training: Lessons from Singapore. Academic Medicine. 2020;**95**:1359-1361

[13] Yuen J, Xie F. Medical education during the COVID-19 pandemic: Perspectives from UK trainees. Postgraduate Medical Journal. 2020;**96**:432-433

[14] Sahi PK, Mishra D, Singh T. Medical education amid the COVID-19 pandemic. Indian Pediatrics. 2020;**57**:652-657

[15] Odedra D, Chahal BS, Patlas MN. Impact of COVID-19 on Canadian radiology residency training programs. Canadian Association of Radiologists Journal. 2020;**71**:482-489

[16] Agarwal S, Sabadia S, Abou-Fayssal N, Kurzweil A, Balcer LJ,

Galetta SL. Training in neurology: Flexibility and adaptability of a neurology training program at the epicenter of COVID-19. Neurology. 2020;**94**:e2608-e2614

[17] Bambakidis NC, Tomei KL. Editorial. Impact of COVID-19 on neurosurgery resident training and education. Journal of Neurosurgery. 2020;**133**:10-11

[18] Crosby DL, Sharma A. Insights on otolaryngology residency training during the COVID-19 pandemic. Otolaryngology and Head and Neck Surgery. 2020;**163**:38-41

[19] DeFilippis EM, Stefanescu Schmidt AC, Reza N. Adapting the educational environment for cardiovascular fellows-in-training during the COVID-19 pandemic. Journal of the American College of Cardiology. 2020;**75**:2630-2634

[20] Ehrlich H, McKenney M, Elkbuli A. We asked the experts: Virtual learning in surgical education during the COVID-19 pandemic—shaping the future of surgical education and training. World Journal of Surgery. 2020;**44**:2053-2055

[21] Gaur U, Majumder MAA, Sa B, Sarkar S, Williams A, Singh K. Challenges and opportunities of preclinical medical education: COVID-19 crisis and beyond. SN Comprehensive Clinical Medicine. 2020;**2**:1992-1997

[22] Sklar DP. COVID-19: Lessons From the Disaster That Can Improve Health Professions Education. Academic Medicine. 2020 Nov;**95**(11):1631-1633. DOI: 10.1097/ACM.0000000000003547. PMID: 32544103; PMCID: PMC7309647

Chapter 24

# "Deaths of Despair" among College Students Amidst COVID-19 Pandemic: A Call for Action

*Kavita Batra and Ravi Batra*


## Abstract

As COVID-19 pandemic gains foothold worldwide, all spheres of life, including daily activities, education, economic, social sectors experienced significant downturns. While COVID-19 affects all population subgroups, college students are particularly vulnerable given their transition to the emerging adulthood surrounded by a broad possibility of future. According to a mounting evidence, college students bear a disproportionate burden of psychosocial morbidities, which can be explained by the uncertainties surrounding the course of the pandemic and the sudden transition to online education. Moreover, many businesses scaled down their recruitment efforts leaving limited employment for students and more competition in the graduate labor market. COVID-19 pandemic has set up a "perfect storm" for students to initiate or relapse of maladaptive behaviors to alleviate their negative feelings. This is where "Deaths of Despair" comes into play. This chapter aims to reflect on the factors contributing to "Deaths of Despair" among college students in the wake of COVID-19 pandemic. Author of this chapter would like to advocate for developing tailored interventions to promote the post-traumatic growth among college students.


**Keywords:** COVID-19, SARS-COV-19, anxiety, depression, mental health, college students, psychosocial, suicide, deaths of despair

## 1. Introduction

COVID-19 pandemic has set up a "perfect storm" for all population subgroups, students are particularly vulnerable due to their transition to the emerging adulthood with a broad horizon of future [1]. A recent meta-analytical evidence reported a higher proportion of psychological cluster of symptoms among college students amidst COVID-19 pandemic [1]. This unprecedented rise in mental health morbidities during COVID-19 contributed to the suicidal ideations among students [2]. According to the Centers for Disease Control and Prevention (CDC), the suicidal ideation and increase in maladaptive behaviors were among the most common reported outcomes by the persons aged 18–24 years [3]. The mortality associated with increased substance abuse and suicide is termed as "deaths of despair," which is a burgeoning public health concern [4]. A report from the Well Being Trust projects nearly 75,000 "deaths of despair" may result from the substance abuse and suicides during pandemic [4]. These projections are concerning and underscore the need of developing targeted interventions to improve mental health outcomes of college students. For this, it is critical to explore all dimensions of "despair" in the context of the COVID-19 pandemic for the conceptual mapping [5], which authors attempt to describe in this chapter.

### 1.1 Despair ("down from hope"): an interwoven concept

Previous studies conceptualized "despair" as a common pathway or triggering mechanism to other causes of mortality at an individual and community level [5]. These pathways may persist for years and may predispose individuals to the diseases of despair, i.e. addiction and suicidal ideation [5]. The mechanism of interplay between individual and community factors is yet to be understood fully [5]. Despair can intersect across multiple interrelated domains, including cognitive, behavioral, emotional, biological, and social networks [4, 5]. More importantly, despair in the community level may predispose individual to the "deaths of despair," which highlights the need of diffusing protective factors, such as social inclusion, behavioral activation, and reappraisals of difficult situations to prevent "deaths of despair" among college students [5]. Social context of despair is critical especially among college students because they may have a shared exposure with others in a circumscribed set of networks, such as school setting [4, 5]. Next, the social comparison is another yet important dimension, which may contribute to the individual-level despair among students [4, 5]. Undoubtedly, COVID-19 pandemic played a significant role in increasing the prevalence of community factors of despair, including the structural inequities, systemic problems, and economic stagnation, which may have permeated into the individual level of despair [1, 4–6].

## 2. Stressors among college students

Stress among students during COVID-19 pandemic may stem from environmental pressure, academic workload, and social or interpersonal pressure [7], which form the basis to understand an interwoven concept of "diseases of despair" [7]. The environmental pressure also includes the factors associated with the micro and macro socio-economic dynamics [6].

### 2.1 Environmental pressure during COVID-19 pandemic

As an overlay effect of COVID-19 pandemic, economic recession is an important dimension of despair to understand micro and macro socio-economic stressors [6]. Given the strong association between economic recession and suicide, it is vital to study financial stressors or economic determinants of COVID-19 among college students [8]. Job insecurity, uncertainties about future, plummeted job opportunities, job loss and difficulty in securing new jobs stemming from COVID-19 contributed to the adverse psychological outcomes among students [1, 9, 10]. In a Texas based study, above 50% students reported financial difficulties experienced by them or by their loved ones [11]. Every 3 in 10 students reported having limited opportunities for the internships or job placements [11]. A significant proportion of students reported changes in the living environment to be more distractive [11]. The majority of students had fear of contagion and expressed their worries about their family members getting infected with COVID-19 [11].

### 2.2 Academic pressure as a stressor

The effects of COVID-19 are far ranging and education is not spared [11, 12]. With the sudden transition to the virtual learning, students experience undue academic pressure and poor emotional health [12–15]. Fear of academic year loss was associated with psychological distress and suicidal ideation among students as suggested by previous evidence [13–16]. Black students reported the greater risk of academic failure compared to their white counterparts [14, 15]. Reduced access to technology and electronic devices may explain the socioeconomic and racial dividends, which highlights the need of addressing structural inequities to prevent "deaths of despair" among students [14].

### 2.3 Social or interpersonal pressure (COVID-19 pandemic: an antisocial event)

With the institution of social distancing mandates, such as lockdown measures, the rates of social isolation and loneliness have surged among students with limited or no face-to-face interactions [16–18]. This social isolation and loneliness have contributed significantly to the suicidal ideations and subsequent "deaths of despair" among students [16–18]. With the reduced opportunities of in-person interactions, students are relying more on the social media and are getting exposed to the false news or "infodemic" which may act as a triggering mechanism for the suicidal behavior and unhealthy behaviors, i.e. substance abuse ("diseases of despair") [18, 19].

## 3. Diseases of despair (DoD)

Not all individuals start from suicidal actions stemming from the feelings of depression, anxiety, and hopelessness, some may develop dependence on noxious substances first in the hope to improve their situations [20, 21]. However, in reality, these behaviors worsen the situations and sets up a vicious cycle to contribute to subsequent depression and suicidal behaviors [21]. This points to the fact that the death of despair is a common pathway to suicides and substance abuse [22]. In a recent survey conducted among nearly 1500 individuals, young adults were twice likely to engage in the substance abuse behaviors and the prevalence of despair among young adults was 20 percent [22]. Reportedly, suicidal ideation increased by over 200% between 2009 and 2018 among young adults aged 18–34 years [23]. This is a complex problem with a multifactorial origin, which stem from the change in social structure and social media [19, 20, 23]. Cyberbullying and sleep problems are also contributing to the adverse mental health outcomes, including psychological distress and suicidal thoughts [19]. Three behaviors, including drug overdose, suicides, and alcoholic liver disease collectively called diseases of despair [19–25], which contribute to the deaths of despair.

### 3.1 Sociodemographic determinants of DoD

Just like other events, gender and race/ethnic disparities do exist in the prevalence of diseases or deaths of despair [22, 23, 26]. As compared to females, males are nearly twice likely to be diagnosed with alcohol and substance abuse related despair diagnoses [26]. However, females have had higher odds of exhibiting suicidal ideations than their male counterparts [26]. These differences in the suicidal attempts can be partially explained by differences in perception, natural coping mechanism, and social expectations among males and females [27]. Females tend to have safety seeking behaviors and are less likely to resort to self-destructive behaviors, such as suicidal attempts [27, 28]. Age was also a significant predictor of DoD, with 18–35 years old being at the highest risk [21, 25, 26]. African Americans, people with lower socio-economic status and less education attainment had the higher rates of despair [22]. Type of insurance was also associated with the higher risk of diseases of despair [26]. People with public insurance and Affordable Care Act (ACA) were significantly more likely to exhibit any diseases of despair diagnoses compared to those with commercial insurance plans [26]. These disparate effects highlight the need of deciphering potential mechanisms of risk based on theoretical frameworks [28].

## 4. DoD through a theoretical lens

DoD can be investigated through a theoretical lens and there are several theories, including cognitive behavior models, Precarious Manhood Theory, and the Interpersonal-Psychological Theory of Suicide, which paints a comprehensive layout to conceptualize psychopathology associated with DoD [28]. The Beck's cognitive model [29] states that the engagement in the self-destructive behaviors occur subsequent to the distortion of the beliefs following trauma. There are two maladaptive cognitions, namely assimilated and overaccommodated cognitions [28, 29], which can easily be described in the context of COVID-19. Assimilated cognitions are related to the feeling of self-blame, for instance self-doubt or regret for not getting the employment. On the other hand, overaccommodated cognitions is linking multiple events to question self-worth [29]. For instance, previous rejections by the employers made one believe that he/she will never find a job [29]. These experiences may trigger the feelings of low self-efficacy and hopelessness leading to the depressive symptoms as explained through the Learned Helplessness Theory of Depression [29, 30]. Hopelessness is a well-established risk factor of "Deaths of Despair," and COVID-19 has created a conducive environment for the hopelessness among college students with regards to the financial hardships and limited job opportunities [29, 30]. Another framework is Precarious Manhood Theory, which is important dimension with regards to DoD. Men feel distressed if asked to engage in "feminine" activities [29, 30] and attempt to engaging in stereotypic masculine coping behaviors to restore their gender-role [29, 30]. All these models explain the potential mechanisms of hopelessness, which drive up the diseases of despair.

### 4.1 Psychological capital and social media

The levels of hopelessness during COVID-19 pandemic were investigated among students. Students reported worries associated with far-ranging impacts of COVID-19 on their academic goals, job security and fear of contagion, which may result in undesirable outcomes, such as DoD [31, 32]. The anxiety and hopelessness were greater among students spending more time on social media [31, 32]. Excessive use of social media predisposes students to the negative coping mechanisms of escapism, thereby reducing their psychological capital [31, 32]. Students with the less psychological capital tend to use self-destructive measures to cope with the negative events, such as COVID-19 pandemic [31, 32]. According to the collective evidence, psychological capital acts as a mediator in the association between excessive use of media (problematic social media use) and mental health issues among college students [31–33].

### 4.2 Social media and suicide

Social media increases the risk of suicidal behavior through cyberbullying [32, 33]. Previous research indicate that victims of cyberbullying were more likely to commit suicides than those who were not victims [32, 33]. Cyberbullying is not a sole predictor of suicidal behaviors among young adults, however, the risk can be increased by preponderance of other psychological and environmental stressors described elsewhere in this chapter [11–15, 19, 32, 33]. Another emerging concern is the media contagion effect [34–36]. Evidence suggested suicidal behavior as a contagion, can be impacted directly or indirectly through media reporting, suicide clusters, and through an exposure to a suicidal peer [37]. These effects are more pronounced among college students due to the social-influence effect on the risk perception of this group [36, 37]. Several reports confirmed that self-harming young adults are more active in social media than those who do not engage in such behaviors [35–38]. Researchers have suggested a U-shaped relationship between social media use and mental health, meaning poor mental being at lower and higher ends of internet use [37, 38]. Social media advertisements expose adolescents to other risky behaviors, which can have a negative influence on their psychological well-being [37, 38].

### 4.3 Social media and risky behaviors

Social marketing may have negative influence on mental health and behaviors among young adults, for instance, alcohol brand promotion advertisements on social media platforms [37, 38]. Alcohol brands are strongly presented over the social media channels, including Facebook, YouTube, and Twitter these days and expose young adults to underage drinking [38, 39]. Unrestricted advertisements are responsible for the mass persuasion and viewers (especially young adults) perceive such behaviors as normative and desirable and are at greater risk of adopting maladaptive behaviors. Another emerging issue, which has a strong association with mental health, substance abuse, and suicidality is sexting and digital abuse [38–41]. Sexting is sharing the sexually explicit messages through messages, emails, and/or internet, and this acts as a moderator of age-inappropriate sexual behavior [40, 41]. Young adults who sexted had higher odds of being engaged in substance abuse, which is one of the diseases of despair [41, 42]. Young adults are highly predisposed to these behaviors due to their propensity towards peer pressure, lack of self-regulation, and technophilic nature [41–43]. The content presented in this chapter point to developing effective mental health and suicide prevention programs to address the unmet needs of the adolescents.

## 5. Public health recommendations: a call for action

A number of micro and macro level strategies can be undertaken to overcome the barriers and challenges in the road of preventing DoD. Microlevel strategies will entail activities to increase personal and social capital of at-risk individuals. Promoting healthy behaviors, and reversing biological depletion through pharmacological interventions will also be included [4, 5]. A sense of belongingness, meaning, and hope can be improved through embedding at- risk individuals in the social activities. In fact, students should be the part of discussion of improving mental health outcomes.

At macrolevel, identification of at-risk students will be critical. Identifying students with early stress symptoms can be beneficial to prevent the progression to the chronic mental disorders. School and community based psychological interventions can help alleviate the diseases of despair among college students [36, 37]. Educating parents to openly communicate with their children will help curbing this crisis [36, 37]. Control of underlying factors associated with DoD is critical, especially in the current crisis of COVID-19 pandemic. For instance, more jobs can be created for the students to alleviate their fears of financial instability during COVID-19 pandemic. Educational institutions can develop some training programs for the students to make them suitable for the competitive markets. Academic institutions need to invest more in building the mental health infrastructure to provide psychological counselling, harm reduction services, and to expand mental health treatment services to the students. Educators can play a role of gatekeeper by identifying behaviors of despair among their students. Periodic assessment of mental health of students is critical. COVID-19 pandemic is a wake-up call for us to take actions for addressing emotional, social, and psychological needs of the adolescents. Access to mental health services should not be driven by gender and race/ethnic status as healthcare is a right for all. Authors of this chapter advocate for the equitable healthcare delivery model to address the systemic inequities already prevailing across the nation.

## 6. Conclusions

COVID-10 has impacted all aspects of life and students are particularly vulnerable. Psychological and economic impacts of COVID-19 are devastating and will leave a lasting thumbprint in the absence of culturally and linguistically appropriate public health interventions. It is critical to take proactive approach to overcome underlying causes of deaths of despair among students. Early identification of at-risk students, promoting parental educations to develop open communications with their young children, building mental health infrastructure at institutional and community level will be critical. Students can be educated to take care of their general health by incorporating healthy lifestyle habits to develop a connection between mind and body. Mindfulness meditation may offer a great strategy not only to relieve stress but also improve memory and focus. Telehealth services can also be employed to overcome the accessibility barriers. Programs to bolster economic, social, and psychological support need to be prioritized and suicide prevention should not be optional.

## Conflict of interest

The authors declare no conflict of interest.

## Notes/thanks/other declarations

None.

## Author details

Kavita Batra[1]* and Ravi Batra[2]

1 Office of Research, Kirk Kerkorian School of Medicine, University of Nevada, Las Vegas, Nevada, United States

2 Department of Information Technology, Coforge Ltd., Atlanta, Georgia, United States

*Address all correspondence to: kavita.batra@unlv.edu

## References

[1] Batra K, Sharma M, Batra R, Singh TP, Schvaneveldt N. Assessing the psychological impact of COVID-19 among college students: An evidence of 15 countries. Healthcare (Basel). 2021;**9**(2):222. DOI: 10.3390/healthcare 9020222

[2] Pandemic increasing suicidal ideation. Inside Higher Ed. 2020. Available from: https://www.insidehighered.com/news/2020/08/17/suicidal-ideation-rise-college-aged-adults-due-covid-19-pandemic. [Accessed: September 1, 2021]

[3] Czeisler MÉ, Lane RI, Petrosky E, et al. Mental health, substance use, and suicidal ideation during the COVID-19 pandemic — United States, June 24-30, 2020. MMWR. Morbidity and Mortality Weekly Report. 2020;**69**:1049-1057. DOI: 10.15585/mmwr.mm6932 a1external icon

[4] Projected deaths of despair from COVID-19. Well Being Trust. 2020. Available from: https://wellbeingtrust.org/wp-content/uploads/2020/05/WBT_Deaths-of-Despair_COVID-19-FINAL-FINAL.pdf. [Accessed: September 1, 2021]

[5] Shanahan L, Hill SN, Gaydosh LM, et al. Does despair really kill? A roadmap for an evidence-based answer. American Journal of Public Health. 2019;**109**(6): 854-858. DOI: 10.2105/AJPH.2019.305016

[6] Oyesanya M, Lopez-Morinigo J, Dutta R. Systematic review of suicide in economic recession. World Journal of Psychiatry. 2015;**5**(2):243-254. DOI: 10.5498/wjp.v5.i2.243. PMID: 26110126; PMCID: PMC4473496. Available from: https://www.ncbi.nlm.nih.gov/pmc/articles/PMC4473496/

[7] DeVylder J, Zhou S, Oh H. Suicide attempts among college students hospitalized for COVID-19. Journal of Affective Disorders. 2021;**294**:241-244. DOI: 10.1016/j.jad.2021.07.058

[8] Kim C, Cho Y. Does unstable employment have an association with suicide rates among the young? International Journal of Environmental Research and Public Health. 2017;**14**(5):470. DOI: 10.3390/ijerph14050470

[9] Bhandari N, Batra K, Upadhyay S, Cochran C. Impact of COVID-19 on healthcare labor market in the United States: Lower paid workers experienced higher vulnerability and slower recovery. International Journal of Environmental Research and Public Health. 2021;**18**(8):3894. DOI: 10.3390/ijerph18083894

[10] Wilson JM, Lee J, Fitzgerald HN, Oosterhoff B, Sevi B, Shook NJ. Job insecurity and financial concern during the COVID-19 pandemic are associated with worse mental health. Journal of Occupational and Environmental Medicine. 2020;**62**(9):686-691. DOI: 10.1097/JOM.0000000000001962

[11] Son C, Hegde S, Smith A, Wang X, Sasangohar F. Effects of COVID-19 on college students' mental health in the United States: Interview survey study. Journal of Medical Internet Research. 2020;**22**(9):e21279. DOI: 10.2196/21279

[12] Clabaugh A, Duque JF, Fields LJ. Academic stress and emotional well-being in United States college students following onset of the COVID-19 pandemic. Frontiers in Psychology. 2021;**12**:628787. DOI: 10.3389/fpsyg.2021.628787

[13] Hasan N, Bao Y. Impact of "e-Learning crack-up" perception on psychological distress among college students during COVID-19 pandemic: A mediating role of "fear of academic year

loss". Children and Youth Services Review. 2020;**118**:105355. DOI: 10.1016/j.childyouth.2020.105355

[14] Luo M, Guo L, Yu M, Jiang W, Wang H. The psychological and mental impact of coronavirus disease 2019 (COVID-19) on medical staff and general public - A systematic review and meta-analysis. Psychiatry Research. 2020;**291**:113190. DOI: 10.1016/j.psychres.2020.113190

[15] Kaurani P, Batra K, Rathore Hooja H, et al. Perceptions of dental undergraduates towards online education during COVID-19: Assessment from India, Nepal and Sri Lanka. Advances in Medical Education and Practice. 2021;**12**:1199-1210. DOI: 10.2147/AMEP.S328097

[16] Cheung T, Lam SC, Lee PH, Xiang YT, PSF Y. International research collaboration on COVID-19. Global imperative of suicidal ideation in 10 Countries amid the COVID-19 pandemic. Frontiers in Psychiatry. 2021;**11**:588781. DOI: 10.3389/fpsyt.2020.588781

[17] O'Connor RC, Kirtley OJ. The integrated motivational-volitional model of suicidal behaviour. Philosophical Transactions of the Royal Society of London. Series B, Biological Sciences. 2018;**373**(1754):20170268. DOI: 10.1098/rstb.2017.0268

[18] Uddin R, Burton NW, Maple M, Khan SR, Tremblay MS, Khan A. Low physical activity and high sedentary behaviour are associated with adolescents' suicidal vulnerability: Evidence from 52 low- and middle-income countries. Acta Paediatrica. 2020;**109**(6):1252-1259. DOI: 10.1111/apa.15079

[19] Sharma M, Batra K, Flatt J. Testing the Multi-Theory Model (MTM) to predict the use of new technology for social connectedness in the COVID-19 pandemic. Healthcare (Basel). 2021;**9**(7):838. DOI: 10.3390/healthcare9070838

[20] Daniels M, Sharma M, Batra K. Social media, stress and sleep deprivation: A triple "S" among adolescents. Journal of Health and Social Sciences. 2021;**6**(2):159-166

[21] Biswas T, Scott JG, Munir K, Renzaho AMN, Rawal LB, Baxter J, et al. Global variation in the prevalence of suicidal ideation, anxiety and their correlates among adolescents: A population-based study of 82 countries. E Clinical Medicine. 2020;**24**(100395):1-9

[22] Copeland WE, Gaydosh L, Hill SN, et al. Associations of despair with suicidality and substance misuse among young adults. JAMA Network Open. 2020;**3**(6):e208627. DOI: 10.1001/jamanetworkopen.2020.8627

[23] Diseases of Despair skyrocket in America. USA News. 2020. Available from: https://www.usnews.com/news/health-news/articles/2020-11-10/diseases-of-despair-skyrocket-in-america. [Accessed: September 1, 2021]

[24] Sex, racial/ethnic disparities apparent among adolescents with suicidal ideation. Healio. 2021. Available from: https://www.healio.com/news/psychiatry/20210614/sex-racialethnic-disparities-apparent-among-adolescents-with-suicidal-ideation. [Accessed: September 1, 2021]

[25] Ohio Deaths of Despair. Ohio University. 2020. Available from: https://878570bd-c4fe-4dfe-8107-669a96dd214b.filesusr.com/ugd/89e8f1_c87f53c4fd3744b3a7445a0cba20b42d.pdf. [Accessed: September 1, 2021]

[26] George DR, Snyder B, Van Scoy LJ, et al. Perceptions of diseases of despair by members of rural and urban high-prevalence communities: A qualitative study. JAMA Network Open.

2021;**4**(7):e2118134. DOI: 10.1001/jamanetworkopen.2021.18134

[27] Rhodes AE, Boyle MH, Bridge JA, et al. Antecedents and sex/gender differences in youth suicidal behavior. World Journal of Psychiatry. 2014;**4**(4): 120-132. DOI: 10.5498/wjp.v4.i4.120

[28] Rehder K, Lusk J, Chen JI. Deaths of despair: Conceptual and clinical implications. Cognitive and Behavioral Practice. 2021;**28**(1):40-52. DOI: 10.1016/j.cbpra.2019.10.002

[29] Beck AT, Emery G, Greenberg RL. Anxiety Disorders and Phobias: A Cognitive Perspective. New York, NY: Basic Books; 1985

[30] Franklin JC, Ribeiro JD, Fox KR, et al. Risk factors for suicidal thoughts and behaviors: A meta-analysis of 50 years of research. Psychological Bulletin. 2017;**143**(2):187-232. DOI: 10.1037/bul0000084

[31] Vandello JA, Bosson JK, Cohen D, Burnaford RM, Weaver JR. Precarious manhood. Journal of Personality and Social Psychology. 2008;**95**(6):1325-1339. DOI: 10.1037/a0012453

[32] Kaplan Serin E, Doğan R. The relationship between anxiety and hopelessness levels among nursing students during the COVID-19 pandemic and related factors. Omega (Westport). 2021:302228211029144. DOI: 10.1177/00302228211029144 [Published online ahead of print, 2021 Jul 4]

[33] Sedgwick R, Epstein S, Dutta R, Ougrin D. Social media, internet use and suicide attempts in adolescents. Current Opinion in Psychiatry. 2019;**32**(6):534-541. DOI: 10.1097/YCO.0000000000000547

[34] Whitlock JL, Powers JL, Eckenrode J. The virtual cutting edge. Developmental Psychology. 2006;**42**(3):407-417

[35] Baume P, Cantor CH, Rolfe A. Cybersuicide: The role of interactive suicide notes on the Internet. Crisis. 1997;**18**(2):73-79

[36] Webb M, Burns J, Collin P. Providing online support for young people with mental health difficulties: Challenges and opportunities explored. Early Intervention in Psychiatry. 2008;**2**(2):108-113

[37] Luxton DD, June JD, Fairall JM. Social media and suicide: A public health perspective. American Journal of Public Health. 2012;**102**(Suppl. 2): S195-S200. DOI: 10.2105/AJPH.2011.300608

[38] Forum on Global Violence Prevention; Board on Global Health; Institute of Medicine; National Research Council. Contagion of Violence: Workshop Summary. Washington (DC): National Academies Press (US); 2013 II.4, The contagion of suicidal behavior. Available from: https://www.ncbi.nlm.nih.gov/books/NBK207262/

[39] Memon AM, Sharma SG, Mohite SS, Jain S. The role of online social networking on deliberate self-harm and suicidality in adolescents: A systematized review of literature. Indian Journal of Psychiatry. 2018;**60**(4):384-392. DOI: 10.4103/psychiatry.IndianJPsychiatry_414_17

[40] Chassiakos YLR, Radesky J, Christakis D, Moreno MA, Cross C. Council on communication and media. Pediatrics. 2016;**138**(5):e20162593. DOI: https://pediatrics.aappublications.org/content/138/5/e2016259

[41] Teen sexting linked to sexual activity, thoughts of suicide. NBC News. 2011. Available from: https://www.nbcnews.com/id/wbna44819455. [Accessed: September 1, 2021]

[42] Gassó AM, Klettke B, Agustina JR, Montiel I. Sexting, mental health, and

victimization among adolescents: A literature review. International Journal of Environmental Research and Public Health. 2019;**16**(13):2364. DOI: 10.3390/ijerph16132364

[43] Ybarra ML, Mitchell KJ. "Sexting" and its relation to sexual activity and sexual risk behavior in a national survey of adolescents. The Journal of Adolescent Health. 2014;**55**(6):757-764. DOI: 10.1016/j.jadohealth.2014.07.012

Section 3

# Economic Impacts

Chapter 25

# Consistency in Leadership during a Pandemic: Managing Academics at a Private Higher Education Institution in South Africa

*Willy H. Engelbrecht*

## Abstract

The Covid-19 pandemic forced leaders to adapt their leadership approaches to the online environment. This chapter reviews the leadership approaches applied by managers at a Private Higher Education Institution (PHEI) in response to the Covid-19 pandemic and examines how these managers ensured that academics perform optimally while working remotely. A qualitative research methodology, combined with semi-structured interviews, enabled the researcher to source rich data from the managers and academics at the PHEI in question. Most managers indicated that only minor adjustments to their leadership approaches were required to work in a remote online environment. Participants also noted that a combination of various leadership approaches in a specific context enhances a leader's efficiency, as it allows them to analyze a situation and consider the impact of proposed approaches on stakeholders before a decision is made.

**Keywords:** leadership, Covid-19, private higher education, academics, South Africa

## 1. Introduction

The novel Coronavirus (referred to as Covid-19) in the rest of this chapter caused major disruptions worldwide during 2020. Industries across the globe have been forced to rethink their operational models to ensure resiliency when faced with disruptions like the Covid-19 pandemic. Organizations have had to get accustomed to conducting business and being profitable despite strict lockdown restrictions imposed by governments, to prevent the rapid spread of Covid-19. In the case of higher education, which services approximately 80% of the student population across 150 countries had to cease in-person learning [1, 2] and transfer to online learning [3, 4] by the end of March 2020. The rapid transfer to online learning resulted in various unexpected costs for institutions, academics, administrative staff, and students [3, 5]. Higher education institutions in South Africa were also impacted by lockdowns, with academics being required to work remotely. Leadership has had to apply a consistent approach in managing academics whilst achieving institutional goals and objectives, by making efficient use of online mechanisms. To date, there has been no evidence indicating which leadership approaches work best for remote teams, especially in the Private Higher Education

(PHE) sector [6]. This chapter focuses on the positive impact of leadership consistency on academics and their mandate to serve all students.

## 2. Private higher education in South Africa and the pandemic

The South African higher education landscape consists of approximately 131 private and 26 public higher education institutions, 50 technical and vocational education and training (TVET) colleges, 9 community education and training (CET) colleges, and 287 registered private colleges [7]. This sector is strictly regulated by the Council on Higher Education (CHE), which is an independent statutory quality council overseen by the Department of Higher Education, Science and Technology (DHET) [8, 9]. A record number of 208,978 students (16% of the student population) enrolled at Private Higher Education Institutions (PHEIs) in South Africa in 2019. This figure increases year on year, as there is an extremely high demand for higher education qualifications [9, 10]. This demand is created by the assumption that a higher education qualification increases job prospects and improves the quality of life [11, 12]. It is, however, important to note that the success of PHEIs in South Africa depends on their ability to deliver graduates with industry-relevant competencies that will enable them to actively contribute to the economy and become global citizens [13].

The Covid-19 pandemic exposed the weaknesses of HEI, including their inability to swiftly move to online learning. This inability is mainly the result of higher education institutions (HEIs) not using online learning management systems (LMSs), like Blackboard, Sakai, and Moodle [4, 13–19]. Some of the most notable challenges that leaders have had to manage to include:

- Academic's resistance to a methodological change in teaching and learning practices through an LMS.

- Time constraints on the development of adequate, skills-focused assessments online and in open-book format to assess students' knowledge competencies [20].

- The ability of academics to incorporate new technological tools and software to enable student learning in the online environment [20]. The lack of technological skills and inability to quickly master online software and technology, which placed further stress and anxiety on academics and students (on top of the shorter academic semester) [19].

- Student engagement, which has proven even more challenging online given the disruption that comes with the use of the technology when teaching through online platforms [21].

The Covid-19 pandemic has been impacting academics and students, with leadership having to find ways to save the academic year without compromising education quality or academics and student wellbeing. The sudden shift to online teaching and learning impacted academics' ability to effectively deliver on deadlines [22]. Leadership teams have had to ensure that students continue their studies whilst academics continue to deliver on the PHEI's mandate. This requires consistency in current leadership approaches with a slight adjustment to the application of the leadership style.

*DOI: http://dx.doi.org/10.5772/intechopen.102858*

## 3. Leadership during a disruption

A unique feature of HEIs in South Africa is each institution's perception of quality and how it should be applied (in conjunction with institutional strengths) to achieve its goals [15]. This creates diversity amongst the various HEIs; each institution views itself as unique and the best in delivering graduates to the market. There is a constant drive to ensure that high-quality graduates gain immediate employment and that business intelligence software is used to identify potential gaps in the learning process. However, the social, economic, and policy/governance conditions [23] in South Africa make it extremely challenging for leadership, especially at PHEIs, to keep academics engaged despite the constant changes in the regulatory and external environment. The biggest challenge since the restructuring of HEIs in the early 2000s has been the transformation into a digital learning community, which was fast-tracked by the Covid-19-pandemic. This fast-tracked shift to online teaching and learning has raised several questions about the equality, accessibility, training, and accountability of academics from a student perspective [4, 24]. HEI leadership had to carefully consider how the sudden shift to online learning would affect PHEI students and academics. As such, leadership has had to remain principle-driven in the decision-making process and ensure that students are at the center of each decision [17]. In addition, leaders in this sector are required to be flexible, adaptable, and reflective in their leadership approaches, especially during times of disruption or change [25–27].

An individual's ability to influence others in reaching a common goal or objective, using a motivation to establish coherence amongst the team [16, 17, 28], is considered leadership. It is the leader's responsibility to continuously monitor the external environment and influence the team's approach in achieving a goal. A leader gives direction when no one else can see the way forward. The Covid-19 pandemic forced HEI leadership teams to reaffirm and showcase their abilities to get teams on board and implement changes as a collective to ensure students successfully complete the academic year [4, 26, 29, 30]. Leadership teams had to ensure that academics, operations, administration, information technology systems, and facilities departments (amongst others) worked together to deliver exceptional service and support to students during the shift to online learning.

With the constant change in HEIs, leaders must constantly adapt to the changes in the external and internal business environments, whilst prioritizing the aim and purposes of the institution [24, 26]. The vision of the PHEI in question is to provide students with a quality higher education experience, focusing on equitable delivery of material and assessments through the institution's LMS. In addition, the PHEI in question aims to leave no student behind and ensure that students become global citizens who, at some point in time, will pay it forward. The vision of the institution has always been its main driver, and this did not change during the hard lockdown (27 March to 21 April 2020). Rather, the institution reaffirmed its vision amongst academics and found solutions to better support students and make its vision a reality. The extent to which leadership teams promoted efficacy amongst their teams was critical to the success of the new working conditions and the delivery of quality higher educational material and assessments to students [31].

**Table 1** provides an overview of the various leadership approaches that exist. Given this chapter's nature and purpose, middle-level managers in a PHEI was the target population. At middle-level management, it is important that leaders focus on achieving the goals and objectives of the PHEI as determined by the senior executive team. The other two leadership categories (contemporary leadership and emerging approaches to leadership) align with lower levels of management and

| Leadership category | Leadership style/approach | Summary |
|---|---|---|
| Contemporary leadership | **Level 5 leadership** | • Has a tier level of managerial capabilities.<br>• Focuses on the leader's ability to be modest in their approach to managing employees.<br>• Leader accepts responsibility for successes and failures in the team and gives credit to employees where it is due.<br>• Organization's success is based on the founding values and principles that drive the organizational culture and influences employee behavior.<br>• Leader is driven to develop the talent in the team and ensure that succession plans are in place.<br>• Professional development of employees in the institution enables growth and success in achieving institutional goals. |
| | **Servant leadership** | • Focuses on resolving social issues and challenges faced by the community.<br>• Ethical behavior and practices drive these leaders to affect change in communities.<br>• Strong focus on the role and purpose of the organization in the community.<br>• There is a shared approach to organizational success, goals and incentives.<br>• Use skills and knowledge to serve others, like non-governmental or non-profitable organizations. |
| | **Authentic leadership** | • High levels of self-efficacy that is supported by strong ethical values and objectivity.<br>• Stay true to what the leader believes in, like moral values and beliefs.<br>• Focus on collaborations and develop others into respected and respectful leaders.<br>• Leader is self-disciplined, establishes relationships, pursues a purpose with passion and commitment, and has solid values. |
| | **Interactive leadership** | • Agreement is reached on a shared goal.<br>• Relationship is personal and not authoritative in nature.<br>• Shows strong signs of humility, inclusion, relationship building, and care for employees and customers. |

*DOI: http://dx.doi.org/10.5772/intechopen.102858*

| Leadership category | Leadership style/approach | Summary |
|---|---|---|
| New leadership paradigm | **Transactional leadership** | • Matches employee needs and organizational objectives.<br>• Sets clear goals and tasks for employees to achieve a specific outcome.<br>• Conforms to organizational structures, policies, and systems within which work has to be executed.<br>• Manages performance through incentives and/or punishment.<br>• Focuses on achieving organizational goals and objectives. |
| | **Transformational leadership** | • Develops relationships with employees to develop the individual in the workplace.<br>• Creates a shared vision that is supported by innovation and creativity.<br>• Recognizes the individual and provides different perspectives on challenges to ensure a positive outcome.<br>• Is collaborative in nature and feedback is key to all goals being reached, with the incentive being personal self-development rather than rewards.<br>• Motivation is mutual and enables higher-order goals to be achieved.<br>• Inspires, empowers, and stimulates followers. |
| | **Charismatic leadership** | • Leader is charismatic and inspires support and acceptance.<br>• Establishes positive relationships by setting specific goals.<br>• Inspires followers to achieve goals by establishing and maintaining strong positive relationships.<br>• Leader has a strong personality, good communication skills, compassion, confidence and demonstrates positive body language.<br>• Leader applies an outcome-based approach, no matter what it takes.<br>• The leader is a visionary and stimulates and motivates others to achieve goals.<br>• Followers are fixed on the ideology of the leader and have similar beliefs showcasing affection and obedience towards the leader with a strong emotional involvement.<br>• Followers are focused on achieving the common goal established by the leader rather than their individual goals. |

| Leadership category | Leadership style/approach | Summary |
|---|---|---|
| Emerging approaches to leadership | **Strategic leadership** | • Leader understands the intricacies of the organization and business environments to lead the organization to succeed.<br>• Leader can only be successful if there is a good foundation of the organization's history, culture, strengths, and weaknesses.<br>• Leader has to be a visionary capable of identifying potential future trends, whilst managing current organizational conditions to have the organization succeed. |
| | **Cross-cultural leadership** | • Leader is able to understand and work with employees from diverse cultural backgrounds.<br>• Leader has affection and respect for other cultures and implements an inclusive organizational culture.<br>• Leader must understand how the various cultures perceive rewards/incentives and work around goal setting and overall organizational performance. |
| | **Ethical leadership** | • Leader establishes ethical practices in the organization.<br>• Important that this leader portrays ethical conduct in a professional and personal capacity.<br>• Focuses on successful implementation of corporate governance practices. |
| | **Crisis leadership** | • This leader can create meaning from a crisis and provide a clear direction on the way forward.<br>• Crisis leaders have exceptional communication skills as it is important to send out transparent messaging during the crisis and keep all employees updated on any changes.<br>• Focuses on a collaborative work environment as crises require employees to often take on more roles and responsibilities to navigate a crisis.<br>• These leaders can adapt their leadership approach during a crisis to steer the organization through the crisis and ensure it remains sustainable and profitable.<br>• Builds solid relationships with all stakeholders (internal and external) and keeps them abreast of developments. |

**Table 1.**
*Summary of leadership approaches [32].*

executive management, respectively. It could, however, be argued that leadership is not just one of these styles, but the ability to analyze situations and apply whichever leadership style is necessary to ensure that a specific goal is reached.

Leaders in the PHE sector must constantly wear two hats: an academic hat and a business hat. It is close to impossible to have these two idealists join in a conversation and agree on matters without significant debate. If the debate aligns with other HEIs, the academia and arguments around it often get a seat at the table. When a disruption like Covid-19 occurs, it becomes difficult to find a solution that will be beneficial to the business (financially and sustainably), and ensure that students continue to receive a quality education during the disruption. This requires that academic leadership teams in PHEIs have a variety of leadership skills while following a consistent leadership approach and successfully marrying business and academia. It takes time and effort to get a workable solution that ensures student-centricity and business sustainability. Consistency in leadership is what ensured the PHEI in question's success and enabled it to guide academics and students through the hard lockdown as well as the enduring pandemic.

**Table 1** shows the variety of leadership styles available. This research emphasizes the characteristics of transactional leadership, transformational leadership, and crisis leadership. All three of these leadership approaches align with the PHEI in question, as it is has remained goal-oriented (transactional) and people-oriented (transformational) throughout the pandemic (crisis). These three approaches will be unpacked in the following. The findings will showcase how a blend of these three theories ensured academic consistency and efficacy in delivering quality higher education to students.

### 3.1 Transactional leadership

Educational leaders applying a transactional approach clearly define individual roles and responsibilities in alignment with organizational processes and procedures, whereafter an agreement is reached on the timeframe within which goals must be achieved [33–36]. A reward or incentive is in most instances attached to an individual's key performance areas (KPAs) and takes the form of performance bonuses, additional leave, salary increase, or (in cases of unsatisfactory performance) disciplinary action [36, 37]. The relationship that exists in this leadership approach is often a leader vs. follower approach, which could be detrimental to individuals wanting to challenge the status quo and bring new ideas to the table. Leaders applying this form of leadership are more focused on achieving organizational goals and objectives than on developing individuals in gaining more skills and improving organizational processes and procedures.

### 3.2 Transformational leadership

Transformational leaders focus on developing and inspiring individuals through a collaborative approach by being proactive about change whilst staying focused on the institutional goals and objectives [33, 35, 37]. These leaders carefully analyze academic's expectations and then influence them and gain their trust. Additional support and guidance are provided to help academics align their personal goals with that of the institution, ensuring that individual and organizational goals and objectives are met [38–41]. Solidarity keeps transformational leaders moving forward, as long as the goals and objectives to be achieved are framed with the collective approach in mind. The problem with transformational leaders is that they can be both charismatic and narcissistic in their approach to transforming others in reaching organizational goals and objectives. Furthermore, these leaders are often ignorant of present challenges and only focus on the future and how the future will look and feel different from the present [35]. This often puts more pressure on academics to achieve the future self, just to arrive there and find that the goalpost has shifted again. Ultimately, the transformational leader is one that inspires, motivates, stimulates, and gives individual attention to academic, making them feel a sense of value and worth [39, 40, 42].

### 3.3 Crisis leadership

The fast reaction required by HEI leaders in South Africa to shift to online teaching and learning leans itself to the preferred leadership style to apply. Given the fast-changing pace of higher education, being flexible, adaptable, and able to predict future changes from the volatile external environment is a key competency for any leader, whether it is related to a crisis or not [43]. There are three key factors that leaders face when leading a team through a crisis, namely: the ability to "improve awareness of the factors that constitute a crisis"; "the ability to clearly explain the experiences associated with the crisis being dealt with"; and "the ability to navigate a crisis" [43]. It is critical that leaders who find themselves in a crisis situation have the ability to clearly direct the attention of academics to where their focus should be and how to resolve the crisis; make sense of the situation and communicate a clear message to the teams so that everyone is on the same page; promote the collaborative work culture until the crisis has been resolved; and engage in adaptive leadership styles to ensure that the ultimate goal of the organization is achieved throughout the crises [4, 24, 44].

It is evident that a mixture of the three leadership approaches enabled the PHEI in question to successfully support students and academics through the hard lockdown and enduring pandemic in 2020. One leadership approach would not have had the same impact as a combination of the three leadership styles, together with consistency. The sudden change of leadership style in a crisis like the Covid-19 pandemic could increase stress for academics and students, confirming the importance of consistency in leadership. What has to be determined is whether or not leaders can follow their leadership approaches remotely using technology in a higher education setting.

## 4. Methodology

The research question focused on determining the impact of Covid-19 on leadership approaches of managers in a PHEI to effectively manage academic performance while they work remotely. The study applied a phenomenology approach in which an inductive qualitative approach enabled the researcher to source rich data on the changes in leadership approaches due to the Covid-19 pandemic [45–48] directly from the managers and academics.

Semi-structured interview schedules were developed, and the managers and academics were asked similar questions. The application of the inductive approach enabled the researcher to ask "what" managers and academics perceived the leadership approach of the manager to be before and during the Covid-19 pandemic. The "how" question came into effect by asking managers their perception of whether their leadership style had changed and how it changed (if at all) [49]. Academics were asked to describe how they perceived their manager's leadership style after the first hard lockdown (27 March to 21 April 2020) when they had to work remotely. The four managers from the four faculties that agreed to participate in this research were all interviewed face-to-face at the PHEI in the question's offices. The academics requested online interviews given that they had to talk about their line managers and were not comfortable doing so in the open-plan offices at the institution where they work. The institution had five faculties at the time of the research being conducted, but only four of the five faculties signed the participant consent form acknowledging their interest in participating in the research. The remaining faculty never responded to any of the email communication that was sent to invite individuals to participate in the research.

The academic parameters included a minimum of 3 years of working experience, the designation of senior academic in their faculty, and at least 3 years of reporting to the relevant line manager. Of the five senior academics who conformed to the parameters at the time, only four academics (one from each faculty, apart from the faculty not participating) indicated their interest in participating in the research. The respondents all agreed to the interviews being recorded and it lasted 45–60 minutes. The interviews took place in November 2020, 8 months after the hard lock down and just before the second wave started in South Africa. This enabled the respondents to reflect on the time that had passed and consider the changes and the effects it had had on them as managers and academics.

The interviews were transcribed, then thematically analyzed by the researcher. The researcher read through the transcribed interviews and identified specific themes identified by each of the managers and the academics. The researcher familiarized themselves with the content of the transcripts, whereafter a coding process followed from which themes were generated. The various themes were reviewed, defined, and written up [50]. The inductive approach enabled the researcher to identify key themes for consideration by managers when it comes to deciding on leadership approaches to apply during a crisis. The credibility and dependability of the data rest on the triangulation of the data from the managers and the senior academic members reporting to the respective managers. This confirmed that the responses from managers are a true reflection of what transpired during the hard lockdown in the respective faculties. The researcher obtained ethical clearance (R. 15,487) from the PHEI to conduct this research.

## 5. Findings and discussion

The findings revealed two core themes, namely consistency during a crisis and the culmination of various leadership characteristics are important. Consistency is critical and it was evident in all the interviews with the relevant managers that minor amendments were made to their leadership style application, but that new styles were not adopted. The academics confirmed this by stating that their managers were "*supportive, approachable; knowledgeable, share information, developmental, provide guidance, trust, collaborative and empowered them*". These characteristics are evident of a unique, good leader [4, 15–17, 25–30]. Furthermore, transformational leadership requires the delegation of responsibilities to develop academics. In two of the faculties where appointments were made during the pandemic, the educational leaders assigned the new employees to senior academic members to conduct training and act as mentors. The senior academic therefore had daily interactions with the new academic. The educational leaders could focus their attention on more pressing matters whilst knowing that the new academics were being trained and supported as per institutional requirements. This showcased leadership's ability to transform academics by delegating training and mentoring roles in the faculty to academics, thereby transforming academics and building more capacity.

The crisis leadership style element manifested in the form of weekly faculty meetings changing to daily meetings (educational managers and academics noted this). One of the academics responded by saying: "*the way in which they [the manager] managed did not change. But the situation called for frequent meetings and it is not about the academic but the situation*". The aim of these daily meetings was to concentrate on academic wellness and delivery of student material, as assessments had to be adjusted to online and take-home assessments in record time, to accommodate students having to write exams. All this had to happen while ensuring that the academic year did not get too far behind schedule. The changes in the external environment necessitated educational leaders to adopt certain crisis leadership principles [43] to navigate the faculties through the pandemic-induced changes in HEIs. One of the educational leaders noted that "*trust is built through collaboration and empowering others*". This refers to the ability of educational leaders to retain their leadership approach, reduce academic's anxiety and establish some sense of normalcy during the pandemic. Academic supported this notion through "*an increase in communication and support*" by educational leaders to navigate the sudden changes. Furthermore, one of the managers noted that another manager had bi-weekly coffee chats with academics, which focused solely on academic wellbeing and not work. This created a supportive working environment in which trust is built.

A statement from one of the academics captured what another academic said, namely that they have "*strong internal locus of control. It is about doing what I do*". The academics all had experience, which added to them being able to work efficiently through the pandemic with their educational leader. It is in these instances that academics felt that their educational leaders manage individual outputs and give them the freedom to work within the parameters of the job specification. The freedom to work within the parameters of a given position and managing academics outputs is one of the key leadership abilities that the PHEI requires from its leadership corps. The leadership approach of most managers aligns with the PHEI vision and goals, which is transactional, yet transformational in nature. The educational leaders must establish a collaborative work environment in which academics develop new skillsets and knowledge about higher education, teaching and learning, quality assessments, and operational delivery of material. Throughout the pandemic, the educational leaders have been communicating the vision and mission of the PHEI and reminding academics of their role within the institution. It is evident that in this case, educational leaders embraced the institutional governance systems and processes to promote the institution's vision and mission while being compassionate and understanding of the socio-cultural circumstances of all stakeholders [32]. The ability of educational leaders to be business-oriented and academically inclined has enabled the institution to successfully navigate the pandemic by ensuring students are serviced and academics' well-being is taken into consideration. One aspect that came out of the interviews, which can be considered either positive or negative, depending on the context, is the amount of training academics had to undergo during the hard lockdown to make changes to assessments. This showed the need for PHEIs to invest more in upskilling academics on digital or online assessment practices. This should not just be for the pandemic but as a means of going forward to become a transformed 4th industrial revolution institution. This finding is important for the PHEI (as it is for any HEI); to be successful it requires leadership that is business and academic thought leaders.

Contrary to the view of the authors [51] the educational leaders embraced the online tools and software to support their leadership style through regular informal check-ins with academics, switching on videos to show their faces, and make time in meetings for academic to share their best practices in dealing with hard lockdown regulations [24–26]. It is clear that educational leaders analyzed the situation and adapted using the relevant tools and software to engage with academics and ensure student material is delivered [52].

## 6. Conclusion

This chapter outlined the challenges that Covid-19 brought to the PHEI sector in South Africa. **Table 1** summarizes the key characteristics of the various leadership approaches. Each leadership approach is unique and has a specific aim. It is important to note that subordinates will not necessarily analyze the leader's performance in different situations or circumstances, but rather look at the extent to which the leader practices consistent, fair, and equitable decision-making within the given circumstances. Future research should be done on the leadership applied within public higher education institutions to determine if there is consistency between public and private institutions of higher education.

## Author details

Willy H. Engelbrecht
The Independent Institute of Education (IIE), Johannesburg, South Africa

*Address all correspondence to: wengelbrecht@iie.ac.za

## References

[1] Sahu P. Closure of universities due to coronavirus disease 2019 (COVID-19): Impact on education and mental health of students and academic. Cureus. 2020;**12**(4):1-7. DOI: 10.7759/cureus.7541

[2] Toquero CM. Challenges and opportunities for higher education amid the Covid-19 pandemic: The Philippine context. Pedagogical Research. 2020;**5**(4):1-5. DOI: 10.29333/pr/7947

[3] Gerwin V. Five tips for moving teaching online as COVID-19 takes hold. Nature. 2020;**580**:295-296. DOI: 10.1038/d41586-020-00896-7

[4] Marshall J, Roache D, Moody-Marshall R. Crises leadership: A critical examination of educational leadership in higher education in the midst of the COVID-19 pandemic. International Studies in Educational Administration. 2020;**48**(3):30-37

[5] Ebner M, Schön S, Braun C, Ebner M, Grigoriadis Y, Haas M, et al. Covid-19 epidemic as e-learning boost? Chronological development and effects at an Austrian University against the background of the concept of "e-learning readiness". Future Internet. 2020;**12**(6):1-20. DOI: 10.3390/fi12060094

[6] Strielkowski W, Wang J. An introduction: Covid-19 pandemic and academic leadership. In: 6th International Conference on Social, Economic, and Academic Leadership (ICSEAL-6-2019). Atlantis Press; 2020. vol. 441. pp. 1-4

[7] Department of Higher Education and Training (DHET). Annual Performance Plan 2021/22 [Internet]. 2021. Available from: https://www.dhet.gov.za/SiteAssets/Planing%2cPolicy%20and%20Strategy/DHET%20202122%20Annual%20Performance%20Plan%20.pdf [Accessed: 31-08-2021]

[8] CHE. Council on Higher Education: The Changing Landscape of Private Higher Education [Internet]. 2018. Available from: https://firebasestorage.googleapis.com/v0/b/che2020c5efd.appspot.com/o/website%2F88wkw4mblr61?alt=media&token=ee01b0c7-3118-4c14-b8dc-d89cba2c2bde [Accessed: 31-08-2021]

[9] Department of Department of Higher Education and Training [DHET]. Register of Private Higher Education Institutions [Internet]. 2020. Available from: https://www.dhet.gov.za/Registers_DocLib/REGISTER%20OF%20PRIVATE%20HIGHER%20EDUCATION%20INSTITUTIONS%2017%20March%202020.pdf [Accessed: 31-08-2021]

[10] Shah M, Nair CS, Bennett L. Factors influencing student choice to study at private higher education institutions. Quality Assurance in Education. 2013;**21**(4):402-416. DOI: 10.1108/QAE-04-2012-0019

[11] Viljoen D. Higher education—a vast and changing future [Internet]. 2018. Available from https://www.fin24.com/Finweek/Featured/higher-education-a-vast-and-changing-future-landscape-20180228 [Accessed: 31-08-2021]

[12] Tjønneland EN. Crisis at South Africa's universities—what are the implications for future cooperation with Norway? [Internet]. 2017. Available from: https://www.cmi.no/publications/6180-crisis-at-south-africas-universities-what-are-the [Accessed: 31-08-2021]

[13] Persichitte KA. Leadership for educational technology context s in tumultuous higher education seas. TechTrends. 2013;**57**(5):14-17

[14] Duemer LS. A history of transactional leadership in academe: A

cautionary tale. Journal of Philosophy and History of Education. 2017;**67**:35-42

[15] Markova M. A model of leadership in integrating educational technology in higher education. Online Journal of Distance Learning Administration. 2014;**17**(4):1-9

[16] Sirin YW, Aydin Ő, Bilir FP. Transformational-transactional leadership and organizational cynicism perception: Physical education and sport teacher sample. Universal Journal of Educational Research. 2018;**6**(9): 2008-2018. DOI: 10.13189/ujer.2018.060920

[17] Zuber-Skerrit O. Leadership development in south African higher education: The heart of the matter. South African Journal of Higher Education. 2007;**21**(7):984-1005

[18] Neuwirth LS, Jović S, Mukherji BR. Reimagining higher education during and post-COVID-19: Challenges and opportunities. Journal of Adult and Continuing Education. 2020;**2**:1-16. DOI: 10.1177/1477971420947738

[19] Rahim A, Ali S, Ali S, Fayyaz H. Online education during COVID-19 pandemic; an experience of Riphah International University Faculty of Health and Medical Sciences. Pakistan Armed Forces Medical Journal. 2020;**70**(2):506-512

[20] Tabatabai S. Simulations and virtual learning supporting clinical education during the Covid-19 pandemic. Advances in Medical Education and Practice. 2020;**11**(1):513-516. DOI: 10.2147/AMEP.S257750

[21] Dhawan S. Online learning: A panacea in the time of COVID-19 crisis. Journal of Educational Technology. 2020;**49**(1):5-22. DOI: 10.1177/0047239520934018

[22] Choudhari R. Covid 19 pandemic: Mental health challenges of internal migrant workers of India. Asian Journal of Psychiatry. 2020;**54**(1):1-4. DOI: 10.1016/j.ajp.2020.102254

[23] Smith BL, Hughey AW. Leadership in higher education—Its evolution and potential: A unique role facing critical challenges. Industry and Higher Education. 2006;**20**(3):157-163

[24] Gigliotti RA. Leader as performer; leader as human: A discursive and retrospective construction of crisis leadership. Atlantic Journal of Communication. 2016;**24**(4):185-200. DOI: 10.1080/15456870.2016.1208660

[25] Azorín Tarab A. Becoming familiar with qualitative research. In: Gupta M, Shabeen M, Reddy KP, editors. Qualitative Techniques for Workplace Data Analysis. Hershey: United States of America: IGI Global; 2019. pp. 1-4. DOI: 10.4018/978-1-5225-5366-3.ch001

[26] Drysdale L, Gurr D. Leadership in uncertain times. International Studies in Educational Administration. 2017;**45**(2):131-159

[27] Sathithada K, Niramitchainont P. Scenarios of sustainable E-leadership for Thai higher educational institutional leaders in 2027. Discourse and Communication for Sustainable Education. 2019;**10**(1):81-90. DOI: 10.2478/dcse-2019-0007

[28] Vigoda-Gadot E. Leadership style, organizational politics, and employee's performance: An empirical examination of two competing models. Personnel Review. 2006;**36**(5):661-683. DOI: 10.1108/00483480710773981

[29] Aston AW, Aston HS. Leadership reconsidered: Engaging higher education in social change [Internet]. 2020. Available from: https://digitalcommons.unomaha.edu/cgi/viewcontent.cgi?article=1122&context=slcehighered [Accessed: 31-08-2021]

[30] Marshall SG. Education middle change leadership in New Zealand: The meat in the sandwich. International Journal of Educational Management. 2012;**26**(6):502-528. DOI: 10.1108/09513541211251361

[31] Van Schalkwyk RD, Davis A, Pellissier R. The impact of leadership practices on service quality in private higher education in South Africa. Journal of Contemporary Management. 2013;**10**(1):223-238

[32] Engelbrecht WH. Leadership Approaches at a Private Higher Education Institution during Covid-19 Pandemic [Dissertation]. Johannesburg: University of Johannesburg; 2021

[33] Antonakis J, Avolio BJ, Sivasubramaniam N. Context and leadership: An examination of the nine-factor full-range leadership theory using the multifactor leadership questionnaire. The Leadership Quarterly. 2003;**14**(3):261-295. DOI: 10.1016/S1048-9843(03)00030-4

[34] Khan N. Adaptive or transactional leadership in current higher education: A brief comparison. The International Review of Research in Open and Distance Learning. 2017;**18**(3):178-183. DOI: 10.19173/irrodl.v18i3.3294

[35] Ma X, Jiang W. Transformational leadership, transactional leadership, and employee creativity in entrepreneurial firms. The Journal of Applied Behavioral Science. 2018;**54**(3):302-324. DOI: 10.1177/0021886318764346

[36] Young P. Leadership and gender in higher education: A case study. Journal of Further and Higher Education. 2004;**28**(1):95-106. DOI: 10.1080/0309877032000161841

[37] Rowold J. Instrumental leadership: Extending the transformational-transactional leadership paradigm. German Journal of Human Resource Management. 2014;**28**(3):367-390. DOI: 10.1688/ZfP-2014-03

[38] Daft RL, Benson A, Henry B. Management. 2nd ed. Hampshire: Cengage; 2020. p. 640

[39] Iszatt-White M, Saunders C. Leadership. 2nd ed. Oxford: Oxford University Press; 2014. p. 369

[40] Lee H-W. Motivational effect of performance management: Does leadership matter? Transylvanian Review of Administrative Sciences. 2020;**16**(59):59-76. DOI: 10.24193/tras.59E.4

[41] Ngcobo T, Mestry R. Introduction to educational leadership. In: Mestry R, Ngcobo T, editors. Education Management and Leadership: A South African Perspective. Cape Town: Oxford; 2018. pp. 1-18

[42] Trépanier S-G, Fernet C, Austin S. Social and motivational antecedents of perceptions of transformational leadership: A self-determination theory perspective. Canadian Journal of Behavioural Science. 2012;**44**(4):272-277. DOI: 10.1037/a0028699

[43] Kayes DC, Allen N, Self N. Integrating learning, leadership, and crises in management education: Lessons from army officers in Iraq and Afghanistan. Journal of Management Education. 2012;**37**(2):180-202. DOI: 10.1177/1052562912456168

[44] Fortunato JA, Gigliotti RA, Ruben BD. Analysing the dynamics of crisis leadership in higher education: A study of racial incidents at the University of Missouri. Journal of Contingencies & Crisis Management. 2018;**26**(4):510-518. DOI: 10.1111/1468-5973.12220

[45] Alvinius A, Ohlsson A, Larsson G. Organizational challenges and leaders' coping strategies: A qualitative study of

Swedish military academic organization. Journal of Military Studies. 2020;**9**(1):24-33

[46] Chan ZC, Fung YL, Chien WT. Bracketing in phenomenology: Only undertaken in the data collection and analysis process. The Qualitative Report. 2013;**18**(30):1-9. DOI: 10.46743/2160-3715/2013.1486

[47] Maggs-Rapport F. Combining methodological approaches in research: Ethnography and interpretive phenomenology. Journal of Advanced Nursing. 2000;**31**(1):219-225

[48] Reiners GM. Understanding the differences between Husserl's (descriptive) and Heidegger's (interpretive) phenomenological research. The Journal of Nursing Care. 2012;**1**(5):1-3. DOI: 10.4172/2167-1168.1000119

[49] Woiceshyn J, Daellenbach U. Evaluating inductive vs deductive research in management studies: Implications for authors, editors and reviewers. Qualitative Research in Organizations and Management. 2018;**13**(2):183-195. DOI: 10.1108/QROM-06-2017-1538

[50] Clark V, Braun V. Thematic analysis. The Journal of Positive Psychology. 2017;**12**(3):297-298. DOI: 10.1080/17439760.2016.1262613

[51] Francisco CDC, Nuqui A. Emergence of a situational leadership Covid-19 pandemic called new normal leadership. International Journal of Academic Multidisciplinary Research. 2020;**4**(10):15-19

[52] Thompson G, Clasø L. Situational leadership theory: A test from a leader-follower congruence approach. Leadership and Organization Development Journal. 2018;**36**(5):527-544. DOI: 10.1108/LODJ-01-2018-0050

Chapter 26

# Measuring the Systematic Risk of Sectors within the US Market via Principal Components Analysis: Before and during the COVID-19 Pandemic

*Jaime González Maiz Jiménez and Adán Reyes Santiago*

## Abstract

This research measures the systematic risk of 10 sectors in the American Stock Market, discerning the COVID-19 pandemic period. The novelty of this study is the use of the Principal Component Analysis (PCA) technique to measure the systematic risk of each sector, selecting five stocks per sector with the greatest market capitalization. The results show that the sectors that have the greatest increase in exposure to systematic risk during the pandemic are restaurants, clothing, and insurance, whereas the sectors that show the greatest decrease in terms of exposure to systematic risk are automakers and tobacco. Due to the results of this study, it seems advisable for practitioners to select stocks that belong to either the automakers or tobacco sector to get protection from health crises, such as COVID-19.

**Keywords:** sectors, Principal Component Analysis, systematic risk, American stock market, COVID-19

## 1. Introduction

According to Sullivan and Sheffrin [1], diversification is the process of allocating capital in a way that reduces the exposure to any particular asset or risk. Fama and Miller [2] state that the Capital Asset Pricing Model (CAPM) introduces the concepts of diversifiable and non-diversifiable risk. Synonyms for diversifiable risk are unsystematic risk and security-specific risk. Synonyms for non-diversifiable risk are systematic risk, beta risk, and market risk. Thus, the CAPM argues that investors should only be compensated for non-diversifiable risk.

According to Pasini [3], the principal Component Analysis (PCA) is a method of multivariate analysis. The idea behind the PCA is to reduce the dimensionality of a dataset in which there are a large number of interrelated variables, to maximize the variance of a linear combination of the variables. It is a method applied to data with no groupings among the observations and no partitioning of the variables into subsets $y$ and $x$. Particularly, the principal components are obtained by applying this method. The first one is the linear combination with maximal variance, the second one is the linear combination with maximal variance in the orthogonal direction to the first principal component and so for the others. Moreover, they are ordered sequentially with the first one explaining much of the variation as it can.

With the help of the PCA, we measure how each sector is affected by market risk, measured by the first component. This article proceeds as follows. The next section presents relevant literature on PCA and the stock market, and the third section describes our methods and data. The fourth section presents the analyses of the findings, and lastly, we present our conclusions in the fifth section.

## 2. Literature review

### 2.1 Systematic risk

Lakonishok and Shapiro [4] conclude that neither the traditional measure of risk (beta) nor the alternative risk measures (variance or residual standard deviation) can explain the cross-sectional variation in returns; only size seems to matter. Gencay et al. [5] propose a new approach to estimating systematic risk (the beta of an asset) and find that the relationship between the return of a portfolio and its beta becomes stronger as the wavelet scale increases. Campbell et al. [6] state that the systematic risks of individual stocks with similar accounting characteristics are primarily driven by the systematic risks of their fundamentals. Xing and Yan [7] indicate that improving accounting information quality causes the systematic risk to decrease, thus having important implications for disclosure decisions, portfolio management, and asset pricing.

### 2.2 PCA and the stock market

Liu and Wand [8] study the Chinese stock market and find that the performance of the BP model integrating PCA is closer to that of the proposed model in a relatively large sample. Hargreaves and Mani [9], using PCA through a perceptual map, provide a clear picture of the winning stocks that should be selected for trading. Wang et al. [10] achieve a good level of fitness, using two-directional two-dimensional PCA and Radial Basis Functional Neural Networks (RBFNN) in the Shangai stock market. Zahedi and Rounaghi [11], studying the Tehran stock exchange, through the usage of artificial neural network models and PCA method, note that prices have been accurately predicted and modeled in the form of a new pattern consisting of all variables. Noby and Lee [12] analyze global financial indices in the years 1998–2012 and indicate that the dynamics of individual indices within the group increase in similarity with time, and the dynamics of indices are more similar during crises. Gao et al. [13] experiment the prediction of the closing price of the stock market with two-dimensional PCA and deep belief networks (DBNs).

Waqar et al. [14] analyze three stock exchanges and show how PCA can help to improve the predictive performance of machine learning methods while reducing the redundancy among the data. Zhing and Enke [15] forecast the daily direction of the S&P 500 Index ETF (SPY) return and show that DNNs using two PCA-represented datasets give slightly higher classification accuracy than the entire untransformed dataset. Nahil and Lyhyaoui [16] show that the structure of the investment decision system can be simplified through the application of kernel PCA. Berradi and Lazaar [17], using both PCA and recurrent neural network model, reduce the number of features from eight to six, giving a good prediction of total Maroc stock price. Cao and Wang [18] compare the performance of both PCA and backpropagation (BP) neural network algorithms and find that the latter has the highest prediction accuracy.

More recently, Wen et al. [19] demonstrate how both PCA and LTSM can accurately predict the stock price fluctuation trend of Pingon Bank. According to Liang et al. [20], using volatility information of grains and softs through PCA and FA, find significant predictive ability in forecasting the RV of the S&P 500. Xu et al. [21], through the use of PCA, investigate the Chinese A-shares market over the 2013–2019 period and find that no matter investor sentiment, stock prices react significantly to rumors as well as when the rumor goes public. Yaojie et al. [22], using PCA and other methods, show the significant ability of the combined international volatility to predict US stock volatility. The literature review shows how PCA has been useful in dimensionality reduction, predicting prices, and other features of the stock market, in particular, this paper applies this mathematical technique in an innovative way, namely measuring the systematic risk in various sectors of the US stock market.

## 3. Methods and data

According to Ross et al. [23], systematic risk is the one that influences a large number of assets, thus having market-wide effects. On the other hand, unsystematic risk is the one that affects a single asset or a group of assets. Since the former cannot be eliminated through diversification is called non-diversifiable risk, whereas the latter is called diversifiable risk because it can be eliminated through portfolio diversification.

### 3.1 Principal Component Analysis

According to [24], PCA is a technique that may be useful where explanatory variables are closely related. In specific, if there are $k$ explanatory variables in the regression model, PCA will transform them into $k$ uncorrelated new variables. To explain, suppose that the original explanatory variables are denoted $x_1, x_2, \ldots, x_k$, and denote the principal components by $p_1, p_2, \ldots, p_k$. These principal components are independent linear combinations of the original data

$$
\begin{aligned}
p_1 &= \alpha_{11}x_1 + \alpha_{12}x_2 + \ldots + \alpha_{1k}x_k \\
p_2 &= \alpha_{21}x_1 + \alpha_{22}x_2 + \ldots + \alpha_{2k}x_k \\
&\ldots\ldots\ldots\ldots\ldots\ldots\ldots\ldots\ldots\ldots \\
p_3 &= \alpha_{k1}x_1 + \alpha_{k2}x_2 + \ldots + \alpha_{kk}x_k
\end{aligned}
\tag{1}
$$

Where $\alpha_{ij}$ are coefficients to be calculated, representing the coefficient on the $j$th explanatory variable in the principal component. These coefficients are also known as factor loadings. The principal components are derived in such a way that they are in descending order of importance. In particular, for this study, we take the first component as a representative of systematic risk, that is, the risk that affects the whole sector and cannot be diversified in a stock portfolio. For this analysis we write a script in Python, particularly we use *sklearn* library to compute the principal components.

We gather all data from yahoo finance, where we include 10 sectors of the US stock market, choosing the biggest five companies per stock by market capitalization (**Table 1**), taking daily log returns of stock prices, and dividing the periods of study into two—the pre-COVID-19 era—January 10 to May 10, 2021.

| Ticker | Company |
|---|---|
| **Insurance** | |
| UNH | UnitedHealth Group |
| ANTM | Anthem Inc |
| MMC | Marsh & McLennon Companies |
| CI | Cigna Corp |
| PGR | The Progressive Corp |
| **Clothing** | |
| BURL | Burlington Stores Inc |
| COLM | Columbia Sportswear |
| SFIX | Stitch Fix Inc |
| BOOT | Boot Barn Holdings |
| ANF | Abercombie & Fitch Co. |
| **Software** | |
| AAPL | Apple |
| MSFT | Microsoft |
| GOOGL | Alphabet |
| ADBE | Adobe |
| CRM | Salesforce.com, Inc |
| **Tobacco** | |
| PM | Philip Morris |
| MO | Altria Group |
| BTI | British American Tobacco |
| XXII | 22nd Century Group |
| UVV | Universal Corp |
| **Restaurants** | |
| MCD | Mc Donald's |
| CMG | Chipotle Mexican Grill |
| YUM | Yum! Brands Inc |
| QSR | Restaurants Brands International |
| DRI | Darden Restaurants Inc |
| **Healthcare** | |
| UNH | UnitedHealth Group |
| CVS | CVS Health Group |
| HCA | HCA Healthcare Inc |
| MCK | Merck |
| ABC | Amerisource Bergen Corp |
| **Banks** | |
| JPM | JP Morgan Chase |
| BAC | Bank of America |
| WFC | Wells Fargo |
| MS | Morgan Stanley |

| Ticker | Company |
|---|---|
| C | Citigroup |
| **Hotels** | |
| MAR | Marriot |
| HLT | Hilton |
| LVS | Las Vegas Sands Corp |
| MGM | MGM Resorts International |
| WYNN | Wynn Resorts Limited |
| **Airlines** | |
| LUV | Southwest |
| DAL | Delta Airlines |
| UAL | United Airlines |
| AAL | American Airlines |
| CEA | China Eastern Airlines |
| **Automakers** | |
| TSLA | Tesla |
| TM | Toyota |
| F | Ford |
| GM | General Motors |
| HMC | Honda Motor Company |

*Source: Yahoo Finance.*

**Table 1.**
*List of sectors/companies.*

## 4. Findings

**Table 2** displays the explained variance per principal component by sector, in specific we consider the first principal component to be representative of the systematic risk, whereas the other two are representative of non-systematic risk, that is, the diversifiable risk. The three principal components embody the majority of the variance, having a range from 86.3% (restaurants), to 95.5% (airlines) during the pre-COVID period, in contrast, during the COVID period, the range goes from 88.1% (clothing) to 97.1% (banks). **Figure 1** shows the overall results for the explained variance by the first principal component of all sectors analyzed. Before the pandemic, the three sectors with the highest systematic risk are—measured by the first principal component—banks, energy, and airlines; and the sectors with the lowest systematic risk are restaurants, healthcare, and automakers. Nevertheless, during the COVID-19, the three sectors that augmented the exposure to systematic risk are the restaurants' sector with an increase of 39.3%, clothing with 22.2%, and insurance with 14.5%. On the other hand, the sectors that presented a reduction of systematic risk during COVID-19 are automakers with 13.2% and tobacco with 10.3%.

The interpretation of the results is that according to our proposed metric of systematic risk, the sectors that are affected the most due to crises such pandemics are the restaurants, the clothing, and the insurance sector; in contrast, the sectors that show reliability during the pandemic are the automakers and tobacco. Due to these results, it seems advisable for practitioners to rely more on stocks that are both in the automakers and tobacco sectors, due to lesser exposure to systematic risk.

| Sector | Pre-COVID | | | | COVID | | | |
|---|---|---|---|---|---|---|---|---|
| | **First component** | **Second component** | **Third component** | **Total** | **First component** | **Second component** | **Third component** | **Total** |
| Insurance | 69.1 | 15.8 | 7.3 | 92.2 | 79.3 | 9.0 | 5.4 | 93.7 |
| Clothing | 45.4 | 22.9 | 19.2 | 87.5 | 55.2 | 25.1 | 7.8 | 88.1 |
| Software | 71.5 | 11.9 | 7.7 | 91.1 | 79.1 | 9.7 | 5.1 | 93.9 |
| Tobacco | 77.9 | 13.0 | 4.6 | 95.5 | 70.1 | 21.7 | 3.5 | 95.3 |
| Restaurants | 56.3 | 17.0 | 13.0 | 86.3 | 78.1 | 9.5 | 5.5 | 93.1 |
| Healthcare | 62.8 | 17.0 | 9.0 | 88.8 | 66.1 | 19.0 | 7.5 | 92.6 |
| Banks | 87.7 | 5.0 | 3.6 | 96.3 | 90.8 | 3.4 | 2.9 | 97.1 |
| Hotels | 77.3 | 10.3 | 6.8 | 94.4 | 84.6 | 6.7 | 5.1 | 96.4 |
| Airlines | 85.0 | 6.1 | 4.5 | 95.6 | 83.1 | 7.3 | 5.3 | 95.7 |
| Automakers | 67.8 | 21.8 | 5.8 | 95.4 | 58.6 | 29.4 | 6.2 | 94.2 |

*Source: Python.*

**Table 2.**
*Explained variation per principal component in percentage by sector.*

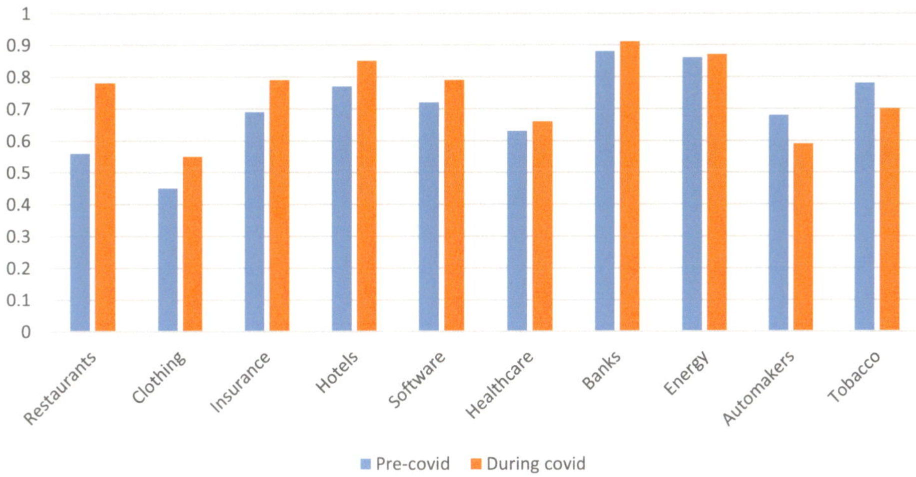


**Figure 1.**
*Explained variance by first component pre-COVID and during COVID by sectors. Source: Own elaboration.*

## 5. Conclusions

The innovation of this research is twofold—first, we apply PCA to measure systematic risk, and second, we discern systematic risk before and during COVID-19. In particular, the sectors that increase the most in terms of exposure to systematic risk are—the restaurants, clothing, and insurance sectors; in contrast, the sectors that show a decrease in systematic risk during the pandemic are—automakers and tobacco sectors, showing resilience during the pandemic. The results indicate that for portfolio managers it is better to pick stocks that belong to sectors, such as automakers and tobacco sectors in times of health crises such as pandemics, enhancing the benefits of diversification, and creating a shield against the increase of systematic risk due to these kinds of shocks. Consequently, further research could use the methodology proposed in this paper to measure systematic risk to better protect against crises such as COVID-19, thus having practical implications around the world (Video, https://youtu.be/o5SIhEHrRW8).

## Author details

Jaime González Maiz Jiménez[1]* and Adán Reyes Santiago[2]

1 Universidad de las Américas Puebla, Puebla, Mexico

2 Universidad de Monterrey, Monterrey, Mexico

*Address all correspondence to: jaime.gonzalezmaiz@udlap.mx

## References

[1] O'Sullivan A, Sheffrin S. Economics: Principles in Action. Upper Sadddle River, New Jersey: Prentice Hall; 2003. ISBN: 013063459X 9780130634597 0130634506 9780130634504

[2] Fama E, Miller M. The Theory of Finance. New York: Holt Rinehart & Winston; 1972. DOI: 10.1080/00137917 308902739

[3] Pasini G. Principal component analysis for stock Portfolio management. International Journal of Pure and Applied Mathematics. 2017;**115**(1):153-167. DOI: 10.12732/ ijpam.v115i1.12

[4] Lakonishok J, Shapiro A. Systematic risk, total risk and size as determinants of stock market returns. Journal of Banking & Finance. 1986;**10**(1):115-132. DOI: 10.1016/0378-4266(86)90023-3

[5] Gencay R, Selcuk F, Whitcher B. Multiscale systematic risk. Journal of International Money and Finance. 2005;**24**(1):55-70. DOI: 10.1016/j. jimonfin.2004.10.003

[6] Campbell J, Polk C, Vuoltccnaho T. Growth or glamour? Fundamentals and systematic risk in stock returns. The Review of Financial Studies. 2010;**23**(1): 305-344. DOI: 10.1093/rfs/hhp029

[7] Xing X, Yan S. Accounting information quality and systematic risk. Review of Quantitative Finance and Accounting. 2019;**52**:85-103. DOI: 10.1007/s11156-018-0703-z

[8] Liu H, Wand J. Integrating independent component analysis and PCA with neural networks to predict Chinese stock market. Mathematical Problems in Engineering. 2018;**2011**:1-15. DOI: 10.1155/2011/382659

[9] Hargreaves C, Mani C. The selection of winning stocks using principal component analysis. Journal of Marketing Research. 2015;**1**(3):183-188

[10] Wang G, Yang H, Miller DJ. A stock market forecasting model combining two-directional two-dimensional principal component analysis and radial function network. Plus One. 2015;**10**(4):e0122385. DOI: 10.1371/ journal.pone.0122385

[11] Zahedi J, Rounaghi M. Application of artificial neural network models in predicting stock prices on Tehran Stock Exchange. Physica A: Statistical Mechanics and its Applications. 2015;**438**(15):178-187 e0122385. DOI: 10.1016/j.physa.2015.06.033

[12] Noby A, Lee J. State and group dynamics of world stock market by principal component analysis. Physica A: Statistical Mechanics and its Applications. 2016;**450**(15):85-94. DOI: 10.1016/j.physa.2015.12.144

[13] Gao T, Chai Y, Tang Y. Deep learning with stock indicators and two-dimensional principal component analysis and deep belief networks (DBNs). In: Proceedings of the 7th IEE International Conference on Software Engineering and Service Science. Beijing, China: Institute of Electrical and Electronic Engineers; March 2016. DOI: 10.1109/ICSESS.2016.7883040

[14] Waqar M, Dawood H, Shahnawaz M, Ghazanfar M. Prediction of stock market by principal component analysis. In: Proceedings of the 13th IEE International Conference on Computational Intelligence and Security. Beijing, China; December 2017. DOI: 10.1109/CIS.2017.00139

[15] Zhing X, Enke D. Predicting the daily return direction of the stock market using hybrid machine learning algorithms. Financial Innovations.

2015;**5**:1-20. DOI: 10.1186/s40854-019-0138-0

[16] Nahil A, Lyhyaoui A. Short-term stock price forecasting using kernel principal component and support vector machines: The case of Casablanca stock exchange. Procedia Computer Science. 2018;**127**:161-169. DOI: org/10.1016/j.procs.2018.01.111

[17] Berradi Z, Lazaar M. Integration of principal component analysis and recurrent neural network to forecast the stock price of casablanca stock exchange. Procedia Computer Science. 2019;**148**:55-61. DOI: 10.1016/j.procs.2019.01.008

[18] Cao J, Wang J. Exploration of stock index change prediction model based on the combination of principal component analysis and artificial neural network. Soft Computing. 2019;**24**:7851-7860. DOI: 10.1007/s00500-019-03918-3

[19] Wen Y, Lin P, Nie X. Research of stock price prediction based on PCA-LSTM model. In: Proceedings of the IOP Conference Series Materials Science and Engineering. Jinan, China; 2019. DOI: 10.1088/1757-899X/790/1/012109

[20] Liang C, Ma F, Li Z, Li Y. Which types of commodity price information are more useful for predicting US stock market volatility? Economic Modelling. 2020;**93**:642-650. DOI: 10.1016/j.econmod.2020.03.022

[21] Xu Q, Chang V, Hsu C. Event study and principal component analysis based on sentiment analysis—A combined methodology to study the stock market with empirical study. Information System Frontiers. 2020;**22**:1021-1037. DOI: 10.1007/s10796-020-10024-5

[22] Yaojie Z, Yudong W, Feng M. Forecasting US stock market volatility: How to use international volatility information. Journal of Forecasting. 2021;**40**(5):733-768. DOI: 10.1002/for.2737

[23] Ross S, Westerfield R, Jaffe J, Jordan B. Corporate Finance: Core Principles & Applications. Penn Plaza, New York: Mc Graw Hill; 2014. ISBN-10: 0077861655

[24] Brooks C. Introductory Econometrics for Finance. United Kingdom: Cambridge University Press; 2019. ISBN: 9781108436823

Chapter 27

# Cases of Principal Leadership Responses in a Volatile, Uncertain and Complex School Environment

*Bongani Sibusiso Mchunu*

## Abstract

The findings of a small-scale qualitative study of school leadership responses to the volatile, uncertain, complex, and ambiguous (VUCA) school environment performed among secondary schools in the Mpumalanga Circuit are presented in this paper. The article looks at how principals were responding to the pandemic's disruptive effects and how they were planning to mitigate the effects on school operations. It employed qualitative, multiple case-study approaches to collect data from to secondary sample schools in Mpumalanga Circuit, using 10 principals as respondents. The findings illustrate how principals dealt with the issues posed by the implementation of the social distance and COVID-19 regulations in a VUCA-oriented school environment. Teacher leave applications contributed to the intricacy, with unexpected results such as teacher shortages and subjects not being taught. Despite these challenges, the principals were able to achieve their goals.

**Keywords:** volatile, uncertain, complex and ambiguity, turbulent, leadership

## 1. Introduction

With the onset of the COVID-19 pandemic, top management has been confronted with changes that have caused volatility, uncertainty, complexity, and ambiguity (VUCA) [1]. For the principals, administering the schools in the face of the coronavirus's marauding torrent has been unfathomable. Principals had to deal with systemic challenges such as deteriorating infrastructure, a lack of basic sanitation, and a politicised school atmosphere. In both primary and secondary schools, the unsustainable redesigned classroom was unable to handle the staggered phasing in of all grades. Existing discrepancies between the previous ex-model C and House of Delegates to the township and rural schools added to the woes of the ongoing contestations between the National Education Ministry policymakers and the Joint Teacher Unions, further complicating these complex difficulties. The reports from the Joint Teacher Unions were contradictory.

The responses of school principals in maintaining school functionality in a turbulent, uncertain, and complicated school environment are examined in this research. It looks at how social distancing has affected timetabling, as well as teaching and learning. It examines how each principal in their leadership has chosen the types of models to ensure that all grades are phased in at school. It demonstrates some of the difficulties that schools were confronted with, when teachers or students were infected with the coronavirus. Finally, it highlights the principals' leadership in ensuring that, despite debilitating conditions and the possibility of the coronavirus, programs for recovering lost time were developed at school.

The following are the key research questions:

i. How did principals handle school management and the implementation of policy directives?

ii. How did the principals deal with the loss of control?

We feel that the information gathered while answering all of these questions will be useful in understanding how principals responded to COVID-19's disruptive effects on school operations. It is critical that, before looking for empirically generated answers to these concerns, we review what is currently known in the literature about the pandemic's overall disruptive effect on the educational system.

## 2. Literature on the subject

We conducted a general evaluation of the current literature on COVID-19's disruptive influence on the educational landscape. We looked at the research on the harmful consequences of lockdown policies on the educational system. These included the impact of lost teaching time on student advancement, as well as the impact of social distance measurements on learner accommodation in classrooms and teaching time. We also addressed the mitigation of lost teaching time through the use of catch-up and rehabilitation programs.

Darvasi [2] noted on the unpredictability and unusual nature of the effect of 1–1.5 m of social separation in crowded classrooms. As a result of social distancing, the available school spaces may not be able to accommodate all of the students, as was the case before COVID-19. The screening of teachers and students necessitated the implementation of isolation measures to prevent the potential of retaliation. Catch-up programs, according to Montoya [3], can help schools mitigate the loss of teaching time caused by the COVID disruptive effect. During the first and second terms, most schools did not participate in Easter vacation, winter camps, or Saturday classes as part of their catch-up and recovery programs. Professor Nicky Roberts, an education expert, proposed that the Basic Education Department look into other solutions for students who were having their academic year disrupted by the COVID-19 outbreak [4]. The gap between fee-paying and non-fee-paying students are widening, according to Roberts.

She feared that the 4-week school closure would burden the study of grade 12 students even more [4]. Mthethwa [4] discovered that some grade 12 students were highly concerned about their prospects and preparation for the upcoming National Senior Certificate in his conversation with them. The staggered phasing in was further disrupted as the Joint Teacher Unions put pressure on the Education Ministry to close schools as more evidence emerged that schools had been impacted by the quickly expanding pandemic during the peak period of June to July 2020. President Cyril Ramaphosa has stated that the second term will be adjourned from the 7th to the 12th of August. We must remember that this abrupt shutdown followed a brief period of reopening on June 8th for only grades 7 and 12 as exit classes. Due to these uncertainties and disruptions, policymakers at the National Education Ministry was faced with the difficult task of finalising the school calendar, which resulted in a great deal of academic instability.

After a protracted period of debates about the return and phasing in of the remaining grades, namely grades 1–6 and 8–11 in the primary and secondary schools, finality was reached. After a long period of debates over the return and

| Term | Duration | No. of weeks | No. of school days | Actual no. of school days |
|---|---|---|---|---|
| 1 | (13) 15 Jan–18 March | 10 | (48) 46 | (48) 46 |
| 2 | (01 June) 08 June–07 August | (10) 09 | (50) 45 | (50) 45 |
| 3 | 12 August–23 September | 07 | 31 | 31 |
| 4 | 05 October–15 December | 11 | 52 | 52 |
| Total | Duration | (38) 37 | (181) 174 | (181) 174 |

**Table 1.**
*Amended school calendar.*

phasing in of the remaining grades, grades 1–6 and 8–11 in the primary and secondary phases, respectively, finality was reached. Another factor that affected the substantial alterations to the school the calendar was the pressure from Joint Teacher Unions on the Education Minister to close schools because of an increase in infections during the peak period of July and August 2020. This led to a 2-week hiatus beginning on August 7th and ending on August 12th, when the school reopened for the third term. As a result, depending on how the school organised the phasing in of the other grades, some students were only allowed to return to school on August 12th. The final calendar, as shown in **Table 1**, was approved by all important parties. The third term begins on August 12th. As a result, depending on how the school organised the phasing in of the other grades, some students were only allowed to return to school on August 12th. The final calendar, as shown in **Table 1**, was approved by all important parties. A careful examination of the calendar reveals that the academic year has been pushed into the first 2 weeks of December, something that has never happened before. After the presidential declaration of the movement to go from Level 4 to Level 1 measures on September 19th, there was a sense of stability. Teachers who had previously sought for temporary release based on underlying comorbidities were recalled by the District Offices to resume work on September 21, 2020 [5–7].

The gap in the number of lost teaching days owing to the enforced lockdown from the 16th March to the reopening date on the 8th June 2020 is shown in **Table 1**. The dates in brackets refer to the dates on which teachers were expected to begin their tasks at school before students arrived. Due to the increased spread of the coronavirus, the modified schedule shows a reduction in the number of days available for teaching and learning in schools, particularly in term three. The worst-case scenario was that students in grades 8–11 had to make sacrifices to accommodate grade 12 trial examinations and final examinations in late September and early November, respectively, to the 15th of December. This adds to the problem by causing some schools to lose instructional time for these grades.

## 3. VUCA as the conceptual framework

VUCA refers to how the principals dealt with the unpredictable nature of the school environment from the peak of the COVID-19 pandemic through the end of the final exams, as a conceptual framework that underpins this article. There are several features and emphases of the VUCA world's application that may or may not apply to this paper. However, we will only consider those factors that help to explain the quandary that our schools faced after reopening till the end of the semester. The study examines the principal's management of the school's operations throughout a challenging and uncertain academic year. There are different interpretations and application of the concept VUCA.

Volatility has a connotation for meaning an unstable change, where information is available and the situation is understandable, however change is characterised by being frequent and unpredictable. Uncertainty pertains to a situation where the lack of knowledge may be considered to be not showing any relation between cause and effect. What makes the situation look complex is the multiple parts that are interconnected, whereas ambiguity is the nature of doubt that comes into play in understanding whether there is a cause and effect relationships [8].

Certain groups agree that in a VUCA-oriented school climate, leadership is thrown out the window. In terms of their leadership and management of the schools, the principals were unable to cope with such a high level of unknown, unpredictable, and complex issues, which could not have been learned in any recent educational leadership textbook. The purpose of this article is to learn how these secondary school principals dealt with these problems in a tumultuous school climate. Complexity in this paper refers to the interconnectedness and interdependence of numerous components in the educational system that points to the school's functionality [1]. When it comes to intricacy, scholars must bear this in mind. Because of the non-linear interaction and interdependencies among diverse actors, as well as the complex activities and interactions at the school, the outcomes of a consciously managed settings are surprising.

## 4. Data presentation and methodology

The goal of the study on which this report is based was to examine how principals used their leadership skills in response to the interruptions to school operations caused by the COVID-19 outbreak. The study used a case study methodology to conduct a qualitative investigation. It incorporated both quantitative and qualitative information. The Mpumalanga Circuit Manager, who supervises the 10 secondary principals, cleared all of the initial ethical issues with the Kwazulu-Natal Department of Education, Office of the Director in Pinetown District and the Chief Education Specialist (CES) at Umhlathuzana Circuit Management Centre. Participating principals were handed questionnaires with informed consent letters from these authorities, who were asked to sign their letters of consent to participate in the study. To protect their identity, schools were given pseudonyms. All the 10 selected secondary schools are located in the Mpumalanga Township across the circuit. The Mpumalanga Circuit has 32 schools, 10 of which are secondary schools, whilst 22 are primary schools. Amongst the 10 selected there are only two female principals, whilst the rest of the eight are males. The Mpumalanga Township is located outside of the EThekwini Metro.

The enrolments from the 10 selected secondary schools range from 350 to 940 learners. Their quintiles range from 1 to 4, and six of them are no fee schools, although all are provided with the feeding scheme for learners.

Closed and semi-structured questionnaires were used to collect quantitative data, while free-form interviews were used to obtain qualitative data. During the peak of the epidemic, questionnaires were sent to 10 secondary schools in the Mpumalanga Circuit through email. When collecting a big amount of quantitative data, the respondents are advised [9]. Short face-to-face interviews with principals supplemented the semi-structured and closed questionnaires to gain clarification on how they performed trials examinations, catch-up programs, and pre-planning for the final upcoming assessments. After the pandemic's tremendous storm had passed, 10 secondary school principals participated in free attitude interviews.

As part of following the research protocols, pseudonyms were allocated to the names of the schools and principals. Attitudes that are free interviews allow people to express themselves freely. This guarantees that participants are treated with respect rather than being marginalised [10]. Audio recordings of free attitudes interviews were made and subsequently transcribed verbatim into themes. As part of the investigation, questionnaires were circulated using emails to 10 secondary schools in the Mpumalanga Circuit during the peak of the pandemic. Questionnaires are recommended for the collection of a large volume of quantitative data [9]. The semi-structured and closed questionnaires were supplemented by short face to face interviews with principals to seek clarity on how they conducted trials examination, the catch-up programmes and preplanning for the final oncoming examinations. Free attitudes interviews were conducted after the great storm of the pandemic was over with 10 secondary school principals. The pseudonyms were assigned to the names of the schools and principals as part of observing the protocols for research. Free Attitudes Interviews enable the participants to freely express themselves. This ensures that participants are respected and not undermined [10]. Free attitudes interviews were audio-recorded and then, they were transcribed verbatim into themes. We read each transcript numerous times to ensure that we were comfortable with the interview facts in general [11]. We then extracted ideas from each transcript and analysed them. Then, using descriptive codes, we came up with topics and categories [12]. We also noticed ethical principles including non-maleficence, participant autonomy as evidenced by voluntary engagement, informed consent, confidentiality, and anonymity [9, 13]. The questionnaires' analysis showed several features of the schools' functionality. These were analysed, and the results are given in the following tables as part of the paper's quantitative findings. Open-ended questions were provided to clarify some of the replies from the questionnaires, and content analysis was utilised to analyse them.

These were analysed, and the results are listed in the following tables as part of the paper's quantitative findings. Open-ended questions were posed to clarify some of the responses from the questionnaires, and content analysis was used to analyse them. The scope of this paper was narrowed because school functionality is a broad aspect that contributes to a conducive environment for teaching and learning. It was limited to the reengineering of classrooms and their configurations, the implementation of COVID-19 policies, revision planning, catch-up and recovery programs, and final examination planning. We present the analyses and comparative tables based on the responses from the 10 secondary schools, and how they contribute to the functionality of the school. In the reviewed literature we investigated the disruptive effect of the COVID-19 on school functionality, teaching and learning and timetabling and the reconfigured classroom.

The pseudonyms allotted to each of the secondary schools are presented in **Table 2**. These are the pseudonyms of the 10 secondary schools in the Mpumalanga Circuit.

| | | | |
|---|---|---|---|
| 1 | uMasingana | 6 | uLwezi |
| 2 | uNdasa | 7 | uNtulikazi |
| 3 | uMbasa | 8 | uNcwaba |
| 4 | uNhlaba | 9 | uMandulo |
| 5 | uNhlangulana | 10 | Zibandlela |

**Table 2.**
*Pseudonyms of schools.*

## 5. Data presentation

The COVID-19 Committee activities, the staggered phasing period, assessment and revision plans, and catch up programs are among the issues that emerged from this research. These are deliberately recognised as significant characteristics of the school's functionality to better understand how principals coped in a highly VUCA-oriented educational environment. These features of school functionality may not be congruent with existing literature because no literature on the subject was available at the time. However, in such a chaotic school climate, school leadership and management may not contradict the construct and conceptual literature on VUCA.

### 5.1 Activities of the COVID-19 Committee

The number of coronavirus cases reported and the number of days lost to teaching and learning are shown in **Table 1**. The KZN Circular No 41 of 2020 has been followed by all principals whose schools were affected. The principal of Umasingana indicated that the circular had been misinterpreted in terms of its implementation, particularly the method to follow for teachers with underlying illnesses. Principals were unsure whether or not the teachers who had applied had to wait for the approval. However, due to the circuits' high level of unionism, many of the teachers who applied stayed at home without permission. The Umbasa principal described how he bargained with teachers who had underlying illnesses to attend school and teach within the periods allotted to them rather than leave the school grounds. This flexibility guaranteed that all subjects were covered and that the needs of the teachers were met.

All 10 principals reported incidents of teachers who tested positive for the coronavirus, whether it was identified during the school day or the summer vacation. In some circumstances, the circuit manager came to visit schools where positive cases had been reported solely to clarify the protocol to be followed and to de-escalate the issue. This meant that provisions had to be taken for the isolation and quarantine of those teachers and students who were infected by the coronavirus. It also meant that schools would be closed for 3 days as the classrooms were fumigated. The procurement of a service provider to fumigate Ulwezi's school has been delayed, according to the school's principal. As a result of the reported service delay, the school lost 5 days of non-teaching and learning time. The method requires that the national policy direction be followed.

It is obvious that most schools were impacted in some way by the cases of sick teachers. However, as the policy procedures became more explicit, a great deal of ambiguity was avoided. Undasa and Umbasa were forced to wait nearly 14 days before the District found a service provider to complete the fumigation at the school. Teachers were initially forced to quarantine for 14 days, however, this was eventually reduced to 10 days. Principals claimed that several teachers used their medical aids to conduct their COVID-19 assessments at the new private hospital. In this way, the private hospital's results and feedback were faster than the local health clinics'.

### 5.2 Untaught subjects

The principal of Umbasa stated that there was a high level of fear and worry among the workers. Due to a shortage of available counselling services within the Kwazulu-Natal Department of Education, the schools were not receiving any counselling. According to the Principal of Umasingana, four teachers were granted exemption based on underlying sicknesses. The policy was announced in June 2020 until the announcement of the Level 3 measure in September 2020, which forced them to return to their respective schools. Furthermore, five teachers at uMasingana were admitted to the hospital, adding to the school's burden of altering the timetable and subject allocation. There were no substitute teachers assigned to fill in for these gaps in subject instruction. The principal of Umasingana stated that at a school with 32 students, Maths Lit, Maths, Religion, Business Studies, English First Additional Language (FAL), Zulu Home Language in grade 10 and English FAL in grade 11, were not taught to teacher shortages. The principal of Uncwaba claimed that there were no teachers for Life Science and Mathematical Literacy in grades 10 and 11. Considering that Zibandlela is a Small school, there were numerous issues with teacher shortages as well.

Accounting in grades 10 and 11 and physical science in years 10 and 11 were the topics that were not taught. Due to the small number of students, the school was in the process of lowering the number of topics offered.

The comparison in the number of reported cases and the effect this had on the number of school days lost is shown in **Table 3**. This added to the numerous days that had already been lost due to the Level 5 and 4 lockdowns. The COVID Committees were in charge of overseeing the daily operations at each of the 10 schools. All of the principals were in charge of fostering a positive learning environment. The level of volatility and unpredictability caused by the epidemic, on the other hand, crippled teaching and learning. The loss of 14 days in Umbasa owing to a lack of systems to obtain the services of organisations responsible for fumigation of those impacted areas schools areas is an uncommon situation worth noticing. The National COVID-19 policy guideline created a number of loopholes that contributed to school dysfunction. Another factor is the lack of coordination of services at the level of the Pinetown District in providing the required service providers to fumigate the schools.

| No. | School | No. cases | No. of days lost | Intervention |
|---|---|---|---|---|
| 1 | Umasingana | 1 | 5 | Kitchen: closed for 1 week; the service provider fumigated the school premises |
| 2 | Undasa | 1 | 14 | Service provider fumigated the school after 14 days |
| 3 | Umbasa | 8 | 3 | Service provider fumigated school after 14 days lost |
| 4 | Unhlaba | 1 | No closure | It was still early days, as a result there were no systems and structures and policies to service providers to fumigate the school |
| 5 | Unhlangulana | 1 | 3 | Service provider fumigated the school |
| 6 | Ulwezi | 4 | 10 | Service provider conducted fumigation |
| 7 | Untulikazi | 2 | School vacation | Service provider conducted during school vacation |
| 8 | Uncwaba | 2 | 10 | Service provider conducted fumigation |
| 9 | Umandulo | 1 | 4 | Service provider conducted fumigation |
| 10 | Zibandlela | 1 | 10 | No fumigation was done |
| | Total | 21 | | |

**Table 3.**
*Reporting on cases and interventions.*

### 5.3 Period of staggered phasing

**Table 4** shows the various ways taken by the 10 schools studied to accommodate phasing in grades 8–11 when they returned to school. A closer examination of the data reveals that there were additional teaching time losses as a result of the phasing in grades 8–11, as will be seen. The incident occurred as the principals attempted to use the juggling effect to fit the remaining grades into the available classrooms. The majority of schools preferred the alternate and bi-weekly approaches, while one school employed a mixed strategy. Due to a lack of classrooms, the grades used an alternate strategy in which they alternated days in terms of class attendance. The bi-weekly model means that some of these grades would go to school for 1 week and then not return until the following week.

### 5.4 Assessment and revision plans

The principals reported that the abrupt closure of schools on the 16th March 2020, disturbed some of the Term 1 assessments. Normally secondary schools would conduct extra tuition for a week during the end of the first term as part of their catch up and recovery programmes. After the partial reopening on the 8th of June for grade 12, the principals managed to finalise the Term 1 assessments to have a record of the results for purposes of the Continuous Assessment programme (CASS). At the time of conducting the face to face interviews with the principals, all

| No. | School | Grade and no. of days attended per week | | | | Model explained |
|---|---|---|---|---|---|---|
| | | 11 | 10 | 9 | 8 | |
| 1 | Umasingana | 3 | 2 | 2 | 2 | Alternate; 10 days cycle; weeks 1 and 2; grades alternate 3/2 days/ week |
| 2 | Undasa | 3 | 2 | 2 | 2 | Alternate; grades 8 and 9 divided into two groups; A and B: alternate Monday (A); Tuesday (B); Wednesday (A); Thursday (B) |
| 3 | Umbasa | 5 | 1 | 1 | 1 | Biweekly; grades 8–10 were coming only 1 day/week |
| 4 | Unhlaba | 2 | 2 | 1 | 1 | Alternate days allocated to grade 11 (2 days); grade 10 (2 days); grade 9 (1 day); grade 8 (1 day) |
| 5 | Unhlangulana | 2 | 1 | 1 | 1 | Alternate; grade 11: (Monday and Wednesday); grade 10: Tuesday; grade 9: Thursday; grade 8: Friday |
| 6 | Ulwezi | 5 | 2 | 2 | 2 | Biweekly; grade 8–10; grade 11 (5 days a week) |
| 7 | Untulikazi | 5 | 3 | 2 | 2 | Biweekly: grade 10: 1st week; grade 11: 2nd week; Monday; Wednesday and Friday; grade 9: Tuesday and Thursday; grade 8: Tuesday and Thursday; 2nd week: grades alternate days |
| 8 | Uncwaba | 2 | 1 | 1 | 1 | Alternation: (Monday and Tuesday; grade 11; grade 10) Wednesday; grade 9: Thursday; grade 8: Friday |
| 9 | Umandulo | 3 | 2 | 3 | 2 | Alternate days; 10 days cycle; week 1 and 2; grades alternate 3/ 2 days/week |
| 10 | Zibandlela | 3 | 3 | 2 | 2 | Alternate days for attendance grade 8; 9; 10; grade 12 learners ceded to nearby secondary school due to post provisioning norm (PPN) challenges |

**Table 4.**
*Staggered phasing models.*

the secondary schools had just finished the Trial Examinations for grade 12 that were held in the last 2 weeks of September. It also meant that the principals were arranging the revision plans for grade 12 learners during the 1 week vacation as part of the catch-up and recovery programme. In all the 10 secondary schools the principals and Senior Management Teams were finalising the preplanning for both the internal and external assessments. By internal assessments we mean the final examinations for grades 8–11 and by external we mean the National Senior Examinations (NSC) for grade 12.

Social distancing had a knock-on effect on the types of examinations that schools required to prepare to fit the current grade, 12 students in 2020, into the available classrooms. The 2020 NSC examinations were unique in that due to the cancellation of the June Part-time NSC tests, part-time grade 12 learners and repeaters of grade 12 had to be accommodated at these adjacent schools for their examinations. According to all 10 principals, they were obligated to provide seats for three groups of students. The present grade 12 students, part-time students, and repeaters who required to write certain topics were divided into three groups. This created a lot of difficulties when it came to interpreting the schedule. Let alone the impact it had on an already tumultuous academic year caused by social isolation. The current NSC examinations were accommodated by principals for the final NSC tests.

The disruption led to some classes closing early to make room for these final exams. The early closure for grade 8–11 students also meant they were hardly getting enough time to be taught because they were either using the alternate or bi-weekly model. Five principals reported that they were bound to start grade 8–11 internal final examinations earlier than the requirements specified in the provincial circular. In other cases, the principals adopted the platoon technique due to adequate planning, which allowed some of these students to write in the afternoon sessions or alternately in the morning when the grade 12 NSC examinations were not seated according to the timetable. As a result, final internal evaluations for grades 8–11 were held in four secondary schools from early October to late October, before the start of the NSC final examinations on November 5th.

The disruptive effect it caused meant some of the classes needed to open the space for these final examinations, and therefore early closure for the grade 8–11 learners who hardly got enough time to be taught as they were either using the alternate or bi-weekly model. In the five secondary schools, the principals were bound to start early the internal final assessments for grades 8–11. In other instances due to proper planning, the principals used the platoon method, which meant some of these learners could write in the afternoon sessions or alternately in the morning when the grade 12 NSC examinations were not seated in terms of the timetable. As a result in four of the secondary schools, the final internal assessments for grades 8–11 were conducted early in October till late October before the commencement of the NSC final examinations on the 5th of November.

All 10 principals said they were juggling a lot of things and making a lot of adaptations to fit internal and external exams into the available learning spaces. Ulwezi school grade 11 students wrote the Isizulu and English Paper 1 and 2 earlier on the 7th and 8th of October to free up classroom space. As these were regarded to be language papers, this would allow teachers to complete their marking. The principle of Umbasa had written to the circuit manager, requesting that the grade 8 and 9 students be kept at home at the end of the third term to make room for grades 10–11 internal examinations. The principal at Umbasa wanted to make sure that grade 10–12 students shared lessons for both internal and external NSC exams.

At the time of some of the interviews, all 10 secondary schools had just completed the Trial Examination at the end of September, and teachers had just begun marking to provide feedback to students at the start of the fourth term. The input and results of the trial exams for grade 12 students helped teachers plan and prepare focused areas that would impact revision plans for the 1 week of holiday. The grade 12 revision program, which began on October 26th and ended on October 30th, was designed by all 10 principals. This included attending Saturday courses as part of the final stretch of preparation for the final examinations, which began on the 5th of November and ended on the 15th of December. After grade 12 students had completed their exams, just nine secondary schools began a 3-week revision program.

As part of the ongoing catch-up programs, the principal of Uncwaba reported that two teachers were delivering Maths and Physical Science lessons at the Provincial Ukhozi Radio program. Uncwaba's principal was sure that the school would be able to make up for lost time and meet the goals set before the COVID-19 delays. The Undasa principal's grade 12 review technique was to divide students into groups based on their performance to prevent a one-size-fits-all approach that failed to address the risky students. The principals of Ulwezi and Uncwaba participated in networking, team teaching, and exchange programs to capitalise on the talents of the teachers, particularly in Math and Physical Science, respectively.

### 5.5 Programs for a catch-up and recovery

The principals only conducted the catch-up program as a final push before the final NSC examinations at nine schools. Because Zibandlela School did not have enough teachers for the other subjects, the grade 12 students were sent to Unhlaba School. The Mpumalanga Circuit's only rescue strategy was to keep the school open and avoid more problems with children who were unable to find teachers due to the PPN (**Table 5**).

| No | School | Saturday classes | Revision plans (3 weeks) | Spring school (1 week) |
|---|---|---|---|---|
| 1 | Umasingana | Yes | Yes | Yes |
| 2 | Undasa | Yes | Yes | Yes |
| 3 | Umbasa | Yes | Yes | Yes |
| 4 | Unhlaba | Yes | Yes | Yes |
| 5 | Unhlangulana | Yes | Yes | Yes |
| 6 | Ulwezi | Yes | Yes | Yes |
| 7 | Untulikazi | Yes | Yes | Yes |
| 8 | Uncwaba | Yes | Yes | Yes |
| 9 | Umandulo | Yes | Yes | Yes |
| 10 | Zibandlela | No | No | No |

**Table 5.**
*School catch up programmes.*

## 6. Findings

The conclusions touch on a variety of topics related to the school's operation. We have condensed these for this study to concentrate on the most important points. The findings suggest to early confusion in the system and structures that administrators had set up to apply the defined policies and procedures, particularly when there were reports of both teachers and students being infected with the coronavirus. The COVID Committees did their screening and cleaning tasks at all 10 schools, reporting any irregularities to the administrators. As the system and structures became more stable, the principals followed the procedures and reported to the circuit managers, which enhanced alignment with the local health clinics. Principals were pressured by the South African Democratic Teachers Union (SADTU) to close schools at the height of the pandemic to put pressure on the National and Provincial governments [14].

Second, due to the early closure of schools from August 7 to 12, the staggered phasing-in method for grades 8–11 was delayed and disrupted. It was more of a case where we decided that a slice of bread was preferable to not having even half a loaf. To accommodate the phased grades 8–11, Principals and SMTs had to juggle subject allocation and change the timetables.

Finally, studies show that principals' troubles were exacerbated by their preparation for the trial and the final NSC examinations. Due to the need to prepare for trials and NSC exams, principals prioritised grade 12 students. For grades 8–11, the unanticipated consequences meant more missed time for teaching and learning. The administrators were optimistic that the grade 12 students would meet their goals, given the effectiveness of the catch-up programs, notwithstanding some concerns.

Finally, the catch-up programs that were scheduled once the school reopened benefited only grade 12 students. These catch-up programs aided grade 12 students in their preparation for the Trial exams. The catch-up programs also helped students feel more secure about sitting for final exams, which began on November 5th and ended on December 15th. The principals were successful in guiding the schools through both internal and external assessments, but with significant compromises in teaching and learning for students in grades 8–11.

## 7. Conclusions

We can make conclusions from the above discussion. In terms of lost interaction time between teachers and learners, the staggered phasing-in method had a negative impact. However, proclaiming that grade 8–11 students would be required to stay at home until the next year became the worst-case scenario.

Second, because neither the biweekly nor the alternate day's models were imposed on the teachers, they were accepted. The principals and staff made decisions based on what was appropriate and practical in their situation.

Third, we may deduce that some of the disciplines that were not taught will negatively affect those learners in terms of content and skills as they go through the grades and even to the level of tertiary education entrance due to a lack of specialism in specific areas. We can say that there will be students who are taken into consideration.

Fifth, it is understandable that some of the lost teaching time could have been prevented if our schools did not have such a strong union culture. On the other hand, if active unionism had not existed, school instructors and students would have been forced to work in surroundings that would have become epicentres for the coronavirus pandemic, The school-level reactions to the pandemic have educated and prepared principals for the delayed opening of schools in February 2021, yet the most concerning element was the amount of casualties caused owing to the new form of the virus.

We feel this study is unable to make any claims, but it does have the potential to do so. We feel that while this study cannot make any claims, it can add to the expanding body of knowledge that informs school administrators, policymakers, researchers, and teachers about how to plan for the coming academic year. Finally, the study may inform stakeholders about the pandemic's approaching effects and the necessity for collaboration among people interested in education. The findings may contribute to filling some of the identified gaps in the literature study in terms of the primary leadership in handling pandemic concerns, therefore allowing for the implementation of VUCA studies.

## A. Annexure No. 1

The Principal

____________________School

Dr. BS Mchunu: Topic: Cases of principal leadership responses in a volatile, uncertain and complex school environment

Dr. BS Mchunu: is conducting a study on the experiences of Principals in managing teaching and learning in the midst of COVID-19 Pandemic. The study explores the experiences of principals in implementing DBE COVID Sector Plan and other KZN Circulars No 44 and 57 as a policy guideline to manage teaching and learning in the face of the challenges posed by the corona virus. We hereby request your experiences in implementing such and to understand the challenging situation on ground. The name of the Principal and School will not be used, rather a pseudonym (anonymous name) will be allocated. Responses are strictly confidential and anonymous. There is no right or wrong answer. The researcher will give an opportunity to the respondents to check the responses before publication.

Thank you for your time and consideration.

Yours in education

Dr. Bongani S. Mchunu (0828321936: mchunudoctor2016@gmail.com)

Kindly fill the questionnaire and survey by opening this site attached:

This questionnaire is examining the experiences of Principals in responding to the volatile, uncertain and complex school environment caused by the disruptive effect of the pandemic at Mpumalanga Circuit.

NB: Questionnaire to the principals

1. Indicate below the number following information as part of the school profile

| Learners acc. grades | Grade R | 1 | 2 | 3 | 4 | 5 | 6 | 7 | Total |
|---|---|---|---|---|---|---|---|---|---|
| No of learners | | | | | | | | | |
| Estimate the average prior to COVID | | | | | | | | | |
| Estimate the average with COVID (social distancing) | | | | | | | | | |
| Estimate the average prior to COVID | | | | | | | | | |
| Estimate the average with COVID (social distance) | | | | | | | | | |

2. Indicate the number of classrooms (teaching space available) for conducting teaching and learning prior to social distancing and during the observation of social distancing.

| No. classrooms | Grade 8 | 9 | 10 | 11 | 12 | Total |
|---|---|---|---|---|---|---|
| (Prior to COVID) | | | | | | |
| Social distance | | | | | | |

3. Indicate the number of shortages of classrooms (teaching space) in keeping with social distancing

| No. classrooms | Grade 8 | 9 | 10 | 11 | 12 | Total |
|---|---|---|---|---|---|---|
| No. required for social distance | | | | | | |
| Shortage due to social distance | | | | | | |

4. Indicate which one of these steps has been taken by the school in managing the social distancing in classrooms after the Phasing in of the other grades at school (indicate against applicable model X)

| | Methods applicable | Comment and explain in details how it works |
|---|---|---|
| a | Bi weekly approach (1 week attendance rotation of grades) | |
| b | Alternate day approach (some grades attending on some days) | |
| c | Platoon model (some learners attending in morning others in afternoon) | |
| d | Maintenance of the status quo (small schools attending normally) | |
| e | Combination of two of the above | |
| | Explain the option you have chosen/how is working. | |

5. Explain the model the school is using to give more clarity on how it is working at school.

6. Indicate the number of subjects in terms of grades that are not taught due to teacher shortages.

| Grade | 8 | 9 | 10 | 11 | 12 |
|---|---|---|---|---|---|
| | | | | | |
| Subject names not taught due to teacher shortages | | | | | |

7.1 Indicate the number of support staff that was allocated and that is available to ensure Implementation of the DBE Sector COVID-19 Plan.

| | |
|---|---|
| • **Screening of learners** | |
| • Screening of teachers | |

| |
|---|
| • **Screening of learners** |
| • Sanitisation of leaners at entry points |
| • Cleaning and sanitisation of classrooms |
| • Handling of food by kitchen handlers |

7.2 Provide the details below:

| | **Comment in details** |
|---|---|
| 7.3 Do you have an isolation room: Yes/No | |
| 7.4 What is the school using as an isolation room? | |
| 7.5 Have you ever used for isolation purposes? YES/No | |
| 7.6 What is inside the isolation room? | |

| |
|---|
| 8. Explain some of the actions that were taken based on the following: |
| 8.1 Explain how did you report the cases of affected teachers/leaners? |
| 8.2 How did you notify the Circuit Manager when cases of affected teachers/learners were identified? |
| 8.3 How did you notify the local clinic whenever there identified cases? |
| 8.4 What was the procedure for the closing of the schools? |
| 8.5 How long did it take to get the school fumigated? |

9.1 Indicate the number of teaching staff on the basis of the following factors below.

| **Post provisioning norm (PPN) allocation** | **No. of teachers present** | **No. of teachers applied for risk management due to underlying comorbidities** | **No. teachers on sick leave** | **No. teachers on quarantine** |
|---|---|---|---|---|
| | | | | |

| **9.2 Explain the effect of the teacher applications for leave on subject teaching** | | | |
|---|---|---|---|
| **Subjects not taught** | **Grade 10** | **11** | **12** |
| | | | |

10. Indicate how you have taken any action in terms of the following procedures as part of the protocols in Circulars 44 and 57 respectively for implementation at school.

(Yes/No)

| **Provisions and procedures in circulars** | **Yes/ No** | **Clarify how action was taken** |
|---|---|---|
| 1. To isolate a learner with symptomatic signs high temperature, cough, etc. | | |
| 2. Isolate a teachers with symptomatic high temperature, cough, etc. | | |

| Provisions and procedures in circulars | Yes/ No | Clarify how action was taken |
|---|---|---|
| 3. Notify Local Health Department of identified positive case(s) | | |
| 4. Notify district/circuit manager of your intended action | | |
| 5. Forced school closure | | |
| 6. Decontamination of the school after closure | | |

11. Indicate the number in terms of the following factors below since the schools reopened.

| No. of reported cases of learners | No. of reported cases of teachers | No. of days school closed | No. of teachers in quarantine | Subjects affected whilst teacher/s on quarantine of teachers |
|---|---|---|---|---|
| | | | | |

12. Indicate how the prevalence of factors that informed the School Recovery Plan/Curriculum Catch Up programmes prior to COVID-19 and after COVID-19.

| | | Prior to COVID Yes/No | COVID period Yes/No | Comment how is worked/how long |
|---|---|---|---|---|
| s1 | Grade 12 morning classes | | | |
| 2 | Grade 12 afternoon tutorials | | | |
| 3 | Saturday classes | | | |
| 4 | Sunday classes | | | |
| 5 | Evening classes/study | | | |

13. Indicate the level of support for a Curriculum Catch Up programmes amongst teachers for the following during this COVID-19 period.

Very High (10); High (8); Moderate (6); Low (4); Very Low (2)

| Changing of timetables adjustment of examinations |
|---|
| Working on afternoon teaching programmes |
| Working on morning teaching programmes |
| Working on Saturday morning teaching |

14. Indicate the level of confidence by the school in achieving its set targets prior to COVID-19 by giving an estimate of the expected number in term of the factors below.

Very High (10); High (8); Moderate (6); Low (4); Very Low (2)

| Grade 12 pass rate in 2019 | Bachelor | Diploma | Higher certificate | Overall pass/ target |
|---|---|---|---|---|
| Estimated grade 12: set target (2020) prior to COVID-19 | | | | |

| Grade 12 pass rate in 2019 | Bachelor | Diploma | Higher certificate | Overall pass/ target |
|---|---|---|---|---|
| Estimated grade 12 target (2020) with COVID-19 disruption period | | | | |

15. What is the level of confidence in terms of the following factors?

(Very High; High; Moderate; Low; Very Low)

| |
|---|
| 1. Completing tasks (ATPs) |
| 2. Catch up programme implemented |
| 3. Assessment tasks completed |
| 4. All grade 12 learners returning to school |
| 5. Teachers completing ATPs in other grades |

Thank you for your inputs.

End of questionnaire and questions to Principals

## Author details

Bongani Sibusiso Mchunu
KwaZulu-Natal Department of Education, Pietermaritzburg, South Africa

*Address all correspondence to: mchunudoctor2016@gmail.com

## References

[1] Rimita K, Hoon SN, Levasseur R. Leader readiness in a volatile, uncertain, complex, and ambiguous business environment. Journal of Social Change. 2020;**12**(1):2

[2] Darvasi P. How designing accessible curriculum for all can help make online learning more equitable. 2020

[3] Montoya S. Impact of School Closures on Learning can be Curbed with Adequate Catch-up Strategies. UNESCO Institute for Statistics; 2020

[4] Mthethwa A. Being in matric is not easy; doing it in the middle of a pandemic is not for the fainthearted. Daily Maverick. 2020

[5] Collective Agreement No 1 of 2020-Concession for Educators

[6] HRM Circular No 24 of 2020. ELRC Agreement 1 of 2020-Concession process to follow for employees with comorbidity (COVID-19)

[7] HRM Circular No 31 of 2020. Implementation of ELRC Collective Agreement No 1 of 2020. Concession profess to follow for employees with comorbidity (COVID-19)

[8] Bennett N, Lemoine GJ. What a difference a word makes: Understanding threats to performance in a VUCA world. Business Horizons. 2014;**57**(3):311-317

[9] Cohen L, Manion L, Morrison K. Research Methods in Education. 8th ed. London & New York: Routledge; 2018

[10] Netshandama V, Mahlomaholo S. The role of community engagement in higher education: Focus on the discourse relating to knowledge development. In: The Intellectual: A Phenomenon in Multidimensional Perspectives. Brill; 2010. pp. 109-117

[11] De Vos, A.S. 2010. Scientific theory and professional research. In A.S. De Vos, H. Strydom, CB Fouche, Delport CSL, editors. Research at Grassroots: For the Social Sciences and Human Service Professionals. 3rd ed. Pretoria: Van Schaik Publishers

[12] Saldaa J. The Coding Manual for Qualitative Researchers. Vol. 2. Los Angeles, CA; 2013

[13] Creswell JW. Qualitative Inquiry and Research Design: Choosing among Five Approaches. 2nd ed. Thousand Oaks, CA: SAGE Publications; 2007

[14] C-19 People's Coalition. No society is not ready to safely reopen schools and education centres. 17 June 2020

Chapter 28

# Challenges and Futures of Long-Term Care Industry after COVID-19 Pandemic

*Jia Yu*


## Abstract

COVID-19 pandemic has affected people's daily life dramatically since December 2019. More than 211 million cases and 4.42 million deaths have been reported and confirmed all over the world. Long-term care facilities are taking the biggest hit during this pandemic, even after the spread-out of the vaccines. Globally, residents in long-term care facilities have experienced disproportionately high morbidity and mortality from COVID-19. Elderlies residing in long-term care facilities have the greatest susceptibility to COVID-19 and the poorest outcomes from infections. This chapter overviewed the insight, impact, and challenges of COVID-19 on the residential care homes in UK, US, and Australia and provided possible implications for the long-term care market post-pandemic.


**Keywords:** long-term care facility, COVID-19 pandemic, residential aged care facility, nursing homes, post pandemic

## 1. Introduction

COVID-19 pandemic has affected people's daily life dramatically since December 2019, since it was firstly discovered in Wuhan, China, in December 2019. The pandemic has already spread out to the entire world since March 2020. More than 211 million cases and 4.42 million deaths have been reported and confirmed all over the world. The COVID-19 pandemic has already become one of the deadliest pandemics in human history.

Globally, residents in long-term facilities have experienced disproportionately high morbidity and mortality from COVID-19. Across Europe, almost all countries have struggled to protect vulnerable people in long-term care facilities, no matter their relaxed or strict strategies. Despite the difficulties arising from differences in definitions, in almost all countries where there have been deaths linked to COVID-19, a substantial proportion of those deaths were among care home residents [1]. Based on the same report from International Long Term Care Policy Network, the current average of the share of all COVID-19 deaths that were care home residents is 46% (data from 21 countries). Take an example of May 2020, in Belgium, 51% of the country's 9,052 fatal COVID-19 cases were reported from long-term care facilities [2]; there were 7,469 reported cases from long-term care facilities in France, including 66% from nursing homes and 34% from other facilities [3]; Germany had reported 22,071 infections related to institutions caring for the elderly (long-term care facilities and nursing homes), disabled people, homeless



IntechOpen

people, migrants, or those in prison [4]. In the US, COVID-19 also has been shown to affect the elderly (aged 65 years and older particularly severely, with this demographic having the highest COVID-19-associated hospitalization rate around 600 per 100,000 cases based on the date in 2020 [5].

Given that older adults experience a greater number and severity of chronic diseases and disabilities, it is inevitable that COVID-19 will disproportionately affect this population [6]. Thus, it is not surprising that elderly people residing in long-term care facilities, such as nursing homes, care homes, have the greatest susceptibility to COVID-19, as well as the poorest outcomes from infections. This Chapter would like to overview the insight and impact of COVID-19 on the care homes in the UK, US, and Australia, and provide possible implications for the long-term care market post-pandemic.

## 2. The care homes in the United Kingdom

### 2.1 COVID-19 in care homes

The UK government publishes daily statistics on COVID-19 related cases and deaths. The detailed reports about care homes across the UK were published in different ways in each separate sub-section.

In England, the Office of National Statistics (ONS) started publishing data on all care home resident deaths on April 11$^{th}$, 2020.29,511 care home residents in England died from COVID-19 or related causes up until July 23$^{rd}$, 2021, which is 22% of all England COVID-related deaths. The lower percentage of deaths in 2021, compared with 2020, also relatively shows the effectiveness of the vaccines.

In Scotland, the Care Inspectorate Scotland (CIS) has reported weekly data on confirmed COVID-19 related death of care home residents since May 25$^{th}$, 2020. There are 10,505 COVID-19 related deaths in Scotland overall as the date of August 16$^{th}$, 2021, 3,317 care home deaths (32%) are included. However, even there's a lower number of deaths in Scotland, the percentage of COVID-related nursing home deaths in 2021 is higher than that in 2020. The elderlies living in care homes (nursing homes) are still the group that has been hit the most.

In Wales, Care inspectorate Wales (CIW) reported weekly data on notifications of deaths of care home residents. A total of 1,932 care home residents' COVID-19 related deaths have been reported to the CIW, since the first confirmation on March 16$^{th}$, 2020. There are 24% of overall COVID-related deaths in Wales happened in care homes (nursing homes).

The Department of Health of Northern Ireland released daily statistics on COVID-19 cases and deaths since April 19$^{th}$, 2020. By the date of August 26$^{th}$, 2021, there are 2,337 COVID-19 related deaths in Northern Ireland. Of those, 439 occurred in residential/care homes, and 1,859 were confirmed in hospitals [7]. During Fall 2020, 437 care home residents died from suspected or confirmed COVID-19, i.e., around 81% of all COVID-19 care home resident deaths occurred within the care home [8]. Therefore, the total care home resident deaths make up 14% of all COVID-19 deaths in Northern Ireland (**Table 1**).

### 2.2 The structure of the care homes in UK

The UK care home market is a relatively fragmented sector. The structures of care homes are from large corporate operators providing in excess of 10,000 beds to sole traders with one or two homes. Most of the care homes are operated by charities

| | Total deaths (2021) | Care home deaths (2021) | % | Total deaths (2020) | Care home deaths (2020) | % | Total death percentage |
|---|---|---|---|---|---|---|---|
| UK Total | 65,276 | 12,353 | 19% | 89,243 | 22,836 | 26% | 23% |
| England | 57,137 | 10,263 | 18% | 75,782 | 19,248 | 25% | 22% |
| Scotland | 3,762 | 1,320 | 35% | 6,686 | 1,997 | 30% | 32% |
| Wales | 3,002 | 663 | 22% | 4,945 | 1,269 | 26% | 24% |
| Northern Ireland | 1,255 | 107 | 9% | 1,830 | 322 | 18% | 14% |

*Source: Office of National Statistics; Care Inspectorate Scotland; Care Inspectorate Wales; Department of Health of Northern Ireland.*

**Table 1.**
*The COVID-19 statistics about care homes in the UK (July 2021).*

and other not-for-profit organizations. The care home industry, as a whole, is a vital social service. The independent (non-public sector) operators, such as the 10 largest for-profit providers, dominated a quarter of the market. Smaller groups made up around 38% of capacity, with the remainder owned by operators with one or two homes [9]. According to the Grant Thornton report in 2018, in recent years, a two-tier market has emerged based on payment methods, including public pay and self-paying. The operators whose income is mainly from public supports, such as local authority or NHS usually achieves significantly lower profits than those with self-paying.

Like many other countries, the UK's age structure is shifting towards older ages. In 1999, around 15.8% of people were 65 years and over, this increased to 18.5% people in 2019 and is projected to reach around 23.9% people by 2039 (**Figure 1**) [10].

The increasing number and percentage of an aging population will be a large group requiring access to care services, such as residential care, care home services, and nursing homes. However, although the growth rate in the 65+ population is forecast to accelerate over the next decade, the absolute number of long-term residential accommodations has declined by 4.4% between 2001 and 2016 [9]. In 2017, 14.8% (estimated) of 85 years and older were in elderly residential accommodation, compared with 25.2% [9].

There are two types of payments for elderlies, one is from local authorities (i.e., public payment), the other one is self-pay. According to Grant Thornton's research in 2018, around 25% of care homes have over 75% of residents placed by local authorities. Average fees covered by local authorities were 10% less than the total cost of providing care, approximately a 200 million pounds to 300 million pounds shortfall in funding. To counteract this, self-funders have to pay around 40% more out of pocket to care homes, compared with the UK council-funded patients. Even though, the self-pay market is still growing at a fast rate.

### 2.3 The challenge of the care homes in UK

The biggest challenges of care homes in the UK, before the COVID-19 pandemic, are three aspects: decreasing potential demand due to the switching payment methods; increasing population size with limited bed numbers; declining qualified staff and nurses in care homes. These challenges, under the outbreak of COVID-19, become much tougher and more difficult to deal with.

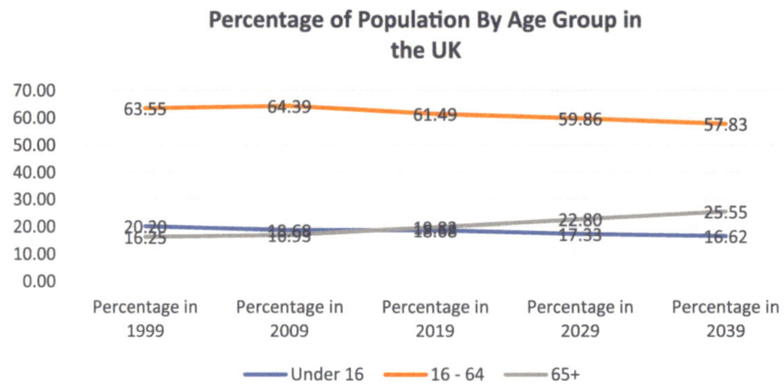


**Figure 1.**
*Percentage of Population by Age Group in the UK. Source: Office for National Statistics (January 2021).*

Before the COVID-19 pandemic, the potential demand for care homes have already decreased due to the switching payment methods. Self-funders become the new focus of the market after several care home closures that focused on local authority-funded payers [9]. Without the support from the local authority, not every single elderly, who is eligible for residential care homes, has sufficient ability to self-support his/her stay and other further expenses. After the pandemic, due to the high numbers of confirmed cases and deaths, a proportion of potential consumers would start to question care homes and reconsider their options after retirement. The demand for care homes may have an even sharp decline during the post-pandemic period.

The residential care home industry has experienced dramatic changes due to the pandemic. With the drastic hit from COVID-19, residential care homes would have to face many potential problems, such as social distancing bed arrangement, more inputs on disinfection supplies, etc. The capacity of the care homes dropped because of the limitation of room and space, to protect patients and follow the pandemic safety rule. Piling inputs on disinfection supplies may cause declining investment in other aspects (such as staffing, daily operation supplies, etc.), which possibly affect the daily routine or even the operation model. The percentage of net earnings[1] among care home providers falls from 32.8% in 2006/07 to 25.2% in 2016/17, which has been attributed to increased food and property costs, the freezing of local authority fee rates in real terms, and higher wage costs before COVID-19 [9]. After the pandemic, the care homes may face an even lower percentage of net earnings due to the increasing investment in preventive and disinfection supplies and higher hiring costs for qualified staff.

Hiring a qualified and satisfying staff was one of the biggest challenges for the care homes in the UK before the pandemic. It is estimated that 1.22 million social care workers will be needed between 2016 and 2036 [9]. The increase of national living wage (NLW) and national minimum wage (NMW) has raised the real wages and the original costs of each care home. However, the pandemic completely changed the story of nursing education, which may turn the staffing situation in UK in a different direction. According to the data from the Universities and Colleges Admission Services (UCAS), there has been a total 37,635 nursing students accepted onto the course in 2020, comparing 30,395 in 2019. It includes 29,740 students placed in England, 4,785 in Scotland, 1,985 in Wales, and 1,125 in Northern Ireland. There was a significant fall in nursing students in England in 2017 due to the

[1] Net earnings mean the earnings before interest, tax, depreciation, amortization, rent, and central management costs.

removal of the NHS bursary. This 2020 number shows a new faith and understanding of the nursing world during pandemic. Even though, the Health Foundation warned the government's pledge for 50,000 more nurses by 2025 would be insufficient to meet growing demand, especially during the coronavirus pandemic. The pandemic may still have potential to shrink this gap by encouraging more people to pursue careers in medical field.

## 3. The nursing homes in the United States[2]

### 3.1 COVID-19 in nursing homes

The COVID-19 pandemic in the United States has already confirmed more than 39.1 million cases, with more than 639,000 deaths, which make the United States the most of any country, and the 24 highest per capita worldwide. COVID-19 has been shown to affect the elderly (aged 65 years and older) particularly severely, with this demographic having the highest COVID-19-related hospitalization rate in the US of around 600 per 100,000 cases [5]. Given that older adults experience a greater number and severity of chronic diseases and disabilities, it is inevitable that COVID-19 will disproportionately affect this population [6]. Thus, it is not surprising that elderly people residing in long-term care facilities, such as nursing homes, have the greatest susceptibility to COVID-19, as well as the poorest outcomes from infections.

Using state and federal data, the COVID Tracking Project (CTP) estimates that as of March 2021, about 8% of people who love in US long-term care facilities have died of COVID-19 (nearly 1 in 12), and nearly 1 in 10 for nursing homes alone. According to CTP, throughout the COVID-19 pandemic, a third of all US COVID-related deaths were long-term-care facility deaths, which include nursing homes, assisted living, and other long-term care facilities.

### 3.2 The structure of nursing homes

Nursing homes in the US are aiming to provide care to those with permanent disabilities rather than to 'cure' [12]. According to the Centers for Disease Control and Prevention 2016 statistics, there are approximately 15,600 nursing homes in the US, with around 1.7 million beds and over 1.3 million residents. There are also 12,200 home health agencies, providing care in the patient's own home and serving 4.5 million patients each year. Other types of long-term care contain hospice care agencies, residential care communities, and adult day service communities, the latter two of which provide able patients assistance (**Table 2**).

The nursing home industry contains a relatively large number of nursing homes, with fees being affected by numerous factors, including consumer demand and government regulations. As a result, it is a highly competitive industry [13].

The COVID-19 pandemic may affect consumers' preferences regarding the long-term care facilities they choose. Before the substantial rise in COVID-19 cases among the general population in July 2020, nursing homes and assisted living facilities made up the majority of US COVID-19 cases, with a fatality count of more than 50,000, comprising over 43% of the total deaths in June [19]. This high death rate and the following struggle to ensure patient safety and transmission control in nursing homes may deter potential service users from selecting residential care.

[2] Majority of this part is from the paper I published with my student, Amber Schultz [11].

| | Nursing homes | Home health agencies | Hospice care agencies | Residential care communities | Adult day services centers |
|---|---|---|---|---|---|
| Number of facilities | 15,600 | 12,200 | 4,300 | 28,900 | 4,600 |
| Number of beds | 1,700,000 | N/A | N/A | 996,100 | N/A |
| Number of residents | 1,300,000 | 4,500,000 | 1,400,000 | 811,500 | 286,300 |

*Source: National Center for Health Statistics, CDC, 2019.*

**Table 2.**
*Statistics about Long-Term Care Facilities in the US (2016).*

This scenario may lead to a demand shifting on the long-term care services market, from nursing homes to home care.

### 3.3 The challenge of nursing homes

The conduct of nursing homes relates to various external factors, which impact the behavior of long-term care providers, such as government regulations, policies, and property rights (for-profit or not-for-profit). And not all patients were always treated and cared for equally.

Throughout the pandemic, all residential care facilities were following the same government COVID-19 regulations and protocols to the best of their ability, such as maintaining social distancing rules in a public area, separating and quarantining COVID-19 patients, emphasizing strict facial mask rules, etc [14]. All the regulations and rules caused another layer of the financial burden for most residential care facilities. Some small facilities, or those that lack strong financial support, may struggle to implement these changes, and therefore must face tough competition from other nursing homes with greater financial means, as well as from other substitutes for long-term care.

To assess the overall performance of the long-term care industry, several measures are usually examined, including expenditure on long-term care, private insurance for long-term care, the price of nursing home care, and the relative use of nursing homes, home healthcare, and hospice services [13]. Long-term care facility costs comprise the largest share of annual direct spending by those receiving Medicare beneficiaries as a result of age (>65 years) or disability status [15]. Long-term care expenses, such as nursing homes and assisted living facilities, are the number one category for out-of-pocket payment, followed by home healthcare [16]. In 2020, nursing homes cost an averagely of $6,844 monthly, or $82,128 per year, which is higher than the median household income in the US. Given the scale of the financial costs, the additional risk of COVID- 19 infection, and the restrictions on visiting could turn potential consumers away from all this type of long-term care, especially with inexpensive other forms of care. For example, home healthcare costs an average of roughly $4,000 a month [17].

Before the pandemic, nursing homes were usually the prioritized choice for elderlies, because of trustworthy performance, regarding the quality of care, group living, and partial insurance coverage [18]. However, even prior to 2020, the average annual growth in demand for home healthcare was greater than that of nursing home facilities (**Table 3**) [19]. With the additional influence of the

| NHE, billions | 2009 | 2010 | 2011 | 2012 | 2013 | 2014 | 2015 |
|---|---|---|---|---|---|---|---|
| Nursing care facilities and continuing care retirement communities | 134.9 | 140.0 | 145.0 | 147.4 | 149.2 | 152.6 | 158.8 |
| Home health care | 67.3 | 71.0 | 73.8 | 77.1 | 80.0 | 83.6 | 88.8 |
| Annual Growth, % | | | | | | | |
| Nursing care facilities and continuing care retirement communities | 3.5 | 3.8 | 3.6 | 1.6 | 1.3 | 2.3 | 2.7 |
| Home health care | 8.3 | 5.5 | 4.0 | 4.4 | 3.7 | 4.5 | 6.3 |

*Source: Centers for Medicare and Medicaid Services (CMS), Office of Actuary, National Health Statistics Group.*

**Table 3.**
*National Health Expenditure (NHE) amounts and annual growth for nursing home and home health care.*

pandemic, it is reasonable to observe that more people will start to choose home healthcare over nursing home care as the most appropriate, safe, and affordable option for their later lives.

## 4. The residential aged care facilities in Australia

### 4.1 COVID-19 in residential aged care facilities

The COVID-19 pandemic was confirmed to have reached Australia on January 25$^{th}$, 2020. Until now, there were 56,565 positive cases and 1,019 deaths confirmed in Australia. The Australian Government Department of Health reported positive cases and COVID-associated deaths on daily basis. The elderly account for a staggering 697 of those deaths. 61% of deaths occurred in residential aged care facilities. People who had picked up the infection in the nursing home where they were supposed to feel safe. **Table 4** here illustrated the positive cases overall and in residential aged care facilities for each subarea in Australia.

In the ACT, Northern Territory, South Australia, and West Australia, there're no active reported positive cases or death available in nursing homes. In other subareas, the number of positive cases and deaths is not as high as UK or US, but the percentage still may prove the severity of the outbreak at the residential aged care facilities. In Victoria, almost 80% of COVID-related deaths are from residential aged care facilities (**Figure 2**).

### 4.2 The structure of nursing homes in Australia

Aged Care in Australia is the provision of services to meet the unique requirements and needs of elderlies in Australia, which includes in-home care, residential care in aged care (nursing) homes, and short-term care such as respite care [20]. The aged care industry provides older Australians with a range of different services, allowing them to access appropriate and affordable care when and where they need it. In Australia, many aged care services are government-subsidized to help keep costs manageable and affordable [21]. Australians, who are eligible for government subsidies, will still be expected to contribute to the cost of services if they can afford to.

| | Total cases | Total deaths | Total cases in residential aged care facilities | Total deaths in residential aged care facilities | Percentage deaths in residential aged care facilities |
|---|---|---|---|---|---|
| Australia | 85,629 | 1,162 | 2,338 | 710 | 61.15% |
| Australian Capital Territory (ACT) | 742 | 3 | — | — | — |
| New South Wales (NSW) | 51,986 | 295 | 345 | 53 | 17.97% |
| Northern Territory | 204 | — | — | — | — |
| Queensland | 2,016 | 7 | 1 | 1 | 14.29% |
| South Australia | 898 | 4 | — | — | — |
| Tasmania | 235 | 13 | 1 | 1 | 7.69% |
| Victoria | 28,456 | 831 | 1,991 | 655 | 78.82% |
| Western Australia | 1,093 | 9 | — | — | — |

*Source: Australia Government Department of Health (09/19/2021).*

**Table 4.**
*COVID-19 in Australia (09/19/2021).*

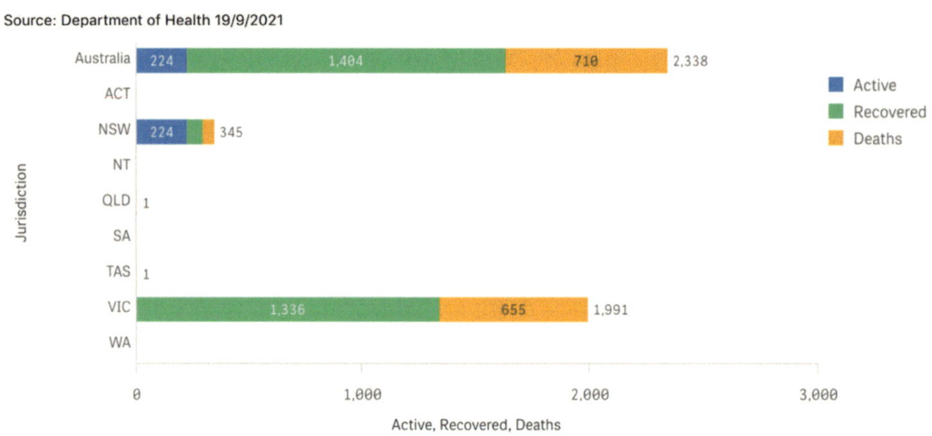


**Figure 2.**
*COVID-19 in Australia's nursing homes (September 2021).*

The Australian aged care sector is large and complex. According to the Aged Care Financing Authority, the aged care industry is one of Australia's largest service industries, including over 350,000 employees, over one million consumers, and around 2,000 service providers. The aged care industry is essential to elderlies in providing a variety of care options for their later stages of life. In 2016/17, aged care services made up $17.8 billion of Commonwealth expenditure, which is a significant public involvement [22].

There are over 2,000 aged care services in Australia, supplying three different types of aged care services: home and community care (HCC); home care; and residential care. HCC provides entry-level basic support for older people who need assistance to live independently. Home care contains 4 levels of care provided to elderlies living at home, ranging from basic to high-care needs. Residential care provides accommodation and support for those who choose to live within residential care facilities, which is the one we focus on in this chapter. In 2013/14, residential care facilities generated 82% (14.8b) of total revenue and received 73% ($9.8b) of total Commonwealth funding to the aged care sector, while residential aged care places represented only 18% (189,283) of total aged care places (**Table 5**).

A combination of for-profit, not-for-profit, and government service providers contributed to these three types of aged care services. Across all three types, not-for-profit providers supplied most aged care services, with the market share of these providers ranging from 52% in residential care to 74% in HCC [22].

Looking at the recent patterns and prominent factors, the growth of the aged care industry is a given without the hit of COVID-19. Apparently, the pandemic warned people to make a smart choice about their aged life. The aged care facilities, especially the residential aged care facilities, face quite big challenges before and after the COVID-19 pandemic.

### 4.3 The challenges of the nursing home industry

The first challenge is the changes of demands of the Baby Boomers. As Baby Boomers move into old age, this trend is set father greater momentum over the next three decades. Baby Boomers are a sizable cohort, accounting for nearly 5.6 million Australians [23]. The proportion of people aged 65 years or over is projected to increase from 13% in 2010 to 23% by June 2050 (**Figure 3**) [24].

Given that the number of seniors is continuously climbing and potential consumers are now exercising more control over the care packages and facilities, policymakers and service providers should focus on creating a sustainable system that supports the increasing volume of the elderly [25]. Compared with the new generations, Baby Boomer tends to be cautious and rational on consumption behavior. With the hit from COVID-19, it is possible to switch Baby Boomers' decision-making process and affect the demand of aged care facilities. Aged care service providers can consider investing in technologies such as Augmented Reality, Virtual Reality, Artificial Intelligence, Video Calling, CRM solutions and more to suit the varying demands of seniors.

The second challenge is the lack of skilled staffs and how the aged care facilities attract them. The Aged care sector is heavily dependent on the skills of the workforce. From the population perspective, for every couple of retirement age, there were 15 people in the working-age population in 1970. This number dropped to 10 by 2010 and is projected to decline to 5 by 2050 [26]. Apparently, the number of skilled workers leaving this industry is rising. Increasing workload and stress, less career growth opportunities, extended working hours and dissatisfaction from the remuneration are some of the main reasons responsible for the drain of skilled employees [25].

| | HCC | Home care | Residential care |
|---|---|---|---|
| Number of providers | 1,676 | 504 | 1,016 |
| Number of places | 775,959 | 66,149 | 189,283 |
| Commonwealth funding | $1,701m | $1,271m | $9,814m |
| Total revenue | $1.8b | $1.3b | $14.8b |

*Source: Deloitte Access Economics [22].*

**Table 5.**
*Basics about the Aged Care Facilities in Australia.*

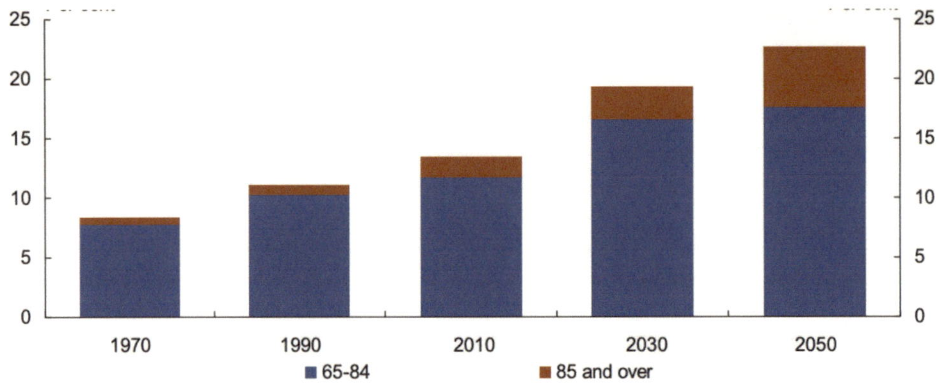


**Figure 3.**
*Estimates about the percentage of elderlies by 2050. Source: Australian Government [24].*

The COVID-19 pandemic is possible to make this situation even worse. According to a survey of the Australian nursing, midwifery, and care worker workforce, which was completed by Rosemary Bryant AO Research Centre in May 2021, around half of the survey respondents were moderately or extremely concerned about having adequate staff (53.18%), the welfare of their colleagues (52.15%) and having the right skills mix in the workplace (51.43%). The workload for nurses has significantly increased since the pandemic. During the pandemic, working at an aged care facilities means the highest levels of workplace demand, role conflict, work-life conflict, and lowest job satisfaction, as well as the lowest clarity compared to other workplace groups [27].

Another problem is to attract qualified and skilled workers. Recruitment of a skilled workforce such as certified care givers and nurses for the aged care facilities is also a big challenge as well. Under situations with high workloads and low job satisfaction during the pandemic, attracting a qualified workforce becomes even harder. The aged care service provider may invest in some high-quality technology solutions and create a robust infrastructure to manage the situation. For example, they can offer the remote working options or proper transport facilities by arranging private vehicles or an appropriate bus facility [25].

## 5. Conclusion

Starting from the early months of the COVID-19 pandemic, the long-term care facilities have experienced an extremely tough period all over the world. Suddenly, the nursing home industry, which has been long operated out of public view, finds itself at the center of scrutiny. During a crisis like this pandemic, it becomes especially critical to preserve the necessary functions for long-term care facilities. It is essential for aged care centers to maintain their size, the number of beds, recourses, manage external emergency circumstances, and also boost the potential demands. Based on our findings from the UK, the US, and Australia, we can say that the COVID-19 outbreak will likely push potential or existing residents and their families to question and reconsider whether the residential long-term care facilities, such as nursing homes, senior centers, or aged care facilities, are the best or safest options for them to be.

The pandemic challenged and changed the way of operations for almost all the long-term care facilities all over the world. Even the number of elderlies is rising in the future, the diverse format of retirement life care and the decreasing trend of public financial supports have already dropped the demand for residential long-term care facilities before the COVID-19 pandemic. Due to the rising number of confirmed COVID cases and deaths in nursing homes, not only the potential patients, but also the qualified staffs and workers may have second thoughts about continuing their works in nursing homes. Meanwhile, the entire long-term care industry has been lacking qualified and skilled staffs and nurses all the time even without the pandemic. Although, in some countries (such as UK), potential students who may dedicate their will to become a nurse or font-line medical workers after seeing and understanding the meaning and importance of medical-related work. Unfortunately, this is not happening in most of the countries.

After the COVID-19, for potential elderlies or demanders who may need residential care, there're many other new options that can provide sufficient and affordable care. All options for later-life care, including assisted living facilities, home healthcare, and community-based care, need to be reviewed and re-evaluated after COVID-19. As the major financial supporters of long-term care, each government may also need to consider how to adjust the residential aged care facilities and adapt them into the new business norm after COVID-19. And also, potentially speaking, home- and community-based care are highly possible to become the new dominants for the post-COVID long-term care industry.

## Conflict of interest

The authors declare no conflict of interest.

## Author details

Jia Yu
Southern Connecticut State University, New Haven, CT, USA

*Address all correspondence to: yuj4@southernct.edu

## References

[1] Comas-Herrera A et al. Mortality associated with COVID-19 in care homes: International evidence. In: International Long Term Care Policy Network. 2020

[2] Sciensano. Coronavirus COVID-19, Overall Epidemiological Situation 2020. 2020. Available from: https://covid-19.sciensano.be/fr/covid-19-situation-epidemiologique

[3] Sante Publique France. The COVID-19 epdemic in France. 2020. Available from: https://www.santepubliquefrance.fr/dossiers/coronavirus-covid-19

[4] Robert Koch Institut. Aktueller Lage-/Situationsbericht des RKI zu COVID-19. 2020. Available from: https://www.rki.de/DE/Content/InfAZ/N/Neuartiges_Coronavirus/Situationsberichte/Gesamt.html

[5] Elflein, J. Rate of COVID-19 Hospitalization in the US as of Septermber 26, 2020, by Age Group. *statista.com.* 2020. Available from: https://www.statista.com/statistics/1122354/covid-19-us-hospital-rate-by-age/

[6] D'Adamo H, Yoshikawa T, Ouslander JG. Coronavirus disease 2019 in geriatrics and long-term care: The ABCDs of COVID-19. Journal of the American Geriatrics Society. 2020;**68**(5):912-917

[7] Department of Health of Northern Ireland. COVID-19 Deaths by Setting. 2021. Available from: https://app.powerbi.com/view?r=eyJrIjoiZGYxNjYzNmUtOTlmZS00ODAxLWE1YTEtMjA0NjZhMzlmN2JmIiwidCI6IjljOWEzMGRlLWQ4ZDctNGFhNC05NjAwLTRiZTc2MjVmZjZjNSIsImMiOjh9

[8] Comas-Herrera A et al. Mortality associated with COVID-19 in care homes: International evidence. In: International Long Term Care Policy Network. 2021

[9] Smith D et al. Care Homes for the Elderly: Where are We Now? Grant Thornton; 2018

[10] Office of National Statistics. Overview of the UK Population: January 2021. Office of National Statistics; 2021

[11] Schultz A, Yu J. "No more nursing homes?" Consumers' preference changes on long-term care facilities selection after the COVID-19 pandemic. British Journal of Healthcare Management. 2020;**26**(11):276-280

[12] Scanlon WJ. A theory of the nursing home market. Inquiry. 1980;**17**:25-41

[13] Santerre RE, Neun SP. Chapter 15: The long-term care industry. In: Health Economics: Theories, Insights and Industry Studies. South-West: Cengage Learning; 2010. pp. 497-537

[14] Centers for Disease Control and Prevention. Interim Infection Prevention and Control Recommendations to Prevent SARS-CoV-2 Spread in Nursing Homes. *COVID-19.* 2021. Available from: https://www.cdc.gov/coronavirus/2019-ncov/hcp/long-term-care.html?CDC_AA_refVal=https%3A%2F%2Fwww.cdc.gov%2Fcoronavirus%2F2019-ncov%2Fhcp%2Fnursing-homes-responding.html

[15] Cubanski J et al. How Much Do Medicare Beneficiaries Spend Out of Pocket on Health Care? Kaiser Family Foundation; 2019 Available from: https://www.kff.org/medicare/issue-brief/how-much-do-medicare-beneficiaries-spend-out-of-pocket-on-health-care/

[16] Mendoza, Michelle. Out-of-Pocket Spending for Senior Care: The Harsh

Reality. Amada Senior Care. 2019. Available from: https://www.amadaseniorcare.com/2019/03/out-of-pocket-spending-for-senior-care/

[17] National Council for Aging Care. In-Home Cost Breakdown. *Aging.com.* 2020. Available from: https://aging.com/in-home-care-costs-breakdown/

[18] Kane RL, Kane RA. What older people want from long-term care, and how they can get it. Health Affairs. 2001;**20**:114-127

[19] Centers for Medicare and Medicaid Services. National Health Expenditure 2019 Highlights. Centers for Medicare and Medicaid Services; 2020

[20] McTaggart, Debbir. Must-know aged care terms. Your Life Choices. 2017. Available from: https://www.yourlifechoices.com.au/aged-care/mustknow-aged-care-terms/

[21] Health Direct. Aged Care Services. Health Direct. 2016. Available from: https://www.healthdirect.gov.au/aged-care-services

[22] Deloitte Access Economics. Australia's Aged Care Sector: Economic Contribution and Future Directions. Deloitte Access Economics; 2016

[23] Yu S. Modelling Demand Driven Provision of Aged Care to Baby Boomers in Australia. University of Canberra; 2015 https://researchprofiles.canberra.edu.au/en/studentTheses/modelling-demand-driven-provision-of-aged-care-to-baby-boomers-in

[24] Australian Government. Australia to 2050: Future challenges. Australian Government; 2010

[25] Trivedi, Vivek. Five Challenges Faced by the Australian Aged Care Industry. ExigoTech. 2019. Available from: https://exigotech.com.au/five-challenges-faced-by-the-australian-aged-care-industry/

[26] McCrindle Research. Demand vs Supply: The Aged Care Puzzle. McCrindle Research; 2014

[27] Adelson P et al. COVID-19 and Workforce Wellbring: A Survey of the Australian Nursing, Midwifery, and Care Worker Workforce. Rosemary Bryant AO Research Centre; 2021

Chapter 29

# Companies and Covid-19: Emerging Challenges and Recovery Strategies through Technological Upgrading

*Adalberto Rangone*


## Abstract

This work aims to outline the emerging challenges that businesses are facing as a result of the pandemic spread of Covid-19 and possible solutions for rapid recovery of production and commercial activities. Studies show that the pandemic situation clearly combines with an evolutionary process already underway (revolution 4.0) that requires a reformulation of business models in a digital key. Through the explanation of the concept of *techno-corporate gap*, a term we coined, in this work it is shown how the "micro" initiatives of companies in adopting innovative systems have "macro" repercussions on the whole, influencing the well-known process of technological gap of an entire country with respect to others. Investments in innovation and business upgrading, therefore, are observed not only as a means to implement recovery strategies but also as a specific contribution that companies can give to make their country more competitive. Moreover, through the description of what we have called "Strategy Poker," we explain how, during an extremely delicate situations such as the current one, companies must "to raise" rather than "to fold" in order to maintain the trust of all stakeholders and regain market share.


**Keywords:** corporate strategy, innovation, investments, techno-corporate gap, strategy "poker", business administration

## 1. Introduction

After the great economic and financial crisis of 2007, the Covid-19 pandemic is posing one of the greatest economic and social challenges humans have ever faced. From a health and humanitarian point of view, the extent of this impact has already been understood by everyone, thanks to the daily data attesting to a continuing pandemic spread throughout the world, even as procedures aimed at combating the virus have been launched. As far as the social and economic effects are concerned, direct understanding has come about as a result of regulatory impositions that have restricted not only transport and travel but also economic activities, inevitably slowing down the entire economic system.

But can we claim to have fully understood the effects of this scale on companies and business?

This new climate in which both businesses and private citizens have found themselves can really be considered as unexplored, although there have been similar experiences in the last century [1]. The pandemic has induced profound negative effects throughout the global economy [2] affecting mainly the key points of companies' operational management—first of all the supply chain—together with the way companies have to relate to clients and consumers. Initially, the negative influences led to the closure of simple units, then of business units, and finally, for the companies in trouble, of the entire business. This was induced by multiple factors:

- the prolonged suspension of certain production and service activities;
- supply chain disruption and tighter regulation;
- the severe reduction in business sales;
- the liquidity problems of companies and organizations due to the blockage of activities;
- legal disputes over delays in orders and services

All this was accompanied by the payment of extraordinary costs for adjustments to business structures required by governments to continue operations using precautionary health measures to contain the pandemic spread.

Therefore, the costs that companies have had to bear have paradoxically increased, but at the same time sales volumes and capacity utilization have decreased.

According to CERVED data, nearly one in four businesses closed at a loss in the first year of the pandemic. The study shows that in 2020, the revenues of the companies in the sample analyzed collapsed by 10.7%, compared with the 3% growth they had achieved in 2019, the last year of a positive trend that began in 2013 [3].

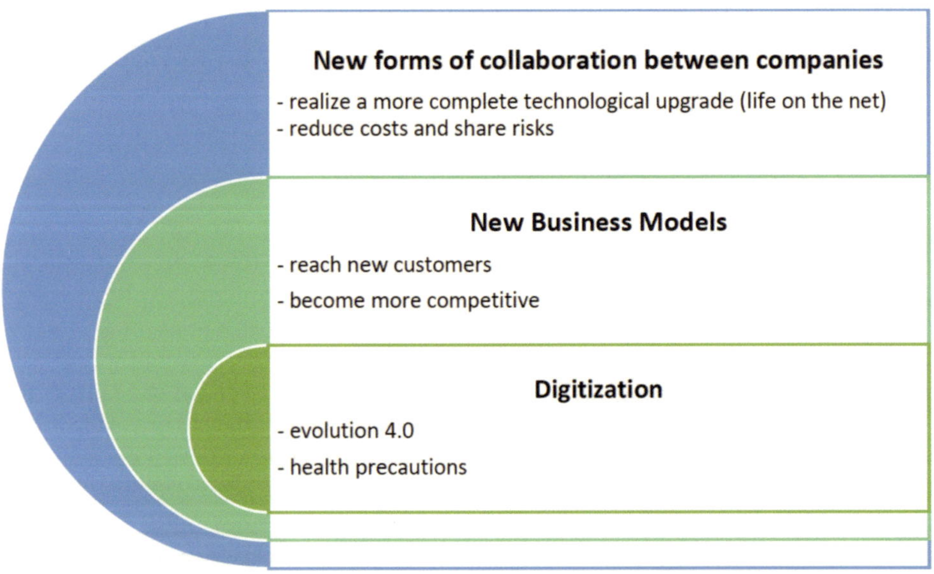


**Figure 1.**
*Scenarios induced by the pandemic crisis and the revolutionary process 4.0. Source: author's elaboration.*

These irrefutable data make it possible to outline and hypothesize new trends and possible scenarios induced by the pandemic (**Figure 1**).

The inability to individually ensure the smooth running of business operations and the provision of required services will increasingly induce companies to operate collegially in a network rather than continue with individualistic models. The perception of common problems will lead to the creation of business alliances aimed at stabilizing supply chains and formulating new models capable of achieving cost efficiency and maximizing performance.

However, this need will be realized in an increasing context of digitization. The impressive digital framework already underway will become so large that it will be able to absorb most of the investments made by companies to satisfy the new desires and upcoming needs of customers who are increasingly operating on the Internet.

Therefore, we are driven to argue that all those companies now considered *traditional* that, by inability or desire, will not want to adapt to such a change will be inexorably expelled from a system of advanced interconnection and operation 4.0.

## 2. Emerging challenges for business after the pandemic

As in any crisis situation, it has to be said that, even in the case of the Covid-19 pandemic spread, entrepreneurial ability, adaptability, and business dynamism will make the difference.

Although this principle is already widely expressed in the "classic" texts of business administration and economics [4, 5], it remains more valid than ever today and should not be disregarded.

In fact, it is possible to see that weak companies risk becoming weaker, while those that are already strong have the opportunity to become even stronger. The case of Amazon is a more than obvious example. It holds an entrenched business model aimed at providing online services, has exponentially increased its revenue and stock market value [6], and today demonstrates a high ROE of 25.6% compared with 19.9% for the industry sector [7]. In the analysis of the status quaestionis, it should be stressed at the same time that the income and wealth gap between households and individuals will also increase. This factor is by no means to be underestimated if we consider that in countries such as Italy, Spain and Greece—by way of example—the entrepreneurial fabric is made up for the most part of micro-small enterprises with family or unipersonal governance systems [8–10].

These perspectives therefore suggest how specific scenarios are emerging, harbingers of new needs and concerns but also the need for new bold actions by equally bold entrepreneurs.

The analysis of the trends outlined above in the introductory section demonstrates, therefore, some needs and challenges experienced by businesses today and can be summarized as follows:

- Companies are experiencing rapid obsolescence in their business models.
- Internal communication and organizational systems, toward and from employees and collaborators, are being reformulated in an innovative way.
- A deep and wise investment in smart asset is essential.

Only by implementing a real trend reversal, thus trying to satisfy these three points as best as possible, companies will be able to adapt not only to the change related to the current pandemic but equally to the 4.0 revolution already underway [11].

## 2.1 Toward a radical restructuring of the corporate business model

Among the main needs highlighted by companies and the imminent challenges to be faced, we note first of all the radical restructuring of the traditional business model. One must then ask: why? What are the motivations behind this important choice? And again, what are the criteria for achieving this in the best possible way?

Motivations can have internal and external connotations. These include the following:

- goods or services require a different formulation in order to be accepted by clients and consumers who express new preferences, as they are influenced by new trends;
- threats from new market entrants;
- the product life cycle has reached a stage of maturity, which, if not reformulated and properly managed, risks leading to a phase of decline;
- corporate compliance to a new regulatory environment;
- particular market events and changed economic conditions.

Analyzing the current economic environment in which businesses operate today as a result of the pandemic spread, it is practically possible to find both the validity and contextuality of all the conditions.

The drama is inherent in the fact that all these conditions are interconnected.

In fact, as graphically depicted in **Figure 2**, Covid-19 resulted in changing economic and market conditions due to the disruption of business operations with concomitant bankruptcy of many firms. In this case, in addition to the individual businesses, the entire supply chain was affected.

This situation was certainly supported by the regulatory impositions that limited the firms' activities during the lockdown. The same sanitary constraints, however necessary, have resulted in a real limitation in customer relations, leading to a distancing of the company from consumers. For many companies, particularly manufacturing companies, the business model tied to a traditional product has become obsolete. It has reached maturity because social distancing as well as the propensity to save has led to a change in the outlook of customers, who are more oriented toward online services and avoid products of secondary importance. These new needs, together with the specific tax benefits promoted by governments, have fomented the birth and spread of new companies (or the further imposition of large companies) aimed at filling the gap of traditional companies, not very accustomed to implement processes and offer technologically advanced services.

Consequently, the continuous and constant change in the articulation of processes and services has led to the imposition of new trends, with the need for *traditional* companies to adopt new systems in order to be competitive or, even more, to survive in a fierce evolutionary context.

It is, however, worth pointing out that the demand for services and products related to a *smart* business reality was not born with the pandemic. Covid-19 simply enhanced a process that was already underway, speeding up its deployment time but exaggerating the potential side effects for companies not yet involved.

Through the restructuring of the business model, the company must try to use its resources more efficiently, making management and operational processes more effective and simpler (**Figure 3**).

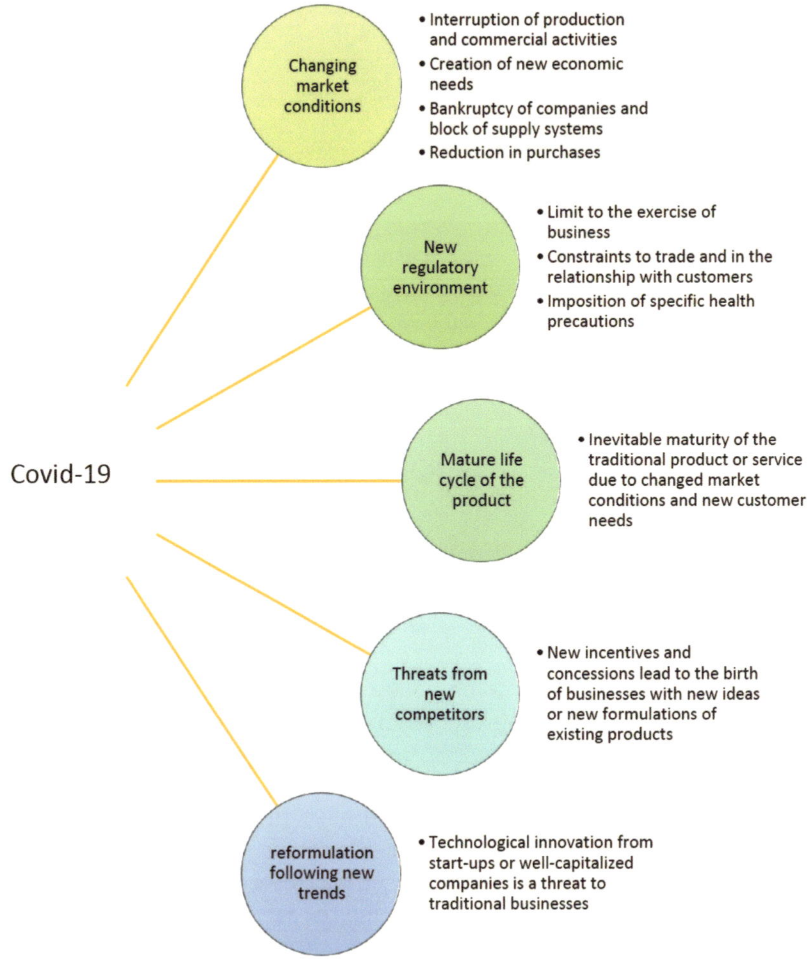


**Figure 2.**
*Relationship between pandemic spread from Covid-19 and conditions for implementation of business model restructuring. Source: author's elaboration.*

But above all, precisely in light of the current needs induced by the pandemic spread, the restructuring of the business model must succeed in placing the company in a new context; we refer here to a new era of 4.0 operations that places the company in a new relationship with customers and employees.

## 2.2 New logic of work and new internal communication systems

Together with the need to reformulate the product or service, the way it is obtained and the way it is offered to the customer, in the era of digitalization it is essential to define new scenarios for the relationship with employees and collaborators.

The 4.0 revolution and even more so the Covid-19 pandemic have given a strong and well-defined impetus on the future of work within the company.

There are still many debates and uncertainties surrounding the issue of *smart* work, but it is also true that, without it, many activities would have come to a complete standstill.

For some years now, several countries around the world have been evaluating and attempting to implement new, more sustainable work systems, aimed at better respecting the private needs of workers and thereby increasing company performance.

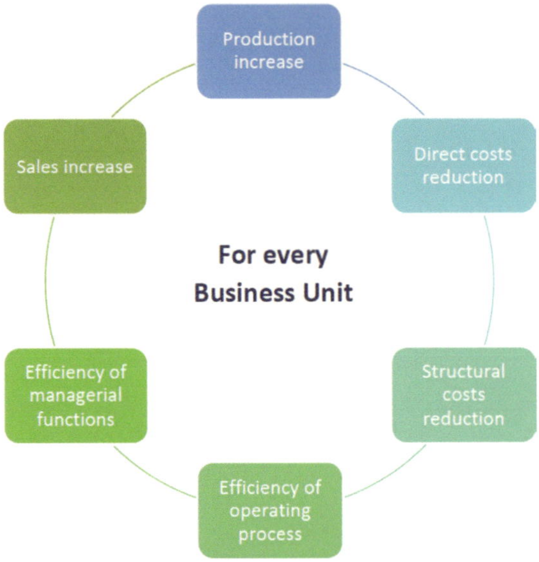


**Figure 3.**
*Internal key points to be met in the reformulation of the business model. Source: author's elaboration.*

The so-called "short week" is an obvious experiment in this regard.

In Japan, the government has promoted initiatives to experiment with a 4-day work week for corporate employees.

In France, the working week has been reduced from 39 hours per week to 35.

The Netherlands (29 hours), Norway (33 hours), and Denmark (33 hours) also have weeks with a reduced number of hours.

Between 2015 and 2019, a 4-day work week was tested in Iceland in the public sector with successful results, without reducing the salary of operational employees in schools, companies, and hospitals [12].

This is leading to a reformulation of the level of effort required of the human resources employed in the company, considering that more careful attention to the needs of individual employees can actually lead to greater efficiency in the workplace.

Unilever was one of the very few multinationals (along with Microsoft in Japan) to have tested the short week system in 2020 on a group of operational employees at its New Zealand headquarters.

Through the words of the CEO, Alan Jope, the company itself claims in fact that:

> *"Traditional employer-employee dynamics are no longer fit for either individuals or businesses. People are increasingly looking for more personally and professionally satisfying work. They want to move beyond the traditional 40-hour/40-week/40-year employment contract to something more flexible that's tailored to their needs and stage of life. Older and more experienced workers are increasingly choosing to work for longer; and younger people are after meaningful jobs with more flexibility. And Covid-19 forced us all to think differently about how and where we worked. We see a hybrid future of work, where people might spend a couple of days in the office and two or three days at home or working remotely. This has unlocked tremendous productivity and flexibility in the Unilever team" [13].*

This vision is certainly forward-looking. It envisages innovative paradigms and "hybrid formulations" aimed at providing new stimuli for the HR working in the company.

As analyzed with the empirical case provided by Unilever, the smart model is certainly the most suitable solution to pursue this objective. However, the digitization of the workplace and of communication systems, which allow information to be exchanged immediately but at a distance, is a prerequisite for applying this principle. Traditional models are not compatible with an initiative that has clear 4.0 traits.

The company should prepare a cost–benefit analysis to determine the impact that a new logic at the workplace may have on efficiency and performance.

*Smart* work should then achieve some specific objectives:

- Achieve a new level of communication with employees. The dramatic experience of Covid-19 should be used to establish new forms of communication with employees. It is critical to understand their needs in a time of crisis in order to identify how their role can be made efficient.
  The management class must be prepared to respond as best they can to the concerns and issues of employees and contractors that have arisen as a result of the pandemic.
  Sessions of meetings with staff can certainly allow the company to find out information about human resources and then define a new work organization strategy by introducing specific task forces or work units set up according to specific skills.

- Establish a sustainable level of optimized work. Transparency, Ductility, and Willingness should become the key words to allow employees to define new horizons of collaboration with the company.
  Compatible with business needs, introducing a *smart* work system allows companies to choose the best options in order to optimize their time at work. Merely as an example, the closure of schools during the pandemic greatly affected the organization of employees with children, especially in the case of single working women.

  The most recent reference literature [14] has defined the need for greater inclusion in the corporate environment not only as an ethical tool but for the purpose of value creation. It may therefore be strategic to ask employees on which time slots or days they prefer a reduction in their hours. Transparency must then emerge through an information system that leverages the company's website and social media. These tools need to be updated daily.

  Obviously, it is essential that the company imposes logging and activity management systems to monitor productivity remotely.

- Achieve a new level of customer relations. Work-at-home arrangements do not mean absence from the workplace, but rather optimization of time, peace of mind, and availability. All features that can be turned into an added value.

  Working remotely must be able to enhance digital sales potential. This can be achieved:

a. defining greater interaction with customers through the use of digital and social devices. Result achieved: customer loyalty;

b. enhancing the online services offered. Result achieved: better monitoring and control of operations and services offered.

## 2.3 The need for an innovative company upgrade

Referring the reader to our specific paper entitled *Managing Corporate Innovation. Determinants, Critical Issues and Success Factors*, published by Springer (2020) for any in-depth study of the topic, we find it interesting to highlight the key features of what we have called the *Techno-corporate Gap*.

Could we ever think that Italy, one of the founding countries of the European Union but above all a destination symbol of good living, is today one of the European countries with a very high rate of *techno-corporate gap*?

According to a 2018 study [15], traditional companies, i.e., those that do not use 4.0 technologies nor have future interventions planned, correspond to 86.9% of the total.

The Center-North confirms itself as the main promoter of investments in innovation, while the South shows a very low propensity to change. As part of the transformation toward Industry 4.0, a greater propensity for process innovation is also considered, together with product innovation connected to a decisive research and development activity. From this point of view, large companies express a much higher potential and show a propensity to invest in both production and data technologies, while small companies (micro-small) prefer the specific use of data technologies [15].

If we consider the investments in a more general way, it emerges that the discriminating element among the different profiles is not to be found in the presence of a mere renewal of the physical capital, but rather in the willingness to act on the human capital together with the investment in ICT technologies. In fact, in order to satisfy their needs, companies resort mainly to human capital training (43.6%) and to the acquisition of external services (37.7%).

Analyzing this aspect also from the point of view of size, some substantial differences emerge, since the larger enterprises resort mainly to staff training and new hires, while micro and small enterprises, in addition to training, resort to a relatively greater extent to the purchase of services and external collaborations [15]. While on the one hand, such a policy may seem appropriate by virtue of a considered *make-or-buy* principle, it is worth stressing how much this situation can actually push toward a constant subjugation of micro-small companies to the wishes of service providers.

The Italian business context therefore shows a situation of enormous diffidence toward the use of technologies to support processes and products.

These data, which can be considered extremely dramatic if contextualized in an international economic system already largely centered on technological development, in our opinion clarify the presence of a limited *Company Logic* [9], in Italy still largely linked to traditionalist preconceptions. In spite of ourselves, this view is not only the expression of a *techno-corporate gap*, but as a whole it contributes to exalting an even more worrying technological gap with other European countries, as expressed by the indicators of the Global Innovation Index [16].

### *2.3.1 The techno-corporate gap*

The statistical results achieved by MET [15] provide us with a very important tool to understand not only the renewal objective of companies but especially the strategy inherent in such processes on which the success of the investments themselves depends. Analyzing the raising of capital for reengineering from a qualitative point of view, it is possible to argue that the planning of a digitization process of the company is largely related to the governance structure. If we want to reason in systemic terms [17, 18], this assumption is expressed by the following relation:

$$\textit{Innovation} \propto \textit{Technology} \propto \textit{Management} \propto \textit{Corporate Governance}.$$

This concatenation is intended to underline how the ability to achieve innovation is closely linked to and depends on the technological skills of the company's scientific team; in turn, the know-how of a company is bound to the managerial choices in terms of development of a new product, research of new and specific technical skills to better face the market competition or more generally for the needs of company reengineering. However, the management is conditioned by the eternal debate on the creation of value for shareholders [19–23] or in small companies by the convictions of the founding owners (still linked to an artisan culture) and is largely conditioned by them. In order to avoid unnecessary misunderstandings, we believe it is useful to underline that when we talk about Corporate Governance, we do not refer to the simple shareholder structure but to the type of structure of the top management (shareholders and top managers) and the way they relate to each other and to their stakeholders [10].

In fact, governance establishes medium-long term objectives (in this specific case, the investment in innovation), but it is also constantly influenced by external dynamics that can be cultural (customs and traditions of the territory in which the company operates or the competence of the shareholders themselves and of the top managers), social (massive influence of stakeholders such as the mass media or political forces that discourage certain types of development), and even market (development of private equity initiatives, support of the banking system, high competition) (**Figure 4**).

Therefore, even if indirectly, the change in the governance structure and the perspectives connected to it can concretely act on the result in terms of innovation: recognizing the need to look for new managers specialized in innovation (innovation coach), approving new investments in the scientific sector, welcoming in its capital new partners to undertake new business initiatives and thus mitigate the risks, etc.

By using the "control theory" in terms of innovation creation, it is possible to identify different levels and levers that the company can use. The *techno-corporate gap*—understood as the margin due to the ability of firms to create innovation (here expressed by the deviation between the target variable Y* and the effect variable Y)—can therefore be reduced thanks to countless strategic choices taken by governance (XN levers) that can be adopted individually or in combination:

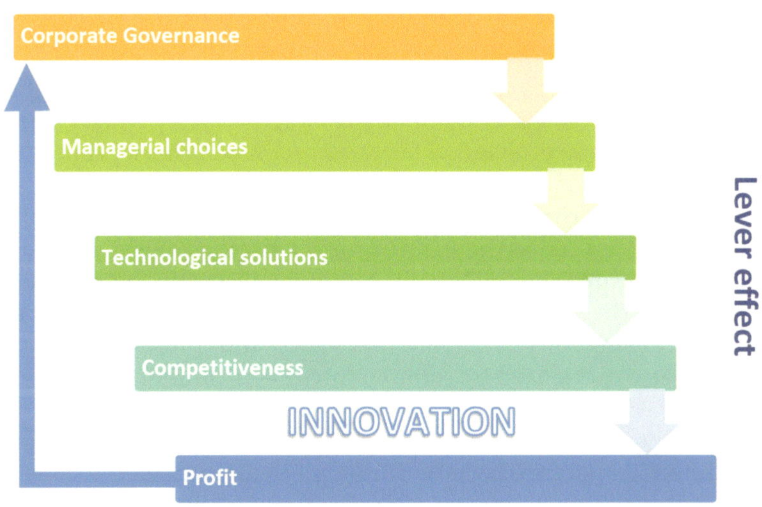


**Figure 4.**
*Cause-effect correlation system between corporate governance and innovation. Source: author's elaboration.*

- maintaining a high control governance structure capable of producing innovation technology internally (having experienced managers, internal R&D areas, with own or borrowed capital);

- search for new partners who will contribute capital by way of equity or contribute assets aimed at achieving new technology (logic of shared enterprise—open governance structure);

- development of strategic partnerships aimed at joining forces exclusively for joint development projects (typically found in the creation of joint ventures);

- membership of enterprise networks;

- drafting of technical agreements in order to be able to develop the technology internally without necessarily making investments (**Figure 5**).

In the light of the strategic solutions adopted, a series of causal diagrams [24, 25] will take shape, which will positively or negatively influence the achievement of an adequate level of innovation. As mentioned earlier, however, it is up to the system thinker or manager to be able to best identify the boundaries of the system being examined.

If we accept the systemic thinking according to which the variation of a simple variable has a cumulative effect on the entire system, and how the loops in which the variables act are repetitive and recursive, then, from the results obtained in the field of innovation and data relating to the level of openness of corporate governance, this correlation becomes clear, homogeneous in all its aspects. Applying the reasoning of System Thinking [17] to Control Theory [26], we can consider systems in terms of variables (input, state, output), and we can evaluate the way in which they are interdependent within the company system also for the purpose of pursuing innovative processes. But the company system is a simple element when considered within a larger context with which it constantly interacts and from which—as we have seen—it receives important influences. It is therefore useful to understand how these dynamic processes are also set in relation to the community, therefore, how the micro systems (or the micro behaviors) interact with the macro ones. To accomplish such an approach, it is possible to make use of the doctrine of Combinatory Systems [18].

This theory starts from the assumption that the collectivity is made up of elements or agents that, operating individually, adopt micro behaviors but as a whole are able to determine macro behaviors.

From **Figure 6**, it is therefore possible to observe the way in which the *techno-corporate gap*—understood as the inability of the firm to achieve innovation—becomes a crucial expression of "micro" behavior; if multiplied countless times, it can characterize the "macro" behavior of a community, which in our specific case consists in the inability to achieve innovation and, therefore, to increase the technological gap experienced by some countries—including Italy—compared with others. It is represented here how the propensity to innovate, stimulated by the different governance structures of a firm (micro effect), can express a general innovation potential when considered in its complexity. Collective investment in innovation has macro effects in terms of increasing or reducing the technological gap between countries and others. Let us consider first of all

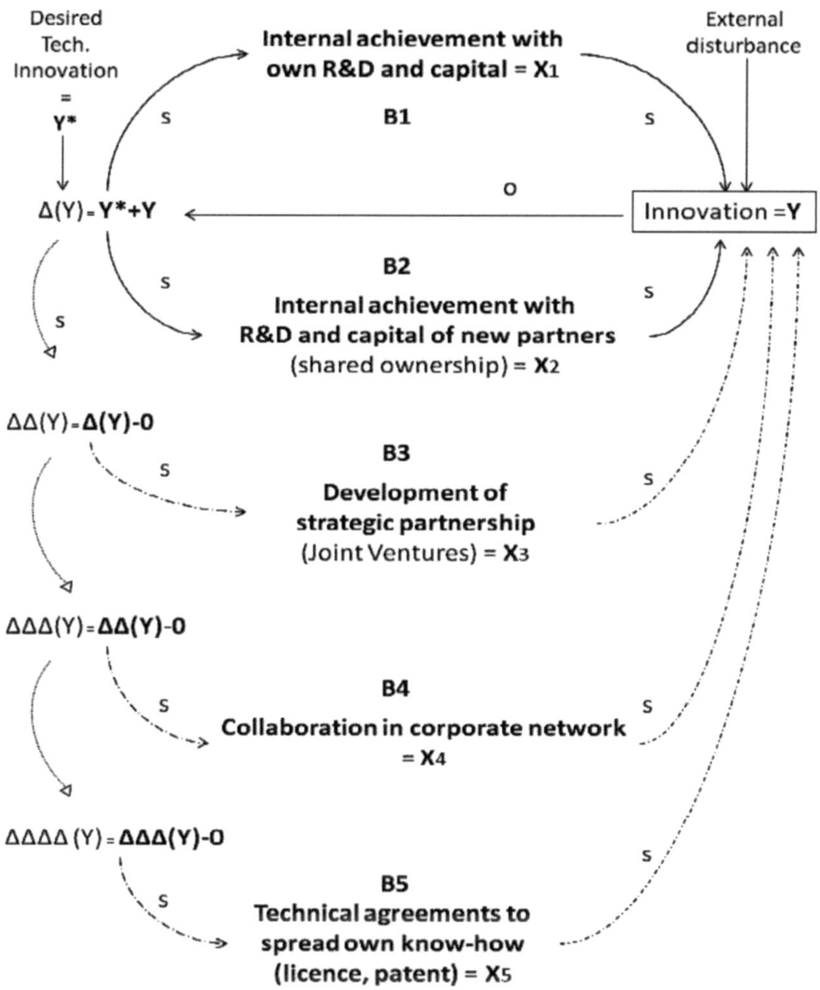


**Figure 5.**
*Innovation control system with multiple levers and levels. Source: Rangone [8].*

that every company can achieve innovation according to the type of investment made or strategies adopted. Therefore, thanks to the numerous levers, the top management can consider to open the capital to new partners or follow new partnerships achieving a specific development strategy, and consequently, top managers can take decisions that spur the company to achieve specific objectives in the technological field. The particular governance structure that characterizes companies in a specific geographical area can therefore be a winner or a critical factor. We must not forget that a territory can be considered developed if the companies and bodies operating within it are efficient and not simply because of the ability of a single company—however large—to produce efficiently. The result is that the ability to open up to innovation of every single company in a specific territory, together with similar micro behaviors, will influence and compose the collective behavior in terms of technological development; the latter factor will be the source of macro effects that translate into a technological gap with neighboring areas, regions, and, as a consequence, competing countries, if we look at the process in macro terms. The core of the problem then lies at the heart of the company and must be analyzed there.

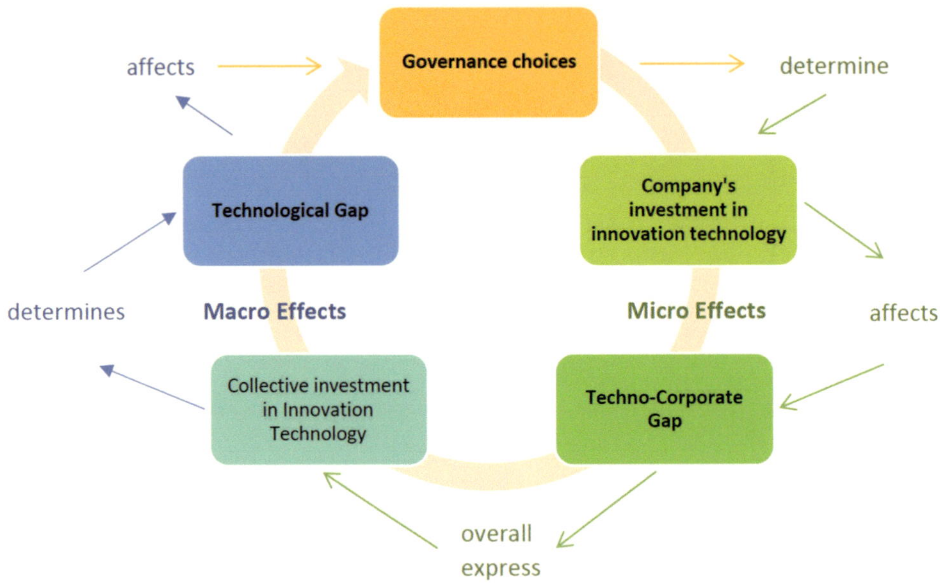


**Figure 6.**
*Micro and macro effects in terms of investment in innovation technology. Source: author's elaboration.*

## 3. Technological upgrading and competitiveness: define a strategy

### 3.1 Sectors and perspectives: is there a common line?

In identifying a strategy that can enable businesses to recover optimally from an economic and financial point of view after the pandemic spread, it should first be pointed out that not all sectors have been adversely affected by the crisis. Wanting to subdivide the company sectors between those that have received a positive impact and those that have suffered enormously from the pandemic crisis, it is possible to consider the summary scheme proposed in **Figure 7**, which provides a subdivision that is certainly not exhaustive but still useful to have a general idea:

- The sectors least affected or even benefiting from this situation are those related to the satisfaction of basic needs, such as food and health, but also those that have a close connection with digital activity. We are therefore talking about online service platforms, online market places and the delivery sector (against online orders).

- On the contrary, most of the sectors that do not fall into these macro-areas have suffered heavy setbacks. Restrictions on travel and fears of an increase in contagions have imposed a real freeze on the tourist industry.

- The fashion industry has received backlash as it is not an expression of basic needs. The restaurant industry suffered the full impact of the lockdown by keeping their businesses closed for several months; moreover, when they reopened, the businesses had to make some important choices:

    a. primarily incurred expenses in retrofitting their facilities in light of government-mandated health criteria;

    b. secondly, they had to choose between different levers aimed at recovering immediate losses or dealing with impending difficulties:

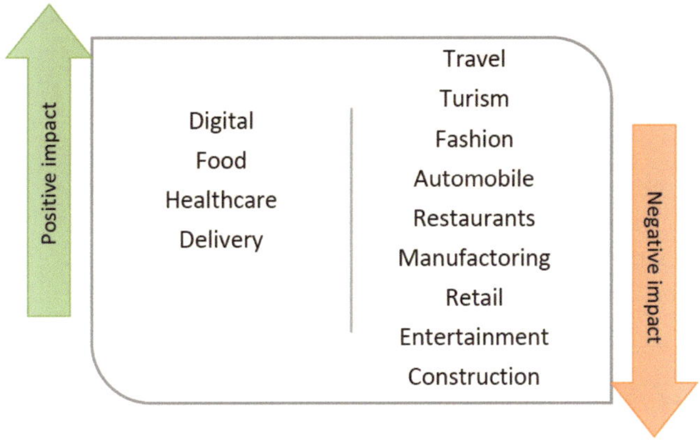


**Figure 7.**
*Sectors affected and sectors that have benefited from the current situation. Source: author's elaboration.*

- reduce staff;
- give up a portion of the profits;
- raise prices;
- increase table rotation.

All this considered, it is our belief that short-term strategic solutions are certainly a *modus operandi* aimed at sustaining the business in a short period of time, but they are not a solution that can really help businesses affected by the pandemic to break the deadlock.

Today, more than ever, we need recovery strategies that are the expression of a medium-long term vision and that are aimed at helping companies regain a specific position in the evolutionary context we are experiencing.

Sudden difficulties have led companies to shelve long-term projects, therefore, to suspend the expansion and value projects that produce the true profit margin. Today, companies aim to carry out short-term interventions, perhaps pending public subsidies and aimed at reducing costs as much as possible and obtaining flexibility.

The opportunity is actually great to definitely understand the company status. Paradoxically, if the repercussions of the crisis have been.

*slight = previous good company status > use of strategic levers in the short term.*
*acute = previous weak corporate status > use of m/l-term strategic levers.*

In the latter case, it is certainly appropriate to use levers that provide immediate economic and financial relief, but a thorough analysis of the status of the company is urgently needed to allow radical changes in the company in order to offer a new and attractive product or service. This can be done by making estimates as soon as possible that define:

- changes in the company's market positioning (trends by year and economic and financial variances);
- the margins resulting from the adoption of a new business model depending on the different scenarios;

- the costs of investments in new company assets and innovative know-how;
- the timing of the change and the company's ability to sustain such pace considering current operational needs.

We can therefore conclude these reflections by stressing that there is no common line or common strategy. There is only the solution that can be identified by the individual company in light of the backlash received during the pandemic and the company's awareness of its status and positioning on the market.

However, it is our conviction that there is a common need to pursue smart innovation processes, dictated by a constantly evolving economic and social context.

In the light of these forecasts, let us see which specific innovation-related strategic lines can be pursued and in the light of which specific criteria they can best be implemented.

### 3.2 Strategic lines and operating criteria

The experiences of the nearly 2 years since the pandemic spread of Covid-19 have taught a key lesson: businesses will never return to their former reality. Profound changes have been imposed both internally and externally on businesses. There is therefore a totally new dimension that requires new approaches to business and, therefore, new models. The companies that over the years have been able to ride the technological wave, anticipating the dramatic moment we are living today, are certainly prepared for the ongoing evolution and to meet the needs of customers by offering innovative services and products. In the short to medium term, these companies will always be able to acquire new market shares. In the presence of new rules, new needs, and new forms of customer relations, it is our belief that companies must set their recovery strategy along the following lines (**Figure 8**).

#### *3.2.1 Study the new trends and tastes of the digital consumer*

Understanding business after the Covid-19 pandemic means observing the mutations that have characterized consumption trends in the Business-to-Consumer and Business-to-Business spheres and understanding which path the national but above all the global market is taking.

In the digital age, it is not possible to focus only on national trends. Global trends inevitably condition national trends, perhaps not in the immediate term but certainly in the medium to long term. The vision of the entrepreneur must therefore be attentive to what is evolving at international level, always drawing new ideas not only to stay in step with the times but also to anticipate the potential repercussions of foreign competition.

In a post-pandemic period, it is worth considering that not all consumer groups have been affected. Like companies, which as we have observed above can be distinguished between positively and negatively influenced, the consumer market also responds with its own particularities.

Employees working in positively influenced business sectors are certainly able to maintain a consumption trend equal to the pre-pandemic period. Lockdowns and restrictions on transport and communications, as well as on leisure, initially saved resources that can now be put back into the economic circuit. Not to mention that the weakness of the markets is also a lure for investors and speculators interested in setting up new businesses.

All of this is obviously part of an evolutionary context defined by new digital approaches.

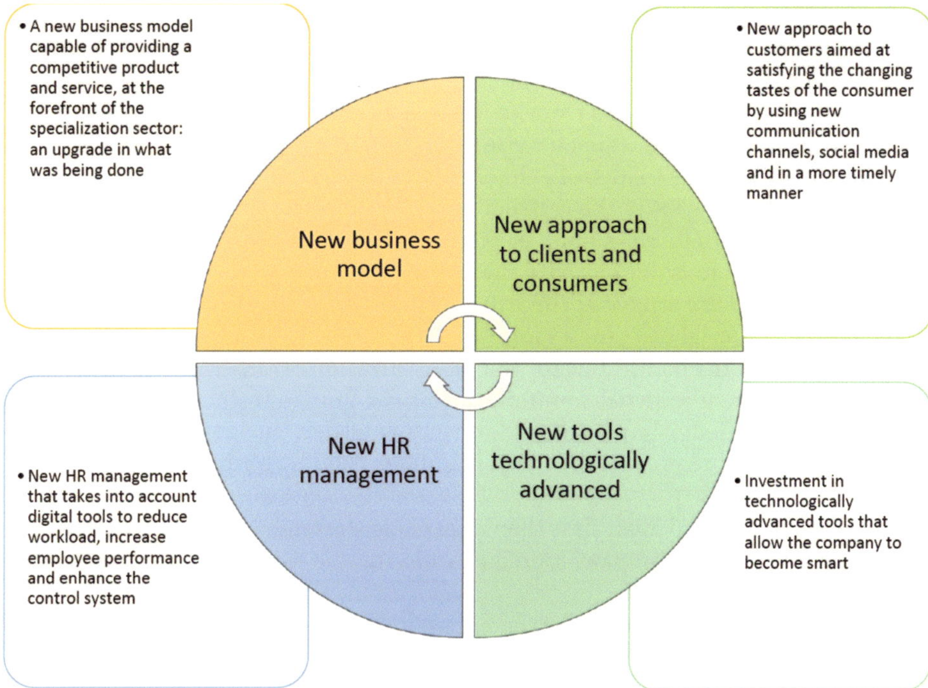


**Figure 8.**
*Elements of intervention for the implementation of a recovery strategy. Source: author's elaboration.*

The transformation of the consumer goes hand in hand with the transformation of companies. Therefore, since the consumers will spend more and more time online and will direct their consumption interests more to products on the web, companies must be able to identify the digital tools available today to understand the new paradigms of consumption, the trends that draw the attention of customers, but above all they must be ready to define solutions that can build consumer loyalty [27].

### *3.2.2 Set up an upgrade or transformation of the business model*

Digital innovation must become an imperative for any business. The business needs to follow innovative protocols, looking to achieve an upgrade (if the impact of the pandemic has been limited) or a full transformation if the conditioning has been larger. We are not talking here about diversification [28], which often arises from a prospect of enlargement, but of evolution aimed at redevelopment.

In order to make an accurate assessment of the need for such a measure, it is essential to carry out different analyses.

Without wishing to have any claim to exhaustiveness, leaving any further in-depth study on the subject to the vast literature of reference, since the present work aims to investigate the challenges experienced by businesses today, it is possible to summarize some key points:

- calculation of the opportunity and application areas;
- definition of the reallocation of expected profitability;
- monitoring and control of new results.

First of all, it is essential to realize to which specific activity, good, or service has connected the business model to be restructured and for which company needs a real digital upgrade. In the case of small and medium-sized enterprises, there are no complex forecasts from an analytical point of view, whereas in the case of larger enterprises, which have several production lines or a diversified business, it is necessary to identify the activities to be examined and which will be the main beneficiaries of the restructuring. At the same time, the risks must be estimated. The previous risks must be compared with the potential risks following the redevelopment in order to verify the feasibility of the project. From this point of view, the feasibility study is primarily the tool that must provide valid alternatives to the managerial class for a more prudent choice of options. Secondly, it is essential to verify the conditions for the reorganization of the entire operation. The reformulation of internal communication and human resource management—nowadays dedicated to the understanding of new horizons of *smart* working—are very delicate phases, too often misunderstood by both company leaders and employees [29, 30].

A third fundamental analysis is then referred to the reallocation of profitability expected following the company reorganization and the reconversion of production and services.

How will corporate value be distributed? What will be the new horizons and prospects promoted by the achievement of corporate value?

These are just some of the fundamental questions that the company must ask itself in order to define the strategic lines aimed at pursuing a correct reformulation of the business model. The answers to these questions come in part from the monitoring and control of the performance achieved, which must take place in a constant manner and always keeping in mind that the evolution today must take place in a "responsible" and "sustainable" key [31].

A few different examples of intervention may be eloquent in this regard (**Table 1**).

Then, both in the event of a good corporate status and in the event of a compromised economic-financial situation, traditional businesses must approach a conversion of their offering models in a *smart* and *lean* way.

Although outlined in their essential points, these steps and macro-areas of intervention are a valid point of reference for companies wishing to draw up well-considered plans to restructure their business in order to respond to the new challenges of the market, to contain the impact of an increasingly ruthless international competition, and still to regain a relationship with customers and collaborator lacerated by the global pandemic and an incessant evolution in a digital key.

| Sector | Firm's status | Type of intervention | Specification |
|---|---|---|---|
| Restaurant | good; strong | upgrade | online order; smart profile; social management |
| | recessionary | trasformation | delivery; ghost kitchen |
| Manufactoring | good; strong | upgrade | e-commerce; smart company |
| | recessionary | trasformation | sale on marketplace; from B2C to B2B; consulting |

**Table 1.**
*Example of interventions according to firm's status and sectors. Source: author's elaboration.*

### *3.2.3 Investing in digital and innovative tools for a firm 4.0*

Investing in digital assets means first of all understanding what digital means, studying its impact on the business model and on the relationship with the customers. Digital technology not only enhances socialization as it amplifies opportunities for relationships, but above all it removes the constraints of space and time. Let us think of a company engaged in agribusiness that has to take care of monitoring the fields, checking the health of the crops.

This requires the use of staff, more or less specialized, and time (full days if the company is of medium or large size). If major forces, such as storm events, come into play, these tasks can be made even more complex and sometimes completely obstructed.

The technology that makes the company *smart* or 4.0 can facilitate this through information systems that make the entire production and control process interconnected with each other [32].

Traceability throughout the supply chain makes supply processes clearer, providing an additional service of transparency to the consumer in addition to a quality product on time.

We've been talking about digital and the *smart company* for several years now, yet the number of businesses benefiting from such systems is really limited.

We believe that this is an opportunity to accelerate those renewal projects that had already been planned and that today join, indeed strengthen, the strategic solutions to combat the emergency.

It's time for businesses to become visible, join the network, and benefit from a renewed digital image.

But in order to do this, a major investment in 4.0 tools is needed.

Investing in digital assets means having a previously described upgrade or transformation plan well in mind.

Now is the time to verify the applicability of new technologies in the company and design innovation processes, thus reducing the *techno-corporate gap* that limits the expansion potential of the company.

In fact, *smart* innovation makes it possible to achieve a quality product, making the most of the resources available to the company (thus reducing costs for raw materials, capital goods, and HR) in a working environment that is not only safer but also leaner (**Figure 9**).

And in a post-pandemic context what better opportunity could there be to provide the consumer with that peace of mind when consulting and purchasing.

In a time of health uncertainty, there is no greater impact factor than transparency that provides peace of mind by increasing trust.

And this trust can be ensured thanks to 4.0 tools along the entire supply chain, during the production phase, the service provision phase, up to the moment of purchase by the consumer.

Giving peace of mind and security to the consumer is in itself a qualifying factor that helps businesses stand out in the market environment to win the competition.

## 3.3 Raise or fold? How to relaunch the company according to the "strategy poker"

Once we have defined the criteria and key elements for understanding the context of a corporate relaunch aimed at facing the countless challenges that everyday life brings, we like to conclude this work with some singular but far from trivial reflections. Apologizing in advance to "pure" theorists for the association proposed

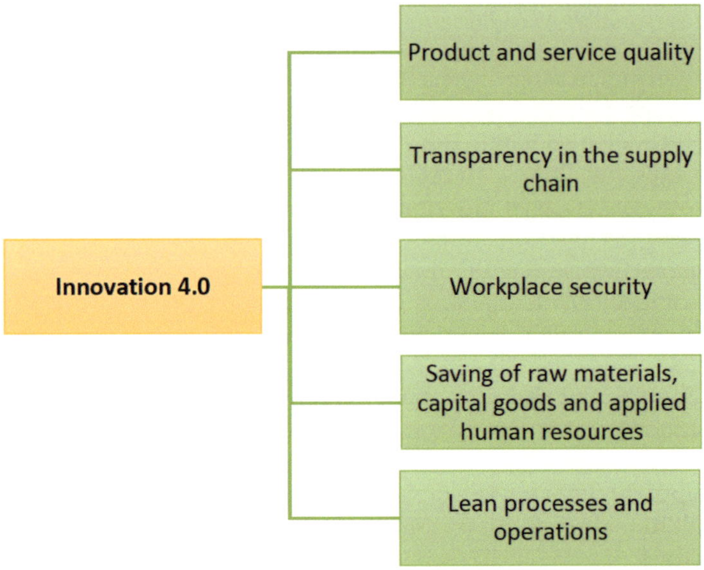


**Figure 9.**
*Strengths of an investment in technology 4.0. Source: author's elaboration.*

here, we think it is really interesting to share many common aspects between business strategies and strategies adopted in the game of Poker that can help us to understand the *forma mentis* adopted by an entrepreneur—or a board of directors—in certain situations.

In poker as in business life, players and companies face a probabilistic challenge to the success of their initiative or investment, whether initial or mid-course. It is true that in the corporate world there are countless systems for risk forecasting, but it is always good to remember that the company is created by man to work among men. Therefore, there are no exact formulas for predicting the future but mathematical conjectures as close to the truth as possible that must be confronted with the human psyche, with the changing moods of man (tastes and tendencies), and with the many unforeseen events such as natural disasters, pandemics, collapses of governments, etc.

Those who are familiar with this card game will not miss the choice of "raise," which defines an aggressive, proactive playing strategy clearly in opposition to "fold." In fact, the fold solution determines a choice aimed at buffering, thus limiting potential damage or losses. The player knows he does not have any winning cards and, intimidated by the probabilistic weight, throws his cards on the table, thus giving up the pot and proceeding with the next pot.

But how long can such a policy continue?

The *fold* solution is then associated with and compared with cases in which companies—in order to cope with impending difficulties—choose:

- the downsizing strategy
- the sale of business branches
- the disposal of assets

If left unchecked, these strategies can lead to a worrying corporate weakening.

This point of view is inherent not only in economic and financial principles but also in social and environmental ones. Living in an economic and social context in which reputation plays an increasingly relevant role [33], a company that adopts *fold* tactics demonstrates loss of control, weak governance, thus demonstrates an image that is likely to heavily intimidate investors, sponsors, and stakeholders.

On the contrary, a "raise" strategy demonstrates confidence in what company does, but also it demonstrates business strength and robustness even in those cases (such as the current post-pandemic one) where business status has been heavily weakened, but it is appropriate not to demonstrate it (*bluff* technique).

The *raise* strategy includes solutions such as:

- turnaround
- leverage
- investment in new assets or initiatives
- mergers
- joint venture

This technique scares competitors, reducing the likelihood of takeovers, implicitly increasing the potential investors and sponsors.

Stakeholders are also induced to work better or to continue the collaboration with a proactive and relaunching company rather than with a submissive company that focuses on downsizing.

Human resources, especially those who can make a significant contribution to business progress, are qualified to work in a company that aims for growth and relaunch rather than *fold* solutions.

With all this, we do not want to emphasize that cost containment strategies or the sale of unused or obsolete assets are to be avoided.

Here we want to link the *raise* strategies that can support companies instead of intimidating them to the principle of transformation or upgrade 4.0.

In this work we do not want to advise the company to constantly live in *bluff*, deceiving the customer or the entire category of stakeholders.

We want to emphasize that the strategies must consider the potential repercussions that a *fold* policy can entail, especially in certain situations such as the current ones.

Innovation in 4.0 key can therefore constitute a real proof that allows the company to experience a dramatic post-pandemic and constantly evolving reality.

Given the requirements of this work, we will still have the opportunity to further deepen these affinities between the corporate strategy and the strategies adopted in Poker in subsequent works.

## 4. Conclusions

The experiences that companies are having today show that the emerging challenges due to the pandemic spread of Covid-19 converge extraordinarily with an evolutionary path already started and due to the so-called 4.0 revolution.

The prospects for businesses are manifold and are determined by the economic and financial status with which companies have had to face the pandemic.

This work wanted to emphasize the fact that, contrary to what one might think, the time has come for companies that have received the greatest repercussions to take a bold step. The time has come to relaunch the business with decisive investments aimed at giving the company a new face.

Today exists a substantial literature aimed at demonstrating the multiple positive effects for companies that adopt technologically advanced systems. This is certainly a point of reference to try to understand the potential solutions and, therefore, in support of the thesis set out in this work.

The new company profile must have 4.0 traits and must allow the company to offer innovative, fast, and competitive services using the technology available on the market today.

This is further demonstrated by the fact that, unlike the most affected companies, those that have not received particular setbacks have been able to benefit from already innovative business models or are part of already digital sectors.

The time has come for "traditional companies" to take the next step, what we have considered a technological upgrade, while those that have remained completely away from technological innovation criteria should carry out a real transformation of the business model.

Decisions in this sense, however, must come from corporate governance, the only real driving force for achieving innovation and aimed at reducing the so-called *techno-corporate gap* with respect to competing companies.

Besides through the description of the relationship between the *techno-corporate gap* and the technological gap, this strategic solution has been analyzed through the description of what we have called "Strategy Poker." With this principle we have defined a clear will to relaunch the company through propositive solutions that influence the image stakeholders have of the company and aimed at acquiring new assets in a digital key.

Obviously, this being the first appearance and description of the concept of *Strategy Poker*, we leave to the following works a greater study of this theory.

## Author details

Adalberto Rangone
University G. D'Annunzio of Chieti-Pescara, Pescara, Italy

*Address all correspondence to: adalberto.rangone@unich.it

## References

[1] Casella N. Covid-19 e influenza spagnola del 1918: Analogie, differenze e lezioni del passato valide anche per il presente. 2020. Available from: https://www.pharmastar.it/news/primo-piano/covid-19-e-influenza-spagnola-del-1918-analogie-differenze-e-lezioni-del-passato-valide-anche-per-il-presente-31859

[2] MacKinsey & Company. COVID-19: Implications for business. 2021. Available from: https://www.mckinsey.com/business-functions/risk-and-resilience/our-insights/covid-19-implications-for-business

[3] Piana L. Colpite ma non affondate. I numeri a sorpresa delle imprese: Ricavi deboli ma debiti sotto controllo. La Repubblica. 2021. Available from: https://www.repubblica.it/economia/affari-e-finanza/2021/08/30/news/colpite_ma_non_affondate_i_numeri_a_sorpresa_delle_imprese_ricavi_deboli_ma_debiti_sotto_controllo-315769052/

[4] Zappa G. Il reddito di impresa. Scritture doppie, conti e bilanci di aziende commerciali. Milano: Giuffrè; 1939

[5] Schumpeter JA. Capitalism, Socialism, and Democracy. London: George Allen and Unwin; 1954

[6] Borsa Italiana. Amazon Market Data. 2021. Available from: https://www.borsaitaliana.it/borsa/azioni/global-equity-market/scheda/US0231351067.html?lang=it

[7] Nasdaq. Is Amazon.com, Inc.'s (NASDAQ: AMZN) Stock's Recent Performance Being Led By Its Attractive Financial Prospects? 2021. Available from: https://www.nasdaq.com/articles/is-amazon.com-inc.s-nasdaq%3Aamzn-stocks-recent-performance-being-led-by-its-attractive

[8] Rangone A. Managing Corporate Innovation. Determinants, Critical Issues and Success Factors. Contributions to Management Science. Cham: Springer; 2020

[9] Rangone A. La Logica di Impresa. Fenomeni e relazioni di influenza nell'attuale contest economico. Roma: Aracne Editrice; 2018

[10] Rangone A. International Perspectives on Corporate Governance: Doctrines, Models and Empirical Investigation concerning the Foundations of Banking Origin. Roma: RIREA; 2017

[11] Schwab K. The Fourth Industrial Revolution. New York: Crown Business; 2017

[12] Dall'Ansén JM. Islanda, la settimana lavorativa di 4 giorni è «un successo travolgente»: i risultati dei test, durati 4 anni. 2021. Available from: https://www.corriere.it/economia/lavoro/21_luglio_08/islanda-settimana-lavorativa-4-giorni-un-successo-travolgente-0810f1cc-dfbb-11eb-b24b-5a8781b79240.shtml

[13] Jope A. Future Workplace. 2021. Available from: https://www.unilever.com/planet-and-society/future-of-work/future-workplace/

[14] Areiqat AY, Hamdan Y, Zamil AMA, Aldabbagh I. True workplace diversity: A key ingredient for business success, regardless of the industry or company size. Talent Development & Excellence. 2020;**12**(2):2304-2314. Available from: https://www.researchgate.net/profile/Issam-Aldabbagh-2/publication/344726486_True_Workplace_Diversity_A_Key_Ingredient_for_Business_Success_Regardless_of_the_Industry_or_Company_Size/links/5f8c26a7299bf1b53e2f274e/True-Workplace-Diversity-A-Key-

Ingredient-for-Business-Success-Regardless-of-the-Industry-or-Company-Size.pdf

[15] MET. La diffusione delle imprese 4.0 e le. politiche: Evidenze 2017. 2018. Available from: https://www.mise.gov.it/index.php/it/198-notizie-stampa/2038333-imprese-etecnologie-4-0-online-risultati-indagine

[16] Cornell University, INSEAD, WIPO. Global Innovation Index. Ithaca: Energizing the World with Innovation; 2018

[17] Senge P. The Fifth Discipline: The Art and Practice of the Learning Organization. Last and enlarged ed. New York: Doubleday Currency; 2006

[18] Mella P. The combinatory systems theory. In: Contemporary Systems Thinking. New York: Springer International; 2017

[19] Kang HC, Anderson RM, Eom KS, Kang SK. Controlling shareholders' value, long-run firm value and short-term performance. Journal of Corporate Finance. 2017;**43**:340-353

[20] Mella P, Velo D. Creazione di valore, corporate governance e informativa societaria. Milano: Giuffrè Editore; 2007

[21] Lazonick W, O'Sullivan M. Maximizing shareholder value: A new ideology for corporate governance. Economy and Society. 2000;**29**(1):13-35

[22] Prahalad CK. Corporate governance or corporate value added? Rethinking the primacy of shareholder value. Journal of Applied Corporate Finance. 1994;**6**(4):40-51

[23] Rappaport A. Creating Shareholder Value: The New Standard for Business Performance. New York: Free Press; 1986

[24] Ishikawa K. Education and Training of Quality Control in Japanese Industry. JUSE: Reports of Statistical Application and Research; 1969. pp. 85-104

[25] Ishikawa K. Guide to Quality Control. Tokyo: Asian Productivity Organization; 1976

[26] Mella P. The magic ring. Systems thinking approach to control systems. In: Contemporary System Thinking. New York: Springer International; 2021

[27] Cachero-Martínez S, Vázquez-Casielles R. Building consumer loyalty through e-shopping experiences: The mediating role of emotions. Journal of Retailing and Consumer Services. 2021;**60**:25-47

[28] Xie Z, Wang J, Miao L. Big data and emerging market firms' innovation in an open economy: The diversification strategy perspective. Technological Forecasting and Social Change. 2021;**173**:1-14

[29] Iannotta M, Meret C, Marchetti G. Defining leadership in smart working contexts: A concept synthesis. Frontiers in Psychology. 2020;**11**:1-11. DOI: 10.3389/fpsyg.2020.556933

[30] Menshikova M, Fedorova A, Gatti M. Introducing smart-working in the conditions of digital business transformation: Analysis of an employee's experience. In: Zaramenskikh E, Fedorova A, editors. Digital Transformation and New Challenges. Lecture Notes in Information Systems and Organisation. Vol. 40. Cham: Springer; 2020. DOI: 10.1007/978-3-030-43993-4_6

[31] Beniulytė D, Šeinauskienė B, Rūtelionė A. Perceived influence of corporate social responsibility on consumer loyalty: The role of ethical ideology. Entrepreneurship and Sustainability Issues. 2020;**8**(1):291-300

[32] Rangone A. Innovative agribusiness. Which strategy for a dynamic

development? Agribusiness and Information Management. 2019;**11**(2):5-15

[33] Rangone A. On the relationship of liability action and reputational risk: An empirical analysis. International Journal of Business and Social Science. 2021;**11**(5):25-56

Chapter 30

# Deciphering Economic Effects of COVID-19

*Fitzgerald Witika*


## Abstract

The novel coronavirus disease (COVID-19) has led to tremendous positive and negative effects in various economies across different countries worldwide. Nonetheless, despite the difference in economic structures of countries, the major effects of COVID-19 on economies are similar but tend to vary in magnitude depending on the level of development and climatic conditions in different countries. In this respect, this chapter is aimed at providing a critical approach to understand the nature of the positive and negative effects of COVID-19 on economies using the aggregate supply and aggregate demand (AS-AD) model in contemporary economics. The basis for this approach is to decipher the economic effects of COVID-19 on economies worldwide with reference to the theoretical literature in economics on the operationalization of market forces illustratable with the AS-AD model. Be that as it may, comprehensive discussions regarding the economic effects of COVID-19 on economies will also encompass contemporary findings in empirical studies on COVID-19. As such, the chapter will demonstrate how contemporary theories pertaining to the AS-AD model can be applicable in explaining the economic effects of COVID-19.


**Keywords:** coronavirus, aggregate, demand, supply, economies, lockdown, pandemic, countries, effect, increase, decrease, market, Price, quantity, equilibrium

## 1. Introduction

The novel coronavirus (COVID-19) is known to be a zoonotic virus classified to be a ribonucleic acid (RNA) virus in the family coronaviridae of the other Nidovirale. Pertaining to this, coronavirus is considered a family of viruses that cause respiratory infections, which were first isolated in 1937 and designated coronaviruses, because they have a crown-like appearance under microscopy in 1965 [1]. Ever since COVID-19 became a pandemic; its existence has led to many economic effects in various countries. Some of the effects can be considered as positive effects on the economy whereas other COVID-19 effects can be considered as negative (detrimental) effects on the economy.

Nonetheless, just as the magnitude of the effect of COVID-19 on individuals is found to vary depending on how strong an individual's immune system is, the extent to which economies are positively or negatively affected by COVID-19 effects also varies depending on the level of development of different economies in different countries. There are so many studies done to assess the effect and impact of COVID-19 on the economy using different quantitative and qualitative approaches to analyzing the effects. However, this chapter provides a graphical analytical approach to the economic effects of COVID-19 with reference to contemporary economic principles and theories. This approach, unlike others, is meant to demonstrate how economic phenomena in theoretical literature are applicable to the resulting effects of COVID-19 on economies. Nonetheless, discussions will also be linked to findings in empirical studies to support the basis of inferences deduced from the graphical analysis.

## 2. Aggregate demand and supply model in the COVID-19 era

Socioeconomic effects of COVID-19 can be viewed from both the aggregate demand side and supply slide of the goods market. With regard to this, aggregate demand is basically a function of different levels of expenditures in the economy. In this respect, aggregate demand comprises consumption (C), investment (I), government expenditure (G), exports (X), and imports (I) in an open economy [2]. This can be mathematically written, as shown in Eq. (1).

$$AD = C + I + G + X - M \quad (1)$$

where AD = f (C, I, G, X, M).

Henceforth, in contemporary economics, the aggregate demand curve is represented by a downward-sloping curve that indicates an inverse relationship between prices and quantities of goods in the market. With a view to this, **Figure 1** shows a graphical presentation of phenomena pertaining to the AD.

Therefore, note that in **Figure 1**, the y-axis measures the level of prices of goods and services demanded in the economy and the X-axis measures the quantity of goods and services demanded in the economy. On the other hand, the aggregate supply model is basically a function of the natural rate of output ($Y_N$) and the difference between the actual price level (P) and the expected price ($P_E$) level. This is shown in Eq. (2).

$$AS = Y_N + a(P - P_E) \quad (2)$$

where $AS = f(Y_N, P, P_E)$

Moreover, $a$ measures how much output (Y = AS) responds to unexpected changes in prices (P). As such, since aggregate supply (AS) is basically the total

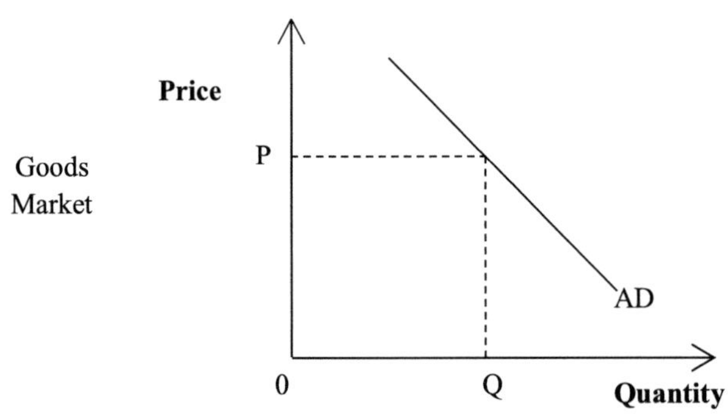


**Figure 1.**
*Aggregate demand (AD) model. Source: F Witika (2021).*

supply (or output) of goods and services in the economy, we can let Y = AS, as shown in Eq. (3).

$$Y = Y_N + a(P - P_E) \tag{3}$$

Similarly, since aggregate demand (AD) is basically the total demand (or output) of goods and services in the economy, we can also let Y = AD, as shown in Eq. (4).

$$Y = C + I + G + X - M \tag{4}$$

Hence, in Eq. (3), Y denotes total output supplied whereas, in Eq. (4), it denotes the total output demanded in the economy. Therefore, the graphical presentation of the aggregate supply curve is shown in **Figure 2**.

Where LRAS indicates the long-run aggregate supply curve and SRAS indicates the short-run aggregate supply curve. Therefore, the combination of the aggregate supply (AS) and aggregate demand (AD) model leads to the derivation of the aggregate supply and aggregate demand model (AS-AD model), as presented in **Figure 3**.

Note that (in **Figure 3**), point E denotes the market equilibrium point where the quantity of goods and services supplied in the economy is equal to the quantity of goods and services demanded in the economy at which the short-run aggregate supply (SRAS) curve, long-run aggregate supply (LRAS) curve, and aggregate demand (AD) curve intersect. Using the AS-AD model, we can assume that before COVID-19, in the short run, economies on the global perspective were operating at the market equilibrium point E where the level of the price of goods supplied and

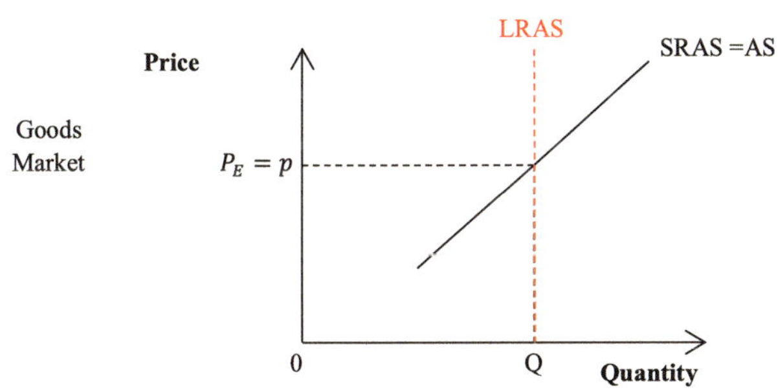


**Figure 2.**
*Aggregate supply (AS) model. Source: F Witika (2021).*

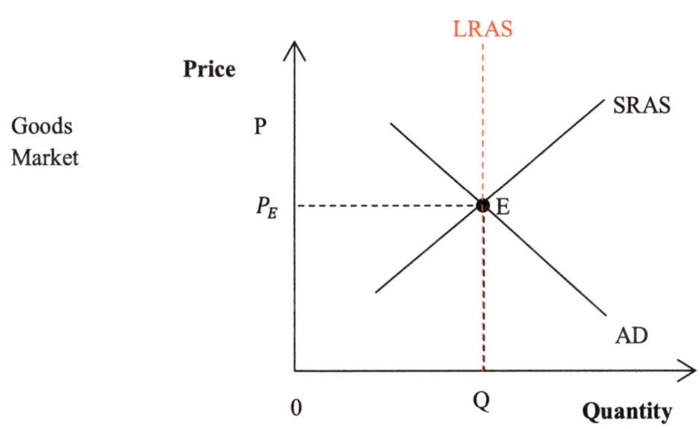


**Figure 3.**
*Aggregate supply and aggregate demand (AS-AD) model. Source: F Witika (2021).*

demanded was at P and the quantity of goods and services supplied and demanded was at Q. With regard to this, according to a study done by the World Health Organization (WHO) aimed at investigating the number of deaths exhibited as a result of COVID-19 infections and providing estimates of the excess morality from a global perspective, on January 30, 2020, COVID-19 was declared a public health emergency of international concern (PHEIC) with an official death toll of 171. Nonetheless, by December 31, 2020, this figure stood at 1813, 188 deaths. Notwithstanding, preliminary estimates postulate that at least 3 million is the magnitude of global deaths attributed to the COVID-19 pandemic in totality. Hence, this represented about 1.2 million deaths than what was reported officially [3].

Therefore, the immediate socioeconomic effect of COVID-19 upon its emergence was high rates of death which had a direct negative effect on the short-run aggregate supply curve through its reduction of the labor force population in the short run as both some people that were actively seeking employment and others who were already employed became infected and lost their lives. Henceforth, the reduction in the labor force due to numerous deaths reported in daily cases shifted the short-run supply curve to the left, as shown in **Figure 4**.

In consequence, the shift of the short-run aggregate supply curve (SRAS) to the left as presented in **Figure 4**, in panel (A), indicates the immediate reduction in natural output ($Y_N$) as a result of the reduction in the labor force population due to increased numbers of deaths owing to COVID-19 spreading infections. As such, the immediate reduction in the labor force population led economies to move from the market equilibrium point E (before COVID-19) to the market equilibrium point $E_1$ after COVID-19. With a view to this, the reduction in the natural level of output ($Y_N$) in economies triggered an increase in expected prices from $P_E$ to $P_{E1}$ as presented in **Figure 4**, in panel (A), because consumers or people began to expect that prices would go up due to lower productivity as a result of the reduced labor force population which indirectly would lead to higher costs of production and consequently, higher prices as firms intend to cover for the loss of labor incurred due to higher death rates perpetuated by COVID-19 infections. Besides that, the reduction in the natural level of output from $Y_N$ to $Y_{N1}$ implied that goods that were produced more efficiently before COVID-19 at the market equilibrium point E became scarce at the new market equilibrium point $E_1$ associated with a lower demographic structure due to COVID-19 deaths. As such, the scarcity of goods and services made most consumers expect increases in prices from $P_E$ to $P_{E1}$, as shown in **Figure 4**, in panel A. Moreover, the decrease in the short-run aggregate supply (SRAS) from SRAS to $SRAS_1$ implied a shift in the long-run aggregate supply curve from LRAS to $LRAS_1$ as a result of the immediate decline in the labor force population in the country.

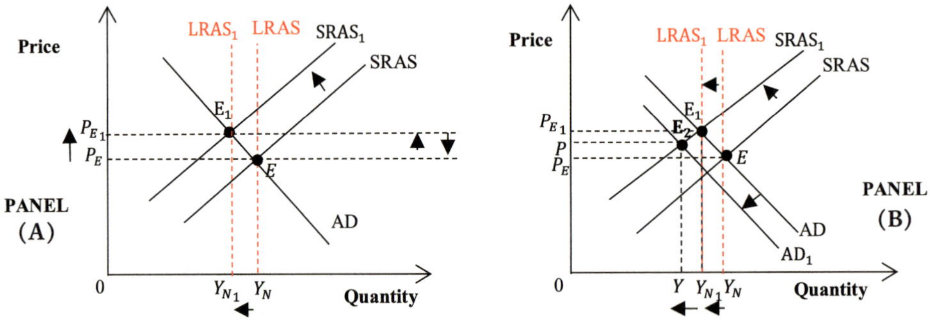


**Figure 4.**
*AS-AD model after COVID-19. Source: F Witika (2021).*

Furthermore, the decrease in the labor force population due to severe COVID-19 deaths shifting the supply curve to the left and leading to a fall in the natural level of output also implied a decrease in the demand for goods and services indicated by the shift to the left in aggregate demand from AD to $AD_1$, as presented in **Figure 4**, in panel (B). This is essential because the reduction in the labor force population and perhaps other people outside the labor force population also imply that domestic consumption expenditure (C) reduced as some potential consumers in the labor force and outside the labor force that were infected with COVID-19 ended up dying as significant losses that formed part of the overall demand for goods and services in the economy. In this regard, the loss in potential supply and potential demand due to exhibited COVID-19 death rates in countries is indicated by both the shift in aggregate demand and aggregate supply to the left.

Consequently, in the medium run, economies moved from the market equilibrium point at E to $E_1$ and later to $E_2$ where the actual output (Y) produced in economies became far less than the natural level of output before COVID-19 ($Y_N$) and moderately less than the new natural level of output after COVID-19 ($Y_{N1}$). Hence, at the market equilibrium point $E_2$, the actual price of goods and services set by firms after COVID-19 was greater than the expected price of goods and services before COVID-19 (P $> P_E$). However, the actual price of goods and services set by firms after COVID-19 was less than the expected price of goods and services by consumers during the COVID-19 era (P $< P_{E1}$). This is because, immediately, COVID-19 led to high death rates in the short run and medium run, firms did not respond quickly to changes in the demand for goods and services considering the fall in the overall demand due to high death rates. As such, what consumers were expecting to be the price in the short run and medium run was higher than the actual price firms had set in the short run and medium run. However, in the long run, economies moved to the market equilibrium point $E_1$, were they begun producing at the natural level of output during the COVID-19 era at which the actual prices (P) firms were charging was adjusted to the magnitude of prices (equal to $P_{E1}$) greater than consumer's expected prices ($P_E$) before the COVID-19 pandemic (at $E$). Notwithstanding, the natural level of output produced after COVID-19 at the market equilibrium point $E_1$ was not greater than what was initially produced at $E$ before COVID-19 led to a change in countries' overall population which affected the demand and supply side in the short run, as presented in **Figure 4**, in Panel (B).

Moreover, according to Yoon and Lee [4], demographic change is one of the most important determinants of the future economic and social landscape. Numerous studies conducted by different researchers in the world have taken a step to investigate the effect that changes in the composition and size of the economy's population may have on macroeconomic outcomes. In consequence, the majority of researchers postulate that demographic changes tend to affect economies through their influence on investment behavior, marginal propensities to save, labor market decisions, and aggregated demand and supply responses. Pertaining to this, in the medium to long run, Yoon and Lee [4] postulated that the aggregate supply of an economy can be altered significantly as a result of the propensity of changes in both the labor supply and productivity either considered to be exogenous or caused by changes in demographics. Therefore, due to the propensity to affect amounts and combinations by which an economy's factor inputs are utilized, changes in demographics consequently affect economic growth. Over the short term, demographic transitions are likely to affect aggregate demand (AD) given the amount of consumption (C) and investment (I) which may depend critically on structural changes in the population's age earning profiles [4]. This supports the basis for the phenomenon of the immediate economic effect of COVID-19, as illustrated in **Figure 4**.

When the COVID-19 disease became a pandemic, among the first, COVID-19 government restrictions were the lockdown implemented to reduce the spread of the virus. In consequence, the lockdown measure led to an immediate supply shock due to its negative effect on production activities, especially in manufacturing industries where 90% of operations rely on production activities. For other businesses, such as restaurants and those in the tourism sector, the lockdown meant a complete shutdown of their operations which in consequence led to a loss of huge amounts of profit in firms. Besides that, farming businesses were also heavily affected by the COVID-19 restriction of the lockdown as farmers were forced to abandon all farming activities. Moreover, in developing countries, such as Zambia where farmers mainly depend on daily farming activities to generate income for survival, the lockdown forced farmers to end up beginning to consume their farm produce to survive. This led to an increase in food insecurity and lower productivity of goods and services in developing countries. As such, in the short run, the immediate effect of the COVID-19 lockdown was a decrease in the natural level of output from $Y_{N1}$ to $Y_{N2}$ (shown in **Figure 5**) which consequently led to an increase in the expected price of goods and services as consumers speculated that the decrease in the quantity supplied would lead to scarcity which in turn would induce firms to increase prices. Pertaining to this, the fall in the supply of goods and services after the COVID-19 lockdown is presented by the shift in the aggregate supply curve to the left from $SRAS_1$ to $SRAS_2$ (as shown in **Figure 5** in panel (C)) following the movement of the economy from the market equilibrium point $E_1$ (before the lockdown) to $E_3$ (after the lockdown).

More than that, the shift in the short-run aggregate supply curve to the left from $SRAS_1$ to $SRAS_2$ also imply a shift in the long-run aggregate supply curve to the left from $LRAS_1$ to $LRAS_2$ due to the reduction in the production capabilities after the implementation of the COVID-19 lockdown, as presented in **Figure 5,** in panel (D). In this regard, the economy moved from the market equilibrium point $E_1$ to the new market equilibrium point $E_3$. However in the medium run, as the natural level of output decreased in many countries from $Y_{N1}$ to $Y_{N2}$, due to the scarcity and shortage of goods and services during the lockdown as companies closed down, the demand for goods and services by people in the economy increased; firms that could still provide some goods and services even during the lockdown whilst maintaining taking into consideration of other COVID-19 restrictions increased their prices as their output decreased and in response to the increased demand. With a view to this, the increase in the demand for goods and services during the

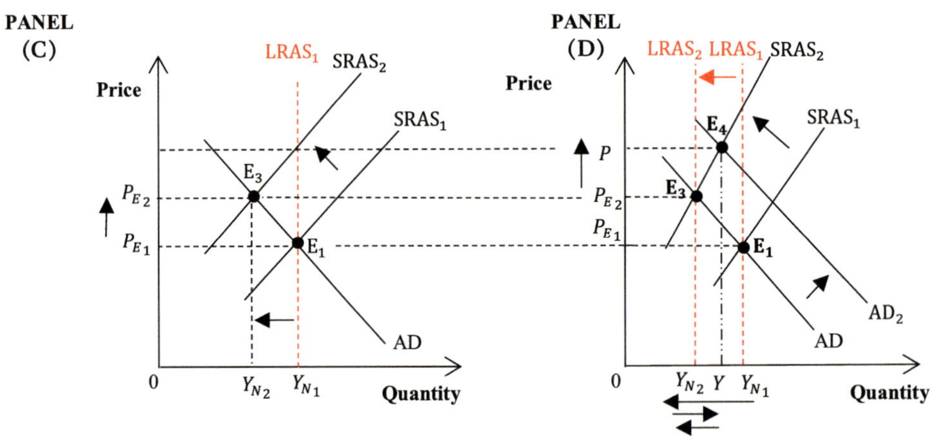


**Figure 5.**
*AS-AD model after COVID-19 government restrictions source: F Witika (2021).*

COVID-19 lockdown imply there was a shift in the aggregate demand curve to the right from AD to $AD_2$ as the economy moved from the market equilibrium point $E_3$ to $E_4$ in the medium run, as shown in **Figure 5**, in panel (D).

In consequence, at the new market equilibrium point $E_4$ during the COVID-19 lockdown, the actual price set by firms denoted as P of the actual level of output supplied at Y was greater than the expected price by consumers (as shown in **Figure 5**, in panel (D)). Hence, in the medium run, firms charged prices that were higher than what consumers expected. Moreover, due to the higher demand for goods and services during the lockdown and other COVID-19 restrictions, some firms whose operation was not completely shut down increased their output such that the level of actual output produced at Y became higher than the natural level of output at $Y_{N2}$ in the medium run but not greater than the natural level of output firms could produce before the COVID-19 lockdown and other restrictions at $E_1$ denoted by $Y_{N1}$ (as shown in **Figure 5**, in panel (D)). Nonetheless, in the long run, economies returned to the market equilibrium point $E_3$ at which they were producing at the natural level of output denoted by $Y_{N2}$ (shown in **Figure 5**). As such, the expected price by consumers charged by firms became equal to the actual price charged by firms during the lockdown and other COVID-19 restrictions. Be that as it may, the expected price by consumers during the lockdown and other COVID-19 restrictions at the equilibrium market point $E_3$ was higher than the expected price by consumers at the market equilibrium point $E_1$ before the COVID-19 lockdown and other restrictions, as illustrated in **Figure 5**, in panel (D).

In relation to the graphical analysis in **Figure 5**, according to the UNDP revised business survey report in Zambia, COVID-19 has adversely affected business operations with 71% of the respondents indicating that they were partially closed while 14% of businesses were totally closed. Only 15% reported having maintained normal operations. More than that, the study found that COVID-19 has caused a number of challenges to enterprises, with the most significant challenges being the loss of customers rated 77.3% of the total responding enterprises. Other reported challenges include supply chain cuts at 37.7%, high commodity prices or material prices reported at 36.0%, and problems with late payments at 32.3% among others. These challenges are expected to affect operating revenue for enterprises [5].

According to classical economics, in the labor market, the number of individuals in the economy willing to work and others working in the labor force is indicated by the supply of labor (denoted by $S_{labour}$ in **Figure 6**). In this regard, people in the labor force are suppliers of labor in the market whereas firms are buyers of labor supplied by individuals in the market. As such, the demand curve denoted by $D_{Demand}$ in **Figure 6** measures the amount of labor demanded by firms in the market. More than that, in **Figure 6**, $W_1$ and $W_2$ denote the wage rate whereas $Q_1$ and $Q_2$ denote the amount of labor demanded and supplied in the economy. As such, the quantity of labor demanded by firms and supplied by individuals in the market indicates the magnitude to which there is employment and unemployment in the economy.

Therefore, assuming that economies were operating at the labor market equilibrium point $E_1$ before the COVID-19 pandemic, the amount of labor supplied by individuals in the market and the amount of labor demanded by firms in the market was at $Q_1$ (as shown in **Figure 6**). Besides that, firms were willing to pay workers at the wage rate of $W_1$ and workers were also willing to work at that particular wage rate. However, after the COVID-19 pandemic and government restrictions, such as the lockdown, social distancing, and work at home policies, due to the lower productivity exhibited during the lockdown and work at home policies, the demand for labor by firms decreased. With regard to this, the decrease in the demand for labor by firms during the COVID-19 lockdown and work at home policies led to a

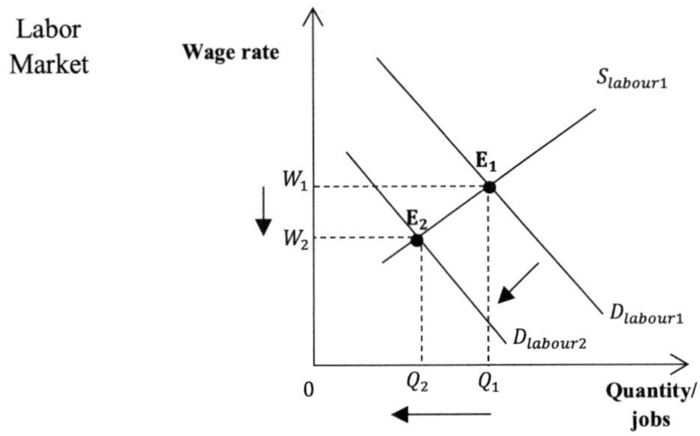


**Figure 6.**
*Labor market model after COVID-19 government restrictions. Source: F Witika (2021).*

decrease in the amount of labor used by firms indicated by the decrease in the quantity of labor from $Q_1$ to $Q_2$ and the corresponding decrease in the wage rate from $W_1$ to $W_2$ as economies moved from the labor market equilibrium point $E_1$ (before COVID-19) to $E_2$ (after COVID-19), as shown in **Figure 6**. Henceforth, the decrease in the quantity of labor from $Q_1$ to $Q_2$ indicates an increase in unemployment due to lower productivity exhibited in the COVID-19 era.

Besides, according to the UNDP revised survey report, some businesses in Zambia have begun disseminating information to employees about layoffs and issues to do with reducing salaries. This situation was reported by 37.3% of the total responding enterprises in Zambia and primarily done by businesses to keep up with the negative consequences of COVID-19 on business operations. In addition, 33.6% of the reports in Zambia were based on flexible shifts and working from home activities undertaken by businesses whereas 22.8% and 16.9% were reports received with regards to enterprises that completely shut down operations and those that exhibited resumptions of work and productivity, respectively [5].

The global coronavirus pandemic (COVID-19) dramatically slowed economic activity as governments implemented lockdown measures; individuals reacted by reducing both their mobility and economic activity, and firms' production processes were disrupted. These broader shifts in the economy affected both firm's demand for labor and workers' ability and willingness to work. In developed countries where data are readily available, market impacts varied considerably across countries, depending on initial economic and labor market conditions and variations in policy responses [6].

The emergence of COVID-19 as a pandemic led to some positive and negative effects. With regards to this, in the goods market, due to COVID-19 restrictions, such as the restrictions on movements and immigrations, which in consequence led to the closure of borders across countries, the aggregate demand in countries declined following the reduction in exports ($Y=C+I+G+(\downarrow X)-M$). Hence, countries exhibited supply shocks in international markets which also led to a reduction in prices and loss of foreign exchange. In **Figure** 7, this is indicated by the shift in the aggregate demand (AD) curve in the goods market from $AD_1$ to $AD_2$. Pertaining to this, as economies moved from the market equilibrium point $E_1$ to $E_2$, their output decreased from $Q_1$ to $Q_2$ as prices declined from $P_1$ to $P_2$ (as presented in **Figure** 7). A comprehensive study was undertaken to investigate the impact of COVID-19 on least developed countries conducted by the United Nations in 2021 found that due to the COVID-19 pandemic, the majority of least developed countries exhibited a reduction in external (or foreign) demand. In addition, LDCs also experienced a decline in prices of important commodities, such as oil and a large

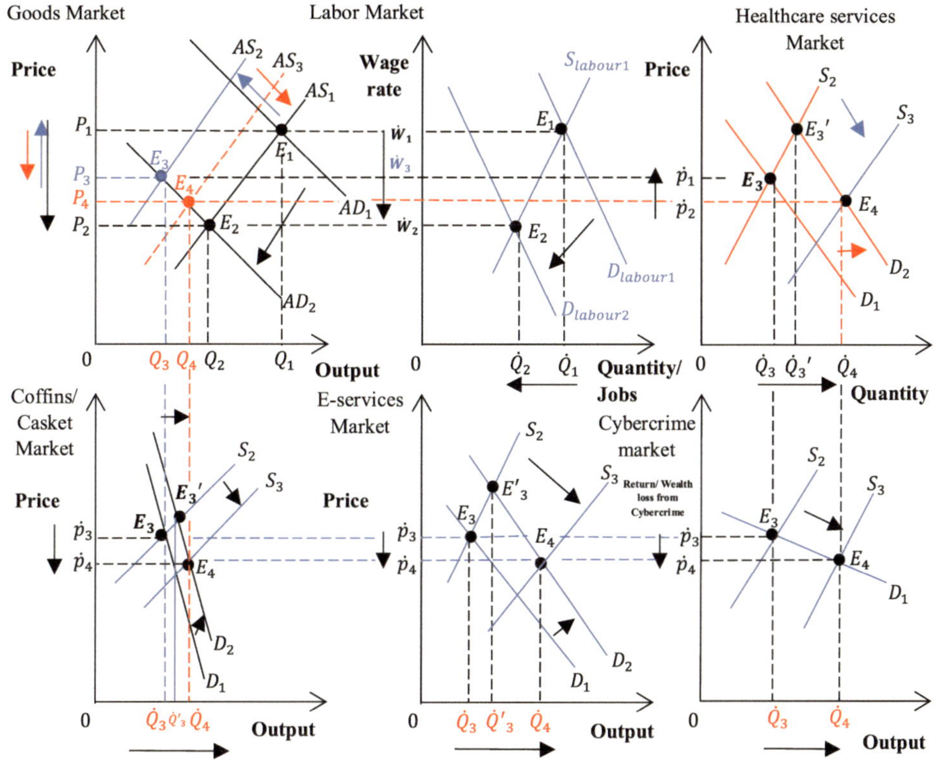


**Figure 7.**
*Positive and negative effects of COVID-19 and government restrictions. Source: F Witika (2021).*

decrease in tourism demand. In consequence, this led to a decline in foreign direct investment, challenges with regards to debt payments and remittances were highly expected to fall [7].

Furthermore, due to the lockdown measures and work at home policies aimed at reducing the spread of COVID-19 infections, the closure of many businesses and other organizations in the economies led to lower productivity. As such, the decline in productivity negatively affected the production capacities of firms in economies which led to lower economic output indicated by the shift in the aggregate supply curve from $AS_1$ to $AS_2$ (in **Figure 7**). With a view to this, the decrease in the supply of goods and services in the goods market as economies moved from the market equilibrium point $E_2$ to $E_3$ led to an increase in the general price level from $P_2$ to $P_3$, as shown in **Figure 7**. Pertaining to this, World Bank conducted an assessment in 2020 to establish effects of COVID-19 in the East and Pacific (EAP) region and found that the negative effects of COVID-19 on firms in East Asia and Pacific (EAP) region were extremely high. With a view to this, the sales of firms and employment in the regions highly declined due to the COVID-19 pandemic. Particularly, the sales of firms in some EAP countries exhibited a 38–58% decrease in sales during the period between April and May in 2020 relative to the time period between the same months in 2019. Besides that, World Bank postulated that small and medium-sized enterprises (SMEs) were the most negatively affected entities by the COVID-19 pandemic. More than that, World Bank further proposed that the pandemic is likely to have a negative lasting impact on productivity and consequently deter growth due to high indebtedness by firms and increased uncertainty which are detrimental to the magnitude of investments. Besides that, World Bank also suggested that firm closures and high unemployment exhibited during the COVID-19 era will lead to a loss of valuable intangible assets [8].

Subsequently, after the COVID-19 pandemic and government restrictions pertaining to the lockdown and stay at home policies, as economies moved from the labor market equilibrium point $E_1$ to $E_2$ (as presented in **Figure** 7), due to lower levels of productivity as a result of the disruption in normal working activities, the demand for labor by firms reduced from $Q_1$ to $Q_2$ and firms became willing to pay workers lower wagers from $\dot{W}_1$ to $\dot{W}_2$ (as shown in **Figure** 7). With a view to this, the decrease in the demand for labor during the lockdown and work at the home policy is indicated by the shift in the demand curve for labor from $D_{labour1}$ to $D_{labour2}$ assuming that the supply for labor remained constant as indicated by the unchanged supply curve for labor (shown in **Figure** 7). In relation to this, the global coronavirus pandemic dramatically slowed economic activity as governments implemented lockdown measures that restricted mobility and firm production processes. As such, the shifts in such dimensions of economic activity consequently had tremendous effects on both the demand for labor by firms and the ability and willingness of people to work [6].

Notwithstanding, government expenditure and private consumption on healthcare services directed toward the ultimate goal of treating COVID-19 infections increased in the healthcare services market in economies around the world. With a view to this, the increase in government expenditure and private consumption of medical facilities or services during the COVID-19 pandemic, in **Figure 7,** is represented by the shift in aggregate demand from $D_1$ (Y = (C) + I +(G) + X-M) to $D_2$ (Y = (↑C) + I + (↑ G) + X-M) as economies moved from the healthcare services market equilibrium point $E_3$ to the new healthcare services market equilibrium point $E_3'$ after the COVID-19 pandemic (as shown in **Figure** 7). However, due to the increase in the demand for healthcare services during the COVID-19 era, firms such as hospitals, clinics, and medical centers increased the supply of healthcare services to meet the unexpected increased demand from $\dot{Q}_3'$ to $\dot{Q}_4$ as the economy moved from the healthcare services market equilibrium point $E_3'$ to $E_4$ indicated by the shift in the supply curve from $S_2$ to $S_4$, as shown in **Figure** 7. Though not socially viewed as a positive effect of COVID-19 on economies, the increased private consumption and government expenditure on healthcare services is a positive economic effect in the sense that it led to more income generated from the purchase or expenditure on COVID-19 prevention materials, such as ventilators, face masks, hand sanitizers, and other COVID-19 prevention tools. In addition, other expenses on healthcare services include investment in COVID-19 vaccinations worldwide; all these forms of expenditure led to an increase in output in economies which contributed to the increase in quantity supplied in the goods market indicated by the shift in aggregate supply to the right, from $AS_2$ to $AS_3$ as the output of healthcare services and products supplied and demanded increased from $Q_3$ to $Q_4$ (as shown in **Figure** 7).

The rapid spread of COVID-19 renewed the focus on how health systems across the globe are financed, especially during public health emergencies. In 2019, during the first periods after the outbreak of COVID-19, it was reported that spending on health care services increased to $8.8 trillion or $1132 per person. However, it was noticed that there were variations with regard to healthcare expenditures within and across different income groups and geographical regions. Moreover, it was estimated that an amount of $54.8 billion was disbursed in 2020 with the ultimate goal of investing in health to assist countries worldwide. Pertaining to this, $13.77 billion was directed toward projects put in place to deal with COVID-19 cases, issues, or health-related problems. Contemporary issues regarding the magnitude of income spent on health have long been of interest with the considering of good health as a fundamental force of human life which is part of social and economic objectives countries intend to achieve. Moreover, the realization of the importance of health worldwide also forms the basis for the ultimate goal of providing assistance in health services globally to attain universal health coverage. However, the COVID-19 pandemic has led to a revolution with regards to the interest toward health financing in the past, present, and the future partially due to the fact that the propensity to respond to the COVID-19 pandemic has been and continues to be tremendously costly globally [9].

More than that, due to the increased number of deaths in many countries as a result of COVID-19 infections, there was an increase in the number of coffins or caskets supplied to meet the unexpected increase in the demand for coffins or caskets; other countries exhibited a shortage in the number of coffins supplied relative to the demand for coffins. As such, in the short run, the increased number of COVID-19 cases of deaths led to an increase in the demand for coffins indicated by the shift in the demand curve for coffins from $D_1$ to $D_2$ as economies moved from the coffins or casket market equilibrium point $E_3$ to $E_3'$ (as shown in **Figure 7**). In consequence, firms were induced to supply more coffins or caskets to meet the unexpected demand for coffins in the market. As such, the increase in the supply of coffins or caskets from $\dot{Q}_3'$ to $\dot{Q}_4$ is indicated by the shift in the supply curve from $S_2$ to $S_3$ (in **Figure 7**). From an economic perspective, the increase in the supply of coffins or caskets was a positive effect on the economy because it led to significant contributions to the overall output produced in the economy from $\dot{Q}_3'$ to $\dot{Q}_4$ (as shown in **Figure 7**). Nonetheless, from a social perspective, the increase in the supply of coffins due to the increased demand for coffins was an indication of the loss of lives which is negative to the welfare of society.

Moreover, in an article titled, "Coffin production in South Africa" written by Kizzi Asala in 2020, it was postulated that South Africa was the most affected country by the COVID-19 pandemic on the African continent with 1.3 million confirmed cases and over 40, 000 deaths, based on latest data from the country's health development indicators. Besides that, the funeral industry has been under great pressure following high death rates exhibited which in consequence have been prompting coffin makers and undertakers to respond to the unexpected increase in demand for coffins or caskets while navigating a mini-crisis of production shortages in the market. Pertaining to this, many people had resorted to expressing their concerns on social media regarding the delay in making funeral arrangements because of the coffin shortages. While coffin makers have been working double shifts to make up for the shortfall, the deputy president of the National Funeral Directors Association, Dr. Lawrence Konyana postulated that the shortage was particularly evident in the Western and Eastern Cape, which had recorded the most deaths. Subsequently, there was an unexpected increase in the number of COVID-19 cases in South Africa from 3000 daily cases in December to more than 20,000 daily COVID-19 cases by the end of December. As a result, there was a shift in the magnitude of the productivity of coffins or caskets such that one manufacturer that could make about 2000 coffins within a week began to produce between 3000 and 4000 coffins per week in response to the unexpected increase in the demand for coffins [10].

While the majority of businesses exhibited a complete shutdown with regards to their operations during the COVID-19 pandemic following government restrictions pertaining to the lockdown intended to reduce the spread of the COVID-19 disease, the coffin-making factory remained in operation particularly in the town of Jussey in northeastern France but could hardly keep up with meeting the demand for coffins in the market. With regards to this, nearly 60,000 COVID-19 cases were confirmed in France with 5387 deaths exhibited on a Friday. As such, this was recorded as the fourth highest tally in the world.

Furthermore, with the ongoing COVID-19 pandemic, the magnitude of the rate at which coffins were been produced increased to 50 coffins a day. Notwithstanding, another coffin-making factory located near ALPs in Eastern France was producing coffins of about 114, 000 a year which made it to be ranked as the country's biggest producer of coffins or caskets. Unfortunately, it was found that a town lying between Paris and the east of France with about 1, 600 inhabitants around the regions at the epicenter of the COVID-19 pandemic accounts for more than 50% of the country's death toll. With regard to this, in 2020, Garret postulated that it is clear that in terms of economic activity, the market for coffins or caskets is where the demand is now strongest. He further claims that in a coffin-making factory, about120 employees beaver away assembling coffins that usually sell for between 700 euros ($756) and 5, 000 euros a piece [11].

Furthermore, due to the COVID-19 lockdown and work at home policies, there was an increase in digital networking, online business marketing, online transactions, online game consumption, and income generated by social media platforms due to more online activities. With a view to this, there was an increase in the consumption of electronic services (E-services) on the internet. This is mainly because the lockdown led to little or no physical activity but more online activity as the internet happened to be a safer place where individuals had nothing to worry about wearing masks, social distancing, or other COVID-19 restrictions. As such, most individuals were forced to transition from doing their daily business activities physically to using online platforms on the internet. Therefore, the increase in the demand for E-services, such as social media, online marketing, online business transactions, and digital networking, is represented by the shift in the demand curve for E-services from $D_1$ to $D_2$, as presented in **Figure 7,** as economies moved from the E-services market equilibrium point $E_3$ to $E_3'$ along the supply curve $S_1$. However, to meet the demand in the market, software engineers, computer scientists, and other entrepreneurs in web designing and software development became more motivated to supply more E-services that can be accessed by consumers indicated (in **Figure** 7) by the shift in the supply curve to the right from $S_2$ to $S_3$ as economies moved from the E-services market equilibrium point $E_3'$ to $E_4$ leading to an increase in output from $Q_3'$ to $Q_4$ and decrease in prices due to competition in the market from $P_3$ to $P_4$.

Additionally, the United Nations Conference on Trade and Development (UNCTAD) conducted a study to assess how COVID-19 triggered the digital and e-commerce turning point and concluded that in years to come, 2020 will be viewed as the moment that changed everything. In this respect, UNCTAD argues that there has never been a time anywhere in the world when unprecedented and unforeseen growth occurred in digital and e-commerce sectors like it has occurred during the COVID-19 pandemic following government restrictions and other COVID-19 preventive mechanisms. In this regard, the COVID-19 pandemic is postulated to have fostered technological advancement with regard to e-commerce and digital transformation. As such, this COVID-19 effect on e-commerce and digital transformation can be viewed as another positive effect of the COVID-29 pandemic on economic activity. During the lockdown as a result of the COVID-19 pandemic, the majority of businesses and consumers resorted to utilizing more digital and online services to provide and purchase more goods and services when the lockdown became the new normal. In consequence, this led to a significant rise in the share of e-commerce across the globe with regards to retail trade from the magnitude of 14% in 2019 to the magnitude of 17% in 2020. Moreover, these results and other findings are presented in a new report produced by UNCTAD titled "Covid-19 and e-commerce." At an event to release the report, UN general assembly president Volkan Bozkin postulated that the trend toward e-commerce is likely to continue throughout the recovery from COVID-19 [12].

Nonetheless, the increase in the demand for E-services due to the lockdown and work at home policies also motivated criminals to venture into cybercrime activities, such as hacking, online shopping fraud, vishing, and mobile money fraud among a few. Therefore, in the market of cybercrime, the supply of cybercrime increased from $S_2$ to $S_3$ along with the demand ($D_1$) or measure of cybercrime tolerance by people accessing E-services (as shown in **Figure 7**). From an economic perspective, the impact of an increase in cybercrime as either positive or negative on economies is subject to debate; it can be positive if criminals use the stolen income to invest in businesses that end up yielding significant contributions to economic growth. In this regard, the only negative outcome would lie in the transfer of resources from those who deserve and own them to those who do not deserve and own them (criminals) illegally. However, depending on how criminals may decide to use the stolen income, their activities may have positive or negative effects on the economy. Nonetheless, from the social perspective, the increase in the supply of cybercrime during the COVID-19 lockdown and stay-at-home policies is negative as it implied an increase in the probability for individuals to lose resources online via scams, hacking, vishing, or mobile money fraud.

In conventional markets, prices serve as a wealth transfer instrument that regulates the exchange of goods and services. In the case of cybercrimes, wealth is moved between the defender and the hacker. For example, when a hacker breaches a company's server to steal customer information, the company offers a loss in terms of reputation damage, customer redness, compensation, or fines payable to regulatory agencies. The hacker can benefit from fame, selling valuable customer information such as credit data or directly using the data for fraudulent behaviors or exploitations, such as email scams or business process compromises. If hacking increases, the defender's loss of wealth and the defender's tolerance (demand) for cybercrime decreases, and they will have a greater incentive to reduce the loss by spending more protection, such as conducting security audits to reduce system bugs or cyber security awareness training [13].

With a view to cybercrime, an INTERPOL assessment of the impact of COVID-19 on cybercrime has shown that cybercriminals have transitioned from targeting only individuals and small businesses to major big corporations, governments, and critical infrastructure. With organizations and businesses rapidly deploying remote systems and networks to support staff working from home, criminals are also taking advantage of increased security vulnerabilities to steal data, generate profits, and cause disruptions. In one to four-month periods (January to April), some 907, 000 spam messages, 737 incidents related to malware, and 48, 000 malicious URLs, all related to COVID-19 were detected by one of INTERPOL's private sector partners. According to INTERPOL's assessment of the cybercrime landscape in relation to the COVID-19 pandemic, cybercriminals entice victims into providing their personal data and downloading malicious content. Around two-thirds of member countries that responded to the global cybercrime, the survey reported significant use of COVID-19 themes for phishing and online fraud ever since the COVID-19 pandemic [14].

## 3. Conclusion

Inasmuch as the COVID-19 pandemic had led to both positive and negative effects on economies worldwide, the magnitude of negative effects of COVID-19 on economies outweighs the magnitude of positive effects. On average, the supply side with regard to economic activities in countries was largely affected which in consequence also negatively affected consumers (on the demand side). To recover from the negative impacts of COVID-19 on economies, it would be fundamental for all countries worldwide to adopt new contemporary policies regarding the use of vaccinations to reduce the spread of COVID-19 rather than government restrictions, such as the lockdown, work from home policies, restrictions on immigration and exports, which have greatly contributed to negative effects of COVID-19 on the economic performance across countries.

## Conflict of interest

The author declares no conflict of interest.

## Author details

Fitzgerald Witika
Research Expert Solutions, Lusaka, Zambia

*Address all correspondence to: fitzgerald.mcdonald.witika@gmail.com

## References

[1] De Oliveira Lima CMA. Information about the new coronavirus disease (COVID-19). Radiologia Brasileira. 2020;**53**(2):v-vi. DOI: 10.1590/0100-3984.2020.53.2e1

[2] Rode S. Advanced Macroeconomics. Denmark: Ventus Publishing; 2012. ISBN: 978-87-403-0156-4

[3] WHO, "The true death toll of COVID-19: estimating global excess mortality," World Health Organization, 2021, 2121 [Online]. Available at: https://www.who.int/data/stories/the-true-death-toll-of-covid-19-estimating-global-excess-mortality.

[4] Yoon J-W, Kim J, Lee J. Impact of demographic changes on inflation and the macroeconomy. IMF Working Papers. 2014;**14**(210):1. DOI: 10.5089/9781498396783.001

[5] Z. Enterprises, "Business Survey Report," Bus. Surv. Report- impact Covid19 Zambian Enterp., p. 76, 2020, [Online]. Available at: https://www.google.com/url?sa=t&rct=j&q=&esrc=s&source=web&cd=&ved=2ahUKEwjy5L6z6ID2AhWOHOwKHZE9CRUQFnoECAkQAQ&url=https%3A%2F%2Fwww.zm.undp.org%2Fcontent%2Fdam%2Fzambia%2FUNDP%2520Revised%2520Business%2520Survey%2520Report%252003-07-2020%2520CLEAN.pdf&usg=AOvVaw3ZuG-19QLGSZs5-xCGyG7o

[6] Khamis M, Prinz D, Newhouse D, Palacios-Lopez A, Pape U, Weber M. The Early Labor Market Impact of COVID-19 in Developing Countries: Evidence from High-Frequency Phone Surveys. Vol. 582021. Washington DC, USA: International Bank for reconstruction and development/The World Bank. DOI: 10.1596/35044

[7] United Nations Committee for Development Policy, "Comprehensive Study on the Impact of COVID-19 on the Least Developed Country Category," no. April, 2021

[8] De Nicola F, Mattoo A, Timmis J, Tran TT. Productivity in the Time of COVID-19: Evidence from East Asia and Pacific. Vol. 462021. Washington DC, USA: The World Bank; 2021

[9] Micah AE et al. Tracking development assistance for health and for COVID-19: A review of development assistance, government, out-of-pocket, and other private spending on health for 204 countries and territories, 1990–2050. Lancet. 2021;**398**(10308):1317-1343. DOI: 10.1016/s0140-6736(21)01258-7

[10] Asala K. News COVID-19 Deaths in South Africa Put Coffin-Makers under Pressure. Lyon, France: Africanews; 2021

[11] Fuentes G, Irish J. Business Booms for Coffin-Makers in Coronavirus-Hit France. London: Reuters; 2021

[12] UNCTAD. How COVID-19 Triggered the Digital and e-Commerce Turning Point. Geneva, Switzerland: UNCTAD (United Nations Conference on Trade and Development); 2021. pp. 1-7, [Online]. Available at: https://unctad.org/news/how-covid-19-triggered-digital-and-e-commerce-turning-point

[13] Kai-Lung H, Jiali Z. Munich Personal RePEc Archive the Economics of Private Digital Currency. Vol. 558242014. Germany: MPRA (Munich Personal RePEc Archive)

[14] Jürgen Stock, "INTERPOL report shows alarming rate of cyberattacks during COVID-19," Interpol, p. 2021, 2020, [Online]. Available at: https://www.interpol.int/en/News-and-Events/News/2020/INTERPOL-report-shows-alarming-rate-of-cyberattacks-during-COVID-19

Chapter 31

# Perspective Chapter: Impact of the COVID-19 Pandemic on the Field of Orthopedics

*Chia-Hao Hsu, Chung-Hwan Chen and Hsuan-Ti Huang*

## Abstract

During the COVID-19 pandemic, countries all over the world suffered from different kinds of service disruption or reduction in the field of orthopedics with or without lockdowns. The consequences include no restriction, partial disruption, overburden of medical services and complete shutdown of clinical practices. This chapter systematically reviews the current published literature on the global impact of COVID-19 on the field of orthopedics through multiple aspects, including educational impact, service volume impact, workload impact, personal practice change, psychological impact, and impact on orthopedic research. The rates of all surgeries and elective surgeries decreased by 15.6%–49.4% and 43.5–100%, respectively. The overall impact was attributable to the staff redeployment in response to the pandemic. Therefore, it is important to maintain a flexible allocation of manpower and more sufficient and reservable staffing measures in case of emergency staff shortages. Orthopedic surgeons are suggested to prepare proper preventive strategies and set up special equipment and places for regular telemedicine for virtual consultations or virtual teaching. It can be expected that the integration of the different experiences of global countries from the impact of COVID-19 may help us to face possible similar impacts in the future.

**Keywords:** COVID-19, pandemic, impact, lockdown, restriction, orthopedics, education, orthopedic service, clinical practice, workload, psychological effect

## 1. Introduction

The World Health Organization declared the 2019 coronavirus disease (COVID-19) as a worldwide pandemic on March 12, 2020. COVID-19 cases were first found in Wuhan, China, in December 2019 [1], possibly owing to the purchase, slaughtering, and consumption of exotic live animals in the Huanan seafood and animal market. COVID-19 is an infectious disease that can cause pneumonia. It has spread rapidly and has infected numerous individuals globally. A cumulative millions of cases have been confirmed, and thousands to millions of people have died of this disease, seriously impacting the global economy. Under this pandemic situation, the global orthopedics field was of course inevitably impacted and the impact was comprehensive.

The COVID-19 pandemic and related lockdowns or restrictions have greatly changed the daily lives of populations worldwide. It forced the healthcare system to undergo dramatic changes in response. A large number of COVID-19 cases in some regions have forced hospitals to reorganize their departments to have the capacity to treat infected patients. Certain administrative or preventive epidemic strategies have caused many restrictions, such as separation of employees, reduction in the number of outpatient clinics, delayed or suspension of elective surgeries, and cancelation of non-emergency consultations or referrals to reduce the infection risk among patients and orthopedic staff.

In this chapter, the relevant publications from various countries in the world were sorted out and extracted their important research results based on different aspects, and provided readers with a comprehensive understanding of the impact of the pandemic. Because of the different infection situations in different countries, with different early responses, different infection control measures and different administrative management strategies, many of the results may not be suitable for a direct comparison. Therefore, this article mostly presented the results in an itemized, organized and narrative manner, avoiding unfair rankings among countries. All publications presenting comparable data, including reduction percentage of all surgeries and reduction percentage of elective surgery, were compared.

## 2. Global research trend of COVID-19 impact on the field of orthopedics

A comprehensive literature search was conducted covering a period from January 1, 2020, to September 1, 2021, to include all possible matching articles since the appearance of the new coronavirus. PubMed served as the database for the literature search. If all the subspecialties of orthopedics were included, the number of searched publications will be too large, so we limit the search to the title that contains "orthopedic" or "orthopedic". The search was performed using the following search items for the title: "impact" AND "COVID-19" AND "orthopedic" (20 search results) plus "impact" AND "COVID-19" AND "orthopedic" (38 search results). One search result was excluded because it was a letter to the editor. In total, 57 studies were identified (**Table 1**). In terms of the regions of these publications, the most are in Europe, followed by Asia and North America.

## 3. Various aspects affected in the field of Orthopedics

Research on the impact in the field of orthopedics can be subdivided into education, clinical service volume, changes in clinical practice, workload, psychological factors, research work, etc. The essence of each peer-reviewed publication was listed in a sorted manner. The remaining few studies, focused on a single or some specific index of orthopedics for analysis, were not discussed in this article.

## 4. Educational impact

Most research on the impact of education comes from the United States, which may also reveal that the pandemic has disrupted their education system to a greater extent. Routine orthopedic education and training are still more or less affected or even suspended in most countries. The source of the impact may come from the interference of lockdowns or restrictions and various infection prevention measures including social distancing.

### 4.1 Impact on application

A perspective/narrative study in the United States discussed and provided potential strategies to understand the impact of COVID-19 on the orthopedic

| No | Year | Study | Country | Region | Focus | Study method |
|---|---|---|---|---|---|---|
| 1 | 2020 | Aiyer *et al.* [2] | USA | North America | Education/Residency Application | Perspective/Narrative |
| 2 | 2020 | Alyami *et al.* [3] | Saudi Arabia | Middle East | Service/Education | Perspective/Narrative |
| 3 | 2020 | Andreozzi *et al.* [4] | Italy | Europe | Service/Orthopedic Trauma | Retrospective |
| 4 | 2020 | Bernstein *et al.* [5] | USA | North America | Education/ Intern, resident training | Perspective/reflection |
| 5 | 2020 | Chang *et al.* [6] | South Korea | Asia | Education/Residency | Questionnaire survey |
| 6 | 2020 | Clement *et al.* [7] | UK | Europe | Surgical Risk Assessment | Multicenter, retrospective |
| 7 | 2020 | Costa *et al.* [8] | Italy | Europe | Prevention measures | Retrospective |
| 8 | 2020 | Danford, *et al.* [9] | USA | North America | Education/Residency Application | Questionnaire survey |
| 9 | 2020 | Dattani *et al.* [10] | UK | Europe | Education/Trainees | Perspective/Narrative |
| 10 | 2020 | Elhalawany *et al.* [11] | UK | Europe | Service/Orthopedic emergency | Retrospective |
| 11 | 2020 | Ghermandi *et al.* [12] | Italy | Europe | Service/Orthopedic oncology and spine | Retrospective |
| 12 | 2020 | Gonzi *et al.* [13] | UK | Europe | Education/Trainees | Four-nation questionnaire survey |
| 13 | 2020 | Haffer *et al.* [14] | Germany | Europe | Service/Orthopedic and Trauma Surgery | Nationwide questionnaire survey |
| 14 | 2020 | Mackay *et al.* [15] | UK | Europe | Surgical Risk Assessment | Retrospective cohort |
| 15 | 2020 | Maniscalco *et al.* [16] | Italy | Europe | Service/Emergency Room and Orthopedics | Retrospective |
| 16 | 2020 | Maryada *et al.* [17] | India | Asia | Service/Orthopedic Trauma | Multi-centre retrospective |
| 17 | 2020 | Megaloikonomos *et al.* [18] | Europe | Europe | Education/Trainees | 23 European countries questionnaire |
| 18 | 2020 | Murphy *et al.* [19] | UK | Europe | Workload / Orthopedic | Retrospective |
| 19 | 2020 | Ong *et al.* [20] | Hong Kong | Asia | Service/Education/Research | Perspective/Experience |
| 20 | 2020 | Park *et al.* [21] | UK | Europe | Workload / Orthopedic trauma | Retrospective |
| 21 | 2020 | Phillips *et al.* [22] | N/A | N/A | Orthopedic care | Review |
| 22 | 2020 | Richardson *et al.* [23] | USA | North America | Education / medical student | Perspectives |

| No | Year | Study | Country | Region | Focus | Study method |
|---|---|---|---|---|---|---|
| 23 | 2020 | Sahu *et al.* [24] | India | Asia | Psychological /orthopedic surgeon | Questionnaire survey |
| 24 | 2020 | Sheridan *et al.* [25] | Ireland | Europe | Education / Trainees | Questionnaire |
| 25 | 2020 | Sugand *et al.* [26] | UK | Europe | Workload / Pediatric orthopedic trauma | Multi-centre retrospective |
| 26 | 2020 | Teo *et al.* [27] | Malaysia | Asia | Practice Change/Surgeon | Nationwide questionnaire survey |
| 27 | 2020 | Upadhyaya *et al.* [28] | India | Asia | Education/Trainees | Questionnaire survey |
| 28 | 2020 | Wallace *et al.* [29] | UK | Europe | Trauma and orthopedic surgery | Perspectives |
| 29 | 2020 | Wong *et al.* [30] | Hong Kong | Asia | Service / Orthopedic and Trauma | Retrospective cohort |
| 30 | 2020 | Wong *et al.* [31] | Singapore | Asia | Psychological/orthopedic outpatient setting | Questionnaire survey |
| 31 | 2021 | Barahona *et al.* [32] | Chile | South America | Service/Orthopedic surgery | Retrospective |
| 32 | 2021 | Blum *et al.* [33] | N/A | N/A | Service/Orthopedic and Trauma Surgery | Review |
| 33 | 2021 | Chatterji *et al.* [34] | N/A | N/A | Miscellaneous | Rapid Review |
| 34 | 2021 | Garcia *et al.* [35] | Spain | Europe | Personal Practice Change/ Orthopedic Surgeon | Questionnaire survey |
| 35 | 2021 | Gibbard *et al.* [36] | N/A | N/A | Personal Practice Change/Pediatric Orthopedic Surgeon | Global (45 countries) questionnaire survey |
| 36 | 2021 | Giordano *et al.* [37] | N/A | N/A | Financial, Psychosocial/Orthopedic Trauma surgeon | 14 Latin American countries questionnaire survey |
| 37 | 2021 | Green *et al.* [38] | UK | Europe | Length of stay/total hip and knee arthroplasty | Retrospective cohort |
| 38 | 2021 | Heaps *et al.* [39] | USA | North America | Service/multi-subspecialty | Retrospective cohort |
| 39 | 2021 | Howles *et al.* [40] | UK | Europe | Service/One-stop minor injuries unit | Retrospective cohort |
| 40 | 2021 | Jain *et al.* [41] | India | Asia | Personal Practice Change/Orthopedic Surgeon | Nationwide questionnaire |
| 41 | 2021 | Khan *et al.* [42] | UK | Europe | Personal Practice Change/Orthopedic Surgeon | Nationwide questionnaire |
| 42 | 2021 | Ma et al. [43] | Taiwan | Asia | Screening/trauma at emergency department | Retrospective cohort |
| 43 | 2021 | Maleitzke *et al.* [44] | Germany | Europe | Service/Orthopedic trauma | Retrospective cohort |

| No | Year | Study | Country | Region | Focus | Study method |
|---|---|---|---|---|---|---|
| 44 | 2021 | Moretti *et al*. [45] | Italy | Europe | Psychological/gender-specific | Nationwide Questionnaire |
| 45 | 2021 | Oguzkaya *et al*. [46] | Turkey | Asia and Europe | Orthopedic fracture characteristics | Multi-center retrospective |
| 46 | 2021 | Paul *et al*. [47] | USA | North America | Practice Change/Elective procedures, telehealth and income | Nationwide Questionnaire |
| 47 | 2021 | Peebles *et al*. [48] | USA | North America | Education/Sports Fellowship Application | Perspective/Narrative Review |
| 48 | 2021 | Probert *et al*. [49] | Australia | Australia | Service/Orthopedic trauma | Retrospective |
| 49 | 2021 | Qian *et al*. [50] | China | Asia | Service/Orthopedic trauma | Retrospective |
| 50 | 2021 | Rachuene *et al*. [51] | South Africa | Africa | Service/Orthopedic trauma | Multicenter retrospective |
| 51 | 2021 | Ribau *et al.* [52] | Portugal | Europe | Service /Orthopedic trauma | Retrospective |
| 52 | 2021 | Shah *et al*. [53] | Canada | North America | Education/Residency application | Perspectives/Narrative Review |
| 53 | 2021 | Sharma *et al*. [54] | India | Asia | Psychological/Practice Change | Questionnaire |
| 54 | 2021 | Shih *et al*. [55] | Taiwan | Asia | Psychological/Service | Retrospective |
| 55 | 2021 | Unterfrauner *et al.* [56] | Switzerland | Europe | Complications/deep surgical site infections | Retrospective |
| 56 | 2021 | Van Heest *et al*. [57] | USA | North America | Education/Orthopedic Graduate Medical Education | Review / Symposium summary |
| 57 | 2021 | Vasiliadis *et al*. [58] | Greece | Europe | Service | Retrospective |

**Table 1.**
*Characteristics of relevant publications.*

residency application process. Because COVID-19 may have an impact on the matching of residents, there is a great demand for insights into the inevitable changes in the application process and how medical students can adapt. In addition, the procedure is likely to ask the applicants how they spent the time they were not in the hospital due to COVID-19, and the applicants should be prepared to provide meaningful answers [2]. A questionnaire survey was conducted in the United States for medical students. Women stated that they are "unlikely" to apply for orthopedic residents due to the pandemic (14.9% vs. 5.5% for men, $P < 0.001$). Students identified as black/African American stated that they were "unlikely" to apply (16.9% compared with 8.8% of non-Hispanic whites, $P < 0.001$). The students stated that they had "slightly fewer" or "much less" opportunities to fully engage in orthopedic surgery training to make professional application choices (88.9% of students) [9].

### 4.2 Impact on training

A perspective study in the United States shared the thoughts of 3 orthopedic interns in different levels of a single training program. Although they are all trainees, the difference in training years is crucial to clarify different sources of professional stress. Everyone has their own sources of stress and response to ongoing crises [5].

A questionnaire survey was performed in South Korea for orthopedic residents. The average working time of 72.7 hours/week before the pandemic was reduced to 65.6 hours/week during the pandemic ($p < 0.001$). During the pandemic, educational time for lectures and clinical case discussions were reduced (both, $p < 0.001$). While reducing the use of traditional teaching methods, the use of online teaching methods has been increased ($p < 0.001$). However, compared with traditional teaching methods, the satisfaction of online teaching methods is significantly lower. The average quality of life score before the pandemic was 68.9 out of 100, which dropped to 61.7 during the pandemic ($p < 0.001$). The most stressful factor for orthopedic residents during the pandemic is family/relative health, followed by their own health and residency plan [6].

A perspective/narrative study in UK described the reductions in trainees' surgical exposure, cancelation of exams and courses, and revisions to professional recruitment and annual evaluations. This group of trainees is witnessing new methods of providing orthopedic services [10]. A four-nation questionnaire survey of orthopedic trainees was conducted in UK. 23.1% (23/101) of the trainees were redeployed to non-surgical positions. A total of 42.9% (42/101)% of the trainees did not have the fracture clinic training on the schedule, 53% (53/101) of the trainees had assigned operating theater training once per week, and 63.8% (64/101) of the trainees did not feel that sufficient experience has been gained in the affiliated subspecialties and preferred repeating training [13].

A questionnaire survey of orthopedic trainees was conducted in 23 European countries. Most trainees retained their usual clinical roles (59.8%), but quite a few were redeployed to COVID-19 units (20.9%). 52.1% stated that teacher-led education was restricted, 46.3% pursued self-directed learning, and 58.6% stated that surgical training was severely impaired. 58.2% of participants expressed concern about achieving the annual training goals, while 25.0% of participants expected an additional year of training [18].

A perspective study in the USA believe that the following suggestions may be helpful to students seeking alternative supplementary learning methods: [1] read major orthopedic journals, [2] contact orthopedic surgeons in the field of interest, [3] contact program coordinators or directors to have the opportunity to participate in their education courses in a virtual way, [4] attend online lectures, and [5] use practice kits to practice suture techniques [23].

A questionnaire survey in Ireland found the average total number of operations per trainee in 2019 was 40.6, and reduced to 18.3 during the 2020 pandemic ($p = 0.043$). Moreover, 7.69% ($n = 3$) of the trainees were infected with COVID-19 [25].

A questionnaire survey in India revealed that 65.1% of the post-graduate trainees stated that no clinical courses are currently offered. Most (94%) confirmed that COVID-19 has affected their surgical and clinical training. A large number (71.6%) encountered problems when completing the thesis, and 96% were worried about their mental health [28].

## 5. Global service impact

Through major publications in different regions, we can understand the real impact of COVID-19 on the volume of clinical services. Generally, the service volume was inevitably reduced in all aspects, except for a few specific items. Even in a country where there was no lockdowns or restrictions, there was still a small reduction, which may also be influenced by psychological factors.

### 5.1 Europe

A study in Italy during lockdown revealed the average age of the COVID-19 group is 51.9 +/− 24.8 years, which is significantly higher than the pre-COVID-19 group (41.4 +/− 25.7) ($p < 0.0001$). The most common injury was fracture (45.1% in 2019; 62.7% in 2020) ($p < 0.0001$). The most severely injured anatomical location during COVID-19 lockdown was the hand (14.2%), while in the pre-COVID-19 group, the most common type of injury was multiple injuries (22.8%) [4]. Another study in Italy focused on orthopedic oncology and spine had a unique result. During the lockdown period, by managing urgent and non-delayable spinal diseases with a low COVID-19 infection rate (3.9%), surgical activities have increased instead [12]. The other study in Italy showed a reduction of emergency room visits (−18.0%). The increase in the number of deaths in the emergency room was equal to +220%. The orthopedic pathway dropped by −26.8%. Trauma at home increased (+19.1%) [16].

A nationwide questionnaire survey in Germany showed only 7 respondents (13.7%) fully agreed or quite agreed with the authorities' support for orthopedics and trauma surgery. Major financial and personnel changes had taken place, resulting in an average reduction in operating room capacity of 49.4% and an estimated loss of income of 29.3%. In addition, 14.7% of doctors were redistributed [14]. Another study in Germany focused on emergency departments during the 35-day lockdown. The daily total number of patient cases (lockdown and control, 106.94 and 167.54) and orthopedic trauma cases (lockdown and control, 30.91 and 52.06) declined with an increase in the incidence of home injuries, bicycle accidents, domestic violence, and acute/conventional drug abuse [44].

A study in the UK focused on orthopedic emergencies, during lockdown, showed that patient visits had a decrease of 58.6%. The orthopedic presentations in 2020 and 2019 were 736 (37.2%) and 1729 (36.2%), a decrease of 57.4% [11]. An orthopedic team in the UK set up a 7-day "One-Stop" clinic for minor injuries/ambulatory patients. Approximately 700 patients who were supposed to be treated in the emergency room changed to minor injuries unit, reducing the pressure on the emergency room. Seventy-one percent of patients were discharged after the initial appointment, and only 9 patients (1%) needed to make an appointment for a fracture clinic within 72 hours. A total of 15 patients (2%) revisited the clinic with concern, and only 4 of them required additional intervention [40].

### 5.2 Asia

A multi-center study in India revealed that the total number of traumas during lockdown period was significantly reduced by 1266 cases, a reduction of 62.7% ($p < 0.01$). Road traffic accident is the main cause of trauma in all age groups except the elderly, and a 77.9% reduction in cases was found during the lockdown period ($n = 1343$ vs. $n = 298$) [17].

A study in Hong Kong showed orthopedic surgery decreased by 44.2%, from a weekly average of 795 ± 115.1 to 443.6 ± 25.8 ($p < 0.001$), and the ratio of emergency surgery to elective surgery increased from 1.27:1 to 3.78:1. Surgery for treatment of upper and lower limb fractures was reduced by 23% (from 98.5 ± 14 to 75.9 ± 15.2 per week; $p < 0.001$) and 20% (from 210.6 ± 29.5 to 168.4 ± 16.9 per week) 16.9 times; $p < 0.001$), while elective joint replacement and ligament reconstruction surgery decreased by 74–84% ($p < 0.001$). The number of hospitalizations decreased by 41.2% (from 2365 ± 243 to 1391 ± 53 per week; $p < 0.001$), while the number of clinical outpatient visits decreased by 29.4% (from 11,693 ± 2240 to 8261 ± 1104 per week; $p < 0.001$, 30).

A study in Taiwan showed that the COVID-19 pandemic resulted in a 22%–29% and 20%–26% reduction in outpatients, 22%–27% and 25%–37% reduction in inpatients, and 26%–35% and 18%–34% reduction in orthopedic operations [55]. Taiwan successfully prevented the spread of COVID-19 without lockdown and adopted many prevention strategies effectively, such as the use of masks in the public [59].

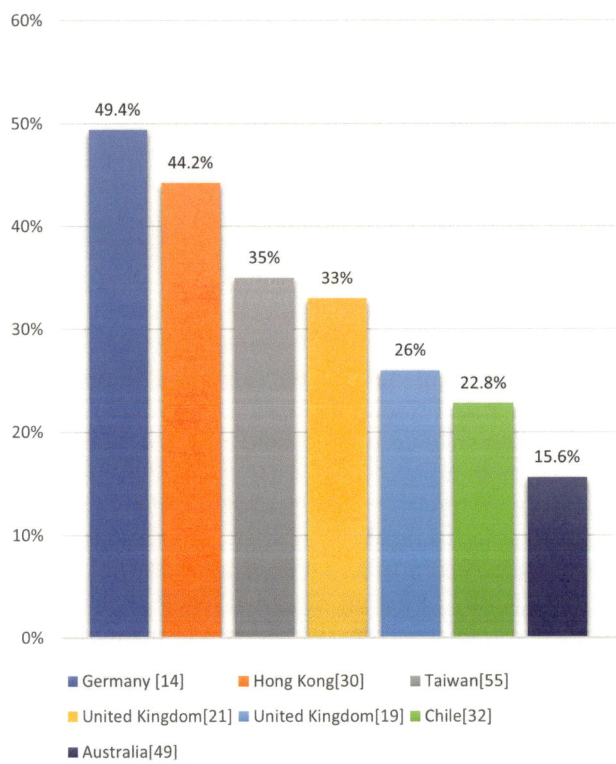


**Figure 1.**
*Reduction percentage of all surgeries.*

### 5.3 North and South America

A study focused on multi-subspecialty in the United States analyzed a total of 2830 (1917 pre-COVID-19 and 913 post-COVID-19) cases. A significant increase in the percentage of hip procedures performed (+3.5 ± 1.1%, p = 0.002), a significant decrease in the percentage of wrist procedures performed (−2.6 ± 0.8%, p = 0.002), and a significant decrease in the percentage of hand procedures performed (−2.1 ± 1.0%, p = 0.027). Foot, ankle, knee, shoulder, elbow, and back procedures showed no significant change [39].

A study in Chile revealed that the number of orthopedic surgeries fell by 22.8%. All surgical procedures were adversely affected, with fracture/traumatic surgery being the least affected. Knee replacement (−64%) had the greatest adverse impact, followed by hip replacement (−41%) and knee ligament reconstruction (−44%). The number of orthopedic surgeries was slightly correlated with the number of COVID-19 cases per month (p = 0.08) and strongly correlated with the country's mobility (p = 0.0001) [32].

### 5.4 Australia

A study in Australia during lockdown revealed the total number of emergency operations performed decreased by 15.6% compared to the same period in 2019. The number of orthopedic hospitalizations decreased by 30.8%. Road trauma accounts for a similar proportion of overall cases; however, bicycle-related

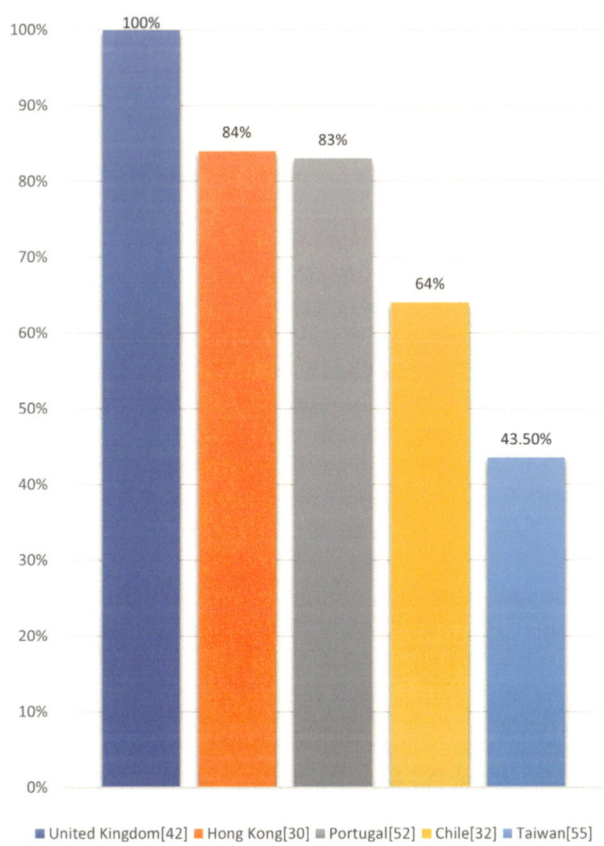


**Figure 2.**
*Maximal reduction percentage of the elective surgeries.*

accidents have increased significantly, accounting for 11% of presentations. During the pandemic, sports injuries, work-related injuries, and multiple injuries have decreased [49].

### 5.5 Comparable reduction percentage of all surgeries and elective surgeries

The reduction percentage in various countries was one of the few parameters that can be compared. However, the data may not be available from some countries. The reduction percentage of the volume of all surgeries was 49.4% in Germany [14], 44.2% in Hong Kong [30], 35% in Taiwan [55], 33% and 26% in the United Kingdom [19, 21], 22.8% in Chile [32], and 15.6% in Australia (**Figure 1**, [49]). Surprisingly, even though there were few COVID-19 cases in the first wave and no serious lockdowns or restrictions in Hong Kong and Taiwan, they still experienced a substantial impact on the number of surgeries. This may be attributable to psychological factors caused by a large flow of people to and from China due to proximity to China.

The maximal reduction percentage of the elective surgery was 100% in the United Kingdom [42], 84% in Hong Kong [30], 83% in Portugal [53], 64% in Chile [32], and 43.5% in Taiwan (**Figure 2**, [55]). The relatively smaller reduction percentage in Taiwan may be attributable to the lack of restrictions or lockdowns [59]. Taiwan prevented the spread of COVID-19 successfully by adopting effective preventive strategies, such as mandatory mask use in public [60].

## 6. Workload impact

Service volume impact represents the entire department or hospital, the workload impact represents individuals. Three studies [19, 21, 26] focused on the impact of personal workload during the pandemic in the UK. A study on the workload in the UK revealed the average number of weekly referrals to the service decreased by 33% ($p < 0.0001$). The number of operations performed each week was reduced by 26% ($p = 0.001$). The number of referrals related to domestic abuse or non-accidental injury had not changed. In addition, the number of hip fractures, periprosthetic fractures, and prosthetic joint dislocations did not change. The number of referrals for simple fractures, natural joint dislocations, wounds, and soft tissue injuries had been significantly reduced. Similarly, in the pediatric population, the reduction in referrals for simple fractures had also been demonstrated [19]. Another study on the workload in UK showed acute trauma referrals decreased almost 50%, with similar distribution between pediatric and adult patients, but the required hospital admissions increased significantly by 19% (RR 1.3, OR 2.6, $p = 0.003$). During the COVID-19 outbreak, the total number of surgical cases fell by a third. The usage of aerosol-generating anesthesia technique was reduced by 14% (RR 0.85, OR 0.20, $p = 0.006$) [21]. A study on pediatric trauma in UK during lockdown revealed that acute pediatric trauma referrals were reduced by two-thirds compared with 2019 ($n = 302$ vs. 97, RR 0.55, OR 0.43) ($p = 0.002$). Outpatient telemedicine was used more, virtual fracture clinics were used more (OR 97, RR 84, $p < 0.001$), and fewer patients received consultation and face-to-face follow-up (OR 0.55, RR 0.05) ($P < 0.001$) [26]. Although for individuals, the reduction in clinical workload during this period may bring more rest time, and the extra free time can also be used for writing, reading or personal research, this also means that the economic income will inevitably decrease accordingly.

## 7. Personal practice change

A nationwide questionnaire survey in Malaysia revealed the majority of respondents are still working (223/235, 94.9%), operating outpatient clinics (168/223, 75.3%), and continuing to perform semi-emergency (190/223, 85.2%) and emergency surgery (213/223, 95.5%). Among surgeons, 11.2% (25/223) did not screen patients for COVID-19 before elective surgery, 30.9% (69/223) did not receive any training on the proper handling of personal protective equipment (PPE), and 84.8% (189/223) made more conservative management decisions due to COVID-19, and 61.9% (138/223) of income was affected. Among surgeons, 19.3% (43/223) started using telemedicine facilities [27].

A questionnaire survey in Spain revealed 85.7% of the respondents had to reduce their surgical activities by 50%–100%. Forty-six percent of them were asked to collaborate in other units or services, and another 43% felt that their work was underutilized. Fifty percent revised the indications for the treatment of various fractures, and there are differences between the center and the community. Thirty percent of the respondents said they were satisfied with the management of the country, and 60% said they were satisfied with the management of their province and center. Seventy percent of the respondents were almost dissatisfied with the training they received on the use of masks and personal protective equipment. Another 80% were not satisfied with the sample-taking training they received. Sixty-five percent of people did not have protective equipment to carry out their work. Forty-six percent refused protective measures to treat patients with suspected or confirmed infections [35].

A nationwide questionnaire survey in India showed most (88.3%) found that trauma surgery and non-traumatic surgery were severely affected (>50%). Significant changes had taken place in individual hospital protocols (91.7%). Most hospitals (74.3%) were equipped with the appropriate personal protective equipment required. Most surgeons (89.5%) did not modify or upgrade the existing operating room infrastructure [41].

A nationwide questionnaire survey in UK showed all 202 respondents reported that their daily practice was disrupted. Ninety-one percent reported that all elective surgeries had been canceled, and only 24% of cases had trauma that continued to be normal. Seventy percent reported interruption of trauma surgery. The capacity of elective clinics was significantly reduced, and there were no elective clinics that were functioning normally. Fifty-five percent reported that their elective clinics were completely canceled, while 38% reported that the operational capacity of elective clinics was reduced and non-emergency appointments were postponed. Only 9% of fracture clinics were operating normally, and 69% had reduced services. Sixty-seven percent of people reported cancelation of teaching and study leave. It is worth noting that 69% of respondents believe that the pandemic will delay the completion of the registrar training program [42].

Finally, a questionnaire survey of orthopedic surgeons received responses from 45 countries. 358 (78.5%) respondents reported the lockdown measures in their area during the survey. Most (n = 337, 94.4%) reported suspension of all elective programs. Surgeons reported that the average number of operations per week has decreased, from 6.89 before the pandemic to 1.25 at the time of the survey. The average weekly number of elective clinic appointments decreased from 67.89 before the pandemic to 11.79 at the time of the survey. A total of 177 (39.4%) surgeons reported using the virtual outpatient appointment model for the first time. Of the 290 surgeons with trainees, 223 (84.5%) reported implementing systems for continuing training, such as webinars or virtual inspections [36].

## 8. Psychological impact

Psychological factors also have a certain percentage of influence. Stress or fear may come from drastic changes in oneself or the external environment. Psychological stress can be individuals or the public.

As for the surgeon's personal psychological pressure, a questionnaire survey in India was completed by 611 orthopedic surgeons from 140 cities in India. 22.5% of orthopedic surgeons said they must be under pressure, and 40.5% said they have mild pressure. With declining age, the percentage of orthopedic surgeons feeling "a lot of stress" had increased. The interruption of life-work balance and the uncertainty of returning to work were other factors closely related to the "absolutely stressed" group [24]. A questionnaire survey in Singapore showed 32 participants (51.6%) had 7 or more positive reactions. "Work adjustments" (74.2%), "changes in personal plans" (72.6%), and "restrictions" (72.6%) received the most positive responses in the questionnaire. On the other hand, "financial issues" received the least positive responses (21.0%) [31].

As for the public panic, it seems more obvious in some countries. As mentioned earlier, even there were few COVID-19 cases and no lockdowns or restrictions initially in Hong Kong and Taiwan, they still experienced an obvious impact on the number of surgeries. This may be attributable to the public's panic because of its proximity to China. At the beginning of the pandemic, exaggeration of the mass media, rumors or false news, and lack of medical resources may also cause widespread public panic. In Taiwan, the COVID-19-related fear seemed to reduce elderly individuals' willingness to undergo elective surgery. Elderly patients carry a higher mortality risk after being infected and they may have postponed their surgeries [55].

## 9. Impact on orthopedic research

A questionnaire survey of orthopedic surgeons received responses from 45 countries. Of the 192 respondents who conducted research, 149 (82.8%) reported continuing research activities during the pandemic, and most of them reported that participant recruitment stopped (n = 75, 64.15%) or decreased (n = 25, 29.9%) [36].

## 10. Conclusions

This chapter provides a comprehensive understanding of the impact of the pandemic on the field of orthopedics globally and aims to review the lessons learned from the impact of the pandemic to prepare for the next possible re-impacts. Although orthopedic surgeons may not be in the front line to fight against COVID-19pandemic, all the fields of orthopedics are still inevitably impacted. Most studies in current literature have reported that the number of cases in all aspects decreased significantly. Education and training, psychological factors, and orthopedic research, which have been less noted, have also been significantly impacted. All the fields of orthopedics were clearly affected by the COVID-19 pandemic. In the future, despite the pandemic, it is important to maintain treatment, especially the surgical care of the patients, to avoid negative effects on the prognosis. Strategies should be developed to enable orthopedic patients to receive timely treatment, even if the pandemic continues. Employees must be properly protected at the same time. This can be achieved by formulating a proper surgical scheduling algorithm for orthopedic patients. Several infection control measures and administrative management strategies may help maintain the normal operation. The implementation of appropriate preventive strategies may aid the scheduling of surgeries during the pandemic, which may, in turn, reassure the patients and prevent the suspension of normal orthopedic surgery practice. It is also important for orthopedic surgeons to prepare emergency response measures under normal circumstances, to deal with the emergency shortage of personnel caused by the redistribution or redeployment of personnel. The overall impact could be attributable to the staff redeployment in response to the pandemic. Therefore, it is important to maintain a flexible allocation of manpower and more sufficient and reservable staffing measures in case of emergency staff shortages. Orthopedic surgeons are suggested to prepare proper preventive strategies and set up special equipment and places for regular telemedicine for virtual consultations or virtual teaching.

## Conflict of interest

The authors declare no conflict of interest.

## Author details

Chia-Hao Hsu*, Chung-Hwan Chen and Hsuan-Ti Huang
Department of Orthopedics, Kaohsiung Municipal Ta-Tung Hospital, Kaohsiung Medical University Hospital, Kaohsiung Medical University, Kaohsiung, Taiwan

*Address all correspondence to: chiahaohsu.ortho@gmail.com

## References

[1] Zhu N, Zhang D, Wang W, Li X, Yang B, Song J, et al. A novel coronavirus from patients with pneumonia in China, 2019. The New England Journal of Medicine. 2020;**382**(8):727-733

[2] Aiyer AA, Granger CJ, McCormick KL, Cipriano CA, Kaplan JR, Varacallo MA, et al. The impact of COVID-19 on the orthopaedic surgery residency application process. The Journal of the American Academy of Orthopaedic Surgeons. 2020;**28**(15):e633-ee41

[3] Alyami AH, Alyami AA, AlMaeen BN. Impact of COVID-19 on orthopedic surgery: Experience from Saudi Arabia. Annals of Medicine and Surgery. 2020;**56**:61-63

[4] Andreozzi V, Marzilli F, Muselli M, Previ L, Cantagalli MR, Princi G, et al. The impact of COVID-19 on orthopaedic trauma: A retrospective comparative study from a single university hospital in Italy. Orthopaedic Review. 2020;**12**(4):8941

[5] Bernstein DN, Greene N, Ibrahim IO. The personal and professional impact of COVID-19 on orthopedic surgery trainees: Reflections from an incoming intern, current intern, and chief resident. Acta Orthopaedica. 2020; **91**(5):547-550

[6] Chang DG, Park JB, Baek GH, Kim HJ, Bosco A, Hey HWD, et al. The impact of COVID-19 pandemic on orthopaedic resident education: A nationwide survey study in South Korea. International Orthopaedics. 2020;**44**(11):2203-2210

[7] Clement ND, Hall AJ, Makaram NS, Robinson PG, Patton RFL, Moran M, et al. IMPACT-restart: The influence of COVID-19 on postoperative mortality and risk factors associated with SARS-CoV-2 infection after orthopaedic and trauma surgery. The Bone & Joint Journal. 2020;**102-B**(12):1774-1781

[8] Costa GG, Fanzone G, Graceffa A, Lauria M, Zocco G, Cassara A, et al. The impact of COVID-19 prevention measures on epidemiology of orthopedic injuries: The outbreak ages fractures! Acta Bio-Medica. 2020; **91**(4):e2020158

[9] Danford NC, Crutchfield C, Aiyer A, Jobin CM, Levine WN, Lynch TS. The impact of the COVID-19 pandemic on orthopaedic surgery residency applicants during the 2021 residency match cycle in the United States. Journal of the American Academy of Orthopaedic Surgeons. Global Research & Reviews. 2020;**4**(11):e20 00103

[10] Dattani R, Morgan C, Li L, Bennett-Brown K, Wharton RMH. The impact of COVID-19 on the future of orthopaedic training in the UK. Acta Orthopaedica. 2020;**91**(6):627-632

[11] Elhalawany AS, Beastall J, Cousins G. The impact of the COVID-19 lockdown on orthopaedic emergency presentations in a remote and rural population. Bone & Joint Open. 2020;**1**(10):621-627

[12] Ghermandi R, Pipola V, Terzi S, Tedesco G, Cavallari C, Bandiera S, et al. The impact of SARS-CoV-2 pandemic on oncologic and degenerative spine surgery department activity: The experience of Rizzoli orthopaedic institute under COVID-19 lockdown. European Review for Medical and Pharmacological Sciences. 2020; **24**(13):7519-7523

[13] Gonzi G, Gwyn R, Rooney K, Boktor J, Roy K, Sciberras NC, et al. The role of orthopaedic trainees during the COVID-19 pandemic and impact on post-graduate orthopaedic education: A

four-nation survey of over 100 orthopaedic trainees. Bone & Joint Open. 2020;**1**(11):676-682

[14] Haffer H, Schomig F, Rickert M, Randau T, Raschke M, Wirtz D, et al. Impact of the COVID-19 pandemic on orthopaedic and trauma surgery in university hospitals in Germany: Results of a Nationwide survey. The Journal of Bone and Joint Surgery. American Volume. 2020;**102**(14):e78

[15] Mackay ND, Wilding CP, Langley CR, Young J. The impact of COVID-19 on trauma and orthopaedic patients requiring surgery during the peak of the pandemic: A retrospective cohort study. Bone & Joint Open. 2020;**1**(9):520-529

[16] Maniscalco P, Ciatti C, Gattoni S, Puma Pagliarello C, Moretti G, Cauteruccio M, et al. The impact of COVID-19 pandemic on the emergency room and Orthopedic Departments in Piacenza: A retrospective analysis. Acta Bio-Medica. 2020;**91**(14-S):e2020028

[17] Maryada VR, Mulpur P, Guravareddy AV, Pedamallu SK, Vijay BB. Impact of COVID-19 pandemic on orthopaedic trauma volumes: A multi-Centre perspective from the state of Telangana. Indian Journal of Orthopaedics. 2020;**54**(Suppl 2):368-373

[18] Megaloikonomos PD, Thaler M, Igoumenou VG, Bonanzinga T, Ostojic M, Couto AF, et al. Impact of the COVID-19 pandemic on orthopaedic and trauma surgery training in Europe. International Orthopaedics. 2020;**44**(9):1611-1619

[19] Murphy T, Akehurst H, Mutimer J. Impact of the 2020 COVID-19 pandemic on the workload of the orthopaedic service in a busy UK district general hospital. Injury. 2020;**51**(10):2142-2147

[20] Ong MT, Ling SK, Wong RM, Ho KK, Chow SK, Cheung LW, et al. Impact of COVID-19 on orthopaedic clinical service, education and research in a university hospital. Journal of Orthopaedic Translation. 2020;**25**:125-127

[21] Park C, Sugand K, Nathwani D, Bhattacharya R, Sarraf KM. Impact of the COVID-19 pandemic on orthopedic trauma workload in a London level 1 trauma center: The "golden month". Acta Orthopaedica. 2020;**91**(5):556-561

[22] Phillips MR, Chang Y, Zura RD, Mehta S, Giannoudis PV, Nolte PA, et al. Impact of COVID-19 on orthopaedic care: A call for nonoperative management. Therapeutic Advances in Musculoskeletal Disease. 2020; **12**:1759720X20934276

[23] Richardson MA, Islam W, Magruder M. The evolving impact of COVID-19 on medical student Orthopedic education: Perspectives from medical students in different phases of the curriculum. Geriatric Orthopaedic Surgery & Rehabilitation. 2020;**11**:2151459320951721

[24] Sahu D, Agrawal T, Rathod V, Bagaria V. Impact of COVID 19 lockdown on orthopaedic surgeons in India: A survey. Journal of Clinical Orthopaedics and Trauma. 2020;**11**(Suppl. 3):S283-SS90

[25] Sheridan GA, Hughes AJ, Quinlan JF, Sheehan E, O'Byrne JM. Quantifying the impact of the COVID-19 pandemic on orthopaedic trainees: A national perspective. Bone & Joint Open. 2020;**1**(10):645-652

[26] Sugand K, Park C, Morgan C, Dyke R, Aframian A, Hulme A, et al. Impact of the COVID-19 pandemic on paediatric orthopaedic trauma workload in Central London: A multi-centre longitudinal observational study over the "golden weeks". Acta Orthopaedica. 2020;**91**(6):633-638

[27] Teo SH, Abd Rahim MR, Nizlan NM. The impact of COVID-19 pandemic on orthopaedic specialty in Malaysia: A cross-sectional survey. Journal of Orthopaedic Surgery (Hong Kong). 2020;**28**(2):2309499020938877

[28] Upadhyaya GK, Jain VK, Iyengar KP, Patralekh MK, Vaish A. Impact of COVID-19 on post-graduate orthopaedic training in Delhi-NCR. Journal of Clinical Orthopaedics and Trauma. 2020;**11**:S687-SS95

[29] Wallace CN, Kontoghiorghe C, Kayani B, Chang JS, Haddad FS. The impact of COVID-19 on trauma and orthopaedic surgery in the United Kingdom. Bone & Joint Open. 2020;**1**(7):420-423

[30] Wong JSH, Cheung KMC. Impact of COVID-19 on orthopaedic and trauma service: An epidemiological study. The Journal of Bone and Joint Surgery. American Volume. 2020;**102**(14):e80

[31] Wong KC, Han XA, Tay KS, Koh SB, Howe TS. The psychological impact on an orthopaedic outpatient setting in the early phase of the COVID-19 pandemic: A cross-sectional study. Journal of Orthopaedic Surgery and Research. 2020;**15**(1):322

[32] Barahona M, Infante CA, Palet MJ, Barahona MA, Barrientos C, Martinez A. Impact of the COVID-19 outbreak on Orthopedic surgery: A Nationwide analysis of the first pandemic year. Cureus. 2021;**13**(8):e17252

[33] Blum P, Putzer D, Liebensteiner MC, Dammerer D. Impact of the Covid-19 pandemic on orthopaedic and trauma surgery - a systematic review of the current literature. In Vivo. 2021;**35**(3):1337-1343

[34] Chatterji G, Patel Y, Jain V, Geevarughese NM, Haq RU. Impact of COVID-19 on orthopaedic care and practice: A rapid review. Indian Journal of Orthopaedics. 2021;**55**(4):839-852

[35] Antolin UGC, Salinas MA, Sanchez DE, Doussoux PC. Survey about the impact of COVID-19 on the traumatology and orthopedic surgery departments in Spain. Journal of Healthcare Quality Research. 2021;**36**(5):253-262

[36] Gibbard M, Ponton E, Sidhu BV, Farrell S, Bone JN, Wu LA, et al. Survey of the impact of COVID-19 on Pediatric orthopaedic surgeons globally. Journal of Pediatric Orthopedics. 2021; **41**(8):e692-e6e7

[37] Giordano V, Belangero W, Godoy-Santos AL, Pires RE, Xicara JA, Labronici P, et al. The hidden impact of rapid spread of the COVID-19 pandemic in professional, financial, and psychosocial health of Latin American orthopedic trauma surgeons. Injury. 2021;**52**(4):673-678

[38] Green G, Abbott S, Vyrides Y, Afzal I, Kader D, Radha S. The impact of the COVID-19 pandemic on the length of stay following total hip and knee arthroplasty in a high volume elective orthopaedic unit. Bone & Joint Open. 2021;**2**(8):655-660

[39] Heaps BM, Ladnier K, Haselman WT, Limpisvasti O, Banffy MB. Epidemiologic impact of COVID-19 on a multi-subspecialty orthopaedic practice. Journal of Orthopaedics. 2021;**25**:151-154

[40] Howles SM, Mahmood T, Lala S, Pearse A, Docker C. Impact of an Orthopedic-delivered 'One-Stop' Clinic for ambulatory trauma on emergency department and fracture clinic pressures during the COVID-19 pandemic. Cureus. 2021;**13**(5):e15207

[41] Jain VK, Upadhyaya GK, Iyengar KP, Patralekh MK, Lal H, Vaishya R. Impact of COVID-19 on clinical practices

during lockdown: A pan India survey of orthopaedic surgeons. Malaysian Orthopaedic Journal. 2021;**15**(1):55-62

[42] Khan H, Williamson M, Trompeter A. The impact of the COVID-19 pandemic on orthopaedic services and training in the UK. European Journal of Orthopaedic Surgery and Traumatology. 2021;**31**(1):105-109

[43] Ma HH, Tsai SW, Chen CF, Wu PK, Chen CM, Chiang CC, et al. Impact of screening COVID-19 on orthopedic trauma patients at the emergency department: A consecutive series from a level I trauma center. Journal of the Chinese Medical Association. 2021;**84**(4):423-427

[44] Maleitzke T, Pumberger M, Gerlach UA, Herrmann C, Slagman A, Henriksen LS, et al. Impact of the COVID-19 shutdown on orthopedic trauma numbers and patterns in an academic level I trauma Center in Berlin, Germany. PLoS One. 2021; **16**(2):e0246956

[45] Moretti L, Vitale E, Bettinsoli M, Bizzoca D, Delmedico M, Papalia R, et al. The psychological and clinical impact of the COVID-19 pandemic on orthopaedic patients: An Italian gender-specific analysis. Orthopedic Reviews. 2021;**13**(1):9005

[46] Oguzkaya S, Misir A, Ozcamdalli M, Eken G, Kizkapan TB, Kurk MB, et al. Impact of the COVID-19 pandemic on orthopedic fracture characteristics in three hospitals in Turkey: A multi-center epidemiological study. Joint Diseases and Related Surgery. 2021;**32**(2):323-332

[47] Paul KD, Levitt E, McGwin G, Brabston EW 3rd, Gilbert SR, Ponce BA, et al. COVID-19 impact on Orthopedic surgeons: Elective procedures, telehealth, and income. Southern Medical Journal. 2021;**114**(5):311-316

[48] Peebles LA, Kraeutler MJ, Waterman BR, Sherman SL, Mulcahey MK. The impact of COVID-19 on the orthopaedic sports medicine fellowship application process. Arthroscopy, Sports Medicine, and Rehabilitation. 2021;**3**(4):e1237-e1e41

[49] Probert AC, Sivakumar BS, An V, Nicholls SL, Shatrov JG, Symes MJ, et al. Impact of COVID-19-related social restrictions on orthopaedic trauma in a level 1 trauma Centre in Sydney: The first wave. ANZ Journal of Surgery. 2021;**91**(1-2):68-72

[50] Qian C, Zheng Y, Meng J, Li H, Wang D. A cross-sectional study on the impact of the prevention and control response of the COVID-19 pandemic on minor's orthopedic trauma in Shanghai. Archives of Public Health. 2021;**79**(1):145

[51] Rachuene PA, Masipa RR, Dey R, Msingapantsi M, Khanyile SM, Phala MP, et al. The impact of COVID-19 national lockdown on orthopaedic trauma admissions in the northern part of South Africa: A multicentre review of tertiary- and secondary-level hospital admissions. South African Medical Journal. 2021;**111**(7):668-673

[52] Ribau A, Vale J, Xara-Leite F, Rodrigues-Pinto R. Impact of COVID-19 pandemic and national lockdown in an orthopaedic and traumatology department-a comparison with the homologous period of 2019. Porto Biomedical Journal. 2021;**6**(1):e109

[53] Shah A, Champagne AA, Del Papa J, Toor J, Larouche J, Nousiainen MT. The unique impact of COVID-19 on orthopedic surgery residency applicants and program directors in Canada. Canadian Journal of Surgery. 2021;**64**(2):E249-EE52

[54] Sharma V, Kumar N, Gupta B, Mahajan A. Impact of COVID-19

pandemic on orthopaedic surgeons in terms of anxiety, sleep outcomes and change in management practices: A cross-sectional study from India. Journal of Orthopaedic Surgery (Hong Kong). 2021;**29**(1):23094990211001621

[55] Shih CL, Huang PJ, Huang HT, Chen CH, Lee TC, Hsu CH. Impact of the COVID-19 pandemic and its related psychological effect on orthopedic surgeries conducted in different types of hospitals in Taiwan. Journal of Orthopaedic Surgery (Hong Kong). 2021;**29**(1):2309499021996072

[56] Unterfrauner I, Hruby LA, Jans P, Steinwender L, Farshad M, Uckay I. Impact of a total lockdown for pandemic SARS-CoV-2 (Covid-19) on deep surgical site infections and other complications after orthopedic surgery: A retrospective analysis. Antimicrobial Resistance and Infection Control. 2021;**10**(1):112

[57] Van Heest A, Brandt AM, Dyer G, Homer CJ, Murray PM. COVID-19: Impact on orthopaedic graduate medical education in the U.S.: AOA critical issues symposium. The Journal of Bone and Joint Surgery. American Volume. 2021;**103**(16):e65

[58] Vasiliadis E, Vlachos C, Papagrigorakis E, Evangelopoulos DS, Lelekis M, Pneumaticos SG. One year later: What was the impact of the COVID-19 pandemic on Orthopedic practice? Cureus. 2021;**13**(6):e16013

[59] Hsu CH, Hsu NC. Impact and strategies on joint surgery Centers without lockdowns during the peak of the COVID-19 pandemic: A Multicenter cross-sectional study. Journal of Clinical Medicine. 2021;**10**(22):5392

[60] Hsu CH, Chen CH, Huang HT, Yang CJ, Chen YH. To safely reopen after a lockdown, masks are crucial: Lessons from Taiwan. Public Health. 2021;**190**:99-100

Chapter 32

# Analysis of the Concept of Deaths per Million in the Impact Assessment of COVID-19 Pandemic in 2020

*Goodluck A.K. Ohanube and Uchejeso M. Obeta*

## Abstract

The pandemic of the Coronavirus disease 2019 has been quite devastating. Assessing the success of the public health measures put in place by different nations has become a herculean task, especially as there is no effective index to determine that. The existing public health indices such as the Case fatality ratio and Mortality rate have not proven efficient in ascertaining the progress made in the early implementation of some public health measures. Hence, the index Deaths Per Million, an estimated mortality rate, is considered an alternative tool to ascertain the progress made at the onset and peak of the pandemic. In this case study, we have compared these three indices to know which best fits the pandemic. We also elucidated when and how deaths per million can be efficiently utilized during a pandemic to know the most appropriate time to impose lockdowns and other public health measures. This is considering the tendency for lockdowns to affect the psycho-social skills of humans and adversely impact economic activities both locally and globally. This work further provided evidence why the index Deaths Per Million is preferred during a pandemic over case fatality ratio and mortality. This was done using statistics from various countries for one year. These countries were selected based on their population and their peculiar nature.

**Keywords:** COVID-19, case fatality ratio, mortality rate, estimated mortality rate, lockdown, basic reproduction number ($R_0$), Herd immunity

## 1. Introduction

The COVID-19 pandemic has led to many unwarranted deaths that could have been averted if the necessary measures had been implemented early enough. The difficulty of implementing these measures at the right time could partly stem from the fact that there were no indices to determine the magnitude of the effects caused by this pandemic at the onset. Hence, many lives were lost, and many governments enacted policies that led to harsh economic situations.

During this early onset, many nations came up with innovative ideas for survival. Some chose to use vitamin C tablets and sources rich in this vitamin [1, 2], and others adopted vitamin D [3, 4]. Nevertheless, the world's major economies plummeted due to the decelerated economic activities, leading to an economic quagmire across the world. This economic woe emanating from the reduced rate of economic activities was partly precipitated by the inability to ascertain how many lives have been badly imparted at this early part of the pandemic leading to a pandemonium of a sort. This is mainly because existing indices such as case fatality ratio (CFR) and Mortality rate (MR) have proven unsuccessful in deciphering the extent of imparting whether by exact figures or approximated figures. Hence a need to propose an index that can be utilized in similar situations so as forestall the grounding of economic activities, which is the nerve activity of every nation.

In this study, which is partly a review, we have compared three terms: case fatality ratio, Mortality rate, and Deaths Per Million, a term introduced during this pandemic by the situation report room of the World Health Organisation (WHO). The period under study is from 1st January 2020 to 31st December 2020. The aim is to evaluate the efficacy of the public health measures of some selected countries using these indices to know the index that is the best fit for the early part of the pandemic.

## 2. A case of covid-19 in 2020

According to the WHO definition, the case fatality ratio **(CFR)** is the proportion of individuals diagnosed with a disease who die from that disease [5]. Thus, it estimates the severity among detected cases:

$$\text{Case Fatality ratio (CFR, in\%)} = \frac{\text{Number of deaths from specific disease}}{\text{Number of confirmed cases of specific disease}} \times 100 \tag{1}$$

Attempts to use this index may not be very feasible, considering its definition and designation. Thus, the mortality rate **(MR)**, which is time or interval-based, is defined as the number of deaths from a specific cause divided by the total number of the population in a state or country multiplied by 100,000 at a definite interval was brought into this context [6]. This can be mathematically represented as:

$$\text{Mortality rate} = \frac{\text{Number of deaths from specific cause (D)}}{\text{Total number of a defined population (P)}} \times 100,000 \tag{2}$$

The use of mortality rate may not also be feasible, as some disease outbreaks may persist beyond a definite time interval, say a year, as is the current case of the pandemic. Hence, the term deaths per million **(DPM)** may be more appropriate. This could be why the WHO introduced the deaths per million, via her situation report room, a term that might be relatively new to neophytes in public health. Thus, the need to analyze this term as a concept via available data from the situation report room of the WHO, using the Coronavirus disease 2019 (COVID-19) pandemic as a case study.

### 2.1 Analysis of the terms using available data

Analyzing the data to elucidate the definition involves studying the trend in which the figures follow. A case study of the trend in this pandemic gives a clue as to why the World Health Organisation adopted the term Deaths Per Million (DPM) during a pandemic. The CFR of 2.317 (see **Table 1**) presents Nigeria with many deaths higher than Russia, whose CFR is 1.430, and Australia, whose theirs is at 1.361 (see **Table 1**). However, Nigeria is known to have fewer deaths than Russia and Australia. This scenario indicates that though CFR could be used to determine

| Countries | Total population | Total number of cases | Total number of deaths | Mortality rate | Case fatality ratio | Deaths per million |
|---|---|---|---|---|---|---|
| Australia | 25,203,198 | 7,641 | 104 | 0.412 | 1.361 | 4.126 |
| Brazil | 211,049,527 | 1,274,974 | 55,961 | 26.516 | 4.389 | 265.156 |
| China | 1,433,783,686 | 85,190 | 4,648 | 0.324 | 5.456 | 3.241 |
| India | 1,366,417,754 | 528,859 | 16,095 | 1.178 | 3.0433 | 11.779 |
| Nigeria | 200,963,599 | 24,077 | 558 | 0.278 | 2.317 | 2.777 |
| Russia | 145,872,256 | 634,437 | 9,073 | 6.220 | 1.430 | 62.198 |
| The USA | 329,064,917 | 2,452,048 | 124,811 | 37.930 | 5.090 | 379.290 |
| U.K | 67,530,172 | 310,254 | 43,514 | 64.436 | 14.025 | 644.364 |
| S/Africa | 58,558,270 | 131,800 | 2,413 | 4.121 | 1.831 | 41.207 |

*A table showing the respective population of countries according to the statistics from the United Nations with their MR, CFR, and DPM as of 28th June 2020. Case Fatality Ratio (CFR) and Deaths Per Million (DPM) of the different countries with the largest population in their continents. India and China were added because India is next in demography, aside from China being the abode of the index case. The UK and South Africa were added due to the emergence of the second variant in these countries [7, 8].*

**Table 1.**
*Total population and the total number of cases per selected country between January and June 2020.*

death rates from diagnosed disease cases, it may not be the most appropriate tool during or after a pandemic, especially in an African setting, due to some factors, including laboratory testing capacity. The erroneous impression given by CFR led to considering the mortality rate as an index [5]. However, the mortality rate, which is strongly influenced by time, may not be appropriate. This makes the data for case fatality ratio and mortality rate in (**Tables 1** and **2**) inaccurate [5, 6]. The inaccuracy presented by these two indices limits their use during a pandemic. Hence, the

| Countries | Total population | Cumulative number of cases | Cumulative number of deaths | Mortality rate | Case fatality ratio | Deaths per million |
|---|---|---|---|---|---|---|
| Australia | 25,203,198 | 28,296 | 908 | 3.603 | 3.209 | 36.027 |
| Brazil | 211,049,527 | 7,448,560 | 190,488 | 90.257 | 2.557 | 902.575 |
| China | 1,433,783,686 | 96,324 | 4,777 | 0.333 | 4.959 | 3.332 |
| India | 1,366,417,754 | 10,187,850 | 147,622 | 10.804 | 1.449 | 108.036 |
| Nigeria | 200,963,599 | 83,576 | 1,247 | 0.620 | 1.492 | 6.205 |
| Russia | 145,872,256 | 3,050,248 | 54,778 | 37.552 | 1.796 | 375.520 |
| The USA | 329,064,917 | 18,648,989 | 328,014 | 99.681 | 1.759 | 996.806 |
| U. K | 67,530,172 | 2,256,009 | 70,405 | 104.257 | 3.120 | 1,042.571 |
| S/Africa | 58,558,270 | 994,911 | 26,521 | 45.290 | 2.666 | 452.899 |

*A table showing the respective population of countries according to the statistics from the United Nations with their MR, CFR, and DPM as of 27th December 2020. Case Fatality Ratio (CFR) and Deaths Per Million (DPM) of the different countries with the largest population in their continents. India and China were added because India is next in demography, aside from China being the abode of the index case. The UK and South Africa were added due to the emergence of the second variant in these countries [8, 9].*

**Table 2.**
*Total population and the total number of cases per selected country between July and December 2020.*

Deaths Per Million (DPM), which estimates the mortality rate irrespective of time, maybe preferred in this context.

According to the World Health Organisation, a COVID-19 death is a death emanating from a clinically compatible illness that is implicitly linked to a COVID-19 case, except when there is a clear alternative cause of death such as trauma which may not be linked to COVID-19 disease. In this case, there should be no gap between the time the patient completely recovers and when the patient dies [7]. This description favours the index called deaths per million (DPM) better than the other two indices. The term DPM could be described as the total number of deaths triggered at any time by the etiology of a pandemic or epidemic per 1,000,000 population of a country. In this instance, deaths from any cause occurring during the pandemic, which follows the description of the WHO, could be attributed to the pandemic [7, 10]. Though it is indicative and not confirmative, the deaths per million remains a crucial indicator of the actual effect of COVID-19 since it is not influenced by the errors in the certification of the causes of death [10]. This index is best fit for monitoring the efficiency of the control measures implemented by countries during a disease outbreak (**Table 3**). It helps to decipher when and where there would be a need for a total or partial lockdown during a pandemic or epidemic. It also helps to verify the progress made in saving lives, despite its limitation of only providing an estimate.

In **Tables 1** and **2**, one would think that the deaths per million (DPM) and the Mortality rate are the same indices or provide the same information. However, the definition of the Mortality rate presents a challenge in its use. Mortality rate, which may be defined as the number of deaths from a specific cause per 100,000 of the population of a state or a country per annum, may not be appropriate in the case of a pandemic, except if this definition is reviewed [6]. Hence the term deaths per million may be the most appropriate considering its flexibility of use.

| Week | Date | Number of cases | Number of deaths | Cumulative difference (deaths) | Deaths per million |
|---|---|---|---|---|---|
| 1 | 1st October | 59,001 | 1112 | 0 | 0 |
| 2 | 8th October | 59,841 | 1113 | 1 | 0.005 |
| 3 | 15th October | 60,982 | 1116 | 3 | 0.015 |
| 4 | 24th October | 61,930 | 1129 | 13 | 0.065 |
| 5 | 29th October | 62,521 | 1141 | 12 | 0.060 |
| 6 | 5th November | 63,508 | 1155 | 14 | 0.070 |
| 7 | 12th November | 64,728 | 1162 | 7 | 0.085 |
| 8 | 19th November | 65,693 | 1163 | 1 | 0.005 |
| 9 | 26th November | 66,974 | 1169 | 6 | 0.030 |
| 10 | 3rd December | 70,669 | 1184 | 15 | 0.075 |
| 11 | 10th December | 71,344 | 1190 | 6 | 0.030 |
| 12 | 17th December | 76,207 | 1201 | 11 | 0.055 |
| 13 | 24th December | 81,963 | 1242 | 41 | 0.204 |
| 14 | 31st December | 87,510 | 1289 | 47 | 0.234 |

*With a total population of 200,963,599, Nigeria had a slight increase in her death toll during the festive period, as seen by her DPM. This could be due to reduced compliance with the COVID-19 protocols [11–13].*

**Table 3.**
*The deaths per million of the number of deaths recorded in Nigeria between 1st October to 31st December 2020.*

The mathematical representation of Deaths Per Million (DPM) is:

$$\frac{\text{Total number of deaths related to the etiology of pandemic (D)}}{\text{Total population of the country (P)}} \times 1,000,000 \tag{3}$$

It is important to note that this term can be applied to areas, regions, or states that have over a million population. For instance, states such as Lagos state in Nigeria, California in the United States, Moscow in Russia, Uttar Pradesh in India, Henan in China, and North-Rhine Westphalia in Germany may be described using DPM. While countries or states that have fewer than a million could be studied using the index such as Deaths Per Thousands (DPT) in a similar style [5].

## 3. Discussion

Understanding the importance of deaths per million as a public health tool is one of the major keys to outliving the pandemic. There are many ways in which this understanding of deaths per million can benefit man. However, this work focuses on its use in invoking lockdowns and in comparing the success rate of countries.

### 3.1 Decision-making process on lockdowns

The estimated mortality rate helps to know when to implement lockdowns. Lockdowns have their benefits; however, lockdowns pose some threats to the psycho-social well-being of man when imposed too frequently. A study done by researchers from the University of Pennsylvania noted that lockdowns led to the number of deaths related to COVID-19 plummeting by 33,000 deaths in the United States, as of 31st May 2020, a number showing 29% improvement in the fight against the virus. As of the same period, 3 million people were out of a job. They opined that implementing lockdowns which does not affect businesses could have saved more lives and a million jobs [14, 15]. The findings of some experts also supported the hypothesis of adverse effects of lockdown in the family. These findings revealed that due to the stress, job losses, anxieties, and other ill experiences are seen among families during the pandemic, restriction of movements (lockdown) could further exacerbate the rate of domestic violence and interpersonal violence, culminating in a spate of child abuse [15–18].

Some authors argued that the aggravation of confirmed cases and mortality rates due to the COVID-19 pandemic negatively impacted mental health during the earlier part of the pandemic; hence, there was a need for a lockdown. These authors believed that the quality of air, water, and aquatic life was drastically improved during the restrictions of human activities. They, however, noted that the restrictions on movements led to economic disaster [19]. At the same time, some researchers think that lockdowns may reduce the rate of exposure to sunlight and alter daily social activities. A scenario that negatively imparts the circadian rhythms, culminating in poor health conditions and diminished psycho-social skills [20].

The importance of using the estimated mortality rate to determine when to call for lockdowns can never be overemphasized; this is because lockdowns create a lacuna in the daily operations and everyday lives of low-income earners. For instance, there was a rise in food scarcity in some parts of America and some countries in Sub-Saharan Africa due to the ill-planned policies on the restriction of movements [15, 21–28]. Domestic violence grew across the globe during these lockdown periods [17, 29–31]. The birth rate in some low-income countries also grew, despite the limited resources [32]. At the same time, complications related to birth increased in some of these countries [32, 33]. Political instability and insecurity aggravated as terrorists, bandits and rogues maximized the opportunity of the lacunae created in the security apparel of nations in sub-Sahara Africa to re-strategize their *modus operandi* in perpetuating heinous activities [34–38]. For instance, the security agencies in Lagos, Nigeria, were overwhelmed with the reports of incessant attacks by criminals in this metropolitan state [39].

Deciphering the appropriate time to implement lockdowns remains a difficult decision for public health officials in many countries, sometimes leading to a debate. This debate could be resolved if one retrospectively analyses the experiences shared by some nations during the early part of the COVID-19 pandemic. For instance, Italy, with a population of 60,376,836, had her index case of COVID-19 in Rome on 31st January 2020 and the first death resulting from this disease on 21st February 2020, and by mid-March 2020, the number of deaths drastically rose, resulting in almost 50% of excess deaths from causes related to COVID-19 in March 2020 [10, 40, 41]. In this case, the total number of new deaths in Italy, which rose from 97 as of 10th March 2020 to 168 as of 11th March 2020, may not cause much panic [42, 43]. However, the statistics of 17th March 2020, which pegs the total number of deaths at 2503 as against the figure of 463 seen on 10th March 2020, calls for grave concern [42, 44]. Hence, ascertaining a weekly outcome may be worthwhile in deciphering the type and stringency of public health measures to be adopted. The estimated mortality rate of Italy presented a clearer picture of the success and compliance rate via this weekly analysis. The DPM of Italy, which was 7.67 as of 10th March 2020, and 41.46 as of 17th March 2020, shows an increase of 6-times fold and over 400% increase, a scenario that required urgent measures.

Considering the case of Italy, one could implicitly say that the DPM should be used to predict the appropriate time for a total or partial lockdown, bearing in mind the epidemic capacity or basic reproduction number ($R_0$) of the microbe. This is especially when the available data shows a 3-times fold and over 200% increase in the space of 7 days [40, 42–44]. Based on the information provided in **Table 3**, lockdowns should be implemented by week 13. This is due to the 270% increase seen between week 12 and week 13, as presented by the case study.

The suspension or ease of lockdowns should be considered when the DPM is closer to the lowest weekly figure, which was observed within 6 to 12 weeks prior to the week of a surge. In this instance, the week with the lowest value and the week when the policy is reviewed should have very little difference. Using **Table 3** as a case study, it would be appropriate to aim at achieving the figures close to that of week 2 or week 8 after there has been a surge in week 14. If the percentage difference in the DPM of both weeks that are compared is between 30% and 100%, the state or country may consider a partial easing of the lockdowns, where only mass gatherings are suspended and public health measures enunciated by the WHO are upheld. If the difference in both weeks is between 2% and 30%, then the lockdown may be fully suspended while maintaining the guidelines of the WHO on non-pharmacological intervention. If the difference between both weeks is between 0% and 2%, then the pandemic may be declared over by the country's public health authorities after reaching a consensus with the WHO. Declaring the pandemic over requires consistency of between 0% and 2% in the cumulative difference of the weekly statistics for 6 to 12 consecutive weeks following the surge in cases. This shows that over 60% of the population of the state or country is already immunized against the virus in line with herd immunity and adaptive immunity.

Whenever it is difficult to ascertain the 0% to 2% fraction of the cumulative difference of DPM between the first time a lockdown is invoked in a country and the weeks preceding the review date, public health officials could make their deductions based on the topography of the country, the season of the year, the population size of the country, the characteristics of the microbes and the route of transmission of this microbial agent. In this case, the pandemic may be declared over only if, after 6 to 12 consecutive weeks, the cumulative difference in the weekly statistics of those still dying from this disease is less than or equivalent to a DPM of 0.01 and less than 2% of the population are reported to be diagnosed of the disease as seen in **Table 3**.

### 3.2 Ascertaining the success of public health measures

The estimated mortality rate helps to determine the success of the public health measures among a population, state, or country. Determining the success of the public health interventions helps instil confidence among the population, a feat that quells the panic attacks, which may obscure the actual situation in the control of these outbreaks [19]. Some health workers who were contacted via Facebook said they felt at ease when they realized that the rate of spread in Nigeria was not as rapid as what was happening in Italy and America as of March 2020. This was evident because, as of 17th March 2020, the DPM of Nigeria stood at zero. As of then, Nigeria had no deaths; Italy had 2503 deaths, making her DPM 41.46, while the United States of America, with 58 deaths, had an insignificant DPM [44].

DPM helps to know if the government and the people are compliant with the proven existing public health measures. India, which was very compliant with the rules in the early part of the pandemic in 2020, was taken unawares when it failed to comply with the public health measures during the second quarter of 2021 [45]. In the last quarter of 2020, Nigeria saw a slight increase in her DPM, when it lost a number of its top health workers partly because of non-compliance to the non-pharmacological interventions in preventing COVID-19 [11]. The data presented by the Nigeria Centre for Disease Control (NCDC) between October and December 2020 gave an insight into the fate of Nigeria, as presented in **Table 3** [12]. The evidence provided in **Table 3** gives credence to the utility of DPM as a veritable public health tool [12, 13].

## 4. Conclusion

The case fatality ratio (CFR) is the proportion of individuals diagnosed with a disease who die from that disease. The mortality rate (MR), which is time or interval-based, is defined as the number of deaths from a specific cause per a hundred thousand of the total population in a state or country. The deaths per million (DPM) is the total number of deaths emanating from a cause related to the etiology of a pandemic per a million of the total number of the population of a state or a country. While these indices all appear similar, the index, deaths per million, has a superior advantage in its use during pandemics; because it is not dependent on an interval, albeit its shortcoming of being an estimated value.

The index Deaths per million, which is an estimated mortality rate, is a relatively new term in the public health domain. It is expected to serve its purpose, especially during pandemics. This is considering how convenient it can be used in place of CFR and MR. Moreover, the use of this index proffers an economic advantage as it guides the public health officials in decision-making processes on movement restriction and monitoring of compliance rate, which influences economic activities. It also helps to determine states or countries that may be considered danger zones to enact the policies of International Health Regulations (IHR). In line with this, it is expected that public health agencies would judiciously utilize this index for the well-being of those they serve both now and in the future.

## Acknowledgements

Special thanks to all the medical and health workers, the public health organizations, and their staff, who strive against all odds to bring succour to Africans during the pandemic.

## Conflict of interest

The authors declare no competing interests.

## Author details

Goodluck A.K. Ohanube[1] and Uchejeso M. Obeta[2*]

1 Department of Biomedical Sciences, University of Applied Sciences, Bonn-Rhein-Sieg, Bonn, Germany

2 Department of Medical Laboratory Management, Federal School of Medical Laboratory Science, Jos, Nigeria

*Address all correspondence to: uchejesoobeta@gmail.com

## References

[1] Ohanube GAK, Obeta MU, Ikeagwulonu RC, Jwanse IR. COVID-19: A case study of using vitamin C enriched plants and ascorbic acid as cure. American Journal of Medical Case Reports. 2020;**8**(11):435-437. DOI: 10.12691/ajmcr-8-11-16

[2] Ohanube GAK, Obeta UM, Ikeagwulonu CR. Case reports in the use of vitamin C based regimen in prophylaxis and management of COVID-19 among Nigerians. Journal of Current Biomedical Reports. 2020;**1**(2):1-4

[3] Griffin G, Hewison M, Hopkin J, Kenny R, Quinton R, Rhodes J, et al. Vitamin D and COVID-19: Evidence and recommendations for supplementation. Royal Society Open Science. 2020;**7**(12): 201912

[4] Ma H, Zhou T, Heianza Y, Qi L. Habitual use of vitamin D supplements and risk of coronavirus disease 2019 (COVID-19) infection: A prospective study in UK Biobank. American Journal of Clinical Nutrition. 2021;**113**(5): 1275-1281

[5] World Health Organization. Estimating mortality from COVID-19: Scientific brief, 4th August 2020. World Health Organization; 2020

[6] World Health Organization. Mortality rate (per 100,000 population). Retrieved 12th November 2020, from https://www.who.int/data/gho/indicator-metadata-registry/imr-details/3130

[7] World Health Organisation Situation report. Coronavirus disease (COVID-19) Weekly Epidemiological Update and Weekly Operational Update for 28th June 2020. Retrieved 20th February 2021, from https://www.who.int/docs/default-source/coronaviruse/situation-reports/20200628-covid-19-sitrep-160.pdf?sfvrsn=2fe1c658_2

[8] United Nations Department of Economic and Social Affairs, Population Division, Population Estimates and Projections Section. Total Population - Both Sexes. World Population Prospects, the 2019 Revision, 2019. Retrieved 20th February 2021 from https://web.archive.org/web/20201015140405/https://population.un.org/wpp/Download/Files/1_Indicators%20(Standard)/EXCEL_FILES/1_Population/WPP2019_POP_F01_1_TOTAL_POPULATION_BOTH_SEXES.xlsx

[9] World Health Organisation situation report. Coronavirus disease (COVID-19) Weekly Epidemiological Update and Weekly Operational Update for 27th December 2020. Retrieved 20th February 2021, from https://www.who.int/publications/m/item/weekly-epidemiological-update—29-december-2020

[10] Alicandro G, Remuzzi G, La Vecchia C. Italy's first wave of the COVID-19 pandemic has ended: No excess mortality in May 2020. The Lancet. 2020;**396**(10253):e27-e28

[11] Premium Times. Buhari mourns 20 Nigerian doctors killed by COVID-19. Premium Times. 26th December 2020. Retrieved on 18th September 2021. Available from: https://www.premiumtimesng.com/news/top-news/433383-buhari-mourns-20-nigerian-doctors-killed-by-covid-19.html

[12] Nigeria Centre for Disease Control. Situation report of the Nigeria Centre for Disease Control (Facebook). Retrieved on 30th December 2020. Available from: https://www.facebook.com/NCDCgov

[13] Nigeria Centre for Disease Control. Situation report of the Nigeria Centre for Disease Control (official website). Retrieved on 30th December 2020. Available from: https://ncdc.gov.ng/

[14] Arnon A, Ricco J, Smetters K. Epidemiological and economic effects of lockdown. Brookings Papers on Economic Activity, 2020

[15] Ganson KT, Tsai AC, Weiser SD, Benabou SE, Nagata JM. Job insecurity and symptoms of anxiety and depression among US young adults during COVID-19. Journal of Adolescent Health. 2021;**68**(1):53-56

[16] Clemens V, Deschamps P, Fegert JM, Anagnostopoulos D, Bailey S, Doyle M, Eliez S, Hansen AS, Hebebrand J, Hillegers M, Jacobs B. Potential effects of "social" distancing measures and school lockdown on child and adolescent mental health. European Child & Adolescent Psychiatry. 2020:1-4. DOI: 10.1007/s00787-020-01549-w

[17] Hamadani JD, Hasan MI, Baldi AJ, Hossain SJ, Shiraji S, Bhuiyan MS, et al. Immediate impact of stay-at-home orders to control COVID-19 transmission on socioeconomic conditions, food insecurity, mental health, and intimate partner violence in Bangladeshi women and their families: An interrupted time series. The Lancet Global Health. 2020;**8**(11):e1380-e1389

[18] Witteveen D, Velthorst E. Economic hardship and mental health complaints during COVID-19. Proceedings of the National Academy of Sciences. 2020;**117**(44):27277-27284

[19] Atalan A. Is the lockdown important to prevent the COVID-19 pandemic? Effects on psychology, environment, and economy-perspective. Annals of Medicine and Surgery. 2020;**56**:38-42

[20] Leone MJ, Sigman M, Golombek DA. Effects of lockdown on human sleep and chronotype during the COVID-19 pandemic. Current Biology. 2020;**30**(16):R930-R931

[21] Headey DD, Oo TZ, Mahrt K, Diao X, Goudet S, Lambrecht I. Poverty, food insecurity, and social protection during COVID-19 in Myanmar: Combined evidence from a household telephone survey and micro-simulations. International Food Policy Research Institute. 2020:1-14

[22] Martinez E. Food insecurity amid the COVID-19 lockdowns in Nigeria: Do impacts on food insecurity persist after lockdowns end? Current Developments in Nutrition. 2021;**5**(Suppl. 2):235

[23] Knuppel A. Diet, lifestyle, and livelihoods during coronavirus disease 2019 (COVID-19)–related lockdowns and the value of web-based nutrition studies. American Journal of Clinical Nutrition. 2021:1-2

[24] Chu IY, Alam P, Larson HJ, Lin L. Social consequences of mass quarantine during epidemics: A systematic review with implications for the COVID-19 response. Journal of Travel Medicine. 2020;**27**(7):taaa192

[25] Arndt C, Davies R, Gabriel S, Harris L, Makrelov K, Robinson S, et al. Covid-19 lockdowns, income distribution, and food security: An analysis for South Africa. Global Food Security. 2020;**26**:100410

[26] McKinney SJ. Covid-19: Food insecurity, digital exclusion and Catholic schools. Journal of Religious Education. 2020;**68**(3):319-330

[27] Andam K, Edeh H, Oboh V, Pauw K, Thurlow J. Impacts of COVID-19 on food systems and poverty in Nigeria. Advances in Food Security and Sustainability. 2020;**5**:145

[28] Adeshokan O. Coronavirus: Food insecurity fallout from Nigeria's lockdown. The Africa Report. Available from: https://www. theafricareport. com/27676/coronavirusfood-insecurity-fallout-from-nigerias-lockdown. [Last accessed on 2020 11th May]. 2020 6th July

[29] Guessoum SB, Lachal J, Radjack R, Carretier E, Minassian S, Benoit L, et al. Adolescent psychiatric disorders during the COVID-19 pandemic and lockdown. Psychiatry Research. 2020; **29**:113264

[30] Gibson J. Domestic violence during COVID-19: The GP role. The British Journal of General Practice. 2020; **70**(696):340

[31] Amusan L, Agunyai SC. The COVID-19 pandemic and the crisis of lockdowns in Nigeria: The household food security perspective. Africa's Public Service Delivery & Performance Review. 2021;**9**(1):10

[32] Ullah M, Moin AT, Araf Y, Bhuiyan AR, Griffiths MD, Gozal D. Potential effects of the COVID-19 pandemic on future birth rate. Frontiers in Public Health. 2020;**8**:893

[33] Ashish KC, Gurung R, Kinney MV, Sunny AK, Moinuddin M, Basnet O, et al. Effect of the COVID-19 pandemic response on intrapartum care, stillbirth, and neonatal mortality outcomes in Nepal: A prospective observational study. The Lancet Global Health. 2020; **8**(10):e1273-e1281

[34] Egunjobi AA. Reflections on the impact of coronavirus pandemic on the political and socioeconomic conditions of African states. International Journal of Advanced Academic Research in Social Sciences, Arts & Humanities. 2020;**6**(8);61-71

[35] Gary A, Hayley P. Terrorism and COVID-19: Actual and Potential Impacts. Perspectives on Terrorism. 2020;**14**(3):59-73

[36] Kruglanski AW, Gunaratna R, Ellenberg M, Speckhard A. Terrorism in time of the pandemic: Exploiting mayhem. Global Security: Health, Science and Policy. 2020;**5**(1): 121-132

[37] De Cauwer HG, Somville F. Health Care Organizations: Soft target during COVID-19 pandemic. Prehospital and Disaster Medicine. 2021;**36**(3):344-347

[38] Akanmu AA, Salisu UO, Daramola OP, Ogunsesan AS, Fasina SO, Adejare JA, et al. The COVID-19 pandemic and insecurity: The furiousness in Nigerian communities. Urban, Planning and Transport Research. 2021;**9**(1):369-407

[39] Emma Nnadozie. LOCKDOWN: Activities of deadly One Million Boys, Awawa gang rubbish police claims in Lagos. Vanguard. 18th April 2020. Retrieved 23rd September 2021. Available from: https://www.vanguardngr.com/2020/04/lockdown-activities-of-deadly-one-million-boys-awawa-gang-rubbish-police-claims-in-lagos/

[40] Remuzzi A, Remuzzi G. COVID-19, and Italy: What next? The Lancet. 2020; **395**(10231):1225-1228

[41] Worldometer. Italy Population (live). Retrieved 16th June 2021. Available from: https://www.worldometers.info/world-population/italy-population/

[42] World Health Organisation situation report. Coronavirus disease (COVID-19) Weekly Epidemiological Update and Weekly Operational Update for 10th March 2020. Retrieved 16th June 2021. Available from: https://www.who.int/docs/default-source/coronaviruse/situation-reports/20200310-sitrep-50-covid-19.pdf?sfvrsn=55e904fb_2

[43] World Health Organisation situation report. Coronavirus disease (COVID-19) Weekly Epidemiological Update and Weekly Operational Update for 11th March 2020. Retrieved 16th June 2021. Available from: https://www.who.int/docs/default-source/coronaviruse/situation-reports/20200311-

sitrep-51-covid-19.pdf?sfvrsn=
1ba62e57_10

[44] World Health Organisation situation report. Coronavirus disease (COVID-19) Weekly Epidemiological Update and Weekly Operational Update for 17th March 2020. Retrieved 16th June 2021. Available from: https://www.who.int/docs/default-source/coronaviruse/situation-reports/20200317-sitrep-57-covid-19.pdf?sfvrsn=a26922f2_4

[45] Kuppalli K, Gala P, Cherabuddi K, Kalantri SP, Mohanan M, Mukherjee B, et al. India's COVID-19 crisis: A call for international action. The Lancet. 2021; **397**(10290):2132-2135